Healing Brain Injury *with*
Chinese Medical Approaches

of related interest

Neuropuncture
A Clinical Handbook of Neuroscience
Acupuncture, Second Edition
Michael D. Corradino
ISBN 978 1 84819 331 4
eISBN 978 0 85701 287 6

Psycho-Emotional Pain and
the Eight Extraordinary Vessels
Yvonne R. Farrell, DAOM, L.Ac.
ISBN 978 1 84819 292 8
eISBN 978 0 85701 239 5

Healing Brain Injury *with* Chinese Medical Approaches

Integrative Approaches for Practitioners

DOUGLAS S. WINGATE

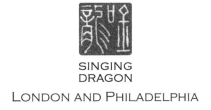

SINGING
DRAGON

LONDON AND PHILADELPHIA

First published in 2018
by Singing Dragon
an imprint of Jessica Kingsley Publishers
73 Collier Street
London N1 9BE, UK
and
400 Market Street, Suite 400
Philadelphia, PA 19106, USA

www.singingdragon.com

Library of Congress Cataloging in Publication Data
Names: Wingate, Douglas S., author.
Title: Healing brain injury with Chinese medical approaches : integrative
approaches for practitioners / Douglas S. Wingate.
Description: London ; Philadelphia : Singing Dragon, 2018. | Includes
bibliographical references and index.
Identifiers: LCCN 2017058482 | ISBN 9781848194021 (alk. paper)
Subjects: | MESH: Brain Injuries--therapy | Medicine, Chinese Traditional |
Integrative Medicine--methods
Classification: LCC RC387.5 | NLM WL 354 | DDC 617.4/81044--
dc23 LC record available at https://lccn.loc.gov/2017058482

British Library Cataloguing in Publication Data
A CIP catalogue record for this book is available from the British Library

ISBN 978 1 84819 402 1
eISBN 978 0 85701 356 9

Printed and bound in Great Britain

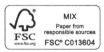

Dedicated to Courtney; without whose support, patience, and own sacrifices this book would have remained just a mess of computer files, internet bookmarks, and piles of notes.

Contents

Introduction

It was during my last year of Chinese medical school that I was first exposed to the dramatic impact a brain injury can have on a person's life. Not in my clinical rounds, but in a neuro-optometrist's office. It was here that I witnessed how much a proper prescription could alter their life for the better following all too common visual problems. People crying within moments of them being placed on their head because the world wasn't blurry or dizzying anymore. It struck me that the topic of brain injury had never been discussed in any of my college studies despite the fact that many of the symptoms people often struggle with can be addressed rather effectively with acupuncture and Chinese herbs. This seemed even more odd as Chinese medicine is quite well suited, and perhaps uniquely qualified, to address some of the complex symptom clusters that occur by proper assessment and diagnosis of pattern differentiation. I thought, surely Chinese medicine's ability to address both root and branch had something to offer in these cases; and indeed it does. The more I involved myself with the brain injury community the more I found the saying "no two brain injuries are the same" to be accurate. Each person is affected slightly (or very) differently. Many who had sustained an injury and experienced cognitive, mental, or behavioral changes would describe themselves as becoming a "different version" of who they were before the injury. A "Mary 2.0" if you will, whereby parts of their preinjury identity, personality, and thought processes remained while other parts changed, whether for what they considered better or worse. For many, recognizing and accepting these changes (or having them recognized and accepted by those close to them) can be among the most difficult parts of recovery. Feelings of depression and isolation can creep in if a good support system seems lacking. But nobody really stays the same anyway. We all have life experiences that change us, whether slowly or suddenly, subtle or dramatic, we all can continue to grow, and all one can do is continue to strive to be the best with the cards we are dealt. Having now attended, spoken at, and been involved in various support groups for those with brain injuries, I have seen how truly helpful it can be for someone to be able to be around others with similar experiences, similar stories of change and perseverance, and to share. Or just listen to others. Despite millions of people in the US living with the chronic after-effects of brain injury, it is strangely a condition that, unless one or someone close is directly affected, seems to get kind of swept under the rug as far as being recognized, discussed, or having ready resources for. It is for this very reason, along with the greatly unrecognized potential that Chinese medicine has to offer to further address it, that I've put this book together. I hope it will both raise further awareness of brain injuries as well as help practitioners have a better and more thorough understanding of what is happening, why, and how to approach it clinically.

Chapter 1

The "Silent Epidemic"

First, some definitions… Brain injuries that are neither congenital, hereditary, degenerative nor induced by birth trauma are collectively referred to as an acquired brain injury (ABI) and are the result of changes in neuronal activity that affect physical integrity, metabolic activity, or functional ability of the nerve cells of the brain. They can occur for a number of different reasons. An acquired brain injury can be placed into two general categories—traumatic and non-traumatic. Causes of each are listed in Table 1.1. Much of the treatment information in this text may be found useful for both, though it is primarily directed to cases of traumatic brain injury (TBI), which is defined as stemming from an external force. Direct impact injuries can be further divided into what are either closed injuries, in which brain lacerations or hemorrhages within the skull cause focal injuries, or open injuries, in which the tissue of the skull or the meninges have actually been breached.

TABLE 1.1 Causes of Brain Injury

Causes of Traumatic Brain Injury	Causes of Non-Traumatic Brain Injury
Falls	Stroke
Assaults	Infectious disease (meningitis, encephalitis)
Motor vehicle accidents	Seizure disorders
Sports and recreational injuries	Electric shock/lightning strike
Abusive head trauma/"shaken baby syndrome"	Tumors (surgery/radiation/chemo)
Gunshot wounds	Toxic exposures (substance misuse, lead ingestion, inhalation of volatile agents)
Workplace injuries	Metabolic disorders (insulin shock, diabetic coma, liver and kidney disease)
Child abuse	
Domestic violence	Neurotoxic poisoning (carbon monoxide, inhalants, lead exposure)
Military actions/blast injuries	Lack of oxygen to the brain (near drowning, airway obstruction, strangulation, cardiopulmonary arrest, hypoxia, anoxia)

Disability from a brain injury can result both from the primary injury (the initial injury itself), and from secondary injuries sustained over time. Components of a secondary injury can include hypoxia, anemia, metabolic abnormalities, hydrocephalus, intracranial hypertension, and hemorrhagic activity. Effects such as the release of excitatory amino acids, oxidative free radical production, arachidonic acid metabolite releases, and disruptions in neurotransmitters such as serotonin and monoamines can also be a delayed result of injury. It is important to keep in mind that a traumatic brain injury is not a single event. Nor is it a final outcome. Rather, it is the beginning of a chronic, potentially progressive, process. A TBI, either acute or chronic, is also not a static process; it may impact multiple organ systems and can both cause and accelerate other pathologies. In some cases, there has been found an accelerated progression of brain deterioration within the white matter of the frontal and temporal lobes. This may be the result of defective apoptotic mechanisms rather than immediate cell death. An individual who has sustained a TBI may be twice as likely to die in other incidences as a non-injured person and there has been a noted reduction in life expectancy of up to seven years.

It is for all of these reasons that it remains very important for the individual and their healthcare providers to be attentive and vigilant in restoring and maintaining the physical, mental, and emotional state of the individual.

The numbers… Annually over 1.7 million people in the US sustain a brain injury. Every day there are 5.4 million people who are living with their residual effects. It is among the leading causes of death and long-term disability. This is made even more staggering when one takes into consideration that the incidence of mild brain injury is generally considered to be greatly underreported. For these reasons, and the relative lack of attention and discussion given to the topic, it has often been referred to as a "silent epidemic." A brain injury can be difficult to understand if one has not been directly impacted by one or close to someone who has. The external initial wounds seemingly heal, while the internal wounds can remain and continue on. A brain injury can result in a range of emotional, behavioral, and/or cognitive impairments. These may include a quickness to anger, loss of executive function, depression, fatigue, emotional lability, socially inappropriate behaviors, or a seeming loss of one's filter when it comes to actions and language. If another person is not aware of the injury these can cause great difficulties in social situations. As it may not seem like anything is physically impaired from an outsider's perspective, knowing or understanding that the individual has been impacted by what can often be very frustrating, and sometimes long-standing, symptoms can be difficult. It is for this reason that those with a brain injury may often also be referred to as the "walking wounded." Over time these difficulties take their toll, not only on the affected person, but stress is placed on their families, friends, caregivers, and social structures. Vocational, educational, and recreational aspects of life can all become affected as the psychiatric components may go unrecognized or misunderstood.

Children aged 0–4 years old have the highest rate of emergency room visits, hospitalizations, and deaths combined when it comes to traumatic brain injury. These primarily result from falls, accidents, or abuse. Abusive head trauma, or "shaken baby syndrome," is a leading cause of death from brain injury in infants and young children. This is followed by adolescents and young adults aged 15–19 years old who tend to sustain an injury due to motor vehicle accidents, falls, and sports injuries. It is estimated that roughly 1.6 million–3.8 million sports-related brain injuries happen annually, including those for which no medical care is sought. It is estimated that, by the age of 25, 38 percent of males and 24 percent of females will have experienced at least one incidence of mild-to-severe brain trauma. Overall, falls have been found to be the leading cause of a traumatic brain injury (35.2%), followed by motor vehicle accidents (17.3%), being "struck by/against" (16.5%), and assaults (10%). At least 156,000 TBI-related deaths, hospitalizations, and emergency room visits happen each year as the result of assault. In the United States women experience about 4.8 million intimate partner-related physical assaults annually, making the potential number of actual occurrences (including those for which medical attention is not sought) significantly higher.

The costs of these incidents add up quickly as well—mentally, emotionally, spiritually, and, certainly, economically. The total lifetime comprehensive costs of fatal, hospitalized, and non-hospitalized traumatic brain injuries among civilians in 2000 alone was estimated to total more than $76.5 billion. This included $14.6 billion in medical costs and $69.2 billion for work-loss costs. An additional $137 billion cost was attributed in value to loss in quality of life.

Fortunately, in recent years, awareness of the impact of brain injuries has begun to grow through exposure relating to national sports leagues and returning service members from recent military operations. Military service members are a high-risk group with at least 325,000 returning US troops estimated to have some form of a brain injury with or without concomitant post-traumatic stress disorder. According to the Department of Defense website, in 2000 there were 10,963 TBI diagnoses. This increased substantially from 2006 to 2009 in which years there averaged 24,074 diagnoses annually and an estimated 11–22.8 percent of deployed service members reported a possible concussion or brain injury.

In light of these statistics, it is apparent that continued research advocacy, and exploration of options for literally millions of individuals affected by a brain injury, is a necessity.

Basic Neuropathology

Many different bodily responses and pathologies can arise from sustaining a brain injury. Some are primary to the injury, while others result secondarily. The degree to which these occur and impact an individual is often defined by location, direction of force, and severity of the injury. The vast majority of brain injuries that are medically treated are considered "mild" (~80%), while ~20 percent fall within the "moderate-to-severe range." Definitions of injury severity can be seen in Tables 1.2 and 1.3. One should not be fooled by the term "mild" however. Even in instances of mild initial symptoms, debilitating long-term results can at times still occur. Definitions and associated differences between these categories are outlined below. Acute symptoms following a mild brain injury (concussion) can include headaches, irritability, concentration/memory problems, sleep disturbance, dizziness, or fatigue. Approximately 43.3 percent of hospitalized TBI survivors in a 2003 study had some form of long-term disability. This risk of long-term disability increases with the age at which the injury is sustained.

TABLE 1.2 Mayo Traumatic Brain Injury Severity Classification System

Moderate–Severe	*One or more of the following criteria apply:*
	Death due to TBI
	Loss of consciousness for 30 minutes or more
	Post-traumatic anterograde amnesia of 24 hours or more
	Worst Glasgow Coma Scale full score in first 24 hours <13 (unless invalidated by review)
	One or more of the following: intracerebral hematoma, subdural hematoma, epidural hematoma, cerebral contusion, hemorrhagic contusion, penetrating brain trauma (dura penetrated), subarachnoid hemorrhage, brainstem injury
Mild	*Does not meet the criteria for severe but presents with one or more of the following:*
	Loss of consciousness of momentary to less than 30 minutes
	Post-traumatic anterograde amnesia of momentary to less than 24 hours
	Depressed, basilar, or linear skull fracture (dura intact)
Symptomatic	*Does not meet criteria for mild or severe but presents with one or more of the following:*
	Blurred vision
	Confusion (mental state changes)
	Dazed
	Dizziness
	Focal neurological symptoms
	Headache
	Nausea

TABLE 1.3 Comparison of Mild Brain Injury with Moderate and Severe Brain Injury

Variable	Mild Brain Injury (Concussion)	Moderate and Severe Brain Injury
Clinical definition	Loss of consciousness for less than 30 minutes Alteration in consciousness or retrograde amnesia lasting less than 24 hours	Loss of consciousness more than 30 minutes Post-traumatic amnesia more than 24 hours Glasgow Coma Scale as low as 3 (see Chapter 2)
Focal neurological signs	None or transient	Frequently present
Imaging (MRI, tomography)	Usually negative or very minor	Diagnostic
Natural history	Usually leads to full recovery Lack of consensus on natural history Evidence of possible prolonged sequelae	Natural history and sequelae are directly related to severity of injury and functional neuroanatomy
Predictors of persistent symptoms or disability	*Consistently associated risk factors*: Psychological factors (depression, anxiety, PTSD) Compensation and litigation Negative expectations and beliefs	Directly related to injury characteristics
Neurocognitive testing	Often inconclusive beyond acute injury period	Essential and valuable component of ongoing clinical case
Neuronal cell damage	Metabolic and ionic processes caused by axonal twisting or stretching can lead to secondary disconnection	Combination of cellular disruption directly related to injury and metabolic and ionic processes
Epidemiological evidence of causation between injury and sequelae	Inconsistent. Debated	Not debated

Mechanistic definitions of a brain injury describe impact, inertial loading, penetrating, and blast injuries.

- *Impact injuries*: Defined by the head making contact with an object and force being transferred to the brain. A rapid acceleration/deceleration as in motor vehicle accidents with head impact, falls, and assaults can create subdural hemorrhages secondary to torn bridging veins. Wider injury to the surrounding axons can also result. If there is significant collateral damage to axons, it is then referred to as a diffuse axonal injury.

- *Inertial loading injuries*: No direct contact with an object is necessary to cause a significant injury to the brain. Here the brain moves within the cranial cavity and is more likely to produce traumatic axonal injury. This can be cases of whiplash in which the brain may sustain both "coup" (movement in the direction of the force) and "contrecoup" (subsequent movement to the opposite side that was hit by the initial force) injuries to multiple injury sites.

- *Penetrating injuries*: When an object passes through the protective covering of the skull, resulting in direct parenchymal damage. Here local tissue necrosis becomes the primary pathology.

- *Blast injuries*: A shock wave from an explosive device can injure the brain parenchyma and have significant microglial and astrocyte activation and brain swelling. This is explored in more detail in Chapter 47.

Intracranial pressure may increase after a brain injury as a result of bleeding and/or hematomas, inflammation, and swelling. Normal intracranial pressure is in the range of 0–10mmHg. Pressures greater than 20 are considered abnormal, over 40 are associated with neurological dysfunction, and over 60 are invariably fatal. If there is diffuse brain swelling, systemic blood pressure will increase in an attempt to maintain cerebral perfusion pressure. However, a point may be reached in which cerebral perfusion pressure drops to such a degree that brain ischemia develops. Neurons are particularly sensitive to this reduction in blood flow and are the first type of cell to be injured. This is especially true for neurons in hippocampal sector CA1 which, as will be discussed in Chapter 7, may cause memory impairments.[1] If there is prolonged ischemia it will begin damaging glial, endothelial, smooth muscle, and other cell types. This damage is not the direct result of hypoxia, but rather a build-up of tissue lactate secondary to the lack of blood. This results in local tissue acidosis and injury. Lactic acid is produced as a normal product of cellular metabolism and generally gets removed via normal blood flow; it is only once blood flow is inhibited that build-up occurs and damage results.

---

1   Margulies, S. and Hicks, R. The combination therapies for traumatic brain injury workshop leaders. Combination therapies for traumatic brain injury: prospective considerations. *Journal of Neurotrauma.* 2009; 26(6): 925–939. doi:10.1089/neu.2008.0794

Brain swelling is common in cases of fatal TBI and may be focal in relationship to contusions, diffuse within one hemisphere of the brain, or diffuse throughout both hemispheres. It may be congestive, secondary to increases in cerebral blood volume, or due to edema. The majority of edema in trauma is cytotoxic swelling adjacent to contusions, which causes physical disruption of the tissues, including to the blood–brain barrier, and a loss of normal autoregulation in local vasculature can occur.

Diffuse traumatic axonal injury contributes to at least 35 percent of mortality and morbidity related to TBI where there are no space-occupying lesions, as well as being an important cause of severe disability and vegetative states. Here forces modify focal sections of axons that result in mechanoporation with an influx of calcium and disruption of the microtubules that impair local axonal transport and swelling. Over time this leads to axonal severing.

Subdural hematomas are most often seen after a head injury, but may also develop secondary to a number of non-traumatic causes. They are estimated to occur in approximately 5 percent of head injuries, the likelihood of such increasing with severity of the injury. Most acute subdural hematomas resolve without the formation of a chronic hematoma, though a chronic hematoma may still form following a relatively trivial head trauma. These are liquid and can spread in the subdural space, producing an accentuation of symptom patterns on the affected side and a flattening of the brain region on the opposite side. As these are mass lesions, the pressure created by them tends to create secondary pathologies.

A subarachnoid hemorrhage is relatively common following a brain injury, but rarely creates significant pathology. However, a primary traumatic subarachnoid hemorrhage (such as due to a single punch just under the mandible) may rupture the vertebral or basilar arteries and carries a high risk of mortality.

Intracerebral hemorrhages are most often seen in the frontal and temporal lobes. Superficial bleeds are most often due to extensive contusional injury, while deeper hematomas tend to occur in instances of greater force such as high-velocity vehicle accidents.

A traumatic brain injury rapidly initiates a series of secondary events that collectively contribute to cell injury and/or repair. These secondary events often create long-term neurological consequences, including cognitive dysfunction. Based primarily on rodent models of TBI, these early events can be divided into three periods, those which arise within minutes after an injury, those that evolve over the first 24 hours, and events that may be more delayed in onset, appearing between 24 and 72 hours postinjury. These acute secondary events are listed in Table 1.4.

TABLE 1.4 Initiation of Acute Secondary Events Following Brain Injury

Within minutes	Cell/axon stretching, compaction of neurofilaments, impaired axonal transport, axonal swelling, axonal disconnection
	Disruption of the blood–brain barrier
	Excessive neuronal activity: glutamate release
	Widespread changes in neurotransmitters: catecholamines, serotonin, histamine, GABA, acetylcholine
	Hemorrhage (heme, iron-mediated toxicity)
	Seizures
	Physiologic disturbances: decreased cerebral blood flow, hypotension, hypoxemia, increased intracranial pressure, decreased cerebral perfusion pressure
	Increased free radical production
	Disruption of calcium homeostasis
	Mitochondrial disturbances
Minutes–24 hours	Oxidative damage: increased reactive oxygen and nitrogen species (lipid peroxidation, protein oxidation, peroxynitrite), reduction in endogenous antioxidants (e.g. glutathione)
	Ischemia
	Edema: cytotoxic, vasogenic
	Enzymatic activation: kallikrein-kinins, calpains, caspases, endonucleases, metalloproteinases
	Decreased ATP: changes in brain metabolism (altered glucose utilization and switch to alternative fuels), elevated lactate
	Cytoskeleton changes in cell somas and axons
	Widespread changes in gene expression: cell cycle, metabolism, inflammation, receptors, channels and transporters, signal transduction, cytoskeleton, membrane proteins, neuropeptides, growth factors, and proteins involved in transcription/translation
	Inflammation: cytokines, chemokines, cell adhesion molecules, influx of leukocytes, activation of resident macrophages
24–72 hours	Non-ischemic metabolic failure

Chapter 2

Standard Assessment and Diagnostics

According to Silver *et al.*[1], a comprehensive assessment of brain injury includes the following:

- Medical history
- Physical examination
- Mental status examination
- "Bedside" cognitive testing
- Neuropsychological testing

- Computer tomography (acute)
- Magnetic resonance imaging
- Functional brain imaging
- Electroencephalogram
- Evoked potentials

Medical History

A thorough medical history should be taken, including a standard review of systems. Knowing the relevent history of preinjury conditions and symptoms is important to aid in gauging proper treatment principles and approaches. Common symptoms are listed in Table 2.1. Utilizing Chinese medical approaches, this includes "the ten questions" along with pulse and tongue diagnosis to form a fuller diagnostic picture and appropriate pattern differentiation(s). Any history of early childhood illness, particularly seizure disorders, previous head injuries, and attention deficit disorder, should be assessed. Those with multiple brain injuries have a poorer prognosis, higher risk of dementia, substance abuse, and atherosclerosis. If cognitive symptoms present, it may be appropriate to inquire into developmental milestones and previous levels of cognitive, intellectual, and attentional functions to form baseline information of the individual's preinjury state.

---

1   Silver, Jonathan, Yudofsky, Stuart, and McAllister, Thomas. *Textbook of Traumatic Brain Injury*. Washington, DC: American Psychiatric Pub. 2011. Print.

Current medications and history of relevant psychotropic or anticonvulsive (for prophylaxis or a continuing seizure disorder) drugs and their efficacy should be noted and considered. Benzodiazepines can impair memory and coordination. Anticholinergic drugs can increase confusion. Food and drug allergies and intolerances should be noted and considered, especially in the case of prescriptions of herbal medications. Potential herb–drug interactions should also be assessed (commonly used pharmaceuticals noted in this text and their potential herb–drug interactions are listed in Appendix D).

Relevant family medical and psychiatric history should be assessed to inform any potential impact on current emotional or psychological abnormalities or concerns. Inquiry into the individual's social history, family dynamic prior to and after injury, and other support structures are all relevant information as these can additionally play into mental–emotional states and the outlook of the individual toward healing. Losses and disruptions in an individual's social dynamic can provide severe additional stress which can act to slow the progress of recovery. Establishing new social connections or participating in leisure activities can become difficult, creating a sense of loneliness. If possible, a referral to a local support group should be considered where it is possible to socially interact with others who have experienced similar life events. Occupational status or pursuits are also of note as they can also be significant stressors.

TABLE 2.1 Traumatic Brain Injury Symptom Checklist

Cognitive	Level of consciousness
	Sensorium
	Attention/concentration
	Short-term memory
	Processing speed
	Thought processes
	Executive function (planning, abstract reasoning, problem solving, information processing, multi-tasking, insight, judgment, etc.)
Emotional	Mood/lability
	Depression
	Hypomania/mania
	Anxiety
	Anger/irritability
	Apathy
Behavioral	Impulsivity
	Disinhibition
	Anger dyscontrol
	Inappropriate sexual behavior
	Lack of initiative
	Change in personality

Physical	Fatigue
	Weight change
	Sleep disturbance
	Headache
	Visual problems
	Balance difficulties
	Dizziness
	Coldness
	Change in hair/skin
	Seizures
	Spasticity
	Loss of urinary control
	Arthritic complaints
Endocrine disturbance	Hypo/hyperthyroidism
	Impaired growth hormone release
	Impaired adrenal cortical function
	Hypopituitarism
	Hypothalamic hypogonadism
	Precocious puberty
	Hyperphagia
	Temperature dysregulation
	Antidiuretic hormone dysregulation
	Diabetes insipidus
	Menstrual irregularities
	Changes in sexual function

Physical Examination

Neurological examinations should be carried out where indicated. Orthopedic and range of motion testing should be carried out and charted where appropriate as well, particularly in pain cases and conditions of spasticity or paralysis. In addition to standard pulse diagnosis, palpatory testing may be done such as abdominal/hara diagnosis (including palpation of the oketsu region to determine Blood stasis as discussed in Chapter 12) and meridian palpation.

Mental State and "Bedside" Cognitive Examination

Common bedside evaluations of frontal lobe operations are listed in Table 2.2. Levels of conscious awareness are frequently gauged according to the Glasgow Coma Scale found in Table 2.3. Recovery stages from a severe brain injury are typically assessed by documenting levels along the Rancho Los Amigos Cognitive Scale found in Table 2.4.

TABLE 2.2 "Bedside" Evaluation of Frontal Lobe Function

Test	Description	Frequent Findings
Clock drawing test	Instruct individual to draw a clock, including all of the numbers, setting the time at 10 past 11 (provide all instructions first, then allow them to begin)	Poor planning (numbers inappropriately positioned, numbers do not fit inside the clock; excess space inside the clock, perseveration, etc.) Incorrect hand placement: hour and minute hands inappropriately placed, "stimulus bound" (hands connecting 10 and 11)
Verbal fluency	Ask individual to list number of words that begin with the same letter or number of animals named in one minute	Unable to name more than ten words, perseveration
Set shifts and sequencing (verbal and written)	Verbal: ask to continue the pattern 1A, 2B, 3C... Written: ask to connect numbers and letters in a sequential and alternating pattern (1A-2B-3C, etc.)	Perseveration; inability to consistently shift sets (e.g. 1A-2B-3C-4C-5C, etc. or 1A-2B-3C-3D-3E-3F, etc.)
"First palm-side"	Ask individual to place their right fist into left palm, the right palm into left palm, then right side of the hand into left palm in a sequential manner	Perseveration of movement
"Go–No Go" test	Ask individual to say "two" when one finger is held up; "one" when two fingers are displayed	Inability to inhibit the visual stimulus (says "one" when one finger displayed)

TABLE 2.3 Glasgow Coma Scale Scores

	Type of Response	Score	Description/Significance
Eye opening	Spontaneous	4	Eyes are open, but this does not imply intact awareness; indicates active arousal mechanisms in the brainstem
	To speech	3	Nonspecific response to speech or shout; does not imply patient obeys commands to open eyes; indicates functional cerebral cortex in processing information
	To pain	2	Pain stimulus is applied to chest or limbs; suggests functioning of the lower levels of the brain
	None	1	No response to speech or pain (not attributable to ocular swelling)

Motor	Obeys commands	6	Can process instructions and respond by obeying a command
	Localizes pain	5	Pain stimulus is applied to supraocular region or fingertip; patient makes an attempt to remove the source of pain stimulus
	Withdrawal	4	Normal flexor response; patient withdraws from painful stimulus with abduction of the shoulder
	Abnormal flexion	3	Abnormal responses to pain stimulus; includes flexion or extension of upper extremities; indicates more severe brain dysfunction. Discortication is manifested by abduction of the upper extremities with flexion of the arms, wrists, and fingers; the lower extremities extend and rotate internally with plantar flexion of the feet; suggests lesions in the cerebral hemispheres or internal capsule
	Extension	2	Decerebrate responses to pain stimulus manifested by abduction and hyperpronation of the upper extremities; the legs are extended with plantar flexion of the feet; includes opisthotonos, indicating damage extending from the midbrain to the upper pontine
	No response	1	Flaccid, fails to respond to painful stimulus
Verbal	Oriented	5	Oriented to person (knows identity); place (knows where he/she is); and time (knows the current year, season, month)
	Confused	4	Responds to questions in a conversational manner, but responses indicate disorientation/confusion
	Inappropriate	3	Intelligible speech (e.g. shouting or swearing), but no sustained or coherent conversation
	Incomprehensible	2	Moaning and groaning; no recognizable words
	No response	1	No verbal response

TABLE 2.4 Rancho Los Amigos Cognitive Scale

I—No response	Unresponsive to any stimulus
II—Generalized response	Limited, inconsistent, and non-purposeful responses, often to pain only
III—Localized response	Purposeful responses; may follow simple commands; may focus on presented object
IV—Confused, agitated	Heightened state of activity; confusion and disorientation; aggressive behavior; unable to perform self-care; unaware of present events; agitation seems related to internal confusion
V—Confused, inappropriate	Non-agitated; appears alert, responds to commands; distractible; does not concentrate on task; agitated response to external stimuli; verbally inappropriate; does not learn new information
VI—Confused, appropriate	Goal-directed behavior, needs cuing; can relearn old skills such as activities of daily living; severe memory problems; some awareness of self and others
VII—Automatic, appropriate	Appears appropriately oriented; frequently robot-like in daily routine; minimal or absent confusion; shallow recall; increased awareness of self and interaction in environment; lacks insight into condition; decreased judgment and problem solving; lacks realistic planning for future
VIII—Purposeful, appropriate	Alert and oriented; recalls and integrates past events; learns new activities and can continue without supervision; independent in home and living skills; capable of driving; defects in stress tolerance, judgment, and abstract reasoning persist; may function at reduced levels in society

Neuropsychiatric Assessment

A brain injury can often be an "invisible injury" whereby effects are not always physical and apparent to observation. The individual may not even be aware of the presence or severity of their impairment. Additionally, standard brain imaging techniques will rarely detect the diffuse axonal injury found in many cases of mild brain injury. For this reason, it is important for a medical professional to do a thorough intake in order to gather as much information as possible about symptoms and details of incidence(s). In addition to performing a thorough review of systems, as is generally used by Chinese medical practitioners during intakes, many of these tools can also be integrated into one's practice to help dig for deeper information or steer (or guide) proper treatment approaches.

Neuropsychiatric manifestations after a brain injury depend on several factors:

- Pre-existing variables: preinjury personality/temperament, family psychiatric history, personal psychiatric, neurologic, medical history

- Psychosocial, economic, and vocational status at time of injury

- Type, location, and severity of injury

- Emotional and psychological responses to brain injury-related disturbances in cognition and behavior

- Impact of these changes on personal and professional roles and relationships, especially family

- Interplay between impairments and community barriers and supports

Sample questions that a practitioner may want to ask to gather a well-rounded clinical picture are included in Table 2.5.

TABLE 2.5 Sample Questions for Assessment of Possible Brain Injuries

Question	Rationale
Have you ever hit your head? Have you ever been in an accident? Have you ever been in or near an explosion?	Probe for car/motorcycle/bicycle/other motor vehicle accidents, falls, assaults, sports or recreational injuries, blast injuries
(If so) did you black out, pass out, or lose consciousness?	Establish any loss of consciousness (verify with witness if possible)
What is the last thing you remember before the injury?	Establish extent of retrograde amnesia
What is the first thing you recall after the injury?	Estimate duration of loss of consciousness and/or post-traumatic amnesia
(If no known loss of consciousness) At time of injury, did you experience any change in thinking or feel "dazed" or "confused"?	Establish change in mentation or level of consciousness
Did you suffer any other injuries during the incident?	Identify related injuries that may contribute to symptom presentation
What problems did you have after the injury?	Delineate postinjury symptoms
Has anyone told you that you're different since the injury? If so, how have you changed?	Detect problems outside of the individual's awareness or those he or she may be minimizing
Did anyone witness or observe your injury?	Identify source of collateral history
Many people who have injured their head had been drinking or using drugs; how about you?	Offer the individual greater "permission" to admit substance use and determine if substances contributed to the altered mental status at the time of injury
Have you had any other injuries to your head or brain?	Identify any previous brain injuries that may increase morbidity from current injury

Neuropsychological Assessment

There are many tests designed to aid medical practitioners in assessing the severity of potential neuropsychological deficits.

Attention and concentration

- Digit Span subtest from the WAIS-III, WMS-III, WAIS-IV
- Spatial Span subtest from the WMS-III
- Spatial Addition subtest from the WMS-IV
- Digit Symbol subtest from the WAIS-IV
- Coding subtest from the WAIS-IV
- Continuous Performance Test
- Paced Auditory Serial Addition Task
- Stroop Color and Word Test
- Digit Vigilance Test
- Consonant Trigrams

Memory and learning

- California Verbal Learning Test, 2nd edition
- Rey-Osterrieth Complex Figure Test
- Hopkins Verbal Learning Test—Revised
- Rey Auditory-Verbal Learning Test
- WMS-III
- WMS-IV
- Benton Visual Retention Test
- Brief Visuospatial Memory Test—Revised

Executive functioning, concept formation, planning

- Booklet Category Test
- Wisconsin Card Sorting Test
- Controlled Oral Word Association Test
- Trail Making Test—Part B
- Delis-Kaplan Executive Function System (multiple subtests)

Language

- Aphasia Examination
- Boston Diagnostic Aphasia Examination
- Multilingual Aphasia Examination
- Western Aphasia Battery
- Boston Naming Test

Visuospatial and visuoconstructional skills

- Visual Form Discrimination Test
- Judgment of Line Orientation Test
- Hooper Visual Organization Test
- Rey-Osterrieth Complex Figure Test
- Block Design subtest from the WAIS-III, WAIS-IV

Intelligence

- WAIS-III
- WAIS-IV

Motor processes

- Finger Tapping Test
- Grooved Pegboard Test

Assessing possible malingering

- 21 Item Test
- Rey 15-Item Memory Test with recognition
- Test of memory malingering
- Word Memory Test
- Portland Digit Recognition Test
- Victoria Symptom Validity Test
- Rey Dot Counting Test

Brief neuropsychological screenings

- Mini-Mental State Examination
- Repeatable Battery for Assessment of Neuropsychological Status

- Shipley Institute of Living Scale

- Barrow Neurological Institute (BNI) Screen for Higher Cerebral Functions

Questions to determine level of orientation and amnesia immediately following injury

What is your name?

When were you born?

Where do you live?

Where are you now?

How did you get here?

What is the first event you can remember before the accident?

Describe in detail the first event you remember after the accident

What time is it now?

What day of the week is it?

What day of the month is it?

What is the month?

What is the year?

Computerized Testing

- *CNS Vital Signs (CNS VS)*: Verbal and visual memory, psychomotor speed, complex attention, reaction time, and cognitive flexibility

- *Automated Neuropsychological Assessment Metrics (ANAM)*: 31 subtests of processing speed, short-term memory, working memory, and resistance to interference

- *Brain Fitness Program*: Auditory Processing Skills Training

Computer Tomography (CT)

CT scans can be used during the acute phase to quickly identify gross brain pathology critical to early head injury management such as hemorrhaging, cerebral edema, and the presence of midline shift. It is also used as a reference to compare to other imaging methods and follow-up imaging studies.

Magnetic Resonance Imaging (MRI)

MRI studies are generally used in the subacute and chronic stages of the recovery process. This helps with outcome expectations and evaluation of potential psychiatric concerns. In order to appear on an MRI, an abnormality needs to be larger than about one cubic millimeter. Small shearing of blood vessels will appear on an MRI as hemosiderin. If there are no other vascular risk factors, this is considered an indicator of diffuse axonal injury. Location and quantity of hemosiderin can also relate to neuropsychological components such as memory and speed of information processing.

Diffuse Tensor Imaging (DTI)

This is a particular method using MRI. DTI imaging is done by assessing water molecules exposed to brief pulses of strong magnetic fields and detectable changes in emitted radiofrequency waves. This is particularly helpful in assessing white matter integrity as the white matter microstructure of myelin sheaths and cell membranes along white matter tracts affect the movement of water molecules. Water molecules tend to move faster parallel to nerve fibers rather than angled or in a perpendicular fashion. This method has been shown to be important in advancing the understanding of how more mild brain injuries affect brain dynamics.

Magnetic Resonance Spectrography (MRS)

This is a spectroscopic assessment of chemical composition which is also done by MRI. Here biochemical information about detectable neurometabolites and mobile lipids can be gathered. Relevant to brain injuries, MRS is able to detect levels of N-acetyl Aspartate, a biomarker of neuronal health, to help in finding subtle abnormalities related to mild brain injury.

Functional Brain Imaging Methods
Single-Photon Emission Computed Tomography (SPECT)

In a SPECT study a radiotracer is injected into an individual's vein. As the tracer decays it emits a photon which is detected and recorded by the SPECT gamma camera. In this way, blood flow can be determined based upon the distribution of the tracer within the brain. Coronal, sagittal, and axial views can be taken as well as three-dimension reconstructions of the brain. This can assess relative cerebral blood flow, but is unable to gather information about absolute cerebral blood flow as can be done with PET imaging.

Positron Emission Tomography (PET)

Using a similar method to SPECT scans, PET imaging uses different radioactive tracers, more precise detection equipment, and greater detail in anatomical imagery. As this tracer decays a positron is released. Once this positron collides with an electron, two photons are produced, traveling away from one another in a straight line at the speed of light. These photons are simultaneously detected by the PET scanner on opposite sides of the scanner. A computerized calculation then determines the location of the positron release. The computer makes a record of these and is able to form a topographic image. These can be assessed visually, but are more often statistically analyzed by computer software.

Functional Magnetic Resonance Imaging (fMRI)

Currently only used for research purposes, fMRI allows for the measurement of activity-related changes in cerebral blood flow without a radioactive tracer. Magnetic qualities of oxygenated and deoxygenated hemoglobin differ in nature. As brain activity increases in a particular area of the brain, so too does its metabolic needs. Blood flow increases to meet this demand to a level just above what is needed to carry out the activity. This higher hemoglobin concentration causes a light increase in magnetic resonance signal intensity and the change is measured by the fMRI. This is then reconstructed by a computer to map areas of increased activation. fMRIs have been carried out in acupuncture research to determine brain regions that appear activated or deactivated upon needle insertion at an acupuncture point. This is discussed further in the next chapter and study results are referenced throughout this text.

Magnetoencephalography (MEG)

A non-invasive method which uses superconducting sensors to measure magnetic fields generated by neuronal activation. These fields pass through the skull without causing distortion to provide data similar to an EEG (discussed below) but with fewer artifacts. Computerized models can then map activation and localized patterns of brain activity. An MEG is able to assess rapid changes in neuronal activity, making it possible to separate components of a cognitive task such as word retrieval or reading.

Electrophysiological Assessment

Electroencephalogram (EEG)

Within the first several hours following a mild TBI there may be a focal slowing and attenuated posterior alpha wave. In mild cases these abnormalities will often resolve within three months following the injury. Approximately 10 percent of individuals will have continued abnormalities at one year postinjury. A low-voltage posterior alpha has been argued to also be the result of postinjury anxiety. As most of the information gathered through an EEG can also be gathered through careful history taking and with abnormalities generally expected to resolve soon after injury, an EEG is recommended to be primarily reserved for the evaluation of suspected post-traumatic epilepsy.

Chapter 3

Treatment Mechanisms of Acupuncture

It is important to understand what exactly is being done and what is occurring in an affected person's body when approaching brain injuries and associated symptoms with Chinese medicine. In this chapter mechanisms of action will be explored along with risks and cautions associated with these treatment approaches. Emphasis will be placed on modern research into physiological mechanisms and responses. The reason for this is twofold: first, classical descriptions of mechanisms are easily accessible in many books on Chinese medicine; second, it is important for a practitioner to understand these physiological responses when communicating with other healthcare professionals unfamiliar with Chinese medical theory/terminology in explaining what care is being provided to a patient. Often those recovering from a brain injury are being treated by a wide group of professionals that may include their primary carer, neurologist, nurses, neuropsychiatrists, speech–language pathologist, occupational therapist, neuro-optometrist, physical therapist, etc.

This is not to dismiss or downplay classical descriptions and actions. In discussing treatment and symptoms later in this text, pattern differentiation, pulses and tongue diagnostics, and treatment principles are essential to treatment and are laid out in accordance with these principles. It is still very important for a practitioner to understand how an individual's organ systems, Qi, Blood, Shen, Fluids, etc. are being affected. These are foundational components of Chinese medicine and arguably the reason it can work so well to address a wide range of symptoms simultaneously and work to reregulate the body system as a whole. However, the onus lies on the Chinese medicine practitioner to be able to bridge any communication gaps and effectively convey what they are doing. This involves using terminology biomedical practitioners are familiar with in order to work together in providing the best care and garner the most benefit for the affected individual.

A significant advantage to the use of Chinese medical treatment approaches is their relative safety and low risk of negative ("side") effects. With acupuncture, the primary risks are minimal and infrequent—mild bruising, numbness, and tingling may occur at the insertion site; hematomas are rare but may also occur. An individual may begin to feel dizzy or light headed during or for a short duration immediately following a treatment. If performed improperly there is a risk of pneumothorax or other organ puncture, nerve damage, or infection due to non-sterile conditions. So long as the practitioner has done adequate and proper training, the likelihood of these occurring is very small. For the patient seeking treatment, however, this is an important reason to make sure their provider has completed adequate training in a full Chinese medical curriculum rather than truncated programs aimed at medical professionals which only teach basic approaches to needling such as exclusively dry needling.

Acupuncture Mechanisms
Local Effects: Pain Reduction, Anti-Inflammatory Effects, Initiation of the Healing Response

The insertion of an acupuncture needle into the skin, in essence, creates a type of microinjury. While this is not enough to cause damage to the area, it is a breaching of the epidermis, which alerts the body to respond in a number of various ways. Upon needle insertion, an "axon reflex" occurs throughout the meshwork of surrounding nerves. This stimulates local muscle fibers including A-delta (also A-gamma and sometimes A-beta) and II and III muscle fibers.[1] Through this there is a triggering of calcitonin gene-related peptide (CGRP), a powerful vasodilator, which opens local capillaries and releases various neuropeptides— prostaglandins, red and white blood cells, glutamate, excitatory amino acids, substance P, and serotonin—from local mast cells. This release downregulates the pain cascade, works to reduce inflammation in the area, initiates the healing response of tissue, fights infections, and increases local circulation. The local tissue cells including arterioles, nerve terminals, and mast cells can stimulate vascular nerve fibers, which triggers nitric oxide (NO) production. Other tissues that may be involved include smooth muscle cells and endothelium cells as a result of NO production which further increases the blood flow and local circulation.[2]

Acupuncture is thought to have its analgesic effect through the release of local endorphin and of the neurotransmitter encephalin, which inhibits the nociceptive pathway as a means of "hyperstimulation." A 2010 study demonstrated acupuncture to effectively trigger a local increase in the extracellular concentration of ATP, ADP, AMP, and adenosine,[3] a key component in energy exchange during metabolic processes. By increasing ATP, the body is better able to create not only a well-recognized analgesic effect but also contribute more usable energy and innate healing potential within the body.

---

1   Filshie, Jacqueline and White, Adrian. *Medical Acupuncture—A Western Scientific Approach.* Edinburgh, London: Churchill Livingstone. 1998. Print.

2   Hsiao, S-H., and Tsai, L.J. A neurovascular transmission model for acupuncture-induced nitric oxide. *Journal of Acupuncture and Meridian Studies.* 2008 Sep; 1(1): 42–50. doi:10.1016/S2005-2901(09)60006-6

3   Goldman, N., Chen, M., Fujita, T. *et al.* Adenosine A1 receptors mediate local anti-nociceptive effects of acupuncture. *Nature Neuroscience.* 2010; 13: 883–888. doi:10.1038/nn.2562

Acupuncture likely has its effect of regulating homeostatic states or the somatic autonomic reflex of both the sympathetic and parasympathetic branches of the autonomic nervous system to reinstate a balanced dynamic between the two. This has been likened to a scientific basis for the concept of the balance between Yin and Yang found within Chinese medical theory. When an acupuncture needle is inserted into the desired acupoint, there are several different peripheral afferent fibers that can be found in the area of insertion. These are the true A-delta, A-beta, and A-gamma fibers in the skin, C-fibers, and II and III muscle fibers that create the neural network underneath the surface. Surface oxygen levels have also been demonstrated to be in higher concentrations at locations of traditional acupuncture points.[4]

Different sensations associated with the phenomenon known as "De Qi" or "Attaining the Qi" in which the patient feels an achy or heavy sensation after needling are directly associated with different neural tracts, with different terminal endings producing different outcomes. These are summarized in Table 3.1.

TABLE 3.1 Classical De Qi Sensation-Associated Nerve Fiber

Soreness	C-fiber
Numbness	A-gamma
Vibration	A-beta
Heaviness	A-delta, III muscle fiber
Achy	IV muscle fiber
Cold	A-delta
Hot	C-fiber, IV muscle fiber
Pinprick	A-delta

Neuromuscular Effects

Muscle motor points, trigger points, and classical Ashi points can all be used to stimulate the neural compartments of the muscle(s). Here the primary afferent nociceptive system which have terminal endings throughout the limbic regions of the brain become stimulated. This may help to "reset" the muscle to a state of relaxation. Gunn[5] uses the term intramuscular stimulation rather than acupuncture when referring to the needling process in which he describes two essential elements of myofascial pain—muscle shortening and neuropathy. The goal of this intramuscular treatment is to release muscle shortening and promote healing.

---

4   Nam, M-H., Yin, C., Soh, K-S., and Choi, S-H. Adult neurogenesis and acupuncture stimulation at ST-36. *Journal of Acupuncture and Meridian Studies*. 2011 Sep; 4(3): 153–158. doi:10.1016/j.jams.2011.09.001

5   Gunn, C.C. *The Gunn Approach to the Treatment of Chronic Pain: intramuscular stimulation for myofascial pain of radiculopathic origin*. 1996. New York: Churchill Livingstone. Print.

In this sense it has been argued that acupuncture may be considered a variation of cortisone injection within myofascial trigger points. In the case of neuralgias and neuropathies, acupuncture stimulation may have a local effect on restoring the diseased nerve by improving the local blood flow and accelerating the metabolism.[6] Table 3.2 shows specific muscle innervations according to the vertebral level at which the nerves exit the spinal cord.

TABLE 3.2 Spinal-Exiting Nerve Muscle Innervation

C1	None
C2	Longus colli, sternocleidomastoid (SCM), rectus capitis
C3	Trapezius, splenius capitis
C4	Trapezius, levator scapulae
C5	Supraspinatus, infraspinatus, deltoid, biceps
C6	Biceps, supinator, wrist extensors
C7	Triceps, wrist flexors
C8	Ulnar deviations, thumb extensors, thumb adductors
T1–T2	Minor innervations of intrinsic muscles of the hand, elbow, forearm, shoulder, scapulae, upper back, and neck
T3–T12	Innervations of the upper torso, as well as posterior and anterior aspects
L1	None
L2	Psoas, hip adductors
L3	Psoas, quadriceps, thigh atrophy
L4	Tibialis anterior, extensor hallucis
L5	Extensor hallucis, peroneals, gluteus medius, dorsiflexors, hamstrings, and calf atrophy
S1	Calf and hamstring, wasting of gluteals, peroneals, plantar flexors
S2	Calf and hamstring, wasting of gluteals, plantar flexors
S3	None
S4	Bladder–rectum

Spinal Segmental Effects: Acupuncture Analgesia and the "Gate Theory"

All primary afferent nociceptive fibers enter the spinal column via the dorsal horn. Varying sensations associated with different sensory fibers are listed in Table 3.3. At the level of

6   Corradino, Michael. *Neuropuncture: a clinical handbook of neuroscience acupuncture.* 2nd ed. London, Philadelphia: Jessica Kingsley Publishers (Singing Dragon). 2017. Print.

the dorsal horn, neurotransmitters—including serotonin and norepinephrine—are released, which have a general depressive effect on dorsal horn activity. This modulates and reduces the signaling of pain, and also inhibits dysfunctional autonomic reflexes of organs and relaxes the smooth muscle of the associated segment. This relaxation inherently releases unnecessary stress on the organ, increases circulation, and aids in enhancing the organ's function. Small intermediate cells are also stimulated, with enkephalin being released to block the transmission of pain in the substantia gelatinosa. Somatic and visceral afferent nerve fibers converge at the dorsal horn, then cross over and travel up the same single spinothalamic tract, passing through the reticular formation into the intralaminar nucleus of the thalamus. Tertiary neurons project to diverse areas of the intermediate and higher brain, including the limbic cortex, insular cortex, and prefrontal cortex.[7]

TABLE 3.3 Peripheral Nociceptors and Sensations

Sensory Fiber	Skin	Muscle	Sensation
Large myelinated	None	I	None
Large myelinated	A-beta	II	Light touch, pressure, vibration
Medium myelinated	A-gamma	II	Numbness
Small myelinated	A-delta	III	Deep pressure, heaviness in muscle, pinprick in skin, cold
Small myelinated	C	IV	Soreness, aching, heat, itching, calmness, burning pain

Acupuncture is theorized to travel along a second channel which terminates the lamina in the spinal cord. Secondary neurons then terminate in various nuclei of the thalamus including the ventroposteriolateral nucleus, dorsomedial nucleus, intralaminar nuclei, and the centromedian nucleus. Major pathways followed include the spinothalamic tract, spinoreticular tract, and the spinomesencephalic tract, which all project to the various cortical areas of the higher brain such as the sensory cortices, limbic and insular cortices, and prefrontal cortex. More importantly, while en route to the thalamus, collaterals of these tracts branch out to terminate at various levels of the brainstem and hypothalamus. At the level of the brainstem, further collaterals branch to the periaqueductal gray and the nucleus locus ceruleus to the nucleus raphe magnus and the nucleus reticularis paragigantocellularis. Monoaminergic neurons here work to inhibit ascending pain signals at the lamina. At the level of the hypothalamus there are two ascending tracts acting on the hypothalamic nuclei

---

7   Cho, Z., Wong, E.K., and Fallon, J. *The Science of Acupuncture and the Brain: brain, nerves, needles, and acupuncture.* Irvine, CA: University of California. 2000. Print.

(the arcuate nucleus) as well as other hypothalamic cells that secrete beta-endorphin. This has been postulated to account for some of the "distal acupuncture" procedures.[8]

Fascia Structure Effects

It has been observed independently by various researchers that the fascia (connective tissue) planes throughout the body form a network that resembles the meridians traditionally described in Chinese medicine. Langevin and Yandow[9] examined the locations of acupuncture points and meridians in gross anatomical sections of the arm of cadavers and found significant correspondences between the locations of acupuncture points and intermuscular or intramuscular connective tissue plane junctions. Yuan *et al.*[10] constructed a virtual human body model, digitally constructing a three-dimensional network of fascial connective tissue areas that resemble the network of meridians and acupuncture points. They hypothesized this network to be a hitherto undiscovered auto-surveillance system in the body that may lead to further explanations of the basic mechanism of acupuncture action. Myers has also explored this correlation in the 3rd edition of his well-received book *Anatomy Trains.*[11]

The nerves within these fascial planes carry signals throughout. It has been suggested that a mechanical signal propagating along these channels may be responsible for some of the therapeutic effects of acupuncture. In essence, when the inserted acupuncture needle impacts connective tissue, it causes the "needle grasp" phenomenon in which the fascia responds and "wraps" around the needle in response to the stimulation/contact with it. This results in a perturbation of mechanical force within muscle tissue which propagates to neighboring muscles. This mechanical signal evokes a response in connective tissue downstream, resulting in adaptive changes in fascia or anti-inflammatory response. Other signals such as the flow of paracrine-signaling molecules[12] and piezoelectric signal conduction throughout the liquid crystalline structure[13, 14] of the fascial network have also been proposed.

8   Filshie, Jacqueline and White, Adrian. *Medical Acupuncture—A Western Scientific Approach.* Edinburgh, London: Churchill Livingstone. 1998. Print.

9   Langevin, H.M. and Yandow, J.A. Relationship of acupuncture points and meridians to connective tissue planes. *The Anatomical Record.* 2002; 269: 257–265. doi:10.1002/ar.10185

10   Yuan, L., Yang, C., Huang, Y., Janos, P., and Bai, Y. Research methods in fasciology: implications for acupuncture meridianology. *Fasciology.* 2011 Jul; 1: 17–30.

11   Myers, Thomas. *Anatomy Trains: myofascial meridians for manual and movement therapists.* 3rd ed. Edinburgh: Elsevier. 2014. Print.

12   Langevin, H., Churchill, D., and Cipolla, M. Mechanical signaling through connective tissue: a mechanism for the therapeutic effect of acupuncture. *The FASEB Journal.* Oct 2001; 15: 353–360.

13   Yang, C., Du, Y., Wu, J., *et al.* Fascia and primo vascular system. *Evidence-Based Complementary and Alternative Medicine: eCAM.* 2015; 2015: 303769. doi:10.1155/2015/303769

14   Gyer, Giles, Michael, Jimmy, and Tolson, Ben. *Dry Needling for Manual Therapists: points, techniques and treatments, including electroacupuncture and advanced tendon techniques.* London: Singing Dragon. 2016. Print.

Endogenous Opioid Circuit (EOC) Effects

The hypothalamus is one of the largest manufacturers of beta-endorphins, our endogenous poly-opioids which reduce pain. As noted above, signals from needle insertion make their way to the hypothalamus. These opioid substances immediately travel to the periaqueductal gray to depress all pain signaling from the periphery. Serotonin is also released in the brainstem and stimulates further serotonin releases, along with norepinephrine within the dorsal horn. Both of these strongly inhibit pain signaling in both directions. Opioid release has been studied extensively in treatment of addiction disorders utilizing electro-acupuncture. Specific millicurrent frequencies have been shown to elicit greater releases of particular endorphins as summarized in Table 3.4.[15]

TABLE 3.4 Lateral Preoptic Nucleus: Lateral Tuberal

Endorphin	Receptor	Frequency/Amperage	Location
Beta-endorphins	Mu	2–4 Hz millicurrent	Midbrain, periaqueductal gray, pituitary
Enkephalins	Delta	2–4 Hz millicurrent	Dorsal horn of the spine
Dynorphins	Kappa	50–100 Hz millicurrent	Brainstem/spine
Orphanin	Mu	2–15 Hz millicurrent	Widespread
NK cells	Immune	4 Hz millicurrent	Widespread
5HTP	5HTPr	20–50 Hz millicurrent	Hypothalamus
Oxytocin	OXTR	2–15/30 Hz millicurrent	CNS
Dopamine	D1	2, 15–30 Hz millicurrent	Prefrontal
NOS	Epithelium	2, 15–30 Hz millicurrent	Widespread

Central Nervous System and Disease Treatment Effects

Endocrinological effects occur through stimulation of the hypothalamus, which influence the anterior pituitary and ultimately the adrenals, having an impact on the entire hypothalamic–pituitary axis (HPA). In this way, endocrine regulation can occur throughout the HPA via acupuncture stimulus arriving at the higher brain centers by passing through the limbic system. This induces the higher brain to initiate the needed commands (possibly from the prefrontal cortex), which passes to the hypothalamus (some through limbic structures) for the final execution of endocrine, autonomic, and other homeostatic tasks. This may include the sensory cortex–multimodal association–amygdala–prefrontal cortex–amygdala–

---

15   Li-Li Cheng, Ming-Xing Ding, Cheng Xiong, Min-Yan Zhou, Zheng-Ying Qiu, and Qiong Wang. Effects of electroacupuncture of different frequencies on the release profile of endogenous opioid peptides in the central nerve system of goats. *Evidence-Based Complementary and Alternative Medicine*. vol. 2012, Article ID 476457, 9 pages, 2012. doi:10.1155/2012/476457

hypothalamus circuitry. ACTH and beta-endorphins are shown to be released, as is 5-hydroxytryptophan (5-HTP).[16]

Immunological influences take place through generalized autonomic changes in the lymphoreticular system of the marrow and spleen. Beta-endorphins are released into the blood stream and there have been demonstrated increases in natural killer cells and changes in gamma-interferon levels.

Primo Vascular Effects

Bong-han Kim, a Korean surgeon, reported observing a novel extensive microscopic duct system distributed throughout the body that may correspond to the meridians. This structure was initially named after its founder as Bonghan ducts, and has since been referred to as the primo vascular system. It has been extensively studied and recently reviewed by others.[17, 18] Observation of the primo vascular system requires special staining. The primo vascular system forms a new circulatory system in the body apart from the blood and lymphatic systems, carrying a liquid that contains, among other substances, hormones, amino acids, and free nucleotides. While holding vast potential in reconciling traditional descriptions of the meridian system, significantly more research is necessary to substantiate the primo vascular system.

Cortical Region Activation and Deactivation Effects

Results of functional magnetic resonance imaging studies have shown that stimulation at a traditional acupuncture point produces a distinct response in specific areas of the brain. This was distinctly different from stimulation at other points on the same spinal segment, and also different from the stimulation at neighboring points on the same meridian.

Neurophysiological studies have also demonstrated point indication specificity. In a meta-analysis of fMRI studies done which mapped areas of the brain influenced by acupuncture, it concluded: "Two third[s] (64%) of 25 studies showed that acupuncture treatments were associated with more activation, mainly in the somatosensory areas, motor areas, basal ganglia, cerebellum, limbic system and higher cognitive areas (e.g. prefrontal cortex). Three studies also showed more deactivation in the limbic system in response to acupuncture."[19] The limbic system is associated with most of the body's emotional processing, and acupuncture's

---

16   Cheng, K. Neurobiological mechanisms of acupuncture for some common illnesses: a clinician's perspective. *Journal of Acupuncture and Meridian Studies.* 2014 Jun; 7(3): 105–114. doi:10.1016/j.jams.2013.07.008

17   Soh, K.S. Bonghan circulatory system as an extension of acupuncture meridians. *Journal of Acupuncture and Meridian Studies.* 2009; 2: 93–106.

18   Stefanov, M. and Kim, J. Primo vascular system as a new morphofunctional integrated system. *Journal of Acupuncture and Meridian Studies.* 2012; 5: 193–200.

19   Huang, W., Pach, D., Napadow, *et al.* Characterizing acupuncture stimuli using brain imaging with fMRI—a systematic review and meta-analysis of the literature. *PLOS ONE.* 2012; 7(4): e32960. https://doi.org/10.1371/journal.pone.0032960

regulatory effect on this region may explain why it can be helpful in mental–emotional concerns following a brain injury such as hypervigilance and anxiety. An example of these brain region activations being point specific was shown in a study finding that the point KI-3, located posterior to the medial malleolus, was shown to enhance connectivity between the superior temporal gyrus and postcentral gyrus, while GB-40, located anterior to the lateral malleolus, enhanced connectivity between the superior temporal gyrus and anterior insula.[20] These studies are limited, however, and further research seems essential to create a thorough map of these influences.

A recent study also demonstrated acupuncture's ability to increase glucose metabolism and improve cerebral blood flow in the brain areas related to cognition and memory by increasing the expression of glucose transporter 1 (GLUT1) which is involved in cellular respiration, regulation of glucose levels, and vitamin C uptake. The laboratory results indicated that upregulation of GLUT1 by acupuncture alleviates ischemia and anoxia-related cognitive impairment.[21]

The Role of Acupuncture in Neuroplasticity and Neurogenesis

Acupuncture has been shown to have a direct influence on neuroplasticity and neurogenesis within the brain. This is the body's ability to create new neural connections and even generate new nerve cells. Until relatively recently it was thought that any neuronal loss due to injury or aging in adults was permanent. It is now known that neural stem cells are still active in certain regions of the adult brain, namely the dentate gyrus of the hippocampus and the subventricular zones. During neurogenesis stem cells are capable of developing into all major types of neural cells: neurons, astrocytes, and oligodendrocytes. While this ability is now known to exist in adults, it is at a significantly slower rate than in children.

A recent study showed acupuncture-induced cell and neuroblast differentiation in the hippocampus, providing evidence that it may be useful as a neurogenesis-stimulating therapy. There has also been a demonstrated effect on cAMP signaling, a transcription factor important in proliferation, differentiation, and survival of neural precursor cells. The regulation of neurotrophic factor which supports the growth, differentiation, and survival of neurons has also been demonstrated. The following acupuncture points have been shown to influence neuronal proliferation:

> ST-36, GV-20, PC-6, HT-7, CV-17, CV-12, CV-6, SP1–10, GV-16, GV-8, LI-11, TW-5, GB-30

One of the most studied and clinically used points among these is ST-36, located on the superior tibialis anterior muscle. Stimulation of ST-36 is used for a wide range of conditions

---

20   Wolters Kluwer-Medknow Publications. Functional magnetic resonance imaging evidence for activated functional brain areas following acupoint needling in the extremities. *Neural Regeneration Research.* 2012; 7(3): 223.

21   Luo, Benhua. Development in study on "qi tonifying, blood regulating, and essence nurturing" acupuncture technique treating vascular dementia. *Chinese Journal of Gerontology.* 2014; 14(139): 4091–4092.

affecting the digestive system, cardiovascular system, immune system, and nervous system, as well as having been widely used for brain disorders. In addition to the above-listed actions, ST-36 was shown to upregulate the expression of neuropeptide Y, which promotes the proliferation of neuronal precursor cells and appeared to lessen the neuropathologic effects of stress in rats.[22]

One study examined the role of acupuncture on brain tissue after cerebral ischemia (loss of blood supply to an area of the brain). This study showed a greater proliferation and differentiation of neural stem cells in the brain and an ability to increase blood flow and decrease cell death. Two points on the head, GV-20 and GV-26, regulated cells which "increase the release of nerve growth factors (NGFs) to make nerve cells survive and axons grow, synthesize neurotransmitters, [and] metabolize toxic substances." Similarly the use of GV-20 and GV-14 was shown to increase neural repair after ischemic damage. These points also activate bodily self-protection and reduction of nerve cell death in and near the site of injury. Needling points along the midline of the torso, traditionally referred to as the conception vessel, were also shown to increase growth factors—basic fibroblast growth factor, epidermal growth factor, and NGF messenger RNA—in the subventricular zones and dentate gyrus.[23]

Scalp Acupuncture

The majority of acupuncture points are located on the trunk and limbs. However, the points along the surface of the head play an important role in addressing sequelae of brain injury with acupuncture. GV-20, located at the top of the head, has been shown to increase cerebral blood flow velocity of the middle cerebral artery and anterior cerebral artery without significant changes in blood pressure and pulse rate.[24] Specific scalp acupuncture systems and protocols are a relatively new, yet promising, method for treating brain injury and its related symptoms.[25, 26, 27] Several scalp "systems" exist, including needling over the sensory–motor humunculi along the parietal and frontal lobes to increase both movement

22   Nam, M-H., Yin, C., Soh, K-S. and Choi, S-H. Adult neurogenesis and acupuncture stimulation at ST-36. *Journal of Acupuncture and Meridian Studies*. 2011 Sep; 4(3): 153–158. doi:10.1016/j.jams.2011.09.001

23   Chen, P-D., Yu H-B. Zhou-xin Yang, *et al*. Research advances in treatment of cerebral ischemic injury by acupuncture of conception and governor vessels to promote nerve regeneration. *Journal of Chinese Integrative Medicine*. 2012 Jan; 10(1): 19–24.

24   Hyung-sik Byeon, Moon, S-K., Park, S-U., *et al*. Effects of GV20 acupuncture on cerebral blood flow velocity of middle cerebral artery and anterior cerebral artery territories, and CO2 reactivity during hypocapnia in normal subjects. *The Journal of Alternative and Complementary Medicine*. 2011 Mar; 17(3): 219–224. https://doi.org/10.1089/acm.2010.0232

25   Tang, W. Clinical observation on scalp acupuncture treatment in 50 cases of headache. *Chinese Medicine*. 2002; 22(3): 190–192.

26   Nakazawa, H. and Averil, A. Scalp acupuncture. *Physical Medicine and Rehabilitation Clinics of North America*. 1999; 10(3): 555–562.

27   Li, J. and Xiao, J. Clinical study on effects of scalp-acupuncture in treating acute cerebral hemorrhage. *Chinese Journal of Integrated Traditional and Western Medicine*. 1999; 19(4): 203–205.

and sensory feedback. Often immediate benefit can be found from this method. A system known as "Yamamoto New Scalp Acupuncture" has a system of reflex points located over the temporal region that have an influence on the functional integrity of the internal organ systems as well as a set of points along the anterior scalp which are noted to correlate to cranial nerve pathology.[28] Future research may be aimed at scalp acupuncture and its effects on the release of neurotransmitters and neurohormones.

---

28   Feely, Richard. *New Scalp Acupuncture: principles and practice.* 2nd ed. New York: Thieme. 2006. Print.

Chapter 4

The Brainstem and Cranial Nerves

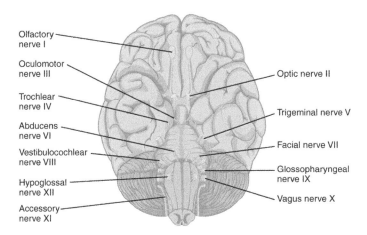

Olfactory nerve I

Oculomotor nerve III

Trochlear nerve IV

Abducens nerve VI

Vestibulocochlear nerve VIII

Hypoglossal nerve XII

Accessory nerve XI

Optic nerve II

Trigeminal nerve V

Facial nerve VII

Glossopharyngeal nerve IX

Vagus nerve X

Functional Overview

The brainstem is the most ancient of brain structures and lies at the root of our ability to survive and maintain life. It can be divided into substructures of the medulla oblongata (myencephalon), pons (metencephalon) and midbrain (mesencephalon), reticular formation, and cranial nerves. Together the brainstem mediates and controls arousal, attention, heart rate, breathing, the sleep cycle, balance, and gross axial movements, as well as coordination of eye, jaw, tongue, and head movement. Visual, somesthetic, gustatory, and auditory perception also fall within its purview. A summary of brainstem structures and roles is found in Table 4.1. These functions operate in an automatic, rhythmic fashion through oscilations of GABA (inhibition) and glutamate (excitation) release that generally do not enter into the conscious mind, requiring neither conscious effort nor the participation of higher cortical structures.

Basic routine motor movements are also controlled by the brainstem such as sucking, chewing, swallowing, swimming, stepping, and walking movements. Brainstem structures, as well as the thalamus, can be activated or inhibited selectively or globally by the frontal lobe so that specific sensory modalities are attended to while others are filtered or suppressed. In this way, selective attention and information processing can occur. If sensory tracts such as the olfactory, auditory, or visual pathways become severed due to an injury, severe lethargy or even apathy can result.

The pons is the most rostal (toward the face) portion of the hindbrain and acts to relay signals from the forebrain to the cerebellum, along with nuclei that deal primarily with sleep, respiration, swallowing, bladder control, hearing, equilibrium, taste, eye movement, facial expressions, facial sensation, and posture. It is hypothesized to also play a role in dreaming, sleepwalking, and sleep paralysis. Somnambulism is presumed to be the result of disinhibition of the brainstem and spinal motor neurons which are normally inhibited during REM sleep. Cranial nerves associated with the pons are nerves V (trigeminal), VI (abducens), VII (facial), and VIII (vestibulocochlear).

The medulla is the most posterior portion of the brainstem which transitions from the spinal cord. Where this occurs, known as the medulla–spinal junction, is the location of the paired medullary pyramids in which the cortico–spinal/pyramidal tracts cross over between the brain and body to exchange information in the hemisphere opposite the side of the body in question. This is the phenomenon of the left hemisphere of the brain controlling the right side of the body and vice versa. Regulation of autonomic functions including breathing, heart rate, and blood pressure occurs within the medulla. Reflex centers control automatic actions such as coughing, sneezing, swallowing, or vomiting. If the lower brainstem becomes injured the patient may become comatose with accompanying cardiovascular and respiratory disturbances. The medulla is associated with cranial nerves IX (glossopharyngeal), X (vagus), XI (accessory), and XII (hypoglossal).

The Midbrain

The midbrain is the smallest portion of the brainstem and is divided into three portions. The tegmentum is the most medial portion which includes dopamine-producing neurons and is an outgrowth of the reticular formation. The ventral segment has descending cortical fibers which pass through it. The tectum is the dorsal segment and includes the superior (visual) and inferior (auditory) colliculi. Between and below the tegmentum lies the substantia nigra which is a major production source of corpus striatal dopamine. The "red nucleus" receives descending motor fibers from the frontal lobe and forms into the rubospinal tract which allows for flexor muscle tone.

The periaqueductal gray is also located within the midbrain and receives extensive input from the amygdala and other nuclei of the limbic system. This brain region is indicated in motor–vocal aspects of emotional expression as well as responses to painful or noxious stimuli. It coordinates the activity of the laryngeal, oral–facial, and both primary and accessory muscles of respiration and inspiration. These pre-programmed motor–vocal operations can produce a wide range of noises that generally reflects an exceedingly negative mood. Plosive sounds such as "puh," "guh," "kuh," etc., which require a strong puff, may also be made. These, however, have no bearing on actual emotional states. That is, negative moods will cause signaling from the forebrain to stimulate the periaqueductal gray and produce these vocalizations, but if the periaqueductal gray is stimulated in isolation or it becomes severed from the limbic system and the emotional signal, the vocalizations will occur without eliciting any particular emotion. So long as the brainstem is active, the individual may still laugh, cry, or howl even if the rest of the brain were completely inactive and lacking consciousness. It is also possible that individuals with injury to regions of the brainstem controlling facial expression may lose control over this faculty and their face may contort in a manner of extreme happiness or grief despite the individual denying experiencing these feelings.

The superior colliculi consist of gray and white layers similar to the cerebral cortex. The superficial layers of these structures receive considerable input from the retinal, temporal, and occipital visual cortices as well as responding to moving stimuli. Deeper layers receive converging motor, somesthetic, auditory, visual, and reticular input. The superior colliculi actually serve as an extension of the reticular formation in which they maintain interconnections with the posterior medulla and the cranial nerves associated with head movement. Both layers receive extensive optical input from the contralateral eye and contralateral visual input for the ipsilateral eye. In this way, the superior colliculi act as a multimodal assimilation area for orienting an individual toward external stimuli and movement. Evolutionarily, in animals such as fish and reptiles, this is likely to help with tracking in the stalking of prey or escaping from potential predators.

The inferior colliculus primarily detects and analyzes auditory stimuli. Before the evolution of the neocortex it acted as the primary source of auditory analysis. Within it, neurons are arranged in a laminar pattern, one atop another, upon which different auditory frequency bands are represented. It is able to respond to auditory signaling from either ear, which allows for the analysis and localization of various sound sources. Fibers from the inferior colliculus carry auditory impulses and extend to the pons, medulla, superior colliculi, spinal cord, and nuclei subserving the neck and face muscles. In this way, a sound may trigger the head or body turning in response to sounds.

Reticular Activating System

The reticular activating system is concerned mostly with generalized and selective arousal and activation of the neuroaxis. Sensory input is received from the skin, muscles, joints, and vestibular system. It then acts to integrate this influx of information. In this way, the reticular activating system is not directly concerned with the arousal itself as much as with the integration and coordination of behavior in response to arousal. This may be movements of the trunk, limb, head, or eyes. Sensory–motor integration is mediated by the excitatory and inhibitory neurotransmitters glutamate and GABA. Modulatory functions which are also carried out are mediated by norepinephrine and serotonin. If there is severe injury to the reticular formation, then forebrain arousal and a permanent comatose state can result in which the individual does not even respond to noxious stimuli.

TABLE 4.1 Structures of the Brainstem

Pons		Sleep, respiration, swallowing, bladder control, hearing, equilibrium, taste, eye movement, facial expressions, facial sensation, posture, and suspected role in dreaming and sleep paralysis
Medulla		Breathing, heart rate, blood pressure, automatic actions such as coughing, sneezing, swallowing, or vomiting
Midbrain	Periaqueductal gray	Motor–vocal aspects of emotional expression, laughing, crying, howling, plosive sounds, facial expressions
	Superior colliculi	Multimodal assimilation area orienting individual toward external stimuli and movement
	Inferior colliculus	Detects and analyzes and localizes auditory stimuli of various sound sources
Reticular formation		Integration of sensory input is received from the skin, muscles, joints, and vestibular system and coordination of responsive behavior

Cranial Nerves
I: Olfactory

The olfactory nerve is not a cranial nerve, in the strictest sense, as it bypasses the brainstem. It is a complex axonal pathway that projects to many structures including the amygdala, entorhinal cortex, hypothalamus, orbital frontal lobes, and dorsal medial cortex. It is, however, associated with many brainstem functions as it receives information regarding smell and taste. The nerve begins in the olfactory endothelium where cells turn over rapidly with a cell's lifespan of only about two days. It then passes through the cribriform plate where it is prone to injury or shearing before reaching the olfactory bulb, then projecting to the amygdala, hippocampus, thalamus, orbital frontal lobes, and insula. If an injury occurs the cribriform plate may fracture, the nerve may be severed, and the meninges may rupture. If this happens an individual may not only lose their sense of smell (anosmia), but may also develop a cerebrospinal fistula in which cerebrospinal fluid drips or gushes into the nose. If anosmia is unilateral then the individual will likely not notice the loss and each nostril should be assessed individually. Dysosmia, or a perversion of the sense of smell, may also occur due to partial injuries to the olfactory bulb or tumor. Olfactory hallucinations are associated with tumors, seizure activity, and head injuries involving the inferior temporal lobes.

II: Optic

All visual impulses from the retina to the brain are transmitted via the optic nerves. Injuries to these pathways create visual defects. If these defects are restricted to only either the right or left visual field they are referred to as homonymous; if bilateral, they are referred to as heteronymous. Heteronymous defects suggest either an injury to both hemispheres of the brain or to the retina or optic nerve before reaching the optic chiasm. Homonymous symptoms indicate the injury can be localized to one side of the optic tract or radiations within one cerebral hemisphere. Complete destruction of the optic tract results in homonymous neglect to the left or right, whereas a partial injury may create a quadratic homonymous defect in which a quadrant of the visual field is affected. Temporal lobe injuries are associated with upper quadrant defects, while injuries to the superior parietal lobe are associated with lower quadrant defects.

III: Oculomotor

Innervation of all ocular rotary muscles, with the exception of the lateral rectus and superior oblique muscles, is provided by the oculomotor nerve. This includes the medial, superior, inferior recti, and inferior oblique muscles. The intraocular and smooth muscles of the pupil (ciliary and pupilloconstrictor muscles) are also innervated by this nerve, as is the levator palprebrae muscle which raises the eyelid. If damaged there may be an inability to rotate the eye upward, downward, or inward. The pupil may also not respond to direct light and there may be ptosis (drooping) of the eyelid due to weakness of levator palpebrae.

IV: Trochlear

Located just caudal to the inferior colliculi, the trochlear nerve innervates the superior oblique muscle of the eye. This allows for depression, abduction, and intorsion of the eyeball so that an individual can look downward or inward. This is the most common cranial nerve to be damaged from head trauma.

V: Trigeminal

The trigeminal nerve is the largest of the cranial nerves. It innervates the trigeminal nucleus within the medulla to control jaw closure, chewing, grinding, and lateral movement of the jaw. In concert with the facial nerve, it impacts muscles involved in facial expression. Pathology of this nerve tract can cause difficulty in chewing. In severe cases, ipsilateral atrophy and complete paralysis of the temporal or masseter muscle(s) may occur. Somatic afferent portions of the nerve mediate general sensory input such as temperature, touch, and pain from the face, teeth, mouth, and mucous membranes of the nose, cheek, tongue, and sinuses. The sometimes intensely painful condition known as trigeminal neuralgia is an instance of this.

VI: Abducens

Primarily concerned with horizontal eye movement, the abducens nerve ascends the brainstem to terminate at the oculomotor complex and innervate the lateral rectus muscle of the eye. This works alongside the pontine center for lateral gaze with eye movements outward to the right or left. It is also linked to the pontine/midbrain center for vertical gaze and is a part of a collection of fibers which form a loop tying into the facial nerve. An injury to the sixth cranial nerve can cause lateral gaze paralysis or paralysis of the lateral rectus muscle which results in horizontal diplopia (double vision).

VII: Facial

The seventh cranial nerve controls motor control of the face. This includes the ability to raise eyebrows, movement of the lips, closure of the auditory canals, and gustatory sensation. The facial nerve also innervates the taste buds of the anterior two-thirds of the tongue, which if injured can cause a loss in taste sensation. The stapedius muscle, which inhibits the movement of the ossicles to dampen excessive sound, is also controlled here. Should the stapedius become paralyzed, an individual may experience sounds as too loud, intolerable, or painful. Other symptoms associated with an injury to this nerve include lip retraction, eyebrow lifting, eyelid closure paralysis (Bell's Palsy), and inability to wrinkle one's forehead, purse one's lips, or show one's teeth. There may also be a drooping of the corner of the mouth.

VIII: Vestibular

The vestibular portion of the eighth cranial nerve innervates the labyrinth of the inner ear and the macules of the saccule and urticle as well as the ampullae of the semicircular canals. The primary function of this nerve is to determine the body's position in visual space in order to maintain equilibrium during movement. Changes of fluid balance within the semicircular canals allow the brain to determine changes in position. As a result, if there is an injury to the vestibular receptors or central connections, an individual can experience abnormal sensations of movement, vertigo, nausea, tendencies to fall, dizziness, and motion sickness. Hearing problems including deafness or tinnitus—which may be described as hearing a buzzing, humming, whistling, roaring, hissing, or clicking sound—can also occur. An individual may feel as though they are being pulled to one side or lean/veer to one side when walking. In order to mediate postural reflexes, the vestibular nerve has rich interconnections with cranial nerves III, IV, and VI, which subserve eye movement. Nystagmus—or difficulty focusing when moving or when an object is in motion—can thus result from injury as well.

IX: Glossopharyngeal

Closely related to the vagus nerve, the ninth cranial nerve receives tactile, thermal, and pain sensations from the tongue and helps to form the gustatory nucleus. It also receives information about carotid artery pressure via fibers from the carotid sinus. All of this information is transmitted to the solitary nucleus which then contributes to the vagus nerve. Together, the ninth and tenth cranial nerves can influence heart rate and arterial blood pressure. Lesions here will usually result in loss of taste and sensation in the posterior third of the tongue, a loss of gag reflex, and carotid sinus reflex. Swallowing or coughing may become intensely painful.

X: Vagus

Actually a complex mix of nerves, the vagus innervates a number of structures including the larynx, pharynx, trachea, esophagus, epiglottis, external auditory meatus, and viscera in the thoracic and abdominal cavities. As such, important bodily functions such as swallowing, breathing, speaking, and movement of the palate, pharynx, and larynx are all within its influence. It is also responsible for the swinging of the soft palate upward to seal off the oropharynx from the nasopharynx when swallowing, whistling, or talking. An injury can cause palate weakness and pseudobulbar palsy. Speech can be severely affected as well if fluids get into the nasal passages, in which case speech will become excessively nasal in nature. Due to its long-reaching influence on a wide range of structures, many other symptoms may develop from injury to the vagus nerve, including gastroparesis, hyperarousal, smooth muscle cramping, IBS, weight gain, depression, bradycardia, chronic inflammation, nutritional deficiencies, and seizures.

XI: Spinal Accessory

Two distinct segments of this nerve exist. The cranial portion, along with the vagus nerve, forms the inferior laryngeal nerve going to the larynx. The spinal portion of this nerve innervates the sternocleidomastoid (SCM) and upper trapezius muscles to help turn the head and elevate the shoulders. As a result, if this nerve becomes injured, one's shoulders may sag on the affected side or the individual may show weakness in turning the head. This is particularly true when performed against resistance.

XII: Hypoglossal

Located in the caudal medulla, the hypoglossal nerve controls movement of the tongue by innervating the relevant skeletal muscle. If the nerve is damaged, the skeletal musculature will not properly move the tongue, and weakness or atrophy can result. Tongue strength can be tested by placing one's tongue on one side of the cheek and pressing against a practitioner's finger when it is placed on the outside of the cheek. Lower motor neuron pathology may cause unilateral atrophy, fasciculation or fibrillation, and paralysis that results in an obvious deviation toward the paralytic side when the tongue is protruded.

A summary of the cranial nerves and their associated symptomology can be found in Table 4.2.

TABLE 4.2 The Cranial Nerves: Pathology and Symptoms

I: Olfactory	Loss of smell/taste, risk of cerebrospinal fluid fistula
II: Optic	Visual defects including blindness, neglect, etc.
III: Oculomotor	Ptosis, pupil unresponsive to direct light, inability to move eye downward, upward, or inward
IV: Trochlear	Inability to move eye in order to look in downward or inward direction
V: Trigeminal	Face pain, difficulty chewing, atrophy or paralysis of temporal or masseter muscles
VI: Abducens	Lateral gaze paralysis, horizontal diplopia
VII: Facial	Bell's Palsy, facial paralysis or flaccidity, eyebrow raising, eyelid closure paralysis, taste loss in anterior two-thirds of tongue, sounds may seem too loud or painful
VIII: Vestibular	Vertigo, nausea, dizziness, leaning or veering to one side when walking, unsteadiness, abnormal sensations of movement, tinnitus, nystagmus, difficulty focusing on objects when they are moving or when walking
IX: Glossopharyngeal	Loss of taste/sensation in posterior third of tongue, loss of gag reflex and carotid sinus reflex, painful swallowing or cough
X: Vagus	Pseudobulbar palsy, difficulty swallowing/dysphagia, slurred speech, palate weakness, gastroparesis, hyperarousal, smooth muscle cramping, IBS, weight gain, depression, bradycardia, chronic inflammation, nutritional deficiencies, seizures
XI: Spinal accessory	Ipsilateral sagging shoulder(s), weakness in turning head (especially against resistance)
XII: Hypoglossal	Tongue weakness/atrophy/deviation

Acupuncture Considerations

A number of points have been demonstrated by fMRI studies to have a correlation to brain activity in the brainstem structure.[1]

---

1   Huang, W., Pach, D., Napadow, *et al.* Characterizing acupuncture stimuli using brain imaging with fMRI—a systematic review and meta-analysis of the literature. *PLOS ONE.* 2012; 7(4): e32960. https://doi.org/10.1371/journal.pone.0032960

Activating

Pons: GB-34, GB-39

Caudate nucleus: GB-34, GB-39

Superior colliculi: GB-37

Deactivating

Basal gyrus: ST-3

George Soulié de Morant[2] notes indications for brain regions according to his extensive studies of the medicine in China prior to the communist revolution. According to his studies, the following points were indicated to influence brainstem structures.

Pons

Tonifying: ST-11, SP-6, SP-9, HT-6, HT-8, KI-6, KI-10, KI-17, KI-19, KI-20, PC-1, GB-20, LR-5

Medulla Oblongata

Tonifying: U-1, LU-7, LI-6, ST-4, ST-14, ST-16, ST-22, ST-32, ST-33, ST-42, ST-44, SP-21, HT-6, SI-8, SI-19, BL-11, BL-51, BL-52, BL-54, BL-66, KI-1, KI-7, KI-21, KI-25, PC-2, TW-19, GB-4, GB-5 (opposite), GB-20, GB-25, GB-26, GB-34, GB-35, GB-37, LR-4, LR-13, CV-9, CV-17, GV-1, GV-10, GV-13, GV-18

Dispersing: KI-2, TW-10, LR-2

Autonomic Nervous System

Sympathetic tonifying: ST-41, PC-8, TW-5, GB-20

Parasympathetic tonifying: ST-21, BL-10, CV-12, GV-20

Parasympathetic dispersing: PC-8

Points in the Brainstem Region

Due to the brainstem lying deep within the skull, there are no acupuncture points which directly lie over the brainstem region. Points in the occipital area below the external occipital protruberance may, however, have an impact.

---

2   Soulié de Morant, George and Zmiewski, Paul. *Chinese Acupuncture.* Brookline, MA: Paradigm Publications. 1994. Print.

Chapter 5

The Cerebellum

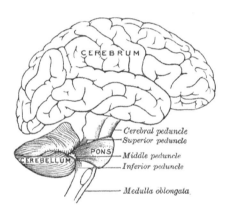

Functional Overview

The cerebellum sits atop the brainstem, straddling the medulla–pontine junction and anchored to the pons through three cerebellar peduncles. It accounts for approximately 25 percent of overall brain volume. It evolved out of the vestibular system over 450 million years ago, before the first vertebrates, as a rudimentary appendage of the brainstem. As more visual, proprioceptive, somesthetic, and complex auditory stimuli were received and demanded additional processing, it gradually increased in size. As species became bipedal, increasingly complex demands were placed on the anterior cerebellum in order to coordinate gait and upper and lower limb movements. This gave rise to the evolution of the neocerebellum (including the dentate gyrus and the cerebellar hemispheres).

While most commonly associated with motor movements and the smoothness with which movements occur, the cerebellum has been implicated in cognitive, emotional, sensory, motor, and speech processing. It communicates with almost all regions of the neuroaxis, with the exception of the striatum. Neuroplasticity has been demonstrated here, as have functions of learning and memory. It has been postulated that this structure may serve as an integrative interface for cognition, emotion, motor functioning, and memory. It has also shown significant influences on autonomic functions, language processing, cognitive agility, discrimination of sensory experiences, classical conditioning, visual memory, and emotional states. A summary and categorization of these functions can be found in Table 5.1.

Structure

The structure of the cerebellum can be subdivided in several different ways. Functionally it can be subdivided into three lobes: the anterior, posterior, and flocculonodular lobes, each of which can be further subdivided into ten lobules. It may also be divided according to three longitudinal zones—the lateral zone, which receives information from the motor and somesthetic cortex via the pons; the medial zone, which receives vestibular, visual, and auditory input; and the intermediate zone, which receives input from the spinal cord and the motor cortex. Divisions may also be made phylogenetically and functionally: the archicerebellum (which includes the flocculonodular lobe); the paleocerebellum (or anterior lobe), which influences autonomic and emotional activity; and the most recently evolved neocerebellum, which includes the posterior lobe and dentate gyrus to influence motor, somatic, and cognitive activities such as neocortical information processing.

Fulton and Dow[1] subdivided the cerebellum in accordance with the symptoms produced when injured:

- *Vestibulocerebellum*: In the vicinity of the flocculonodular lobe, produces symptoms of the vestibular system (e.g. head tilt, circling gait, nystagmus)

- *Spinocerebellum*: In the vicinity of the anterior lobe, produces symptoms of abnormal spinal control over walking (i.e. impaired gait without impaired reaching)

- *Cerebrocerebellum*: In the vicinity of the neocerebellum, produces symptoms of impaired reaching and clumsiness suggesting impairments in voluntary motor control

As noted above, rich connections exist with almost all regions of the forebrain and telencephalon, with the exception of the striatum. These are primarily through a number of feedfoward and feedback loops involving the corticopontine and pontocerebellar thalamocortical pathways. These are partially made up of afferents that convey tactile, auditory, and visual impulses, including those which essentially reconstruct and maintain somesthetic images of the body in different lobules. Most of these signals are carried via "mossy fibers," which are generally excitatory, utilizing glutamate as a neurotransmitter, and connect via synapses with Golgi cells whose axons (parallel fibers) excite Purkinje cells. Purkinje cells are all innervated by climbing fibers from the brainstem, which also uses glutamate as a neurotransmitter. These impulses appear to counter one another and can give rise to long-term potentiation, or long-term depression, which can impact learning capacity.

---

1   Fulton, J. and Dow, R. The cerebellum: a summary of functional localization. *Yale Journal of Biological Medicine.* 1937 Oct; 10(1): 89–119.

In addition, Purkinje cells also receive norepinephrine from the locus ceruleus and serotonin from the raphe nucleus.

Motor Functions

In the regulation of motor control the cerebellum exerts a tonic and stabilizing influence that aids one to coordinate, smooth, fine tune, and maintain timing of motor movements. Neuron firing rates vary during movement, increasing and then decreasing, suggesting that they are modulating these movements. Activity in some deep nuclei, such as the dentate of the neocerebellum, become active prior to movement and prior to activation of the frontal motor cortex. These can fire by just thinking about making a movement. The dentate gyrus controls voluntary actions and direction of movement which involves multiple joints and the upper limbs. Dystaxia, predominantly in the legs, can result from cerebellar dysfunction. This can often appear to others as if the individual is heavily intoxicated. Indeed, in addition to trauma, alcholism and nutritional deficiencies can result in damage to the cerebellum and cause such dystaxia. Motor-related disturbances including tremor, nystagmus, gait disturbances, lack of coordination, and postural instability can be common following an injury.

When an individual acquires new skilled movements, such as when playing a guitar or a piano, it requires conscious control of motor functioning and strong neocortical activity while the cerebellum plays a minimal role. As one practices, less conscious attention and one's "motor memory" become more of a component. The cerebellum receives neocortical signals via the pons and begins to increase its participation and slowly learn the necessary movements. Over time, the cerebellum may begin to acquire primary control over the task, operating subconsciously, with little or no help from the cerebrum and the conscious mind, which are free to do and think about other things. Lesions can abolish the acquisition and retention of conditioned responses. In this, compound movements are more severely affected than simple movements. It has been argued that the cerebellum appears to learn automations and habits, not acting to form actual memories per se. Rather, these are step-by-step motor sequences simply being carried out. This is further substantiated by studies showing that stimulation of the fastigial nucleus, vermis, and superior cerebral peduncle may elicit motor operations such as biting, chewing, and swallowing movements without any actual hunger or food-seeking behavior. The neocerebellum in particular maintains rich interconnections with forebrain motor areas, especially the motor thalamus, which relays these impulses to motor areas four and six in the frontal lobe and the somatosensory areas of the parietal lobe.

The lateral cerebellum appears to be involved in regulating the timing of sequential movements. Injury, as a result, causes difficulty with maintaining timing and rhythm. Abnormalities in the rate, range, and force of movement are demonstrated as deficiencies in finger-to-nose testing. For example, when asked to touch the physician's finger and then their own nose, the patient's arm and hand may sway and miss on both counts. Irregularities in acceleration and deceleration of movement are also common, possibly due to programming errors. Limb extension may be arrested prematurely, such that the target/objective is reached by a series of jerky stop-and-go movements. When asked to touch their nose, they may do it in two stages: by lifting the arm to nose level, then by bringing the fingers to the nose. Movements may become ballistic, being too quick and failing to slow down, or the limb overshoots the mark and the error is corrected only by a series of secondary movements. When asked to make movements as fast as possible, however, they will often do so slower than normal.

Differential Diagnosis in Sensory Abnormalities (Dystaxia)

If the individual performs worse with loss of visual input (closing their eyes) rather than the symptoms worsening with loss of visual guidance (removing visual cues), it is due to insufficient visual and proprioceptive input rather than cerebellar damage. The cerebellum is able to equilibriate only if it has proper proprioceptive information.

In postinjury symptoms, lateralized cerebellar signs limited to one half of the body are due to lesions (infarct, neoplasm, or abscess) affecting only one of the cerebellar hemispheres. Bilateral cerebellar signs are likely a result of toxic-metabolic, demyelating, or other degenerative diseases.

Cerebellar Gait

What is referred to as "cerebellar gait" typically demonstrates as a wide-based gait, steps being characteristically unsteady, irregular, uncertain, and of variable length. If mild, these may only be noticeable when the individual is tired. If severe, the patient may not be able to stand without assistance. Symptoms may include:

- Loss of muscle tone
- Lack of coordination in volitional movements
- Intention tremor
- Minor degrees of muscle weakness
- Being easily fatigued
- Commonly, disorders of equilibrium including nystagmus

Language Functions

The neocerebellum contributes to and is concerned with cognitive functioning, including language. The right cerebellum (interconnected with the left cerebral hemisphere) becomes activated when asked to produce verbs in response to nouns. The cerebellum also becomes activated when reading aloud as opposed to looking at words. Moving the mouth without speaking also activates the cerebellum, whereas internal (silent) speech without motor movement does not.

Those with cerebellar injuries may display disturbances on verbal paired associate tests. With severe injuries some may display an intial mutism. This may be due to brainstem compression involving the periaqueductal gray. They may also be a result of the extensive interconnections between the left cerebellum and the right cerebral hemisphere whereby there are disruptions on neocortical processing and/or afferents as they pass through the brainstem en route to the cranial nerves. It is also possible that these disturbances are due to the complex cognitive processes being performed by and within the cerebellum.

Ataxic Speech

Speech can also be affected and become dysarthric following an injury to the cerebellum. This is particularly true with left-sided damage. If there is a rapid and acute onset, one may become transiently mute. Cerebellar dysarthric speech may be of two types:

- Slowed and slurred, particularly when required to repeat sounds ("ga ga ga")

- Scanning dysarthria with variable intonations as words are broken up into syllables, some of which are explosibly uttered (i.e. ballistic speech).

Vision and Visuo-Spatial Functions

Motor tasks may be inhibited when visual cues generally used to guide movement are eliminated. Lesions in the left neocerebellum (which is interconnected with the right hemisphere) have also been shown to have mild difficulty in performing cognitive–spatial operations in three-dimensional space. This is presumably due to connections with the hippocampus.

Emotional Activity

Injury and electrical stimulation of the cerebellum have shown emotional responses including triggering rage reactions and constant states of hyperactivity. Stimulation of the paleocerebellum will elicit these rage-like reactions, including threat, attack, and autonomic changes such as alterations in arterial pressure, heart rate, piloerection, dilation of the pupils, urination, gastrointestinal changes, and the production of sleep-like EEG spindles. These reactions, however, seem to remain undirected and, at best, semi-purposeful (i.e. "sham rage"). Activation of the anterior cerebellum may also increase blood pressure, heart rate, and respiration, and inhibit gastromotility. The posterior cerebellum has the exact opposite effect. Removal of the cerebellum does not eliminate these or other emotional behaviors, however, and should connections with the amygdala and hypothalamus become severed, cerebellum stimulation ceases to have an influence on these functions.

For these reasons, the emotional responses of the cerebellum tend to be primarily attributed to the rich interconnections maintained between the cerebellum and the limbic system, specifically the amygdala, hippocampus, hypothalamus, septal nuclei, nucleus accumbens, and substantia nigra. It is hypothesized that the cerebellum may exert an inhibitory influence on these nuclei. Fibers from the hypothalamus terminate in all layers of the cerebellar cortex, which in turn project to the lateral, dorsal medial, and anterior hypothalamus, structures implicated in the rudimentary aspects of emotion, including sexuality and control over the autonomic nervous system. Emotional and affective behavior with autonomic changes also appear to be influenced by direct connections with the brainstem. In this regard, it influences and modulates cerebral blood flow, systemic circulation, and metabolism, offering long-term protection of the brain from ischemia. This neuroprotective mechanism has been demonstrated through electrical stimulation—reducing focal cerebral infarction volume by 50 percent due to its dramatic influence on arterial pressure.

"Childhood mania" has been associated with cerebellar dysplasia and, more recently, abnormalities in the cerebellum have also been implicated in the pathogenesis of cases of schizophrenia and autism as well as postinjury/surgery mutism and highly abnormal emotional behavior which often resolves after a few days or weeks. Joseph notes that monkeys reared under deprived conditions displayed abnormal electrophysiological activity in the cerebellum (dentate gyrus) as well as the septal nuclei while also displaying autistic behavior. He notes these findings as significant given the cerebellum is an outgrowth of the vestibular system, and that insufficient social–emotional or physical stimulation may also result in insufficient vestibular activation. Joseph goes on to note that up to 50 percent of patients diagnosed as psychotic or schizophrenic display cerebellar abnormalities, including atrophy of the vermis or tumors, and approximately 50 percent of those who are psychotically depressed show a similar pattern of cerebellar abnormality. Stimulation of the paleocerebellum (i.e. the vermis) can induce electrophysiological desychronization in the thalamus, anterior cingulate, amygdala, hippocampus, orbital frontal lobes, midbrain reticular formation, hypothalamus, and the ventral striatum; nuclei that have been implicated in the genesis of psychotic and emotional disturbances. It has been reported that electrical stimulation of the vermis can relieve chronic and intractable psychotic disturbances in over 90 percent of those treated. Presumably this is due to the effects of cerebellar activity on the limbic system. It has also been reported that cerebellar stimulation may decrease limbic system seizure activity, whereas ablation will result in enhanced limbic system seizures.

TABLE 5.1 The Cerebellum: Pathology and Symptoms

Motor movement	Gait ataxia
	Vertigo
	Hypotonia
	Intention tremor
	Abnormalities in force, accuracy, range, and rate of goal-directed voluntary movements
	Asynergia: lack of motor coordination
	Dysdiachokinesia: inability to make rapid alternating movements of the limbs
	Involuntary motor sequences

Visual and verbal	Disrupted visually guided tracking movements and determination of movement trajectory: past pointing; distances are incorrectly judged
	Dysmetria: falling short or going too far when trying to touch/grasp an object
	Nystagmus: involuntary slow and fast rhythmic lateral eye movements, usually to the side of the lesion
	Dysarthric speech
	Difficulty with paired verbal testing
Emotional	Increased "rage response" (semi-purposeful/"sham")
	Hyperactivity
	Autonomic function dysregulation (heart rate, blood pressure, respiration, gastromotility, etc.)
	Possible schizophrenia psychoses
	Possible autistic-like symptoms

Acupuncture Considerations

A number of points have been demonstrated by fMRI studies to have a correlation to brain activity in the cerebellum.[2]

Activating

Cerebellum general: LR-3, GB-34, GB-39, GB-40, LI-4

Deactivating

N/A

George Soulié de Morant[3] notes indications for brain regions according to his extensive studies of the medicine in China prior to the communist revolution. According to his studies, the following points have been found to influence the cerebellum.

Tonifying

LU-7, LU-8, LU-10, LU-11, LI-6

ST-5, ST-11, ST-15, ST-20, ST-33, SP-6, SP-7, SP-9, SP-21

2   Huang, W., Pach, D., Napadow, *et al.* Characterizing acupuncture stimuli using brain imaging with fMRI—a systematic review and meta-analysis of the literature. *PLOS ONE.* 2012; 7(4): e32960. https://doi.org/10.1371/journal.pone.0032960

3   Sulié de Morant, George and Zmiewski, Paul. *Chinese Acupuncture.* Brookline, MA: Paradigm Publications. 1994. Print.

HT-6, HT-8, SI-3

BL-30, BL-50, BL-56, BL-57, KI-5, KI-6, KI-10, KI-13, KI-17, KI-19, KI-20, KI-22, KI-26

PC-1, PC-2, PC-6, PC-7, TW-6, TW-15

GB-24, GB-32, GB-34, LR-5, LR-8, LR-9, LR-10, LR-13

CV-16, CV-17, CV-21, CV-22, GV-4, GV-6, GV-17, GV-23

Dispersing

LU-5, BL-65, TW-10, LR-2a

Points in the Cerebellar Region

Similar point considerations in the occipital region to those of the brainstem in Chapter 4 may also apply to the cerebellum.

Chapter 6

Occipital Lobe

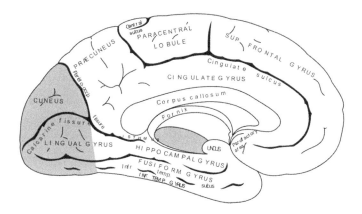

Functional Overview

The occipital lobe is composed of two basic subsections, the primary visual cortex and the visual association area. Simple and complex visual and central/foveal analysis is one of the main functions associated with the occipital lobe; however, neurons also tend to a number of modalities including vestibular, acoustic, visual, visceral, and somesthetic input. These are subdivided into four visual cortices. The primary visual cortex, also called V1, is located predominantly within the medial walls of the cerebral hemispheres and is concerned with the elementary aspects of form perception, transforming information from the retina and lateral geniculate nucleus into a basic code that enables visual information to be extracted by later stages of processing. It is particularly specialized in processing spatial information such as static and moving visual stimuli, colors, and pattern recognition, though the information coming into V1 from the retina is coded as an edge detection rather than discrete optical imagery. A spatial mapping of the subjective visual field with a specific location within V1 is very precise, to where even blind spots may be mapped onto it. This is the most ancient visual portion of the brain and found in most mammals.

From the primary area, information then becomes relayed to the association areas, Brodmann's areas 18 and 19, where complex analysis including form recognition, position, and analysis of depth takes place. Within the visual association area are three subsections, the first of which is the prestriate cortex, or V2, which receives strong connections from V1 and, like V1 neurons, are tuned to simple properties such as orientation, spatial frequency, size, and color. In addition to further processing these qualities, V2 neurons also process more complex properties like orientation of illusionary contours, discrepancies between input from the two eyes, whether objects are part of the foreground or background, and, to a small degree, of attentional modulation. The deepest layer of this area has been found to play an important role in the storage of object recognition memory and the conversion of short-term object memories into long-term memories.

The third visual complex, or V3, is located immediately in front of V2. There is some discrepancy in labels and some subdivide this area even further into dorsal and ventral portions, V3A and V3B respectively. The dorsal V3 region receives input from V1 and V2 and may play a role in global or coherent motion of large patterns. The ventral V3 region has weaker connections from V1 and is more connected with the inferior temporal cortex.

Visual area four, or V4, receives strong input from V2 and some input from V1 and seems to be the first brain region to show strong attentional modulation and selective attention. Similar to V1, V4 responds to orientation, spatial frequency, and color; however, it also processes more complex features such as geometric shapes. It does not process highly complex objects such as faces, which are processed in the inferior temporal lobe. V4 is believed to be the main color center in the brain due to lesions resulting in lack of color vision. Visual area 5 (V5), or the middle temporal visual area (MT), is located in the extrastriate cortex and is specialized for assessing movement of objects. Ninety percent of cells in this region respond to only a single direction of movement and will not respond if movement is in the opposite direction. Damage to this area of the brain can cause an inability to gauge movement or speed. Perception may feel like a series of pictures rather than a fluid experience. Once visual information has been processed by the occipital lobe, it is next relayed to area 7 in the parietal lobe and to the inferior temporal lobule, where higher order analysis and multimodal processing can occur. Damage to the parietal–occipital borders may result in abnormalities involving depth and form perception as well as visual neglect. Destruction of the temporal–occipital regions can give rise to visual agnosias and an inability to recognize complex objects and faces.

The occipital lobes also appear to be lateralized in regard to certain capabilities such as facial recognition. For example, destruction of the right occipital region is associated with prosopagnosia (face blindness), and abnormal activity in this area is more likely to give rise to complex visual hallucinations.

Pathology and Symptoms
Cortical Blindness Prosopagnosia (Face Blindness)

- Occipital lesions, especially of the entire visual cortex

- Ability to discriminate only between different fluxes in luminous energy
  (i.e. lightness and darkness)

If restricted to only one hemisphere, patients will lose patterned vision for the opposite half of the visual field (i.e. a hemianopsia). If only part of the visual cortex is damaged, vision loss is only in the corresponding quadrant of the visual field (scatoma). In cases of partial cortical blindness, patients are able to make compensatory eye movements and are not terribly troubled by their disability. Frequently patients have no awareness that they have lost a quadrant or even half of their visual field. Hence, this should be tested for.

Differential Diagnosis

Right temporal–occipital region:

- Severe disturbance in the ability to recognize the faces of friends, loved ones,
  or pets

- Inability to discriminate and identify even facial affect

- May not recognize themselves in the mirror

Inferior and middle temporal lobe:

- Loss of the ability to recognize faces

- Disturbances in visual discrimination learning and retention

- Visual closure difficulty and recognizing different shapes and patterns and objects
  which differ in regard to size or color

Posterior right temporal gyrus:

- Disrupts visual–spatial memory for faces in general

- Inability to correctly label emotion faces

Visual Agnosia ("Blind Sight")

Visual preservation following primary visual cortex (V1) lesions has been referred to as "blind sight." Although blind, these patients may avoid obstacles and correctly retrieve desired objects and thus appear to have some residual visual functions even though they verbally claim no conscious awareness of sight. This may be due to the preservation of intact subcortical nuclei involved in visual orientation (i.e. area V5). In cases of occipital lesions, complex visual input may still reach the temporal lobe, and may therefore be directed to the auditory areas through a secondary route so that associated "feelings" of seeing something can be communicated and objects can be named, although the patient continues to deny visual perception.

Apperceptive Visual Agnosia

Associated with parietal occipital cortex or bilateral damage to the inferior occipital cortex, this is a disturbance in perceptual and visual–motor integration (difficulty copying or matching objects, failing to draw the complete object). An ability to trace is shown but the individual will not be able to recognize where they started. One cannot synthesize visual details into an integral whole, recognizing only isolated details. If unnecessary lines are drawn across the picture, the ability to recognize the object deteriorates even further.

Associative Visual Agnosia

Associated with left inferior and middle temporal (area 37) occipital abnormalities and parietal occipital cortex, deficit in naming, such that auditory equivalents cannot be matched to a visual perception (may also have alexia—inability to read).

Simultanagnosia

Associated with bilateral superior occipital lobe or superior occipital–parietal region (area 7) lesions—an inability to see more than one thing, or all aspects of an item, at a time.

Impaired Color Recognition Denial of Blindness

While sometimes able to correctly name objects, an individual cannot correctly name, match, and identify or point to colors. Prosopanosia is also frequently displayed.

- Twenty-three percent of those with right cerebral damage and 12 percent of those with left-sided destruction had trouble with color matching

- Some note impairments of color perception are frequently secondary to bilateral inferior occipital lobe damage

- Almost 50 percent of those with aphasia demonstrate deficient color naming and color identification

People with cortical blindness seem initially quite confused, indifferent about their condition, and report a variety of hallucinatory experiences which may be complex or elementary in form. Frequently these patients will initially deny that they experience any blindness and confabulate (Anton's syndrome). It is possible they deny being blind because subcortically they are still able to see. Hence, although at a neocortical level there is no sight, subcortically there remains an unconscious awareness of the visual world.

Visual Hallucinations

When portions of the temporal lobe or occipital lobe are damaged, disconnected from sources of input, or compromised in some fashion, the ability to store information and to draw visual–verbal mnemonic imagery from memory is severely impacted. When artificially or abnormally activated, visual–auditory imagery as well as a variety of involuntary emotional reactions can occur. These may take the form of complex hallucinations, dream-like states, and confusional episodes, or may involve the abnormal attribution of emotional significance to otherwise neutral thoughts and external experiences.

Hallucinations may occur secondarily to tumors or seizures involving the occipital, parietal, frontal, and temporal lobe, or arise following toxic exposure, high fevers, general infections, exhaustion, starvation, extreme thirst, and with partial or complete blindness such as due to glaucoma. Individuals suffering from cortical blindness (i.e. Anton's syndrome) frequently experience hallucinations.

In general, hallucinations secondary to loss of visual or auditory stimuli appear to be the interpretation of neural noise. That is, with a loss of input, various brain regions begin to extract or assign meaningful significance to random neural events, or to whatever limited input may be received. Conversely, hallucinations can occur due to increased levels of neural noise as well. For example, those neurons that subserve facial, word, and object recognition may become simultaneously activated, as well as all associated memories. Consequently, the brain attempts to interpret what it experiences. In the primary regions, neural noise is given a simple interpretation (simple hallucinations), whereas in the association and multi-associational areas, the individual begins to hallucinate via "feature detector" activation, such that they may see faces, chairs, and trees, hear voices and music, and so on, all of which are experienced as a mosaic of something real.

With anterior and inferior temporal abnormalities, the hallucinations become increasingly complex, consisting of both auditory and visual features, including faces, people, objects, animals, etc. This gives rise to the most complex forms of imagery because cells in this area are specialized for the perception and recognition of specific forms. Moreover, structures such as the amygdala and hippocampus become activated, which result in memories and emotions also being evoked, such that the experience may also become personally meaningful to include real individuals and real events that are produced from memory.

Differential Diagnosis of Visual Hallucinations
Middle Temporal Lobe

Tumors or electrical stimulation: associated with the development of auditory and visual hallucinations, dreamy states, and alterations in emotional functioning—particularly as the lesion encroaches on the inferior regions.

Occipital Lobe

Striate cortex (V1, Brodmann's area 17)—simple visual hallucinations such as:

- Sparks

- Tongues of flames

- Colors and flashes of lights

- Objects that seem to become exceedingly large (macropsia) or small (micropsia), blurred in terms of outline or stretched out in a single dimension

- Colors that may become modified or even erased

- Simple geometric forms

Laterality: can be either hemisphere. Usually the hallucination is restricted to the contralateral half of the visual field. Seizure in the right occipital lobe results in the hallucination appearing in the left visual field.

Visual association areas (Brodmann's areas 18 and 19)—complex visual hallucinations such as:

- Images of men or animals

- Various objects and geometric figures

- Liliputian-type individuals, including micropsias and macropsias

- Objects that may seem to become telescoped/far away, or, when approached, objects that may seem to loom and become exceedingly large

Complex hallucinations are usually quite vivid and fully formed and the patient may think what he sees is real. Although usually associated with tumors or abnormal activation of the visual association area, complex hallucinations have also been reported with parietal–occipital involvement, occipital–temporal or inferior–temporal damage, or with lesions of the occipital pole and convexity.

Laterality: complex hallucinations are usually associated with right rather than left cerebral lesions.

Acupuncture Considerations

A number of points have been demonstrated by fMRI studies to have a correlation to brain activity in the occipital lobe.[1]

> Occipital cortex: GB-34 + GB-39

> Occipital lobe: LR-3 left side

---

1   Huang, W., Pach, D., Napadow, *et al.* Characterizing acupuncture stimuli using brain imaging with fMRI—a systematic review and meta-analysis of the literature. *PLOS ONE.* 2012; 7(4): e32960. https://doi.org/10.1371/journal.pone.0032960

Occipital gyrus: ST-36 (ipsilateral effect), LI-4 right side

Middle occipital gyrus: GB-37

Of interest to note, GB-37 is a point that has been specifically indicated for centuries to help with vision disorders and it has now been verified through fMRI to activate the middle occipital gyrus which directly processes visual information.

George Soulié de Morant[2] notes indications for brain regions according to his extensive studies of the medicine in China prior to the communist revolution. According to his studies, points have been found to influence the occipital lobe.

Superior occipital lobe (affecting the instincts): ST-36, ST-37, PC-6, LI-9, GV-22

Inferior occipital lobes (affecting vision): GB-1, GB-12, BL-1, BL-2

Inferior occipital lobe and parietal, temporal, and central lobes: PC-6

Temporal, parietal, and occipital lobes: PC-5

Acupuncture points located over the occipital lobes:

Points physically located over the occipital lobes have a range of indications. Many are beneficial for disorders of the eyes, as well as other concerns. Explanations of these uses can be found in the source texts.[3, 4]

BL-9: Occipital headache, pain from head wind that is difficult to endure, dizziness, pain of the neck with inability to turn head, heaviness of the head and neck, cold sensation in half of the head, cold head with copious sweating, red face, pain of the cheek, bursting eye pain, short-sightedness, nasal congestion, loss of sense of smell, chills and fever, bone pain with chills and fever, vomiting, madness, mad walking, epilepsy, collapse on sudden standing

BL-10: Dizziness, inability of the legs to support the body, sudden muscular contractions, pain of the body, pain and heaviness of the head, headache, head wind, stiffness of the neck with inability to turn head, pain of the shoulder and back, bursting eye pain, redness of the eyes, blurred vision, lacrimation, swelling of the throat with difficulty in speaking, nasal congestion, loss of sense of smell, febrile disease without sweating, mania, incessant talking, seeing ghosts, epilepsy, childhood epilepsy, upward staring eyes

GB-19: Headache, head wind, brain wind, one-sided headache and heaviness of the head, stiffness and pain of the neck with inability to turn the head, dizziness, redness, swelling and pain of the eyes, deafness and tinnitus, pain of the nose, nasal

2   Soulié de Morant, George and Zmiewski, Paul. *Chinese Acupuncture.* Brookline, MA: Paradigm Publications. 1994. Print.

3   Soulié de Morant, George and Zmiewski, Paul. *Chinese Acupuncture.* Brookline, MA: Paradigm Publications. 1994. Print.

4   Deadman, P., Al-Khafaji, M., and Baker, K. *A Manual of Acupuncture.* Hove, East Sussex: Journal of Chinese Medicine Publications. 2011. Print.

congestion, nosebleed, fright palpitations, mania-depression disorder, taxation disorders with emaciation, heat in the body

GB-20: Headache, head wind, one-sided and generalized headache, dizziness, visual dizziness, hypertension, hemiplegia, deviation of the mouth and eye, goiter, lockjaw, insomnia, loss of memory, epilepsy, loss of speech following windstroke, injury by cold without sweating, chills and fever, warm febrile disease with absence of sweating, malaria, painful throat obstruction, swelling of the face, urticaria, redness and pain of the eyes and inner canthus, blurred vision, lacrimation (especially with exposure to wind), night blindness, dimness of vision, nosebleed, rhinitis, nasal congestion and discharge, deafness, tinnitus, blocked ears, stiffness and pain in the neck with inability to turn the head, pain of the shoulder and upper back, pain in the lumbar spine, crooked lumbar spine leading to flaccidity and lack of strength in the sinews of the neck

GV-16: Heaviness of the body with aversion to cold, cold shivering with sweating, swelling and pain of the throat, painful wind obstruction, all types of wind disease, headache, head wind, the hundred diseases of the head, visual dizziness, dizziness, blurred vision, nosebleed, upward staring eyes, sudden loss of voice, sudden inability to speak following windstroke, flaccid tongue with inability to speak, windstroke, numbness of the legs, hemiplegia, hypertension, mania, incessant talking, mad walking and desire to commit suicide, sadness and fear with fright palpitations, difficulty in breathing, heat in the chest, ceaseless vomiting, jaundice, pain of the neck with inability to turn the head, stiff neck

GV-17: Heaviness of the head, head wind, aversion to wind in the head, wind dizziness, swelling and pain of the head, pain of the face, red face, stiffness and pain of the neck, dimness of vision, short-sightedness, eye pain, excessive lacrimation, yellow eyes, jaundice, mania, epilepsy, clonic spasm, lockjaw, loss of voice, bleeding from the root of the tongue, goiter, chills and fever, sweating, pain in the bones

GV-18: Headache, dizziness with agitation, nausea and vomiting of foamy (watery) saliva, stiffness of the neck with inability to turn head, epilepsy, shaking of the head, mad walking, insomnia, mania-depression, clonic spasm

GV-19: Stiffness and pain in the head and neck, one-sided headache, pain of the vertex, wind dizziness, aversion to wind and cold, painful obstruction with sweating, mad walking, insomnia, epileptic convulsions

Chapter 7

The Limbic System

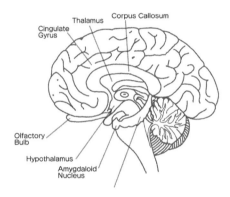

Functional Overview

Buried within the depths of the cerebrum lie several large limbic structures and nuclei which are preeminent in the control and mediation of memory, emotion, learning, dreaming, attention, arousal, and the perception and expression of emotional, motivational, sexual, and social behavior including the formation of loving attachments. The structures of the limbic system are exceedingly ancient, some of which began to evolve over 450 million years ago. Over the course of evolution, these emotional structures expanded in size, some becoming increasingly cortical in response to increased environmental opportunities and demands. In fact, until as recently as 50 million years ago, the brain of the ancestral line that would eventually give rise to humans was dominated by the limbic system. The limbic brain has not been replaced, however, as it is not only predominant in regard to all aspects of motivational and emotional functioning, but is capable of completely overtaking the "rational mind." This is due in part to the massive axonal projections of the limbic system to the neocortex.

The primary structures of the limbic system include the hypothalamus, amygdala, hippocampus, septal nuclei, and anterior cingulate gyrus, structures which are directly interconnected by massive axonal pathways.

Hypothalamus

This could be considered the most "primitive" aspect of the limbic system, despite the functioning of this sexually dimorphic structure being exceedingly complex. A primary function of the hypothalamus is the regulation of the autonomic nervous system. The hypothalamus integrates autonomic responses and endocrine function with behavior to maintain homeostasis of certain systems. Blood pressure and electrolyte composition are maintained by control of thirst and salt appetite. Body temperature is regulated by control of metabolic thermogenesis and behaviors that seek to warm or cool the individual. Energy metabolism is regulated by feeding, digestion, and metabolic rate. Reproduction is regulated through hormonal control. Emergency responses to stress are controlled by regulating blood flow to muscle and other tissues, and by the release of adrenal stress hormones. The medial hypothalamus controls parasympathetic activities (e.g. reduction in heart rate, increased peripheral circulation) and exerts a dampening effect on certain forms of emotional/ motivational arousal. The lateral hypothalamus mediates sympathetic activity (increasing heart rate, elevation of blood pressure) and is involved in controlling the metabolic and somatic correlates of heightened emotionality.

Nearly every region of the cerebrum interacts with the hypothalamus and is subject to its influences. Even more, the hypothalamus utilizes the blood supply to transmit hormonal and humoral messages to peripheral organs and other brain structures. It utilizes the blood supply and cerebrospinal fluid to receive information as well, thus bypassing the synaptic route utilized by almost all other regions of the neuroaxis. It is exceedingly responsive to olfactory (and pheromonal) input. The information received is sensory information from all over the body, which is then compared with biologic set points and, upon detection of deviation from these set points, adjusts autonomic, endocrine, and behavioral responses to return to homeostasis through direct influence on the pituitary gland and hormonal secretion. A summation of subregions in the hypothalamus and their functions can be found in Table 7.1, while Table 7.2 shows various hormones produced by the hypothalamus and their effect on the body.

TABLE 7.1 Regions of the Hypothalamus

Region	Area	Nucleus	Function
Anterior	Medial	Medial preoptic nucleus	Regulates the release of gonadotropic hormones from the adenohypophysis. Contains the sexually dimorphic nucleus, which releases GnRH
		Supraoptic nucleus	Oxytocin release, vasopressin release
		Paraventricular nucleus	Corticotropin-releasing hormone
		Anterior hypothalamic nucleus	Thermoregulation, panting, sweating, thyrotropin inhibition
		Suprachiasmic nucleus	Vasopressin release, circadian rhythms
	Lateral	Lateral preoptic nucleus	Sleep and arousal
		Lateral nucleus	Thirst and hunger
		Part of supraoptic nucleus	Vasopressin release
Tuberal	Medial	Dorsomedial hypothalamic nucleus	Blood pressure, heart rate, GI stimulation
		Ventromedial nucleus	Satiety, neuroendocrine control
		Arcuate nucleus	Growth hormone-releasing hormone (GHRH), feeding, dopamine
	Lateral	Lateral nucleus	Thirst, hunger
		Lateral tuberal nuclei	Feeding and metabolism
Posterior	Medial	Mammillary nuclei	Memory
		Posterior nucleus	Increased blood pressure, pupillary dilation, shivering
	Lateral	Lateral nucleus	Thermoregulation

TABLE 7.2 Hormonal Production and Effects

Hormone	Produced by	Effect
Thyrotropin-releasing hormone (TRH)	Parvocellular neurosecretory neurons	Stimulates thyroid-stimulating hormone (TSH) release from anterior pituitary Stimulates prolactin release from anterior pituitary
Dopamine (DA)	Dopamine neurons of the arcuate nucleus	Inhibits prolactin release from anterior pituitary
Growth hormone-releasing hormone (GRHR)	Neurons of the arcuate nucleus	Stimulates growth hormone (GH) release from anterior pituitary
Somatostatin (SS)	Neuroendocrine cells of the periventricular nucleus	Inhibits growth hormone (GH) release from anterior pituitary Inhibits thyroid-stimulating hormone (TSH) release from anterior pituitary
Gonadotropin-releasing hormone (GnRH)	Neuroendocrine cells of the preoptic area	Stimulates follicle-stimulating hormone (FSH) release from anterior pituitary Stimulates luteinizing hormone (LH) release from anterior pituitary
Corticotropin-releasing hormone (CRH)	Parvocellular neurosecretory neurons	Stimulates adrenocorticotropic hormone (ACTH) release from anterior pituitary
Oxytocin	Magnocellular neurosecretory cells	Uterine contraction Lactation (letdown reflex)
Vasopressin/ antidiuretic hormone (ADH)	Magnocellular neurosecretory neurons	Increase in the permeability to water of the cells of distal tubule and collecting duct in the kidney, thus allowing water reabsorption and excretion of concentrated urine

Possible Symptoms Associated with Lateral vs. Medial Hypothalamic Damage

Lateral lesion:

- Aphagia, adipsia (no motivation to eat or drink)

- Attenuated sense of pleasure and emotional responsiveness

- Pathological laughter and crying

- Passiveness, inability to become aggressive

Medial lesion:

- Hyperphagia, severe obesity (especially ventromedial)

- Pathological laughter and crying

- Aggressive or attack behavior, rage-like outbursts, propensity toward violence

Amygdala

The amygdala has been implicated in the generation of both the most rudimentary and most profound of human emotions including fear, sexual desire, rage, and religious ecstasy. At a more basic level, it aids in determining if something might be appropriate to eat. The amygdala is involved in the seeking out of loving attachments and the formation of long-term emotional memories. It contains neurons which become activated in response to the human face, and which become activated in response to the direction of someone else's gaze. Chemical systems within the amygdala include opiate, leutenizing hormone, vasopressin, somatostatin, and corticotropin-releasing factor. The amygdala can be likened to the chief executive of the limbic system, wielding enormous power over the hypothalamic impulses via the stria terminalis, medial forebrain bundle, and amygdala-fugal pathways. The amygdala is also directly connected to the hippocampus, with which it interacts to contribute to memory storage. In particular it plays a role in the emotional significance of memories. The influence of the amygdala can become so substantial that it is able to overwhelm the neocortex and assume control over behavior when emotions run high.

The amygdala is buried within the depths of the anterior–inferior temporal lobe and consists of several major nuclear groups including the cortical–medial, central, paralaminar, lateral, basal, and accessory basal nucleus which can roughly be grouped as medial and basolateral nuclei. The medial group (or cortico–medial amygdala) is involved in olfaction, sexuality, and motor activity (via its interconnections with the striatum). In females, the medial amygdala is a principal site for uptake of the female sex hormone estrogen, and contains a high concentration of leuteinizing hormone which plays an important role during pregnancy and nursing. In addition, the medial (and lateral) regions are rich in cells containing enkephalins, and opiate receptors can be found throughout the amygdala. As a result, the amygdala becomes exceedingly active when experiencing a craving for pleasurable experiences including addictive drives such as with sex, gambling, and drugs. The basolateral amygdala is the most cortex-like, subserving pleasure circuits and relying on excitatory neurotransmitters (e.g. glutamate), whereas the local-circuit interneurons rely on the inhibitory transmitters (e.g. GABA). This is intimately involved in all aspects of emotional activity and is highly important in analyzing received information and transferring it back to the neocortex so that further elaboration can be carried out at the neocortical level. It is through the lateral division that emotional meaning and significance can be assigned to, as well as extracted from, that which is experienced.

Possible Symptoms Associated with Amygdala Damage

- Docility (hypoactivity)
- Intractable aggression or fear (hyperactivity)
- Inability to recognize faces
- Blunted emotions
- Inability to sing, convey melodic information, or to properly enunciate via vocal inflection (right-sided injury)
- Inability to appropriately respond to social–emotional stimuli (social–emotional agnosia)

- Difficulty maintaining attention
- Lack of emotional speech
- Prolonged, repeated, and inappropriate sexual behavior and/or masturbation
- High-risk behavior, reduced loss aversion (e.g. gambling)
- Memory deficits
- Tendency to react to every stimulus
- Tendency to put objects into the mouth

Hippocampus ("Ammon's Horn" or the "Sea Horse")

The hippocampus is unique in that, unlike other structures, almost all of its input from the neocortex is relayed through the overlying entorhinal cortex which processes direction and spatial mapping. The main body of the hippocampus consists of the dentate gyrus, the subiculum, and sectors referred to as CA1, CA2, CA3, and CA4. It also consists of a number of subcomponents and adjoining structures such as the parahippocampal gyrus, entorhinal and perirhinal cortex, and the uncus (which it shares with the amygdala). Functions include components of memory, new learning, cognitive mapping of the environment, voluntary movement toward a goal, attention, behavioral arousal, and orienting reactions. It plays an exceedingly important role in memory, acting to place various short-term memories into long-term storage. Presumably the hippocampus encodes new information during the storage and consolidation (long-term storage) phase, and assists in the gating of afferent streams of information destined for the neocortex by filtering or suppressing irrelevant sense data that may interfere with memory consolidation. With repeated presentations of a novel stimulus, the hippocampus habituates. Thus, as information is attended to, recognized, and presumably learned and/or stored in memory, hippocampal participation diminishes. Moreover, it is believed that through the development of long-term potentiation, the hippocampus is able to track information as it is stored in the neocortex, and to form conjunctions between synapses and different brain regions which process and store associated memories.

The left amygdala and hippocampus are highly involved in processing and/or attending to verbal information, whereas the right amygdala/hippocampus is more involved in the learning, memory, and recollection of non-verbal, visual–spatial, environmental, emotional, motivational, tactile, olfactory, and facial information. There is minimal hippocampal involvement in emotions, though electrical stimulation has elicited sensations of "anxiety" or "bewilderment." There is evidence that the hippocampus may also work to reduce extremes in cortical arousal by downregulating the reticular activating system or augmenting cortical evoked potential depending on whether cortical activity is high or low respectively.

Possible Symptoms Associated with Hippocampal Damage

- Impaired memory—inability to convert short-term memories into long-term memories (anterograde amnesia)

- Impaired memory for words, passages, conversations, and written material (especially with left-side injury)

- Distractibility

- Hyperresponsiveness—may feel overwhelmed or confused as a result

- Impairment in attention and learning

- Disinhibition of behavioral responsiveness or shifting of attention

- "Input overload"—neuroaxis is overwhelmed by neural noise, disrupting the consolidation phase of memory such that relevant information is not stored or even attended to

Septal Nuclei

The septal nuclei are in part an evolutionary and developmental outgrowth of the hippocampus and the hypothalamus. They link these two structures along with the amygdala, brainstem, and sustania innominata, which is a major memory center that manufactures acetylcholine (ACh), a transmitter directly implicated in memory. There are both lateral and medial segments (i.e. the lateral and medial septal nuclei). Presumably these interconnections allow the septal nuclei to exert modulatory influences on the hippocampus in regard to memory functioning and arousal. The septal nuclei are also interconnected with and share a counterbalancing relationship with the amygdala, particularly pertaining to hypothalamic activity and emotional/sexual arousal. For example, whereas the amygdala promotes indiscriminate contact seeking, and perhaps promiscuous sexual activity, the septal nuclei inhibit these tendencies, assisting in the formation of selective and more enduring emotional attachments. The septal nuclei can also produce extremes of emotion, including explosive violence, known as "septal rage."

Possible Symptoms Associated with Septal Nuclei Damage

- Memory loss due to acetylcholine, norepinephrine, and serotonin depletion in the hippocampus

- Difficulty remembering one's surroundings

- Difficulty with learning and memory due to abolishment of hippocampal theta states

- Increased emotionality or aggression

- "Septal rage"—hyperemotionality, rage, hyperactivity, increased eating

Anterior Cingulate

The anterior cingulate is considered a transitional cortex, or mesocortex. It is intimately interconnected with the hypothalamus, amygdala, septal nuclei, and hippocampus, participating in memory and emotion, including the experience of pain, misery, and anxiety. The evolution and expression of maternal behavior is also directly related to this structure. The anterior cingulate is the most vocal aspect of the brain, becoming active during language tasks, and generating emotional–melodic aspects of speech. These are expressed via interconnections with the right and left frontal speech areas, and the vocalization center in the midbrain periaqueductal gray. As such, the anterior cingulate is implicated in the more cognitive aspects of social–emotional behavior including language and the establishment of long-term attachments beginning with the mother–infant bond. This structure is sexually differentiated, which likely contributes to differences in melodic speech pattern differences between males and females. Joseph also attributes the possibilities of "maternal" vs. "paternal" behavior tendencies to being rooted within these differentiations.

Possible Symptoms Associated with Anterior Cingulate Damage

- Anxiety/panic disorder

- Apathy/blunted emotions

- Depressive symptoms

- Lack of emotional speech

- Social and emotional inappropriateness or unresponsiveness

- Stuttering, word repetition, uncontrollable babbling, or (if severe) mutism

Olfactory Bulb

The olfactory bulb and olfactory system are also implicated in the functioning of the limbic system, the limbic striatum (nucleus accumbens, olfactory tubercle, substantia innominata, ventral caudate, and putamen), and the orbital frontal and inferior temporal lobes, along with the midbrain monoamine system. These systems and structures are also directly connected or separated by only a single synapse, which tend to become aroused not only as a function of emotional arousal, but in reaction to olfactory input. In this way, the olfactory bulb continues to exert profound effects on the human limbic system, and upon human behavior.

Acupuncture Considerations

A number of points have been demonstrated by fMRI studies to have a correlation to brain activity in the limbic system.[1]

Activating

Hippocampus: GB-34, GB-39

Hypothalamus: ST-36

Thalamus: ST-36, GB-34, GB-39

Deactivating

Amygdala: ST-36

Hippocampus: ST-36

Thalamus: LR-3, GB-40

George Soulié de Morant[2] notes indications for brain regions according to his extensive studies of the medicine in China prior to the communist revolution. According to his studies, points have been found to influence the limbic system.

Midbrain

Tonifying: LU-9, ST-23, ST-40, ST-41 (posterior central lobes), ST-43, SI-4, SI-7

BL-10 (anterior), BL-12 (parasymp.), BL-45, BL-54, BL-55, KI-14, KI-23 (anterior/vagus)

PC-2, TW-5, TW-6

---

1   Huang, W., Pach, D., Napadow, *et al.* Characterizing acupuncture stimuli using brain imaging with fMRI—a systematic review and meta-analysis of the literature. *PLOS ONE.* 2012; 7(4): e32960. https://doi.org/10.1371/journal.pone.0032960

2   Soulié de Morant, George and Zmiewski, Paul. *Chinese Acupuncture.* Brookline, MA: Paradigm Publications. 1994. Print.

GB-29, GB-30, GB-36, LR-10

CV-5 (stiopallidum), CV-20 (vagus), GV-3, GV-16 (vagus), GV-20 (anterior), GV-27

Dispersing: BL-60, BL-63

Hypothalamus

Tonifying: ST-21 (anterior), BL-67 (posterior/sympathetic), KI-23 (anterior), GB-20 (posterior), CV-20 (anterior)

Pituitary

Tonifying: LI-1, LI-4, CV-18, GV-14, GV-26

Thalamus

Tonifying: BL-61

Dispersing: TW-10

Chapter 8

The Parietal Lobes

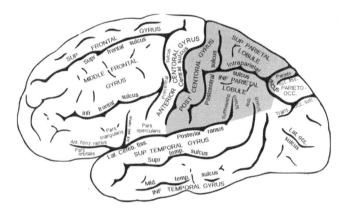

Functional Overview

The parietal lobes act as the senior executive of maintaining an individual's body image and perception of the body within physical and visual space. While commonly associated with the mediation of somesthetic stimuli, they are also concerned with motor and attentional functioning, the perception of spatial relations, including depth, orientation, and location, and the identification of motivationally significant auditory, somesthetic, and visual stimuli. Distinct sensory impressions are received from the entire body providing information about one's surroundings. It is the parietal lobe which guides the movement of the body in space, coordinating body movement while running, walking, climbing, etc. through dense interconnections linking the primary somesthetic with the motor areas in the frontal lobe and impulses transmitted down the cortical–spinal tract. The parietal lobes are also considered the primary cortical structure relating to the hand as it receives sensations from the bones, tendons, muscles, and skin of the hand, then guiding the movement of the hand within visual space. This allows for the ability to reach for and manipulate tools, open and remove bottle caps, and pour the contents into a glass. This is possible through connections with the frontal motor areas and the visual cortex.

The parietal lobes are not a homologous tissue but consist of cells which are responsive to a variety of divergent stimuli, including movement, hand position, objects within grasping distance, audition, eye movement, pain, heat, and cold, as well as complex and motivationally significant visual stimuli.

The inferior parietal lobule of the left hemisphere appears to be the central region concerned with the performance of skilled temporal–sequential motor acts. These engrams assist in programming the motor frontal cortex where the actions are actually executed. If the inferior parietal region is destroyed, the individual loses the ability to perform actions in an appropriate temporal sequence or even to appreciate when they have performed an action incorrectly. This condition is referred to as apraxia.

In contrast, right parietal injuries are associated with severe disturbances of emotion and constructional deficiencies, as well as a host of visual–spatial perceptual abnormalities including left-sided inattention and neglect. For example, with severe lesions in this area there may be a profound inattention to all forms of stimuli falling to their left. When drawing pictures, they may fail to draw the left half of an object; when writing or reading they may ignore the left half of words or the left half of the page. They may fail to perceive and respond to individuals standing to their left, or even the left half of their own body. Largely this condition is secondary to a destruction of neurons which are sensitive to various forms of visual and somesthetic input.

Lesions to the parietal lobe are seldom localized to one particular quadrant, or even restricted to the parietal lobe. Damage may be parietal occipital, parietal temporal, frontal parietal, or even bilateral (in cases of cerebrovascular disease or compression from a tumor). Therefore, an individual may display agraphia but normal reading, stereognosis in the absence of apraxia, or varied mixtures of seemingly unrelated symptoms.

Primary Somesthetic Receiving Areas (Brodmann's Areas 3ab, 1, 2)

This region consists of three narrow strips of tissue (areas 3ab, 1, 2) which differ in sensory input, each maintaining a complete and independent representation of the body.

> *Area 3a*: Receives input from contralateral muscle spindles (group IA muscle afferents) and signals muscle length (flexion or extension)

> *Area 3b*: Receives contralateral cutaneous stimuli

These are semi-independent and organized based on the parts which are most frequently stimulated, creating greater cortical representation in accordance with their sensory importance. The area devoted to the fingers, in fact, is a hundred times larger than the area devoted to the trunk. This information is then relayed to the adjacent areas 1 and 2.

Together these four strips of tissue form a functional unit that is responsive to touch, texture, shape, motion, and the direction of stimulus movement, including temporal–sequential patterning, and can directly monitor the position and movement of the extremities.

> *Area 1*: Maintains an overlapping cutaneous-joint body map

> *Area 2*: Maintains a map of the joint receptors and can signal the position and posture of the limbs based on input from the muscle spindles

The right parietal area is dominant in many aspects of somesthetic information processing. Neurons in this half of the brain appear to be more sensitive and more responsive with a greater ability to monitor events occurring on either half of the body, but particularly the left. The left half of the body exceeds the right in regard to most forms of tactile sensitivity. For instance, the left hand, sole of the left foot, and the left shoulder are more accurate in judging weight as they possess a more delicate sense of touch and temperature. The right parietal lobe appears to have more neocortical space devoted to maintaining images of the body. An awareness of this may well be the reason that in Japanese acupuncture approaches it is instructed to use the left hand when performing palpation.

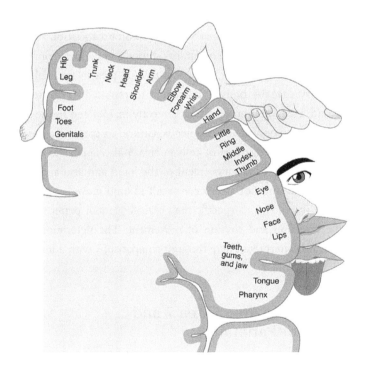

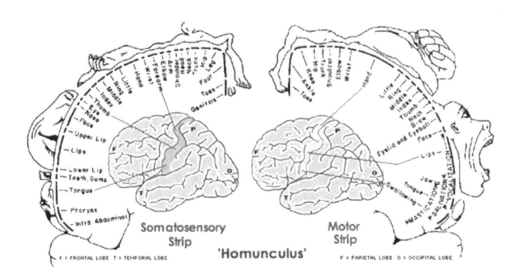

Somesthetic (Supplementary) Association Area

This region has connections stemming from the primary somesthetic cortices, contralateral primary zone of opposite hemisphere (area 5ab only), motor association areas (area 6) in the frontal lobe, and posterior thalamus (i.e. ventral posterior complex). It controls and contains representations of both halves of the body. The trunkal area in particular is represented in this region in a way that the body is bilaterally represented in the secondary sensory areas. This being said, bilateral representation is mostly maintained in the right half of the brain. A detailed representation of the cutaneous surface, in particular the hand and face, is maintained here. A small percentage of cells in area 5 also appear to be concerned with more complex activities such as the movement of the hand and arm and the manipulation of objects. Electrical stimulation of area 5 can result in limb movements. Other neurons in area 5 are especially responsive to specific temporal–sequential patterns of sensation and can determine the direction and rhythm of movement. The determination of positional interrelationships is also interpreted here through comparisons with a more stable image of the body in areas 3ab, 1, and 2.

Polymodal Receiving Area (Area 7 and Superior–Posterior Parietal)

The polymodal receiving area is concerned with the analysis and integration of the highest order visual, auditory, and somesthetic information. Single neurons often have quite divergent capabilities and the ability to monitor many different body parts simultaneously. Through this, it is able to create a three-dimensional image of the body in space. It coordinates/guides gaze and whole-body–positional movement through visual and auditory space, continually updating information of relations between internal and external coordinates. Neurons in area 7 are thought to execute a matching function between the internal drive state of the individual and the object being attended to, that is, responding to signals transmitted from the limbic system (cingulate gyrus) and middle and inferior temporal lobe. These cells guide and monitor eye movement so that the object of interest is fixated on, then exerting motor command functions so that the hand is guided toward the object until it is grasped.

This region has connections via the somesthetic association area, visual-receiving areas of the occipital and middle temporal lobe, motor and non-motor areas of lateral convexity, and the inferior temporal lobe including the parahippocampal gyrus. It also has the ability to receive auditory information to determine sound location. The connection with the parahippocampal gyrus allows for topographic learning. As a result of this information processing, cells are also responsive to, and can determine, a variety of visual-object qualities and interrelationships, including:

- Motivational significance
- Direction of movement
- Distance
- Spatial location

- Figure–ground relationships
- Depth, including discrimination and determination of an object's three-dimensional position in space

Posterior Parietal Areas 5, 7, and Supramarginal Gyrus

Neurons in area 5, as well as those located in the insula, receive direct thalamic input from the ventral and posterior portion of the ventral parietal lobe (VPL). The ventral portion in particular, in addition to somesthetic information, may also convey pain sensation to the parietal lobe. Neurons located in areas 5 and 7 of the parietal lobe demonstrate pain sensitivity, with some area 7 neurons responding exclusively to thermal and nociceptive stimuli and area 5 presumably acting to localize the source of pain.

Inferior Parietal Lobe/Multimodal Assimilation Area (Areas 7, 39, 40)

This portion of the inferior parietal lobule has auditory and (in the left hemisphere) language capabilities. Given its location at the border regions of the somesthetic, auditory, and visual neocortices, and that it is receiving input from all of these regions, there is a multimodal response. A single neuron simultaneously receives highly processed somesthetic, visual, auditory, and movement-related input from the various association areas, incoming visual input which encompasses almost the entire visual field, with some cells responding to visual stimuli of almost any size, shape, or form. The inferior parietal neurons are involved in the assimilation and creation of cross-modal associations and act to increase the capacity for the organization, labeling, and multiple categorization of sensory–motor and conceptual events. This region becomes activated during reading, semantic processing, generating words, and making syllable judgments. It also becomes activated during short-term memory and word retrieval, and highly activated when processing the meaning of words.

Pathology and Symptoms

Because of diverse yet related functions, damage can result in a variety of disturbances depending on which area is involved, including abnormalities in:

- Somesthetic and pain sensation
- The body image
- Visual–spatial relations
- Temporal–sequential motor activity
- Language
- Grammar
- Numerical calculation
- Emotion
- Attention

Attention and Visual Space

Lesions of the superior and inferior parietal lobule and the parietal–occipital junction can greatly disturb the ability to:

- Make eye movements
- Maintain or shift visual attention
- Visually follow moving objects

In the extreme, they can result in oculomotor paralysis.

Emotion

Emotional–motivational functioning may also become altered, alongside body and visual–spatial neglect, clumsiness, and visual–spatial disorganization. Severe right parietal injuries in area 7 may demonstrate initial hypokinesis, with the individual seeming very passive, and inattentive, and unresponsive and taking very little interest in their environment. Moreover, when an individual's symptoms are pointed out (e.g. paresis, paralysis), they may seem indifferent or conversely euphoric. Areas 5 and 7 (and the inferior parietal lobule) receive auditory information and discern the emotional–motivational significance of this information. Differentiation between varied vocal–emotional characteristics are also processed. Hence, when the right parietal region is damaged, there may be difficulty perceiving and differentiating between different forms of emotional speech.

Right vs. Left Lobe Injury of the Parietal Lobes
Left Parietal Injury

- Minimal right-sided neglect—right lobe attends to both halves of the body as well as both halves of visual space
- Impact/control localization only of objects within grasping/manipulation distance

Right Parietal Injury

- Inability to determine location, distance, spatial orientation, and object size

- Compromised visual constructional abilities

- Visual–spatial disorientation, clumsiness

- Defective performance on line orientation tasks, maze learning

- Inability to discriminate between unfamiliar faces

- Inability to filter important visual environment stimuli

- Can result in a complete neglect of the left half of visual space

Right Parietal–Occipital Damage May Also Show

- Deficiency on tasks requiring detection of embedded figures

- Severe problems with dressing (e.g. dressing apraxia)

- Easily lost or disoriented even in the individual's own home

TABLE 8.1 Parietal Regions and Associated Symptomology

Primary Somesthetic Receiving Areas	Somesthetic (Supplementary) Association Area
Elevation of sensory detection thresholds	*Mild*
Loss of position and pressure sense: two-point discrimination and reduced ability to detect movement of the fingers	Impaired movement of the hand and arm and the manipulation of objects
Inability to determine texture, shape, sequential patterning	Deficit will be only manifested when the part of the body represented is examined
Incapable of recognizing objects by touch or to discriminate among different forms or their properties, e.g. size, texture, length, shape	*Severe*
	Abnormalities involving two-point discrimination
Stereognosis significantly attenuated	Position sense
Passive, (non-movement) sensation less impaired	Pressure sensitivity
Motor disturbances such as paresis with hypotonia	May be able to recognize holding something in the hand but unable to determine what it might be (astereognosis)
Ability (or will) to initiate movement may also be reduced	Possible decrease in ability to perform size, roughness, weight, and shape discrimination
Lesions to the parietal lobe which spare the hand area of the post-central gyrus will have continued sensations from their hand, but not from the rest of the body. When testing for parietal lobe dysfunction, not only the face and hands but other body parts should be examined	*Laterality*
	Right: likely to give rise to bilateral abnormalities
	Left: generally affects only the right hand

TABLE 8.2 Parietal Regions and Associated Symptomology

Polymodal Receiving Area	Posterior Parietal Areas 5, 7, and Supramarginal Gyrus
Impaired depth perception	Lack of emotional responsiveness to painful stimuli
Impaired figure–ground analysis	Indifference
Inability to track objects or to correctly manipulate objects in space	Increased pain threshold
Decrease visual fixation	Tolerate pain for an unusually lengthy time period
Inability to direct attention to objects of motivational significance	Failure to respond even to painful threat
Impaired visual grasp/tracking	*Secondary to tumor or seizure activity (primarily right-sided)*
Disrupted attentional functioning	May instead report experiencing pain
Severe	Sensory distortions that concern various body parts due to abnormal activation of the parietal neocortex
Visual neglect—more common with right cerebral lesions, more pronounced for the lower visual fields	
Inferior parietal lobe/multimodal assimilation area	
Anomia (inability to name objects)	
Agraphia	
Pure word blindness	
Conduction aphasia	
Lateralized temporal–sequential function	
Apraxia	
Gerstmann's syndrome	
Finger agnosia	
Acalculia (including number agnosia, alexia, agraphia)	
Right–left disorientation	
Attention and neglect (particularly left-sided neglect) including secondary delusional denial, disconnection, confabulation, gap filling, delusional playmates, egocentric speech	

Gerstmann's Syndrome

When the posterior left parietal lobe is injured, the ability to name objects (anomia), object and finger identification (agnosia), arithmetical abilities (acalculia), and temporal–sequential control over the hands (apraxia) are frequently compromised and collectively referred to as Gerstmann's syndrome. This is most often associated with lesions in the area of the supramarginal gyrus and superior parietal lobule. Some authors have argued that Gerstmann's syndrome is not a syndrome proper as not all symptoms necessarily occur together.

Finger agnosia is not a form of finger blindness, as the name suggests, but rather a difficulty in naming and differentiating among the fingers of either hand and the hands of others.

Lateralized Temporal–Sequential Function

Injuries to the inferior parietal lobe can cause a disruption of visual–spatial functioning and temporal-sequencing ability (e.g. apraxia), as well as logic and grammar, and the capacity to perform calculations, depending on which hemisphere is compromised. Individuals with lesions involving the inferior parietal–occipital border of either hemisphere may have difficulty carrying out spatial–sequential tasks. For instance, when asked to draw a "square beneath a circle and a triangle beneath a square" they may draw the objects in the order described but not in relative spatial position. This is a difficulty in conceptualizing how to place the objects in relation to one another.

Those with left inferior parietal lesions have trouble with more obvious sequential–grammatical relationships such as being unable to understand the question: "John is taller than Jim but shorter than Pete. Who is tallest?" The right brain does not understand grammatical relationships, so a sentence that starts with the name "John" is interpreted by the right parietal area as all about "John," that is, the first word of the sentence is understood as the primary focus regardless of semantics or grammar.

If told "Give me the book after you give me the pencil," the right brain responds to the order of presentation rather than their grammatical relationship and would present the book, then the pencil.

Acupuncture Considerations

A number of points have been demonstrated by fMRI studies to have a correlation to brain activity in the parietal lobes.[1]

Activating

Primary somatosensory area: ST-36, GB-34, GB-37

Secondary somatosensory area: LI-4, LR-3, GB-34, GB-37, GB-40

Supplementary motor area: ST-36

Parietal–temporal cortex: GB-37

1   Huang, W., Pach, D., Napadow, *et al.* Characterizing acupuncture stimuli using brain imaging with fMRI—a systematic review and meta-analysis of the literature. *PLOS ONE*. 2012; 7(4): e32960. https://doi.org/10.1371/journal.pone.0032960

Deactivating

N/A

George Soulié de Morant[2] notes indications for brain regions according to his extensive studies of the medicine in China prior to the communist revolution. According to his studies, points have been found to influence the parietal lobes as well as the temporal lobes as the two are not well differentiated within his work.

Points acting on the temporal-parietal lobes: HT-3, PC-6, LI-9, GV-22

Tonifying: LU-1, LU-3, LU-6, LI-1, LI-7, LI-15
ST-13, ST-25, ST-30, ST-39, ST-42, ST-44
SI-14, SI-15, SI-16, SI-18
BL-4, BL-8, BL-17, BL-18, BL-19, BL-44, KI-18, KI-21
PC-4, PC-9, TW-1, TW-2, TW-7, TW-8, TW-9, TW-21 (Anterior)
GB-8 (Opposite), GB-33, GB-42, GB-44, LR-3, LR-6
CV-13, CV-15, GV-15, GV-21

Dispersing: ST-45

Points physically located over the parietal lobes have a range of indications. Explanations of these uses can be found in the source texts. In addition, the Jiao scalp acupuncture system relies heavily on the structures of the parietal lobes and points lying over them to address many different conditions including voluntary motor movement, sensory and pain conditions, and tremors. Specific body region correlations to be needled roughly follow the neural mapping of sensory–motor cortical regions. This system can be quite effective clinically.

TW-18: Tinnitus, deafness, pain behind the ear, headache, "head wind," vomiting, diarrhea, seminal emission, discharge from the eye, dimness of vision, infantile fright epilepsy, clonic spasm, fright and fear

TW-19: Deafness, tinnitus, ear pain, discharge of pus from ear, itching of the face, redness and swelling in the region of ST-8, headache, heavy head, heat in the body with headache and inability to sleep, dizziness, childhood epilepsy, tetany, fright and fear, childhood vomiting of foamy (watery) saliva, vomiting and drooling, pain of the chest and lateral costal region, dyspnea, seminal emission

TW-20: Tinnitus, deafness, discharge of pus from the ear, redness and swelling of the back of the ear and/or auricle, toothache, tooth decay, swelling and pain of the gums with inability to masticate, stiffness of the lips, dryness of the lips, superficial visual obstruction, stiffness of the nape of the neck with inability to turn the head

GB-3: Deafness, tinnitus, purulent discharge from the ear, dimness of vision, pain of the face, toothache of the upper jaw, stiffness of lips, headache, aversion to wind

---

2   Soulié de Morant, George and Zmiewski, Paul. *Chinese Acupuncture.* Brookline, MA: Paradigm Publications. 1994. Print.

and cold, chills and fever, hemiplegia, deviation of the mouth and eye, lockjaw, tetany leading to bone pain, clonic spasm, weakness of the optic nerve, achloropsia (does not perceive color), hemianopia

GB-4: One-sided headache, "head wind," headache with heat in the body, visual dizziness, pain and redness of the outer canthus, tinnitus, earache, clonic spasm, lockjaw, epilepsy, deviation of the mouth and eye, toothache, sneezing, neck pain, wrist pain, inability to flex the wrist, "joint wind" with sweating, giddiness, "sees nothing"

GB-5: One-sided headache extending to the outer canthus, pain of the outer canthus, headache, toothache, pain, swelling, and redness of the skin of the face, nosebleed, incessant turbid nasal discharge, rhinitis, febrile disease with agitation and fullness, weakness of brain and nerves, excessive thirst, cerebral congestion

GB-6: One-sided headache extending to outer canthus, pain of the outer canthus, sneezing, tinnitus, swelling and redness of the skin of the face, febrile disease with absence of sweating, agitation of the heart with no desire to eat, heat in middle Jiao

GB-7: Headache, swelling of the cheek and submandibular region, lockjaw, loss of speech, deviation of the mouth and eye, vomiting, stiff neck with inability to turn head, shock, depression

GB-8: One-sided headache, heaviness of the head, "head wind," pain in ST-8 region, deviation of the mouth and eye, acute and chronic childhood fright wind [seizure], dizziness, eye disorders, incessant vomiting, cold stomach, "phlegm qi" diaphragm pain, inability to eat, agitation and fullness on eating or drinking, injury by alcohol and vomiting, phlegm dizziness, edema, any kind of intoxication (alcohol, poisons), drug addiction, headache due to drunkenness

GB-9: Headache, tinnitus, damp itching of the ear, toothache, swelling and pain of the gums, goiter, propensity to fear or fright, fright palpitations, epilepsy, tetany, madness; children: cerebral congestion, hemiplegia

GB-10: Headache, heaviness of the head, chills and fever, toothache, deafness, tinnitus, stiffness and pain of the neck, painful throat obstruction, fullness of the chest with dyspnea, chest pain, cough with expectoration of phlegm and foam, pain in the shoulder and arm, inability to raise the arm, flaccidity of the legs with inability to walk, massaging warms opposite limbs

GB-11: Headache, dizziness, eye pain, ear pain, tinnitus, deafness, stiff tongue, bleeding from the root of the tongue, nauseating bitter taste in the mouth, stiffness and pain of the neck, goiter, painful throat obstruction, pain of the lateral costal region, cough, absence of sweating, contraction of sinews of the four limbs, bone taxation, agitation and heat of the hands and feet, cerebral congestion, cerebral hemorrhage, sudden stroke, grinding of teeth

Chapter 9

The Temporal Lobes

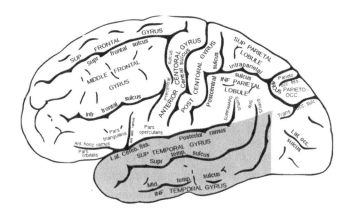

Functional Overview

The temporal lobes are unique in terms of brain regions. They are the only areas of the brain that subserve personalized, subjective emotional and social experience and can store and recall this information from memory. The temporal lobes also have very prominent emotional and cognitive affiliations, encompassing a wide range of emotional states, normal and aberrant. Much of this is in correlation with the limbic system, specifically the amygdala and hippocampus, with which the temporal lobes are intimately connected and are involved in emotion and memory, respectively. This makes sense from an evolutionary perspective as the temporal lobes developed out of the deeper limbic system.

The temporal neocortex can be loosely divided into three subdivisions—superior, middle, and inferior. The superior temporal lobe—also known as the auditory neocortex—acts as the last processing and filtering of sounds before being transferred to Broca's area of the frontal lobe for associations with responsive speaking. In this way, the auditory and language areas of the brain are linked—from the amygdala which houses emotional components to the superior frontal lobe, to the inferior parietal lobe, and to Broca's area and then back again—and may be referred to as the auditory association area. The signals in the superior temporal lobe have already been highly processed and analyzed by the auditory cortices for a number of components such as temporal sequencing and distinguishing non-random sounds from noise. Injury to the superior temporal lobe can show a number of deficits in auditory processing and association with verbal language.

The middle temporal lobe processes visual input. Much of the incoming information has already been processed by older brain structures, in this case the visual cortices. In this manner, the middle temporal lobe groups together many of the previously processed elements into higher order units that include depth, segmenting foreground from background, and integration of information into full gestalts. Damage to this area can result in disorders called agnosias in which certain objects or types of objects cannot be perceived and processed, or there is an inability to associate the information with any meaning or memory. The right lobe is particularly adept at distinguishing speed and direction of objects.

The inferior temporal lobe appears to be involved in the highest level of visual integration and contains highly developed neurons that mediate the perception and recognition of specific shapes and forms. The anterior portion of the inferior temporal lobe can be considered part of the auditory cortex as well as receiving visual input. Strong connections exist with the limbic system, in particular the amygdala and hippocampus. Thus, the inferior temporal lobe responds to auditory, visual, and emotional stimuli. This region is particularly involved in visual attention (the ability to hold focus), other visually guided behaviors, the recognition and learning of visual discrimination, memory of objects, and spatial locations. Cells are sensitive to a variety of components including direction of movement, color, contrast, size, shape, orientation, and the overall processing of three-dimensionality. Damage to this area can result in visual deficits including prosopagnosia, or the inability to discern and recognize faces, visual learning, and in performing visual closure in which the brain "fills in the gaps" when only part of an object is visible.

Hallucinations can develop from injury to the temporal lobes. Type and intensity of the hallucinations vary on the specific regions affected. Less specific auditory hallucinations such as buzzing, clicking, humming, and whispering can be associated with Heschyl's gyrus along the transverse temporal lobe. Abnormal activity in the superior temporal lobe, particularly the right lobe, can develop musical hallucinations including a repetitious melody, singing, or individual instruments playing.

Hallucinations of single words, full sentences, comments, advice, and distant conversations that can't quite be made out are associated with both the right and left superior temporal lobes. The middle and inferior temporal lobes can elicit visual hallucinations when damaged or stimulated. The anterior inferior temporal lobe specifically tends to have the most vivid and complex forms of imagery due to its specialization in recognizing specific forms. When this abnormal activity affects the amygdala and hippocampus, emotions and memories can also be evoked such as involving real people or events from memory. This includes dream-like hallucinations and the feeling of "déjà vu."

The temporal lobes are highly susceptible to injury from a variety of causes, including head injury, stroke, tumor, and epilepsy. In part, this susceptibility is due to the position of the temporal lobe within the skull. With whiplash injuries, or if the skull is struck from the back or the front, the temporal lobes may hit the inside of the skull and be ripped, torn, or sheared. The inferior temporal lobes are also slow to mature, which in turn increases the likelihood that abnormal neural networks may be formed in response to adverse early experience. Hence, abnormal early environmental influences, including profound traumatic stress, can induce language, emotional, and memory disorders such as the repression of childhood experiences and post-traumatic stress disorder. Severe psychiatric abnormalities including schizophrenia and the dissociative phenomenon can implicate the temporal lobes as well as the amygdala and hippocampus.

Pathology and Symptoms

Left Superior Temporal Lobe (Auditory Neocortex)

Difficulty with:

- Perception of real words
- Word lists
- Numbers
- Backwards speech
- Morse code, consonants
- Consonant vowel syllables
- Nonsense syllables
- Transitional elements of speech
- Single phonemes
- Rhyme

Right Superior Temporal Lobe (Auditory Neocortex)

Difficulty with:

- Acoustically related sounds
- Determining location of sounds
- Prosodic–melodic nuances
- Sounds which convey emotional meaning
- Most aspects of music including tempo and meter
- Non-verbal environmental acoustics (e.g. wind, rain, animal noises)

Middle Temporal Lobe

- Associated visual agnosia
- Word-finding difficulty—possible aphasic abnormalities
- Naming deficits
- Abnormalities in maintenance of temporal order and sequence
- Verbal memory impairments
- Reading and naming deficits (phonological alexia)

- Difficulty determining speed and
direction of objects (right lobe)

Note: Individuals with developmental dyslexia have been found to have abnormalities in this region.

Inferior Temporal Lobe

- Difficulty in visual attention/fixation

- Loss of the ability to recognize faces (prosopagnosia)

- Severe disturbances involving visual discrimination learning and retention

- Difficulty performing visual closure and recognizing incomplete figural stimuli (different shapes and patterns and objects which differ in regard to size or color)

Wernicke's Area (Left Lobe)
"Receptive Aphasia"

- Severe comprehension deficits

- Difficulty with expressive speech, reading, writing, repeating, word finding, etc.

- Spontaneous speech may be fluent: increased rate and may seem unable to bring sentences to an end; spoken words may be contaminated by neologistic and paraphasic distortions making them incomprehensible

- Unable to perceive spoken words in their correct order

- Cannot identify the pattern of presentation (e.g. two short and three long taps) and become easily overwhelmed

Inferior Temporal Lobe, Amygdala, Hippocampus

- Memory deficits in short-term emotional, visual, and cognitive memory

- Visual–auditory hallucinations and dream-like mental states

- Temporal lobe epilepsy

- Ability to sing affected (right amygdala)

- Ability to properly intonate altered (right amygdala)

- Anterograde amnesia (hippocampus)

Temporal Lobe Epilepsy

Abnormal electrical activity in the temporal lobe, as in epileptic episodes, does not necessarily include involuntary movements. The individual may simply seem to cease responding to their environment and stare blankly straight ahead. While this may not appear as much externally, internally the person may be going through a wide range of experiences or emotions. Another noteworthy cause may be severe and repeated early emotional trauma which can injure the immature hippocampus and temporal lobe, giving rise to a propensity to develop abnormal neural networks, making individuals more likely to develop psychotic and severe emotional and dissociative disorders.

Automatisms

Occur in 75–95 percent of temporal lobe seizures, about double the rate of any other brain region epilepsy, and may involve the following:

- staring
- searching
- groping
- lip smacking
- spitting
- salivation
- laughing
- crying
- hissing
- picking at one's clothes as if picking at lint

- clenching fist
- confused talking
- screaming
- shouting
- standing
- running
- walking
- kissing
- gritting/gnashing teeth
- etc.

Bodily sensations and/or symptoms may include:

- Numbness, tenseness, pressure, or heaviness
- Visual sensations such as things being very near or far
- Feelings of strangeness or familiarity including déjà vu (~20% of cases, especially right lobe)
- Desire to be alone
- Wanting something but not knowing what
- Olfactory hallucinations: usually quite disagreeable and includes smells like burning meat, fish, lime, acid fumes, burning feces

There may also be gustatory sensations: usually disagreeable with bad and bitter or metallic and sour tastes.

Possible symptoms with amygdala activation:

- Fear or remembrance of a fearful or traumatic memory; déjà vu

- Chest or epigastric sensations including nausea

- Heart palpitations

- Feelings of cold or warmth, shivering

- Pallor or flushing of the face

- Respiratory changes including apnea

- Salivation

- Belching or farting

- Sweating

- Vaginal secretions accompanied by sexual feelings/behaviors

Possible physical and emotional symptoms:

- Laughing (gelastic epilepsy), crying (dacrystic epilepsy), and/or running seizures (cursive epilepsy)

- Fear, anxiety, or depression

- Depersonalization

- Pleasure or displeasure

- Familiarity

- Out-of body experiences: often with feelings of elation, security, eternal harmony, immense joy, paradisiacal happiness, euphoria, and a "completeness"

Possible sexual changes:

- Continuous masturbation, indiscriminate hypersexuality, may expose and manipulate their genitals in public, attempts to have sex with family members

- Amygdala involvement can develop previously absent hyposexuality, hypersexuality, homosexuality, transvestism, confusion over sexual orientation, or may even engage in "sexual intercourse" even in the absence of a partner

Possible "religious" experiences:

- Dissociative states, feelings, and hallucinogenic and dream-like recollections involving threatening men, naked women, sexual intercourse, religion, direct experience of god, demons, ghosts, etc.

- Some report communing with spirits or receiving profound knowledge from the hereafter

Acupuncture Considerations

A number of points have been demonstrated by fMRI studies to have a correlation to brain activity in the temporal lobes.[1]

Activating

Temporal lobe general: PC-6 (electrical acupuncture)

Superior temporal gyrus: LR-3 left side

Inferior temporal gyrus: LI-4 right side

Temporal pole: LI-4 right side

Parietal–temporal cortex: GB-37

Deactivating

Temporal lobe general: LI-4 right side (ipsilaterally)

Superior temporal gyrus: LI-4 left side

Transverse temporal gyri: BL-60, 65, 66, 67 (in combination) right side

George Soulié de Morant[2] notes indications for brain regions according to his extensive studies of the medicine in China prior to the communist revolution. According to his studies, the following points are indicated to influence both the temporal and parietal lobes in conjunction and not individually.

Points acting on the temporal–parietal lobes: HT-3, PC-6, LI-9, GV-22

Points for specific brain centers

Odor-taste affected: LI-20, GV-20

Hearing affected: TW-21, GB-2, SI-19

Language/speech affected: GV-15

---

1   Huang, W., Pach, D., Napadow, *et al.* Characterizing acupuncture stimuli using brain imaging with fMRI—a systematic review and meta-analysis of the literature. *PLOS ONE.* 2012; 7(4): e32960. https://doi.org/10.1371/journal.pone.0032960

2   Soulié de Morant, George and Zmiewski, Paul. *Chinese Acupuncture.* Brookline, MA: Paradigm Publications. 1994. Print.

Points physically located over the temporal lobes have a range of indications. Many are beneficial for disorders of the eyes, ears, and nose as well as other indications. Explanations of these uses can be found in the source texts.

TW-18: Tinnitus, deafness, pain behind the ear, headache, "head wind," vomiting, diarrhea, seminal emission, discharge from the eye, dimness of vision, infantile fright epilepsy, clonic spasm, fright and fear

TW-19: Deafness, tinnitus, ear pain, discharge of pus from ear, itching of the face, redness and swelling in the region of ST-8, headache, heavy head, heat in the body with headache and inability to sleep, dizziness, childhood epilepsy, tetany, fright and fear, childhood vomiting of foamy (watery) saliva, vomiting and drooling, pain of the chest and lateral costal region, dyspnea, seminal emission

TW-20: Tinnitus, deafness, discharge of pus from the ear, redness and swelling of the back of the ear and/or auricle, toothache, tooth decay, swelling and pain of the gums with inability to masticate, stiffness of the lips, dryness of the lips, superficial visual obstruction, stiffness of the nape of the neck with inability to turn the head

GB-3: Deafness, tinnitus, purulent discharge from the ear, dimness of vision, pain of the face, toothache of the upper jaw, stiffness of lips, headache, aversion to wind and cold, chills and fever, hemiplegia, deviation of the mouth and eye, lockjaw, tetany leading to bone pain, clonic spasm, weakness of the optic nerve, achloropsia (does not perceive color), hemianopia

GB-4: One-sided headache, "head wind," headache with heat in the body, visual dizziness, pain and redness of the outer canthus, tinnitus, earache, clonic spasm, lockjaw, epilepsy, deviation of the mouth and eye, toothache, sneezing, neck pain, wrist pain, inability to flex the wrist, "joint wind" with sweating, giddiness, "sees nothing"

GB-5: One-sided headache extending to the outer canthus, pain of the outer canthus, headache, toothache, pain, swelling, and redness of the skin of the face, nosebleed, incessant turbid nasal discharge, rhinitis, febrile disease with agitation and fullness, weakness of brain and nerves, excessive thirst, cerebral congestion

GB-6: One-sided headache extending to outer canthus, pain of the outer canthus, sneezing, tinnitus, swelling and redness of the skin of the face, febrile disease with absence of sweating, agitation of the heart with no desire to eat, heat in middle Jiao

GB-7: Headache, swelling of the cheek and submandibular region, lockjaw, loss of speech, deviation of the mouth and eye, vomiting, stiff neck with inability to turn head, shock, depression

GB-8: One-sided headache, heaviness of the head, "head wind," pain in ST-8 region, deviation of the mouth and eye, acute and chronic childhood fright wind [seizure], dizziness, eye disorders, incessant vomiting, cold stomach, "phlegm qi" diaphragm pain, inability to eat, agitation and fullness on eating or drinking, injury by alcohol and vomiting, phlegm dizziness, edema, any kind of intoxication (alcohol, poisons), drug addiction, headache due to drunkenness

GB-9: Headache, tinnitus, damp itching of the ear, toothache, swelling and pain of the gums, goiter, propensity to fear or fright, fright palpitations, epilepsy, tetany, madness; children: cerebral congestion, hemiplegia

GB-10: Headache, heaviness of the head, chills and fever, toothache, deafness, tinnitus, stiffness and pain of the neck, painful throat obstruction, fullness of the chest with dyspnea, chest pain, cough with expectoration of phlegm and foam, pain in the shoulder and arm, inability to raise the arm, flaccidity of the legs with inability to walk, massaging warms opposite limbs

GB-11: Headache, dizziness, eye pain, ear pain, tinnitus, deafness, stiff tongue, bleeding from the root of the tongue, nauseating bitter taste in the mouth, stiffness and pain of the neck, goiter, painful throat obstruction, pain of the lateral costal region, cough, absence of sweating, contraction of sinews of the four limbs, bone taxation, agitation and heat of the hands and feet, cerebral congestion, cerebral hemorrhage, sudden stroke, grinding of teeth

Chapter 10

The Frontal Lobes

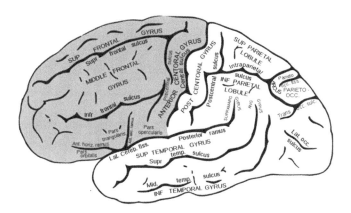

Functional Overview

The frontal lobes are the senior executive of the brain and personality. Over the course of evolution, the frontal lobes have greatly expanded in size, and are largely responsible for qualities that seem uniquely human such as the many achievements in art, culture, music, science, and mathematics. Although the frontal lobes are not the seat of actual intelligence, it is this area of the brain which enables us to utilize our intelligence and to anticipate and plan for future possibilities effectively. Individuals who have had even a significant frontal lobe injury may still score normal on an IQ test as their cognitive ability remains, but may be unable to put to effective use the intelligence they demonstrate.

There are varying theories about the precise essence of frontal lobe function. This includes regulating "cortical tone" with an emphasis on attentional processes; regulating a type of "autonomy" without which the individual becomes dependent on the external environment for cues that are then imitated; providing temporal structuring of behavior which integrates past experience with future plans; and the mediation of self-consciousness which bridges the gap between brain and mind. The frontal lobes act like an intermediary between stimulus

97

and response, allowing for flexible, autonomous, and goal-directed behavior which, in other animals, is much more instinctual and governed by the limbic system and brainstem.

The frontal lobes act to process, integrate, inhibit, assimilate, and remember perceptions and impulses received from the limbic system, striatum, temporal lobe, and neocortical sensory receiving areas. Functions of the frontal lobes broadly include:

- Engaging in decision making and goal formation

- Modulating and shaping character and personality

- Directing attention

- Maintaining concentration

- Participating in information storage and memory retrieval

At the neocortical level, they are also responsible for the vocalization of language, including:

- Organizing and monitoring the processes involved in preparing to speak

- The retrieval of semantic information

- Insertion of syllables

- Translating temporal sequences into auditory output

- Programming and activating the primary motor areas subserving the oral–laryngeal musculature

The right and left frontal lobes appear to differ in their influences over arousal, attention, and sexual, emotional, and memory functioning, including even humor appreciation.

When adults who have been traumatized recall traumatic imagery or when they view combat-related photographs, the right frontal lobe displays increased activity, and the left inferior–orbital region displays reduced activity. The right frontal area mediates emotional and melodic speech. It is dominant for arousal and appears to exert bilateral inhibitory influences over arousal, whereas the influences of the left frontal lobe are more unilateral and excitatory.

The frontal area mediates the syntactical, lexical, semantic, and temporal sequential aspects of speech and is dominant over the right. If the left frontal lobe is injured, cognitive and expressive functions tend to become suppressed and inhibited—a function not only of the injury but of right frontal suppressive influences.

By contrast, right frontal injuries are more likely to give rise to disinhibitory states, including the so-called "frontal lobe personality" discussed below. Due to the bilateral influence of the right frontal lobe and unilateral influence of the left lobe, if unilateral left lobe damage or bilateral damage occurs the individual will express more of a depressed or apathetic affect, whereas only damage to the right lobe will more often result in an excited state. Sadness can reduce right and bi-frontal activity, though in most instances depression is directly attributed to left frontal dysfunction and reduced left frontal activity.

Bilateral damage may show fluctuations between these states and thus resemble something like a bipolar personality trait.

Adults with PTSD have displayed reduced left frontal lobe activity.[1] Major brain areas involved in the pathology of PTSD are the medial frontal prefrontal cortex, anterior cingulate cortex, hippocampus, and the amygdala. The amygdala controls conditioned fear responses, while the medial prefrontal cortex involves the inhibition of such reactions. Injury to the medial prefrontal cortex would therefore lessen one's ability to inhibit fear. It has been theorized that the presence of frontal dysexecutive impairment due to brain injury may increase the perseverative nature of the re-experiencing of trauma.[2] In schizophrenia, lateral frontal gray matter reductions and decreased brain volume and activity have been repeatedly noted.[3]

Pathology and Symptoms
Left Frontal Lobe

- Depression
- "Psycho-motor" stunting
- Tearfulness
- Apathy
- Irritability
- Blunted intellectual and conceptual capability
- Confusion
- Puerility (silliness, childishness)
- Either total or partial unawareness of the environment
- Sometimes characterized as a blunted form of schizophrenia

Right Frontal Lobe

- Disinhibition: speech release, confabulation, lability, and other impulsive disturbances which may wax and wane
- Mania
- Confabulation (unintentional lies, false memories)
- Hypersexuality
- Tangentiality
- Impulsive, labile, disinhibited, and inappropriate social and emotional behaviors

---

1   Silver, Jonathan, Yudofsky, Stuart, and McAllister, Thomas. *Textbook of Traumatic Brain Injury*. Washington, DC: American Psychiatric Pub. 2011. Print.

2   Lash, Marilyn. *The Essential Brain Injury Guide*. 5th ed. Vienna, VA: Academy of Certified Brain Injury Specialists, Brain Injury Association of America. 2016. Print.

3   Silver, Jonathan, Yudofsky, Stuart, and McAllister, Thomas. *Textbook of Traumatic Brain Injury*. Washington, DC: American Psychiatric Pub. 2011. Print.

Motor Cortex

Supplementary motor area:

- Body may become stiff

- Movements tend to be slow, clumsy, and uncoordinated

- Severe agraphia

- Short steps and disturbances of posture, balance, and gait

- May become mute or appear catatonic if severe

Premotor Cortex

- Fine motor function and dexterity affected (e.g. finger tapping)

- Possible grasp reflex (i.e. stimulating the hand it will involuntarily clasp shut)

Primary motor area:

- *Paralysis*: Initially contralateral flaccid hemiplegia, then over several days the muscles develop increased tone and there is resistance to passive movements. Spasticity and hyperreflexia

- Fine movements are usually permanently lost

Occipital Lobe

- Disinhibition

- Hyperactive

- Euphoric

- Extroverted

- Labile

- Overtalkative

- Perseveratory tendencies (repetition of word or phrase)

- Proneness to criminal behavior

- Promiscuity

- Grandiosity

- Paranoia has also been observed

Broca's Area (Left Lobe)

- Loses the capacity to produce fluent speech

- Output becomes labored, sparse, and difficult, and the individual may be unable to say even single words, such as "yes" or "no"

- Immediately following an injury the individual may be almost completely mute and suffer a paralysis of the upper right extremity as well as right facial weakness, and be unable to write, read out loud, or repeat simple words

Frontal Eye Fields

- Abnormalities in fixation

- Decreased sensitivity to stimuli throughout the visual field

- Slowed visual scanning and searching

- Inattention and neglect

- Mislocation of sounds

- Some subgroups of "schizophrenics" have been shown to suffer from smooth pursuit and sacadic abnormalities

The "Frontal Lobe Personality"

With unilateral (primarily left-sided), bilateral, or even seemingly mild frontal lobe dysfunction, individuals may display an initial waxing and waning of abnormalities, including what is referred to as the "frontal lobe personality." This may include the following symptoms:

- Tangentiality, flightiness of ideas

- Silliness or childishness

- Impulsiveness

- Fatuous jocularity

- Lability

- Personal untidiness and dirtiness

- Poor judgment

- Grandiosity

- Irritability, restlessness

- Careless work habits

- Irresponsibility

- Laziness or becoming easily tired

- Hyperexcitability

- Increased sexuality

- Promiscuity

- Extravagent money spending

- Disregard of consequences

- Tactlessness

- Changes in hunger and appetite (usually with weight gain)

- Manic excitement

- Reduction in ability to produce original and imaginative thinking

- Perserveration (repetition of a particular word, phrase, or gesture)

- Compulsive use of utensils and tools (writing an endless letter with mechanical repetition of a certain phrase or word)

With significant frontal lobe pathology:

- Attentional functioning may be grossly compromised

- Behavior may become fragmented

- Initiative, goal seeking, concern for consequences, planning skills, fantasy and imagination, and general attitude toward the future may be lost

- Range of interest may shrink

- May not be able to adapt to new situations or carry out complex, purposive, and goal-directed activities

- Lacks insight, judgment, and common sense

- Shows little to no interest in self-care or the manner in which they dress, or even if they do, their clothes are soiled or inappropriate

A curious mixture of obsessive–compulsiveness and passive–aggressiveness may be suggested by their behavior. Damage to the frontal lobes, the right frontal and orbital frontal in particular, can create symptoms similar to a state of alcohol consumption.

"Medial Frontal Lobe Syndrome"

In medial frontal lobe injury, apathy is the major characteristic. The anterior cingulate gyrus primarily implicated.

- Limited speech

- Akinetic mutism may appear—complete absence of motor activity and speech

- Transcortical motor aphasia (particularly with the left supplementary motor area)

- Lower extremity paresis and gait disturbance can be seen if damage extends to high precentral gyrus

- Sphincteric disturbance (frontal lobe incontinence); the individual tends to be indifferent to this

- Loss of spontaneity and initiative—may seem to lack "free will"

"Dorsolateral Frontal Lobe Syndrome"

This syndrome is characterized by difficulty planning novel cognitive activity and carrying out sequential tasks. Although cognitive abilities such as language, memory, and visuospatial skills are themselves intact, individuals with dorsolateral lesions lack executive control and therefore cannot properly use these skills. This is an instance in which one's "knowledge is divorced from action."

In this syndrome, executive function deficits are paramount, implying the individual may show or be deficient in:

- Planning

- Monitoring

- Flexibility of behavior

- Problem solving involving foresight, goal selection, interference resistance, use of feedback, and sustained effort

- Attentiveness

- Motivation

- Perseveration

- Stimulus-bound behavior (e.g. incorrectly draws hands on a clock at the 10 and 11 positions when asked to show 11:10)

- Echopraxia—involuntary imitation of others' gestures (inhibited personal monitoring)

- Working memory—may overlap with inability for sustained attention

Acupuncture Considerations

A number of points have been demonstrated by fMRI studies to have a correlation to brain activity in the frontal lobes.[4]

Activating

Motor cortex: GB-34+GB-39 (electroacupuncture), ST-36+GB-34 (electroacupuncture)

SMA: ST-36 left side

Middle frontal gyrus: KI-3

Inferior frontal gyrus: KI-3

Deactivating

Medial frontal gyrus: ST-36 left side, LI-4

Dorsolateral prefrontal gyrus: LI-4

Inferior frontal gyrus: LR-3 left side

Middle frontal gyrus: LR-3 left side, [BL-60, 65, 66, 67 right side]

---

4   Huang, W., Pach, D., Napadow, *et al.* Characterizing acupuncture stimuli using brain imaging with fMRI—a systematic review and meta-analysis of the literature. *PLOS ONE.* 2012; 7(4): e32960. https://doi.org/10.1371/journal.pone.0032960

George Soulié de Morant[5] notes indications for brain regions according to his extensive studies of the medicine in China prior to the communist revolution. According to his studies, points have been found to influence the frontal lobes.

Points for the anterior frontal lobe

Insufficiency: Tonify SP-2, SP-3, LR-13, HT-9, GV-24, ST-40, PC-4

Excess: Disperse SP-3, SP-5, GV-24

Points for the posterior frontal lobe: GB-20, GB-27, GB-34, BL-10, PC-6

Points physically located over the frontal lobes have a range of indications. Many are beneficial for disorders of the eyes, ears, and nose as well as other indications more relevant to this chapter's material. For the sake of brevity, I have excluded eye, ear, and nose indications of these points which can easily be found in the source texts.

ST-8: Headache, splitting headache with chills and fever, dizziness, vomiting, dyspnea with agitation and oppression, hemiplegia

GV-22: Chronic headaches, deficiency and cold of the brain, bursting headache due to excessive consumption of alcohol, dizziness, visual dizziness, chronic and acute childhood fright wind, blue–green complexion, red and swollen face, swelling of the skin of the head, dandruff, somnolence, fright palpitations, awakens a response in ST-40, anterior brain, true energy, vitality, Shen, association of ideas, of sensations, of images, concentration, imagination, psychological hearing: hears sounds, but comprehends the meaning poorly. *Insufficiency:* cerebral anemia, rapid fatigue of the brain, moments of weakness, foggy to the point of cerebral confusion, emotional agitation, deranged mind, bluish–white complexion, somnolence, weakness of the blood. *Excess:* cerebral congestion, heat and pain in the brain as if broken, congested face

GV-23: Ceaseless bleeding from the nose and mouth, visual dizziness, redness and swelling of the face, swelling of the skin of the head, head wind, malaria, febrile disease with absence of sweating, mania-depression

GV-24: Mania-depression, ascends to high places and sings, discards clothing and runs around, mimics other people's speech, fright palpitations, insomnia, loss of consciousness, tongue thrusting, upward staring eyes, opisthotonos, wind epilepsy, wind dizziness accompanied by vomiting, vomiting with agitation and fullness, dizziness, head wind, headache with chills and fever, cold sensation of the head, nosebleed, awakens a response in ST-40, psychological and cerebral hyperexcitation, excessive sadness, sobbing, pulls out hair, cannot sleep,

---

5   Soulié de Morant, George and Zmiewski, Paul. *Chinese Acupuncture.* Brookline, MA: Paradigm Publications. 1994. Print.

apprehension, anxiety, jumps up on tables, sings, depression, migraines with photophobia

BL-2: Frontal headache, head wind, dizziness, nosebleed, face pain, red face with cheek pain, infantile epilepsy with upward staring eyes, hemorrhoid pain, manic behavior, loss of consciousness, pain and stiffness of the neck, hyperexcited mind, nightmares, hallucinations, or serious depression to the point of loss of consciousness

BL-3: Headache, vertex headache, dizziness, dyspnea, epilepsy, agitation and fullness of the heart

BL-4: Headache, vertex headache, swelling of the vertex, nosebleed, agitation and fullness of the heart, dyspnea, absence of sweating, agitation, and heat in the body

BL-5: Rigidity of the spine, opisthotonos, upward staring eyes, epilepsy, madness, tetany, clonic spasm, dizziness, headache, pain in the eye and head, heaviness of the head, does not recognize anybody

BL-6: Vertex headache, wind dizziness, deviation of the mouth, vomiting, agitation of the heart with vomiting, febrile disease with absence of sweating

GB-15: Head wind, visual dizziness, pain of the occiput and forehead, pain of the supraorbital ridge, windstroke, epilepsy, loss of consciousness, malaria, pain of the supraclavicular fossa, swelling of the axilla, easy fear, great emotiveness, violent sobbing from shock, trembling, stiffness, painful stretching (particularly at night), depression

GB-16: Headache, swelling of the head and face, toothache of the upper jaw, swelling of the gums, nasal congestion, epilepsy, aversion to cold, chills, and fever with absence of sweating

Chapter 11

Nao: The Brain in Chinese Medicine

Early traditional Chinese descriptions of the brain ("nao") did not give it much attention compared to our modern-day understanding of its functions. It was originally viewed as a canopy situated at the top of the physical body that was thought to attract and receive subtle internal and external emanations of Heavenly Yang. The cranial bone on top was referred to as the "roof of the soul."[1, 2] Daoists viewed it as a transceiver between the mind, body, and the external environment. The Heart organ was primarily associated with consciousness, thought, and regulation of all other organ systems as the "emperor" of the body. The brain essentially acted as a conduit of heavenly influence and information to the Heart organ to be dealt with. The classical texts also referred to an organ called the "Ling Fu" (spiritual depot). It is unclear among scholars whether this is referring to the Heart or the brain, but is said to be a place or mechanism by which the most subtle substances can be joined together for the radiating effect of the spirits. The term "Ling" refers to the revelation of Shen.[3]

Classical texts consider the brain an "extraordinary fu" organ, along with the uterus, gallbladder, the vessels, bone, and marrow.[4] The brain is also described as the "sea of marrow," relating to its close relationship with the Kidney system and its production of marrow. Ling Shu (Chapter 33) makes it known that "Mankind has a sea of marrow, a sea of blood, a sea of Qi and a sea of liquids and grains... [T]he brain is the sea of marrow. Its points are above at the canopy (GV-20)."[5] Marrow is produced by Kidney Jing (essence), which generates and

1   Maciocia, Giovanni. *The Foundations of Chinese Medicine: a comprehensive text*. Edinburgh: Elsevier. 2015. Print.

2   Johnson, Jerry Alan. *The Secret Teachings of Chinese Energetic Medicine*. Monterey: The International Institute of Medical Qigong Publishing House. 2014. Print.

3   Larre, Claude and Rochat de la Vallée, Elizabeth. *The Extraordinary Fu: brain, marrow, bones, mai, gallbladder, and uterus*. Cambridge, England: Monkey Press. 2003. Print.

4   Maciocia, Giovanni. *The Foundations of Chinese Medicine: a comprehensive text*. Edinburgh: Elsevier. 2015. Print.

5   Wu, Jing-nuan. *Ling Shu, or, The Spiritual Pivot = Ling Shu*. Washington, D.C.: Taoist Center. 1993. Print.

ascends up the spine via the governor vessel to nourish and substantiate the brain. Su Wen (Chapter 10) says that "All the marrow is dependent on the brain." The brain is also said to be the fu organ of the "Yuan Shen," or "original Shen," which allows the Shen (mind/spirit) of the Heart and the Hun (ethereal) spirit of the Liver to become active within the upper orifices and the brain to facilitate consciousness, thought, dreaming, and interaction with subtle external influences.[6] The Ben Cao Gang Mu by Li Shi Zhen states that "The Brain is the fu of Yuan Shen (original spirit)" and is the "fu of the spirits, shen, in relation to the origin, yuan."[7]

The brain is considered Yin in nature and it is stated explicitly so in Su Wen (Chapter 81). Its functions were described and limited to controlling one's guiding sense, language, and mental and thinking activities. This is strengthened when Qi and Blood are in abundance. It was also closely correlated to the eyes and their functions. In the Ling Shu (Chapter 10) nao is mentioned in relation to the pathway of the bladder meridian in which it starts at the inner canthus and rises to the top of the head where it has a luo relationship with the brain. The Heart's relationship with the brain is also described to be via the inner eye compared to the Kidney's relationship, which is via the governor vessel. According to difficulty 28 within the Nan Jing (Classic of Difficulties), the Du Mai rises to GV-16 to enter the brain with a shu relationship.[8] A special relationship is said to exist between the Yin Qiao Mai and Yang Qiao Mai with the inner brain. Both of these extraordinary meridians control functions of the eyes and their ability to "open" and "close" which relate to regulation of sleep/wake cycles. While all Yang meridians begin and reach the head, the Liver meridian is the only Yin meridian which is said to ascend to the top of the head where it terminates at the vertex. For this reason, stagnated Liver Qi may flare and ascend upward, causing Liver Yang rising symptoms which influence mental states, including irritability, becoming easily angered, a red face, wind symptoms, and even being "blinded by anger," in which cognitive functions seem to become overtaken.

An excess in the sea of marrow is described as a state in which one is "alert and robust with a lot of strength, one fulfills abundantly the number of years allotted." A deficiency of the sea of marrow is described as "when the brain turns around (vertigo) and the ears buzz, the legs are weak and there is a kind of paralysis and one has visual disturbances. The eye can no longer see. One is slow and lazy and likes to lay down quietly."[9]

Various pathologies can impact the brain. Internally generated heat can damage Yin substances and body fluids. According to Su Wen (Chapter 35), this prevents fluids and essences from nourishing the marrow (and by extension, the brain), and in extreme states is

---

6   Wu, Jing-nuan. *Ling Shu, or, The Spiritual Pivot = Ling Shu.* Washington, D.C.: Taoist Center. 1993. Print.

7   Larre, Claude and Rochat de la Vallée, Elizabeth. *The Extraordinary Fu: brain, marrow, bones, mai, gallbladder, and uterus.* Cambridge, England: Monkey Press. 2003. Print.

8   Larre, Claude and Rochat de la Vallée, Elizabeth. *The Extraordinary Fu: brain, marrow, bones, mai, gallbladder, and uterus.* Cambridge, England: Monkey Press. 2003. Print.

9   Larre, Claude and Rochat de la Vallée, Elizabeth. *The Extraordinary Fu: brain, marrow, bones, mai, gallbladder, and uterus.* Cambridge, England: Monkey Press. 2003. Print.

said to create a condition in which the "brain and marrow are melted." This presents with intermittent fever and disturbances of the orifices (eyes, ears, nose, mouth). Rectifying this condition is said to require restoring Yang Qi movement to the exterior. Su Wen (Chapter 37) also describes a condition in which the Gallbladder transfers heat to the brain, causing severe pain at the nose bridge and a nasal discharge that "seems to come from the abyss" (unclear, continuous). This is said to attack the "liquids in the brain" and, if severe, results in nosebleeds and blood seeping out of pores.[10] Wind is also a major pathological factor that can influence the brain. As stated above, stagnated Liver Qi that has generated heat can stir wind which then, according to Su Wen (Chapter 42), rises to Feng Fu (GV-16) to act as a depot for wind where it is received and can cause wind of the brain.[11] This can lead to unclear thinking, dizziness, vertigo, syncope, or apoplexy. It has also to be stated that "If the brain becomes deficient, then the brain will shrink."[12]

Later texts attributed more function and placed more attention and importance on the brain. This is particularly so relating to memory, with texts stating that "The memory of man is within the brain" and that "the Jing Ji, the spiritual mechanism of the memory, is not in the heart, but in the brain. The heart is the pathway by which the Qi comes in and goes out. How could the heart produce the spiritual mechanism of accumulation and retaining which is called the memory?"[13] "Jin Zheng-Xi explains that 'Man's capacity for remembering lies entirely in the brain.' While Wang Ren-An comments 'when someone wants to remember a past situation, he has to close his eyes or stare upward in order to think. If the supply of Qi to the brain and marrow stops for just a short time, and also if the brain has no consciousness, it will die, regardless of whether the period is short or long.'"[14]

Yi Shu in the 19th century stated in *Art of Medicine*:

When the brain and its marrow is pure and clear, then the spiritual efficacy can find somewhere to stay. But if they are unclear and disturbed, then you have stupidity and bad perception through the sense organs, because they are contrary of clarity and the ability to penetrate, which are the qualities necessary for intelligence, perception, hearing and vision. When one thinks, the Qi of the heart rises in free communication with the skull. When the brain and marrow are in a good state of fullness, then thoughts come easily. But when you think a lot, the fire of the heart burns the brain and the head spins, the vision becomes disturbed and the ears buzz. This shows that the marrow has

---

10   Larre, Claude and Rochat de la Vallée, Elizabeth. *The Extraordinary Fu: brain, marrow, bones, mai, gallbladder, and uterus*. Cambridge, England: Monkey Press. 2003. Print.

11   Ni, Maoshing. *The Yellow Emperor's Classic of Medicine: a new translation of the Neijing Suwen with commentary*. Boston: Shambhala. 1995. Print.

12   Neeb, Gunter and Wang, Qingren. *Blood Stasis: China's classical concept in modern medicine*. Edinburgh: Churchill Livingstone/Elsevier. 2007. Print.

13   Larre, Claude and Rochat de la Vallée, Elizabeth. *The Extraordinary Fu: brain, marrow, bones, mai, gallbladder, and uterus*. Cambridge, England: Monkey Press. 2003. Print.

14   Neeb, Gunter and Wang, Qingren. *Blood Stasis: China's classical concept in modern medicine*. Edinburgh: Churchill Livingstone/Elsevier. 2007. Print.

been injured. The marrow is rooted in the essences for its production, and below it is in free communication with mingmen, the fire of life, and with Du Mai, the governor vessel, which is also present at this place. The fire of ming men or the Yang of Du Mai warm and maintain the warmth of life, and then the marrow, which is in free communication with the essences of the kidneys and with this fire, overflows with power. But if through desires and emotions mingmen is injured, then there will no longer be this rising and warming but a kind of collapse downwards. The brain and marrow are deprived of their nourishment and then they deteriorate.[15]

In considering this information it can be seen that modern understandings of the brain have since informed Chinese medical theory and its approaches to addressing medical issues, while classical descriptions may still offer information on understanding basic mechanisms of essence, Qi, and Blood dynamics relating to brain functions.

---

15   Larre, Claude and Rochat de la Vallée, Elizabeth. *The Extraordinary Fu: brain, marrow, bones, mai, gallbladder, and uterus.* Cambridge, England: Monkey Press. 2003. Print.

Chapter 12

Blood Stasis

While still not well developed in biomedical approaches, the concept of Blood stasis has been long recognized within Chinese medicine, with treatment principles and protocols having been time-tested to show benefit where applicable. Blood stasis refers to a range of conditions in which blood flow has slowed down or been brought to a standstill. This may be systemic or local to a particular tissue, organ system, region, or within the "collaterals" of the body.

Any minor blockage of blood flow may lead to consequences wherein nutrients and oxygen become decreased to all tissues, blood pressure fluctuates or changes, vascular transport becomes impeded, and dysregulation of hormones and messenger substances including waste materials are in need of elimination. The endocrine, metabolic, and immune systems may all be affected by this and demonstrate pathological changes as a result.

Recent biomedical research into the field of hemorheology has been done in which blood fluidity and morphological changes in blood cells have been investigated. Through this, changes in components such as blood viscosity, viscoelasticity, plasma viscosity, erythrocyte aggregation, relative blood cell plasticity, fluidity of white blood cells, and thrombocyte aggregation/adhesion have been shown to impact the development of many chronic diseases.[1] This may include influences on one's risk of stroke, heart attack, diabetes, cancers, acute renal failure, and cor pulmonale, among others found in Table 12.1.

---

1   Neeb, Gunter and Wang, Qingren. *Blood Stasis: China's classical concept in modern medicine.* Edinburgh: Churchill Livingstone/Elsevier. 2007. Print.

TABLE 12.1 Biomedical Diseases Related to Blood Stasis

Cardiology	Heart attack, cardiac insufficiency, angina pectoris, cor pulmonale, arrythmias
Blood vessels and circulation	Arteriosclerosis, thromboses, disseminated intravascular coagulation (DIC), all kinds of hemorrhagic diseases
Neurology and brain	Transient ischemic attack, apoplexies, memory disorders and senile dementia due to vascular ischemia, tinnitus, sudden deafness
Dermatology	Psoriasis, neurodermatitis, seborrhea, ichthyosis, cloasma, etc.
Gynecology	Various menstrual disorders, metrorrhagia, lochial discharges, postpartum disorders
Oncology	All types of tumor formations, especially in the abdomen
Immunology	Low immunity and rheumatic–arthritic diseases
Genitourinary	Acute renal failure, dysuria, prostatitis
Respiratory tract	Dyspnea, asthma, hemoptysis
Mind/psyche	Depression, mania, psychosis, insomnia, senile dementia
Liver/metabolism	Chronic hepatitis, liver cirrhosis, diabetes

Diagnostics

- Blood screening
    - Blood plasma viscosity
    - Slowed sedimentation rate
    - Increased K value
- Nailbed examination (microcirculation)
- Fundus examination (microcirculation)
- CT scan (thrombi, tumors, ischemia)
- MRI (thrombi, tumors, ischemia)
- EMG/sonogram (organ hypertrophies)

Role of Blood Stasis and Traumatic Memories

There has been some interesting research into the use of propranolol, a beta-adrenergic blocker often used for cardiac arrythmia and hypertension, for the treatment of PTSD. This is theorized to act on the tendency for those with PTSD to have heightened noradrenergic (norepinephrine) signaling and elevated activity in the basolateral amygdala (BLA), as well as resistance to extinction learning.[2, 3] The discovery that memories remain plastic, rather than fixed, spurred more research into addressing these components of memory erasure (disrupting reconsolidation) and/or enhancing extinction retention through pharmacological means. A combination of fMRI and probabilistic mapping of intra-amygdalar responses to fearful, neutral, and happy facial expressions found diminished BLA responses and concluded that propranolol modulated norepinephrine both in reactivity and operating characteristics of the BLA via β-noradrenergic receptors.[4] Another study showed that systemic or intra-amygdala-infused propranolol blocks reconsolidation but not consolidation of memories and noted that the influence on the amygdala is particularly pertinent given its role in PTSD.[5] It has also been proposed that propranolol somehow blocks the protein synthesis in the amygdala which would otherwise strengthen the link between a fearful memory and the arousal response. This results in both heightened fear and arousal being either partially erased or unavailable for retrieval.[6]

It has been found that administration of propranolol within hours of a psychologically traumatic event reduced physiologic responses to subsequent imagery or recollection of the event.[7] Giustino *et al.* suggest its effectiveness as a fear-reducing agent when paired with behavioral therapy soon after trauma where psychological stress is high, possibly preventing or dampening the later development of PTSD. They go on to say that for those who have already suffered from PTSD for a significant period of time, this may be less effective at disrupting reconsolidation of strong fear memories but that, when PTSD has already developed, chronic treatment with propranolol may be more effective than the acute intervention given that higher levels of noradrenergic hyperarousal are common in many with PTSD.[8]

Similar results have been demonstrated with prazosin, a brain active alpha-adrenergic receptor agonist often used for blood pressure. Studies found that traumatic nightmares,

2   Giustino, T., Fitzgerald, P. and Maren, S. Revisiting propranolol and PTSD: memory erasure or extinction enhancement? *Neurobiology of Learning and Memory.* 2016; 130: 26–33. http://dx.doi.org/10.1016/j.nlm.2016.01.009

3   Hurlemann, R., Walter, H., *et al.* Human amygdala reactivity is diminished by the β-noradrenergic antagonist propranolol. *Psychological Medicine.* 2010; 40(11): 1839–1848. doi:10.1017/S0033291709992376

4   Hurlemann, R., Walter, H., *et al.* Human amygdala reactivity is diminished by the β-noradrenergic antagonist propranolol. *Psychological Medicine.* 2010; 40(11): 1839–1848. doi:10.1017/S0033291709992376

5   Dębiec, J. and Ledoux, J.E. Disruption of reconsolidation but not consolidation of auditory fear conditioning by noradrenergic blockade in the amygdala. *Neuroscience.* 2014; 129(2): 267–272. http://dx.doi.org/10.1016/j.neuroscience.2004.08.018

6   Gardner, A. and Griffiths, J. Propranolol, post-traumatic stress disorder, and intensive care: incorporating new advances in psychiatry into the ICU. *Critical Care.* 2014; 18(6): 698. PMC. Web. 7 July 2017.

7   Brunet, A., Orr, S., Tremblay, J., Robertson, K., Nader, K., and Pitman, R. Effect of post-retrieval propranolol on psychophysiologic responding during subsequent script-driven traumatic imagery in post-traumatic stress disorder. *Journal of Psychiatric Research.* 2008; 42(6): 503–506. http://dx.doi.org/10.1016/j.jpsychires.2007.05.006

8   Donovan, Elise. Propranolol use in the prevention and treatment of posttraumatic stress disorder in military veterans: forgetting therapy revisited. *Perspectives in Biology and Medicine.* Winter 2010; 53(1): 61–74. doi:10.1353/pbm.0.0140

sleep quality, global clinical status, dream characteristics, and comorbid depression may all respond positively to this drug.[9, 10]

Ethical concerns have been raised by the President's Council for Bioethics about this approach, however, given that propranolol dissociates the state of arousal from the individual's recollection and that this type of therapy disrupts one's sense of self. Others have argued that this point may be moot if the individual with PTSD is otherwise unable to function in society and has therefore essentially already lost their sense of self.[11] These arguments aside, it is interesting to consider the cardiovascular effects of propranolol and its impact on the bloodflow through arteries and veins in light of the Chinese medical view of the memories being stored in the Blood and how herbal approaches using those which impact the Blood may influence psychological as well as physical traumas, as many are indicated to do so. Examples of this include the formula Yu Nan Bai Yao or individual herbs such as San Qi, Dan Shen, and Ru Xiang, which may warrant research into such uses.

Chinese Medical Perspective

In Chinese medicine, Blood stasis has been recognized for hundreds of years as a pathologic process or a contributing factor to a wide range of pathologies. The earliest known mention of such a process is found in the Ling Shu (Chapters 58 and 81) in which it is respectively stated, "Injury resulting from fall produces poor Blood in the interior, which is hard to clear," and "If Ying Qi and Wei Qi stagnate in the channels and vessels, Blood will clot and not move. If this does not move, Wei Qi cannot flow through and starts to accumulate, leading to heat."[12] The most prolific developer in the concept of Blood stasis was the physician Wang Qing-Ren in the 19th century, who developed his theories and treatment protocols after performing the then culturally taboo post-mortem examinations of bodies to expand his medical knowledge of anatomy. Although a good number of his observations turned out to be inaccurate due to blood clotting and pooling that occurs after death, the formulas that were developed from these observations remain relevant and used frequently today for a variety of imbalances in actual pathological Blood stasis cases.

The Chinese medical etiology of Blood in the body is said to be derived from purified food essence following the Spleen organ system sending it to the Lung organ system. Qi gathered from oxygen and the breath then guide it to the Heart organ system where Kidney

9   Raskind, M., Peskind, E., *et al.* A parallel group placebo controlled study of prazosin for trauma nightmares and sleep disturbance in combat veterans with post-traumatic stress disorder. *Biological Psychiatry.* 2007; 61(8): 928–934. http://dx.doi.org/10.1016/j.biopsych.2006.06.032

10   Taylor, Fletcher and Raskind, Murray A. The α1-adrenergic antagonist prazosin improves sleep and nightmares in civilian trauma posttraumatic stress disorder. *Journal of Clinical Psychopharmacology.* 2002 Feb; 22(1): 82–85.

11   Gardner, A. and Griffiths, J. Propranolol, post-traumatic stress disorder, and intensive care: incorporating new advances in psychiatry into the ICU. *Critical Care.* 2014; 18(6): 698. PMC. Web. 7 July 2017.

12   Neeb, Gunter and Wang, Qingren. *Blood Stasis: China's classical concept in modern medicine.* Edinburgh: Churchill Livingstone/Elsevier. 2007. Print.

and Yuan Qi turns it into Blood. Physical trauma causes a local stagnation of Qi or Blood within an area, depending on the severity of the trauma, Blood stasis being associated with more severe cases. Whereas Qi stagnation can develop from emotional factors, there are said to be no emotional states that lead directly to Blood stasis. Qi stagnation from emotions can, however, evolve into further states of Blood stasis.[13]

Causes

- *Injury*: Internal or external bleeding causes acute Blood stasis

- *Qi stagnation*: Liver Qi stagnation is a common cause

- *Qi deficiency*: "Qi is the commander of Blood"

- *Yang deficiency cold*: Faulty warming function allows Blood to become thick and viscous

- *Exogenous pathogenic cold*: Causes contraction as in rheumatic diseases

- *Pathogenic heat*: Consumes body fluids and thickens Blood

- *Blood deficiency*: Blood loss may generate stasis

- *Exogenous dryness or Yin deficiency*: Insufficiency of body fluids thickens the blood

- *Phlegm*: Tenacious and viscous substances that inhibit physiological flow

- *Exhaustion*: Repetitive movements or postures restrict Blood flow

- *Suppressed emotions*: Causes Qi stagnation that can develop into Blood stasis

- *Dietary habits*: Consuming raw or cold food can exhaust the warming function of Spleen Yang

Potential Clinical Symptoms Related to Blood Stasis

- Elevated body temperature

- Heat felt in hands, feet, chest, abdomen, or genitals

- Stabbing pain generally in a fixed location

- All types of blood loss

- Local numbness or sensation as if bitten by ants

- Feeling of pressure or tension in the head, eyes, breast, or limbs

- Epigastric fullness

- Limbs and neck stiffness or difficulty moving

- Itchiness under the skin that doesn't abate with scratching

- Bruises, hemafecia, hemesis, epistaxis

---

13   Maciocia, Giovanni. *The Foundations of Chinese Medicine: a comprehensive text.* Edinburgh: Elsevier. 2015. Print.

- Heavy menstruation with dark or clotted blood

- Dry mouth with disinclination to drink large amounts of water

- Dry hair or skin

- Easily woken up or night terrors with profuse dreams

- Poor memory, difficulty concentrating

- Dark complexion, lips, tongue

- Macules or dots on tongue body

- Dark eye rings

- Engorged sublingual veins

- Throbbing or pulsating sensations in the breast

- Distended abdomen

- Bluish nails

- Distended veins at various body regions

- Easily irritated, very strong emotions

- Palpitations, tachycardia

- Digestive fullness and pain worse with pressure

- Diarrhea/constipation

- Low appetite

- Nausea

- Prolonged respiratory diseases

- Coughing up blood

- Choppy pulse—stagnant and uneven

Differences in pattern differentation and compounded patterns with Blood stasis create different hemorheologic changes,[14] as noted in Table 12.2.

TABLE 12.2 Hemorheologic Changes Associated with Different Pattern Differentiations

Pattern Differentiation	Hemorheologic Changes
Blood stasis with Qi deficiency	Elevated intercellular viscosity of erythrocytes, decreased erythrocyte plasticity
Blood stasis with Yang deficiency	Elevated total blood viscosity, elevated coagulation, elevated plasma viscosity, elevated fibrinogen, elevated hematocrit
Blood stasis with Yin deficiency	Elevated plasma viscosity, elevated hematocrit, elevated K value
Blood stasis with phlegm	Elevated total blood and plasma viscosity, elevated coagulation, elevated fibrinogen, elevated hematocrit, elevated thrombocyte aggregation
General blood stagnation	Elevated shear rate, elevated total blood viscosity, elevated total hematocrit

---

14   Neeb, Gunter and Wang, Qingren. *Blood Stasis: China's classical concept in modern medicine.* Edinburgh: Churchill Livingstone/Elsevier. 2007. Print.

Pattern Differentiation

Blood Stasis with Qi Stagnation

Primary symptoms: Stabbing pain and feeling of oppression in the chest and hypochondrium, palpitations, depression, insomnia, frequent anger, or other emotional factors

Related diseases: Liver and Gallbladder diseases, coronary heart disease, nervous disorders

Treatment principles: Invigorate Blood and move Qi

Acupuncture treatment: ST-36, BL-15, BL-17, SP-10, PC-6, LR-3, LR-14, LI-4, CV-17

Herbal treatment:
Xue Fu Zhu Yu Tang (Anti-stasis Chest Decoction)
[Tao Ren 12g, Dang Gui 9g, Sheng Di 9g, Hong Hua 9g, Niu Xi 9g, Zhi Qiao 6g, Chi Shao 6g, Chuan Xiong 5g, Jie Geng 5g, Chai Hu 3g, Gan Cao 3g]
Guan Xin Fang No.2 (Coronary Decoction No.2)
[Dan Shen 30g, Chuan Xiong 15g, Chi Shao 15g, Hong Hua 15g, Jiang Xiang 15g]

Blood Stasis with Qi Deficiency

Primary symptoms: Weakness, tiredness, shortness of breath, paralysis, chest pain especially under strain, lack of appetite

Related diseases: Coronary heart disease, chronic hepatitis, stroke sequelae

Treatment principles: Invigorate Blood and tonify Qi

Acupuncture treatment: ST-36, SP-6, LR-8, SP-10, BL-17, BL-20, BL-21, CV-4, CV-6

Herbal treatment:
Bu Yang Huan Wu Tang (Five-Tenth Decoction)
[Huang Qi 20g, Dang Gui Wei 6g, Chi Shao 6g, Tao Ren 3g, Chuan Xiong 3g, Hong Hua 3g, Di Long 3g]
Huang Qi Si Wu Tang (Astragalus Four Ingredients Decoction)
[Huang Qi 12g, Ren Shen 9g, Bai Zhu 9g, Fu Ling 9g, Bai Shao 12g, Gan Cao 6g, Dang Gui 12g, Sheng Jiang 6g, Shu Di 12g, Chuan Xiong 9g, Jin Yin Hua 6g]

Blood Stasis with Yin Deficiency

Primary symptoms: 5-palm heat, weight loss, night sweating, tidal fever, dizziness, dry eyes and skin, lusterless complexion

Related diseases: Liver cirrhosis, leukemia, tuberculosis, phlebitis, diabetes, low immunity

Treatment principles: Invigorate Blood and nourish Yin

Acupuncture treatment: KI-3, KI-6, BL-17, BL-23, SP-6, SP-10, CV-4

Herbal treatment:
Xia Yu Xue Tang (Blood Stasis Purging Decoction)
[Tao Ren 32g, Tu Bie Chong 6g, Gan Sui 4g, Da Huang 2g]
Tao Hong Si Wu Tang (Peach Kernal and Safflower Four Ingredient Decoction)
[Sheng Di 15g, Dang Gui 9g, Tao Ren 9g, Chi Shao 9g, Chuan Xiong 6g, Hong Hua 6g]

Blood Stasis with Blood Deficiency

Primary symptoms: Dizziness, insomnia, palpitations, pale complexion, pale lips and nails, dry stools, tinnitus

Related diseases: Anemia, loss of blood sequelae, neurasthenia, cardiac arrhythmias

Treatment principles: Invigorate Blood and nourish Blood

Acupuncture treatment: BL-17, BL-18, LR-3, LR-8, GB-37, SP-10

Herbal treatment:
Si Wu Tang (Four Ingredient Decoction)
[Shu Di 12g, Dang Gui 9g, Shao Yao 9g, Chuan Xiong 6g]
Huo Luo Xiao Ling Dan (Wondrous Pill to Invigorate the Channels)
[Dang Gui 15g, Dan Shen 15g, Ru Xiang 15g, Mo Yao 15g]

Blood Stasis with Pathogenic Cold

Primary symptoms: Strong pain in a fixed location, shortness of breath, heart pain, cold limbs, strong stabbing pain in the limbs, numbness, limb weakness, worse with cold

Related diseases: Postpartum infections, delayed uterine involution, no lactation, retention of placenta, infertility

Treatment principles: Invigorate Blood and dispel cold

Acupuncture treatment: BL-23, GV-4, LU-7, LI-4, BL-17, SP-8, CV-4 moxa

Herbal treatment:

Zhi Shi Xie Bai Gui Zhi Tang (Immature Bitter Orange, Chive, and Cinnamon Decoction)

[Zhi Ke 12g, Huo Po 12g, Gua Luo 12g, Xie Bai 9g, Gui Zhi 6g]

Shen Tong Zhu Yu Tang (Anti-Stasis Pain Decoction)

[Tao Ren 12g, Hong Hua 12g, Dang Gui 12g, Niu Xi 12g, Chuan Xiong 8g, Mo Yao 8g, Wu Ling Zhi 8g, Di Long 8g, Gan Cao 8g, Qin Jiao 4g, Qiang Huo 4g, Xiang Fu 4g]

Blood Stasis with Pathogenic Heat

Primary symptoms: Burning pain in chest area and abdomen, irritability, nervousness, thirst, tendency to bleeding, feeling of heat, dry hard stool, susceptibility to furuncles

Related diseases: Hemorrhagic diathesis (e.g. nosebleed), bronchiectasis, lung abscess, acute hepatitis B, septicemia

Treatment principles: Invigorate Blood and cool heat

Acupuncture treatment: LI-11, LI-4, ST-44, GV-14, BL-17, SP-10

Herbal treatment:

Tao Ren Cheng Qi Tang (Peach Kernel Qi Rectifying Decoction)

[Tao Ren 15pc (pieces), Da Huang 12g, Gui Zhi 9g, Mang Xiao 9g, Gan Cao 9g]

Qing Re Xiao Du San (Cooling Detoxifying Powder)

[Jin Yin Hua 15g, Sheng Di 9g, Shao Yao 9g, Chuan Xiong 9g, Dang Gui 6g, Lian Qiao 6g, Huang Lian 6g, Zhi Zi 6g, Gan Cao 3g]

Blood Stasis with Phlegm

Primary symptoms: Phlegm and sputum in throat and nose, frequent clearing of throat, coughing with phlegm, paralysis, Bi-syndrome in the chest

Related diseases: Bronchitis, coronary heart disease, hyperlipidemia, hemiplegia, epileptiform syndromes, unexplained neurological disorders

Treatment principles: Invigorate Blood and transform phlegm

Acupuncture treatment: ST-40, PC-5, SP-4, SP-10, LI-4, BL-17

Herbal treatment:

Tao Hong Si Wu Tang (Peach Kernel and Safflower Four Ingredient Decoction)

[Sheng Di 15g, Dang Gui 9g, Tao Ren 9g, Chi Shao 9g, Chuan Xiong 6g, Hong Hua 6g]

Xi Huang Wan (Yellow Rhino Pills)
[Mo Yao 30g, Ru Xiang 30g, Huang Mi 30g, She Xiang 4.5g, Niu Huang 1g]

Blood Stasis with Abdominal Masses

Primary symptoms: Abdominal masses and gatherings, goiter and similar conditions

Related diseases: Myomas, ovarian cysts, lymph node swelling, tumors, especially in the vessels, prostatic hypertrophy

Treatment principles: Invigorate Blood and soften masses

Acupuncture treatment: LI-4, LI-11, ST-40, CV-6, ST-36, SP-10, LR-8, BL-17

Herbal treatment:
Gui Zhi Fu Ling Wan (Cinnamon and Poria Pill)
[Gui Zhi 9g, Fu Ling 9g, Mu Dan Pi 9g, Tao Ren 9g, Chi Shao 9g]
Da Huang Zhe Chong Wan (Rhubarb and Eupolyphaga Pill)
[He Shou Wu 40g, Bai Shao 16g, Gan Cao 12g, Huang Qin 8g, Tao Ren 8g, Xing Ren 8g, Mang Qiao 8g, Shui Zhi 8g, Qi Cao 8g, Da Huang 4g, Ti Bie Chong 4g, Gan Qi 4g]

Blood Stasis with Food Stagnation

Primary symptoms: Food accumulation with stomach distension, feeling of distension and accumulation in the abdomen, digestive disorders with delayed digestion or cessation of digestion

Related diseases: Pancreatitis, cholelithesis, acute abdomen with cessation of digestion

Treatment principles: Invigorate Blood and purge

Acupuncture treatment: ST-25, ST-36, SP-4, LI-4, CV-12, BL-17, SP-10

Herbal treatment:
Di Dang Tang (Resistance Decoction)
[Da Huang 40g, Shui Zhi 30pc, Meng Chong 30pc, Tao Ren 20pc]
Tao Hong Cheng Qi Tang (Qi Rectify Peach Kernel and Safflower Decoction)
[Tao Ren 15pc, Da Huang 12g, Gui Zhi 9g, Mang Xiao 9g, Gan Cao 9g]

Blood Stasis with Bleeding

Primary symptoms: Blood heat syndromes, tendency to bleeding, poor blood coagulation, epistaxis, hemafecia, hemuria, metrorrhagia, etc.

Related diseases: All types of hemorrhages

Treatment principles: Invigorate Blood and stop bleeding

Acupuncture treatment: SP-1, LI-11, LI-4, BL-17, SP-10

Herbal treatment:
San Qi Shi Xiao San (Notoginseng Sudden Smile Powder)
[San Qi 15g, Pu Huang 12g, Wu Ling Zhi 12g]

Blood Stasis with Blockage of the Luo Collaterals

Primary symptoms: Blood heat syndromes, tendency to bleeding, poor blood coagulation, epistaxis, hemafecia, hemuria, metrorrhagia, etc.

Related diseases: All types of hemorrhages

Treatment principles: Invigorate Blood and remove obstruction from the Luo collaterals

Acupuncture treatment: Appropriate Luo vessel treatment, plum blossom along luo vessels, pricking appropriate vessels

Herbal treatment:
Huo Luo Xiao Ling Tang (Wondrous Pill to Invigorate the Channels)
[Dang Gui 15g, Dan Shen 15g, Ru Xiang 15g, Mo Yao 15g]
Shen Tong Zhu Yu Tang (Anti-stasis Pain Decoction)
[Tao Ren 12g, Hong Hua 12g, Dang Gui 12g, Niu Xi 12g, Chuan Xiong 8g, Mo Yao 8g, Wu Ling Zhi 8g, Di Long 8g, Gan Cao 8g, Qin Jiao 4g, Qiang Huo 4g, Xiang Fu 4g]

Clinical Notes

- Local points may also be considered to aid in breaking up stasis and moving Qi and Blood in the area. In cases of Blood stasis in the head, several local points may be helpful including GV-16, Taiyang, GB-8, GB-20, GV-20, Si Shen Cong, or ashi points that alleviate symptoms with pressure.

- A practitioner may also consider the use of other acupuncture approaches here including Kiikos Matsumoto's protocols for Oketsu (also known as Blood stasis, "Bad Blood," or "Toxic Blood"), especially if abdominal diagnosis determines the presence of oketsu kai—a palpable lump and pressure pain between KI-15 and ST-27—or other protocols for stagnation of blood in the head, both of which I have found clinically quite useful.[15]

- Another protocol that may be considered is the Korean Sa-Am protocol for Blood stasis in which the Lung tonification pattern is needled: LU-9(+), SP-3(+), LI-11(−), TW-5(−).[16]

Blood Invigorating Medicinals

Blood invigorating herbs can be divided into three broad categories of Blood harmonizing, Blood moving, and Blood stasis breaking medicinals. Recent pharmacological research has shown that many of these medicinals can significantly improve circulation of blood throughout the brain in individuals who have sustained single or multiple infarctions. Blood invigorating herbs are capable of reducing surface activity of erythrocytes, thrombocytes, and coagulation factor VIII as well as thrombocyte aggregation. Plasmin activity is also increased. Some herbs have a particular affinity for affecting the mind including Dan Shen, Chai Hu, Yuan Hu, Su Mu, Ru Xiang, Hong Hua, and Chuan Xiong. Included in Table 12.3 are some of the more common Blood invigorating herbs used in Chinese medicine with pharmacological indications.

15   Matsumoto, Kiiko. *Kiiko Matsumoto's Clinical Strategies: in the spirit of Master Nagano: vol. 2.* Mclean, VA: David Euler. 2014. Print.

16   Youn, Jun Koo. *The Practice of Sa-Am Acupuncture.* Los Angeles, CA: Book and People Pub. 2011. Print.

TABLE 12.3 Common Blood Invigorating Herbs in Chinese Medicine

Blood Harmonizing Herbs	Blood Moving Herbs	Blood Stasis Breaking Herbs
Chi Shao Yao	Chuan Xiong	E Zhu
Dan Shen	Da Huang	Meng Chong
Dang Gui	Hong Hua	San Leng
Hong Jing Tian	Hu Zhang	Shui Zhi
Ji Xue Teng	Niu Xi/Huai Niu Xi	Si Gua Luo (mild)
Mu Dan Pi	Jiang Huang	Tao Ren
Shan Zha	Lu Lu Tong	Tu Bie Chong
Sheng Di Huang	Mao Dong Qing	Xue Jie
	Mo Yao	
	Pu Huang	
	Ru Xiang	
	San Qi	
	Su Mu	
	Wu Ling Zhi	
	Yan Hu Suo	
	Yi Mu Cao	
	Yin Xing Ye	
	Yu Jin	
	Ze Lan	

Blood Harmonizing Herbs
Chi Shao (Red Peony Root)
Pharmacological research:

Blood: Prevents thrombosis formation, antisclerotic and antiplatelet action

Heart: Heart muscle protective function, decreases pulmonary artery pressure, dilates coronary artery, increases resistance to hypoxia

Central nervous system: Calming, analgesic and febrifugal action

Other: Antispasmotic on smooth musculature, antineoplastic, anti-inflammatory and antimycotic

Modern clinical uses: Coronary heart disease, cor pulmonale, acute cerebral thrombosis, acute icteric hepatitis, mycotic dermatitis, acute traumatic sepsis and dermatitis

Dan Shen (Red Sage Root)

Pharmacological research:

Blood: Improves microcirculation, antisclerotic, anticoagulant, and antiplatelet effect, used against thrombocyte aggregation

Heart: Increases heart function and coronary vessel circulation capacity

Central nervous system: CNS suppressant, sedative effect, negates caffeine

Other: Anti-inflammatory, antimycotic, anticarcinogenic, prevents liver damage, ischemic kidney damage, lung damage, antiulcerative, prevents endotoxin-induced shock, captures free radicals, estrogenic action, protects from bronchial asthma, calming effect

Modern clinical uses: Coronary heart disease, bacterial myocarditis in children, high blood viscosity, hemorrhoids, apoplexy, hepatitis, retinal vein thrombosis, whooping cough, nephritis, diabetes, hemorrhagic fever, malignant lymphomas, scleroderma

Dang Gui (Angelica Sinensis)

Pharmacological research:

Blood: Promotes hematopoesis (especially erythropoesis), antithrombic action, prevents thrombocyte aggregation, lowers blood lipid concentration, increases microcirculation and overall circulation by decreasing blood viscosity

Heart: Anti-ischemic, anti-arrhymic action, lowers blood pressure

Immune system: Increases cellular and humoral immune function

Other: Relaxing action, alleviates uterine smooth muscle pain, antibacterial, hepatoprotective, analgesic, anti-inflammatory

Modern clinical uses: Ischemic cerebral apoplexy, thrombophlebitis, cardiac arrythmias, infantile pneumonia, menstrual disorders, uterine prolapse, chronic pelvic inflammation, cor pulmonale, hepatitis, herpes zoster

Hong Jing Tian (Rhodiola Root)

Pharmacological research:

Blood: Blood pressure homeostatic, blood sugar homeostatic, blood lipid antioxidant

Heart: Strengthens heart contractility, reduces ischemic damage

Immune system: Anti-inflammatory, febrifugal, virostatic action

CNS: Strong adaptogen, reduces stress, relaxes

Other: Reduces radiation effects, contractile or relaxing effect on smooth muscle of the small intestine (dose dependent)

Modern clinical uses: Heart insufficiency in old age, reduced physical and memory capacity, anemia, tuberculosis, diabetes, hypotension, impaired mental activity

Ji Xue Teng (Millettia Root)

Pharmacological research:

Blood: Promotes hematopoesis (erythrocytes, thrombocytes, interleukin-2, hemoglobin), counteracts clotting, reduces blood lipid levels

Heart: Reduces oxygen consumption of heart muscles, increases heart rate, lowers blood pressure

Other: Increases phosphate metabolism of kidneys and uterus, calming/sedative effect, uterine stimulant

Modern clinical uses: Thrombocyte insufficiency, mammary gland hyperplasia

Mu Dan Pi (Tree Peony Bark)

Pharmacological research:

Heart: Lowers blood pressure, prevents arrhythmia and ischemia

Blood: Antisclerotic, prevents thrombosis and hemorrhaging in capillaries

Other: Spasmolytic effect in inflammation with inhibition of prostaglandin synthesis calming effect, febrifugal, diuretic, antibacterial, contraceptive, analgesic, sedative, antiseizure, antipyretic, immunostimulant

Modern clinical uses: Prevents bruising, urticaria, pruritis, fever due to infections (appendicitis, cholecystitis, nephritis, etc.), hypertension, allergic rhinitis, amenorrhea, dysmenorrhea

Shan Zha (Hawthorne Fruit)

Pharmacological research:

Blood: Significantly lowers blood pressure and blood lipids, vasodilator

Heart: Increases blood flow and blood quantity in cardiac muscle and protects from damaging effects of ischemia and hypoglycemia

Other: Antioxidative effect, strengthens immune system (T-lymphocytes), antibacterial

Modern clinical uses: Hyperlipidemia, hypertension, CHD, cardiac arrythmias, acute viral hepatitis, infectious colitis, bacterial enteritis, digestive disorders, kidney and renal pelvis inflammations

Sheng Di Huang (Rehmannia Root)

Pharmacological research:

Blood: Lowers blood sugar, stops bleeding, increases T-lymphocyte formation

Heart: Cardiotonic—strengthens contractility

Other: Increases plasma cAMP peak, anti-inflammatory, antibacterial, hepatoprotective, mild laxative and diuretic, increases resistance against lack of oxygen, alleviates radiation damage

Modern clinical usage: CHD, angina pectoris, myocarditis, hypertension, apoplexy, diabetes, anaphylactic shock, hemorrhages, hepatitis, neurodermatitis, measles, retinary phlebitis, otitis media, tonsillitis, externally for all types of ulcers, protects from free radicals

Blood Moving Herbs

Chuan Xiong (Ligusticum)

Pharmacological research:

Blood: Increases microcirculation, increases blood circulation in the kidneys and the brain, lowers brain edema incidences, inhibits thrombocyte aggregation and thrombus formation, anticoagulant

Heart: Dilates peripheral and coronary vessels, lowers blood pressure and vessel resistance, increases coronary blood volume, increases tolerance to hypoxia

Other: Antispasmotic on smooth musculature, nervous system calmative, antibacterial, aids in radiation damage and vitamin E insufficiency

Modern clinical uses: CHD, cardiac insufficiency, cardiac arrythmia, angina pectoris, sudden cardiac arrest, cor pulmonale, cerebral ischemia, brain edema, kidney failure, disseminate intravascular coagulation (DIC), thrombophlebitis, allergic shock, asthma, diabetes, stomach ulcers, dysmenorrhea, psoriasis

Da Huang (Chinese Rhubarb Root)

Pharmacological research:

Blood: Stops bleeding, lowers blood viscosity and blood lipids, increases microcirculation

Heart: Lowers blood pressure and increases force of contractions

Immune system: Anti-inflammatory, antiulcerative, antibacterial, antibiotic, virostatic, inhibits growth of certain cancer cells, antipyretic

Digestive system: Laxative, increases peristalsis, increases colonic water absorption, increases gastric acid, peptides, bile, and pancreatic enzyme secretions

Other: Hepatoprotective, diuretic, estrogenic, anti-aging

Modern clinical uses: Esophageal bleeding, stomach ulcers, stomach bleeding, chronic gastritis, acute pancreatitis, constipation, suppurative appendicitis, lipidemia, kidney failure, hemorrhages of the urinary bladder and other organs, infectious hemorrhagic fever, tonsillitis, parotitis, chronic prostatitis, insecticide poisoning, amenorrhea, cervical tumor

Hong Hua (Safflower)

Pharmacological research:

Blood: Antithrombotic, promotes maturation of T and B-lymphocytes, raises interleukin-2 production

Heart: Lowers blood pressure and blood lipids, increases heart muscle contraction force (small doses only, large doses decrease cardiac output)

Other: Anti-inflammatory, analgesic, calmative, uterine stimulant, CNS suppressant, preventative effect against drug-induced seizures, adaptogenic

Modern clinical uses: CHD, angina pectoris, arrythmias, ischemic and thrombotic apoplexy, cerebral atherosclerosis, thrombophlebitis, nasal polyps, sensorial hearing loss, menstrual disorders, trauma, hemorrhagic fever, duodenal ulcers, neurodermatitis, psoriasis, flat warts, solar dermatitis, erythema multiforme, lupus erythematosus, other dermatological disorders

Hu Zhang (Japanese Knotweed)

Pharmacological research:

Blood: Lowers blood pressure, blood sugar, and blood lipids, improves microcirculation, raises leukocyte and thrombocyte numbers, inhibits thrombocyte aggregation, hemostatic

Other: Antibacterial, virostatic, antitussive, antioxidative, inhibits tumor formation, relaxes digestive tract smooth musculature, hepatoprotective, cholagogue, antidiabetic, antineoplastic (inhibits RNA/DNA synthesis)

Modern clinical uses: Infantile pneumonia, acute viral hepatitis, jaundice, hyperlipidemia, leukopenia, digestive tract hemorrhages, cervical erosion, vaginal mycosis, toothache, stab wounds and burns

Jiang Huang (Turmeric)

Pharmacological research:

Blood: Lowers blood lipids and blood pressure, inhibits thrombocyte aggregation and atherosclerosis

Other: Hepatoprotective, anti-inflammatory, antibacterial, virostatic, anticancer, abortive, contraceptive, antioxidative, captures free radicals

Modern clinical uses: Dysmenorrhea, chest pain, hyperlipidemia, angina pectoris, inflammations, externally for herpes zoster and herpes simplex

Lu Lu Tong (Sweetgum Fruit)

Pharmacological research:

Antiallergenic, externally for antiparasitic actions, hepatoprotective, diuretic, antibiotic

Mao Dong Qing (Ilex Root)

Pharmacological research:

Blood: Prevents clotting (anticoagulant)

Heart: Dilates coronary arteries, increases blood flow to the heart

Other: Lowers blood pressure in the cerebral arteries, anti-inflammatory, antibacterial, antiasthmatic, antitussive, expectorant

Modern clinical uses: CHD, ishemic apoplexy, thrombophlebitis of superficial veins, retinal changes, prostatitis, atropic rhinitis, allergic rhinitis, hemorrhaging fever, wound infections, leprotic leg ulcers, apthae

Mo Yao (Myrrh Resin)

Pharmacological research:

Blood: Lowers blood cholesterol levels

Heart: Increases heart contraction force and tolerance toward hypoxia

Other: Stimulates respiratory center, antimycotic, antihyperlipidemic

Modern clinical uses: Heart pain, high cholesterol, spinal and mammary tuberculosis, menstrual disorders, hemorrhages, ulcers and trauma

Huai Niu Xi (Achyranthes Root)

Pharmacological research:

Blood: Lowers blood pressure, dilates vessels

Other: Promotes protein synthesis (wound healing), diuretic, anti-inflammatory, analgesic, antibacterial, abortive, dilates cervical canal to induce delivery

Modern clinical uses: Epistaxis, infantile pneumonia, painful urination, toothache, functional uterine bleeding, chyluria (galactosuria)

Pu Huang (Cattail Pollen)

Pharmacological research:

Blood: Hemostatic, lowers blood lipids and blood viscosity, protects endothelial cells of the blood vessels, regulates blood clotting, inhibits thrombocyte aggregation, fibrinolytic, increases clotting speed and microcirculation, prevents atherosclerosis

Heart: Improves cardiac capacity, tolerance toward hypoxia, protects heart from ischemic damage, lowers blood pressure

Other: Regulates immune function (cellular and humoral, dose dependent), excites uterine musculature, relaxes bronchial vessels, increases peristalsis, antihyperlipidemic, anti-inflammatory

Modern clinical uses: CHD, hyperlipidemia, ulcerative colitis, all types of hemorrhaging, weeping eczema, labor induction, leukorrhea, insufficient post-partum uterine involution, all kinds of menstrual disorders

Ru Xiang (Frankincense Resin)

Pharmacological research:

Blood: Increases blood clotting speed, lowers thrombocyte aggregation, increases erythrocyte elasticity

Other: Antibacterial, anti-inflammatory, analgesic

Modern clinical uses: Heart pain, intractable hiccups, appendicitis, traumas, rheumatic Bi-syndromes (arthritic conditions)

San Qi (Notoginseng)

Pharmacological research:

Blood: Promotes blood clotting and clotting speed, local vasoconstriction in trauma, if clotting is unnecessary it counteracts thrombocyte aggregation, lowers fibrin and increases fibrinolysis time, lowers blood lipid levels, increases erythrocyte and leukocyte count in peripheral vessels, dilates peripheral vessels and lowers blood pressure

Heart: Increases heart muscle contractions, blood volume, oxygen saturation, and microcirculation, lowers oxygen consumption and pulse rate, anti-arrythmic

Immune system / metabolism: Regulates blood sugar levels, promotes DNA synthesis of kidneys and testes, increases natural killer (NK) lymphocyte and macrophage activity

Other: Protects brain cells from ischemic damage, protects the body from shock, hepatoprotective, stimulates uterine muscles, virostatic, antimycotic, calmative, analgesic, protects from radiation and cancer, significantly increased lifespan of laboratory animals

Modern clinical uses: Angina pectoris, CHD, cardiac arrythmias, hyperlipidemia, hypertension, all types of apoplexy and cranial bleeding, internal and external traumas, all types of hemorrhaging, cancer, hepatitis, liver cirrhosis, acute nephritis, skin diseases, migraine

Su Mu (Sappen Wood)
Pharmacological research:

Blood / Heart: Increases heart contraction force, vasoconstrictive, promotes blood clotting

Other: Calmative, antimycotic, anti-inflammatory, anticarcinogenic (especially leukemia), CNS suppressant, antibiotic

Modern clinical uses: Tetanus, asthma, traumas, vitiligo

Notes: Moves Blood and stops bleeding

Wu Ling Zhi (Flying Squirrel Feces)
Pharmacological research:

Blood: Lowers blood viscosity, elevates erythrocyte sedimentation that is too slow, prevents thrombocyte aggregation, increases microcirculation

Heart: Lowers oxygen consumption of the heart

Other: Strong analgesic, immune regulating, antibacterial, antispasmodic

Modern clinical uses: All acute states of pain, angina pectoris, snake bites, duodenal and gastric ulcers, chronic bronchitis, delayed uterine involution after delivery

Yan Hu Suo (Corydalis Root)

Pharmacological research:

Blood: Lowers blood lipid levels, antiatherosclerotic, improves circulation

Heart: Protects heart from ischemic damage, lowers blood pressure, antiatherosclerotic

Other: Strong analgesic, local anesthetic, increases peristalsis, increases adrenal cortex secretion, reduces gastric secretions, muscle relaxant

Modern clinical uses: All types of pain and neuralgias, insomnia, hypertension, CHD, cardiac arrythmias, angina pectoris, myocardial infarction, gastritis, gastric and duodenal ulcers, acute pancreatitis, acute lower back pain, dysmenorrhea, local anesthetic

Yi Mu Cao (Chinese Motherwort)

Pharmacological research:

Blood: Lowers blood viscosity, reduces clotting and thrombocyte aggregation, also prevents thrombus formation, inhibits agglomeration of antibodies among each other

Heart: Increases circulation and microcirculation of the heart, cardiac muscle protective, lowers blood pressure

Other: Antiatherosclerotic, contraceptive, uterine stimulant, respiratory stimulant

Modern clinical uses: CHD, angina pectoris, cor pulmonale, ishemic apoplexy, hypertension, menstrual disorders, incomplete uterine involution, acute nephritic syndrome, chronic glomerular nephritis, ascites due to liver cirrhosis, diabetes, prostatitis and urinary stones

Yin Xing Ye (Ginkgo Leaf)

Pharmacological research:

Blood/Heart: Increases blood flow to brain tissue, lowers pulse rate and blood pressure, reduces plasma cholesterol, dilates blood vessels

Other: Spasmolytic effect on bronchi and smooth muscles, increases respiratory frequency, antibiotic, uterine stimulant

Modern clinical uses: CHD, angina pectoris, high cholesterol levels, chronic bronchitis, Parkinson's disease, senile dementia

Yu Jin (Curcumin)

Pharmacological research:

> Raises cAMP levels in organ tissues, inhibits lymphocyte maturation, antiatherosclerotic, antimycotic, hepatoprotective, antiarrythmic, increases gastric acid secretion, lowers stomach pH
>
> *Modern clinical uses*: Epilepsy, epistaxis, hepatyitis due to cholecystopathy, heart pain, hematuria, hyperhidrosis, psoriasis

Ze Lan (Bugleweed)

Pharmacological research:

> Inhibits clotting, fibrinogen, and thrombocyte aggregation, increases erythrocyte plasticity, cardiotonic
>
> *Modern clinical uses*: CHD, cor pulmonale, emphysema, chronic hepatitis, jaundice, parotitis, hemorrhoids, postpartum pain, mastitis, female infertility

Blood Stasis Breaking Herbs

E Zhu (Zedoria Root)

Pharmacological research:

> *Blood*: Reduces thrombocyte agglutination time, lowers blood viscosity, improves microcirculation, increases glutamate pyruvate transminase
>
> *Cancer*: Prevents formation of different types of cancer cells—sarcoma, lymphoma, etc.
>
> *Infections*: Wide range antibacterial
>
> *Other*: Contraceptive effect, increases femoral artery blood flow volume, stimulates gastric and intestinal smooth muscle
>
> *Modern clinical uses*: Cancers, CHD, tonsillitis and pneumonia in children, high blood lipid symptoms, stomach ulcers, skin ulcers, neurodermatitis

Meng Chong (Gadfly)

Pharmacological research:

> Dilates blood vessels, increases hypoxia tolerance, activates fibrinolytic system
>
> *Modern clinical uses*: Angina pectoris, cervical tumors, chronic hepatitis, bleeding internal hemorrhoids

San Leng (Burreed Tuber)

Pharmacological research:

Blood: Prolongs clotting time, lowers blood viscosity, reduces thrombocyte aggregation, reduces time and gravity of thrombus, increases blood flow and absorption rate of abdominal blood clots

Other: Antineoplastic, stimulates intestinal smooth muscle

Modern clinical uses: Post-apoplexy hemiplegia, CHD, chronic pelvic inflammatory disease, extrauterine pregnancy, cervical tumors, renal stones

Shui Zhi (Hirudo/Leech)

Pharmacological research:

Blood: Prolongs/prevents thrombocyte aggregation, lowers blood lipids, lowers blood viscosity, thrombus absorption, and flow speed

Heart: Increases Rb-86 assimilation of heart muscle, increases blood volume and microcirculation

Other: Abortive, antihyperlipidemic

Modern clinical uses: Ischemic and hemorrhagic apoplexy, cerebral thrombosis, angina pectoris, CHD, cor pulmonale, hyperlipidemia, thrombophlebitis, liver cirrhosis, polycythemia vera, eye diseases and edema due to kidney dysfunction

Si Gua Luo (Luffa)

Pharmacological research:

Antiasthmatic, anti-inflammatory, analgesic, calmative, antibacterial, cardiotonic, hepatoprotective, mild diuretic

Modern clinical uses: Acute mastitis, bronchial asthma, herpes zoster, chronic nephritis, anal fissures, penile induration, epilepsy, thyroid nodules, uterine prolapse

Tao Ren (Peach Kernel Seed)

Pharmacological research:

Blood: Increases blood flow in cerebral and peripheral vessels, antithrombotic, raises cAMP levels and lowers adenosine diphosphate (ADP) levels in thrombocytes

Other: Antitussive, antiphlogistic, antiallergic, antibacterial, spasmolytic, antioxidative, diuretic, uterine muscle stimulant, hepatoprotective, antiparasitic, delays aging

Modern clinical uses: Hepatitis, liver cirrhosis, CHD, cough, diabetes, skin diseases, trauma, menstrual pain, eye inflammations, chronic laryngitis, loss of voice, tonsillitis, epidemic hemorrhagic fever, acute kidney failure, chronic glomerulonephritis and pyelonephritis, gestational hypertension

Tu Bie Chong (Eupolyphaga/Wingless Cockroach)

Pharmacological research:

Blood: Inhibits blood clotting (antiplatelet), lowers blood lipids

Heart: Improves heart function and increases hypoxia tolerance

Other: Hepatoprotective action, absorbs free radicals, antagonizes cell mutations

Modern clinical uses: Concussion sequelae, CHD, tuberculosis (lung and bone), fractures, hypertension, chest pain following overexertion, acute lower back pain and sciatica, external hemorrhoids, melanoma, nasal cancer, chronic hepatitis

Xue Jie (Dragon's Blood)

Pharmacological research:

Blood: Lowers blood viscosity and thrombocyte aggregation

Other: Analgesic, anti-inflammatory, antibacterial, antimycotic, increases plasma cAMP levels and lowers plasma cGMP value, increases coronary artery blood volume

Modern clinical uses: Internal and external bleeding, traumas, chronic ulcers, coughing of blood, heavy menstrual bleeding, CHD, angina pectoris

Chapter 13

Mild Brain Injury/ Post-Concussion Syndrome

Mild traumatic brain injury (mTBI) or concussions is estimated to represent 75 percent of all TBIs that occur in the United States. This is approximately 1.1 million individuals annually, though there is a high likelihood of this number being significantly higher as those injured do not always report it or seek medical treatment.

Definition

An mTBI is diagnosed solely based on behavioral definitions. It is defined by the American College of Rehabilitation Medicine (ACRM) as a traumatically induced physiological disruption of brain function that includes at least one of the following:

- Loss of consciousness for a period of no more than approximately 30 minutes

- Any memory loss for events before or after the incident no greater than 24 hours

- Any alteration in mental state at the time of the incident (feeling dazed, confused, inability to answer simple questions, etc.)

- Normal brain structure as verified by CT or MRI

Abnormalities shown by imagery would demonstrate a more severe brain injury.

Causes

- Acceleration/deceleration movements

- Head strike

- Blasts/explosions

An mTBI is caused by transfer of kinetic energy into soft tissue, which can lead to chemical/metabolic changes in the brain or direct damage to physical structures such as brain cells. The most common form of damage is diffuse axonal injury. Axonal shearing can also occur in which axons become twisted and disconnected.

The most important chemical change that occurs is a massive release of the neurotransmitter glutamate. Very high levels of glutamate are toxic to the brain as they affect sodium/potassium balances that allow for proper neural signal transmission. ATP, the body's energy currency, also becomes compromised in a concussion by other chemical processes that starves the brain for energy. This may be further impacted by a general constriction of blood flow.

Symptoms

In cases of mTBI most symptoms resolve within a time of about two to four weeks, with only an estimated 10–15 percent of individuals experiencing chronic symptoms. Most symptoms can be categorized as either physical/somatic, cognitive, or behavioral/emotional, as laid out in Table 13.1.

TABLE 13.1 Symptoms Associated with Mild Traumatic Brain Injury

Physical/Somatic Symptoms	Cognitive Symptoms	Behavioral/Emotional Symptoms
Headache	Inattentiveness	Depression
Fatigue	Diminished concentration	Anxiety
Seizure	Poor memory	Agitation
Nausea	Impaired judgment	Irritability
Numbness	Slowed processing speed	Aggression
Poor sleep	Executive dysfunction	Impulsivity
Light/noise sensitivity		"Frontal release": disinhibition, emotional lability, social inappropriateness
Impaired hearing		
Blurred vision, convergence insufficiency		
Dizziness/loss of balance (BPPV, orthostatic hypertension)		
Neurologic abnormalities		

Chronic Traumatic Encephalopathy (CTE)

CTE is a rare, progressively degenerative condition of the central nervous system which typically follows repetitive brain trauma. This may be due to high-risk sports such as football or boxing. Here diffuse axonal injury causes a release of Tau proteins which are changed structurally by the metabolic breakdown of brain cells following trauma to create a chronic inflammatory state that causes a progressive degeneration of the central nervous system.

It has been theorized that cells infiltrated with Tau proteins may affect neighboring neurons, a process that continues to spread over time. Successive brain injuries appear to accelerate this process of spreading Tau proteins in susceptible individuals. Some athletes with repetitive concussive injuries develop amyotropic lateral sclerosis (ALS) in which the brain and spinal cord degenerate.

Differential Diagnosis

There can be many overlapping symptoms that can be the result of concussion, stress, anxiety, depression, or PTSD, as shown in Table 13.2.

TABLE 13.2 Symptom Comparisons and Similarities

	Concussion	Stress	Anxiety	Depression	PTSD
Headache	x	x	x	x	x
Drowsiness	x	x	x	x	x
Irritability	x	x	x	x	x
Depression	x	x	x	x	x
Poor memory	x	x	x	x	x
Attention/concentration	x	x	x	x	x
Fatigue	x	x	x	x	x
Poor sleep	x	x	x	x	x
Nausea	x	x	x	x	x
Worry	x	x	x		x
Dizziness/loss of balance	x		x		
Impaired hearing	x				x
Blurred vision	x				

Chinese Medical Perspective
Relevant Chinese Disease Categories

Tou Tong (head pain), Tou Xuan (dizziness), Jian Wang (forgetfulness), Yu Zheng (depression), Nan Si (difficulty thinking), Shen Si Huang Hu (spirit abstraction), You (anxiety)

Chinese Medical Etiology

External injury to the head results in severing of the channels and vessels in the local region(s). Extravasated blood becomes static, which may obstruct the orifices of the head, resulting in headache, dizziness, unclear thinking and speech, etc. Static Blood also impedes the free flow of Qi, creating symptoms of Qi stagnation. If Qi stagnation becomes too excessive it may lead to ascendant Yang. Qi stagnation may also lead to Spleen deficiency, which can then develop into Heart Blood deficiency. Static Blood may also block essence from the Kidney from filling the sea of marrow (brain).

Pattern Differentiation
Blood Stasis Obstructing the Brain Orifices

Primary symptoms: History of acute head trauma, unclear thinking, cloudiness and haziness of the spirit, unclear speech, headache

Secondary symptoms: Vexation, agitation, restlessness, dizziness, dark facial complexion

Tongue: Dark, purple

Pulse: Wiry (bowstring) choppy or fine choppy

Treatment principles: Free the movement of the orifices and quicken the Blood, arouse the spirit and open the orifices

Acupuncture treatment: GB-20, LI-4, SP-6, GV-16, GV-20, Si Shen Cong

Acupuncture modifications: Insomnia, impaired memory, and unclear speech + GV-24, GB-13
Vexation, agitation, restlessness + KI-1, LR-1
Severe Blood stasis + BL-17

Herbal treatment:
Tong Qiao Huo Xue Tang Jia Wei (Free the Flow of the Orifices and Quicken the Blood Decoction Plus Modifications)
[Chuan Xiong 15g, Bai Zhi 15g, Tao Ren 15g, Di Long 15g, Hong Hua 12g, Chi Shao 9g, Wu Ling Zhi 9g, Man Jing Zi 9g, Sheng Jiang 3 slices, Da Zao 7pc]

Herbal modifications: Insomnia + Yuan Zhi, Suan Zao Ren
Severe headache, unclear thinking and speech + Quan Xie 3g, Wu Gong 3g, Tu Bie Chong 3g
Enduring disease damaging the righteous Qi + Hiuang Qi 15g, Dang Gui 9g

Qi and Blood Stasis

Primary symptoms: Emotional lability, torpor of mind, emotional depression, scanty or no speech, difficult or slow thinking, decreased memory, piercing headache following head trauma

Secondary symptoms: Chest or rib-side distension

Tongue: Dark red with possible macules or spots, white or yellow coat

Pulse: Wiry (bowstring), choppy

Treatment principles: Harmonize the Liver, Move Qi, Quicken the Blood

Acupuncture treatment: GB-20, LR-3, PC-5, GV-16, GV-20, Si Shen Cong

Acupuncture modifications:
Bitter taste in mouth, vexation, agitation, emotional lability + BL-18, BL-47
Pronounced Spleen deficiency with fatigue and weakness + ST-36
Marked cold hands and feet + CV-4 (moxa)
Insomnia, impaired memory, and unclear speech + GV-24, GB-13

Herbal treatment:
Xiao Yao San Jia Wei (Augmented Rambling Powder)
[Pei Lan 15g, Chai Hu 9g, Dang Gui 9g, Chi Shao 9g, Bai Zhu 9g, Fu Ling 9g, Hong Hua 9g, Tao Ren 9g, Pao Jiang 9g, Bo He 6g, Gan Cao 6g]

Modifications:
Severe headache + Quan Xie 6g, Jiang Can 6g
Dizziness, heavy-headedness + Yu Jin 9g, Shi Chang Pu 9g
Spleen deficiency pronounced with fatigue and weakness + Huang Qi 15g, Dang Shen 9g
Yin and Blood deficiency pronounced + Shu Di 12g, He Shou Wu 12g
Cold hands and feet + Gui Zhi 9g

Liver Yang Rising

Primary symptoms: Emotional impetuosity and rashness, vexation, agitation, restlessness, easily angered and irritable, pounding headache

Secondary symptoms: Possible vomiting of white foam or bile following a traumatic head injury

Tongue: Dark red, yellow coat

Pulse: Wiry (bowstring), rapid

Treatment principles: Harmonize the Liver and subdue Yang, quicken the Blood and transform stasis

Acupuncture treatment: GB-20, LR-3, KI-1, GV-16, GV-20, Si Shen Cong

Acupuncture modifications:
Vexation, agitation, restlessness + BL-18, BL-47
Nausea, vomiting, constipation + PC-6, TW-6
Insomnia, impaired memory, and unclear speech + GV-24, GB-13

Herbal treatment:
Ling Jiao Gou Teng Tang Jia Jian (Antelope Horn and Uncaria Decoction Plus Modifications)
[Gou Teng 30g, Sheng Di 30g, Bai Shao 30g, Sang Ye 30g, Ju Hua 15g, Fu Shen 15g, Zhu Ru 12g, Tao Ren 9g, Hong Hua 9g, Zhe Bei Mu 9g, Shan Yang Jiao 9g, Dan Shen 9g, Gan Cao 6g]

Herbal modifications:
Vexation, agitation, restlessness + Tie Lou 12g, Long Gu 12g, Mui Li 12g
Epileptiform symptoms + Quan Xie 6g, Jiang Can 6g, Di Long 9g, Tian Ma 9g
Severe headache + Bai Zhi 12g, Yu Jing 12g, Xia Ku Cao 9g
Mental depression, anger without reason, frequent worry + Dao Zao 15g, Fu Xiao Mai 15g, He Huan Pi 15g, Shi Chang Pu 15g, Bo He 9g

Heart Blood and Spleen Qi Deficiencies with Liver Qi Stagnation

Primary symptoms: Fatigue, forgetfulness, heart palpitations, worry and anxiety, depression, irritability

Secondary symptoms: Possible headache or dizziness, insomnia, pale or sallow facial complexion, pale lips and fingernails, cold hands and feet, possible loose stools

Tongue: Pale, slightly dark, swollen with possible center crack, thin coat

Pulse: Wiry (bowstring), fine, moderate

Treatment principles: Nourish the Heart and fortify the Spleen, rectify Qi and resolve stagnation

Acupuncture treatment: GB-20, LR-3, HT-7, SP-6, GV-20

Acupuncture modifications:
Severe impaired memory and unclear speech + Si Shen Cong
Blood stasis signs + BL-17, BL-18
Depressive heat in Stomach and Heart + PC-7, ST-44
Epileptiform symptoms + LI-4, GV-14

Herbal treatment:
Gui Pi Tang Jia Wei (Restore the Spleen Decoction Plus Modifications)
[Huang Qi 15g, Suan Zao Ren 12g, Dang Shen 9g, Dang Gui 9g, Long Yan

Rou 9g, Bai Zhu 9g, Fu Ling 9g, Yi Zhi Ren 9g, Yuan Zhi 9g, Shi Chang Pu 6g, Mu Xiang 6g, Gan Cao 6g, Sheng Jiang 2 slices, Da Zao 3–5pc]

Modifications:
Blood stasis signs + Tao Ren 9g, Hong Hua 9g, Dan Shen 9g
Liver stagnation pronounced + Chai Hu 9g
Depressive heat in the Stomach + Huang Lian 3–6g
Depressive heat in the Liver + Zhi Zi 9g, Mu Dan Pi 9g

Kidney Qi Debility and Deficiency

Primary symptoms: History of traumatic head injury, essence spirit listlessness, slow and difficult thinking, decreased memory, decreased visual acuity

Secondary symptoms: Dizziness, vertigo, tinnitus, deafness, low back and lower leg soreness and weakness

Tongue: Pale, thin coat

Pulse: Fine, weak

Treatment principles: Supplement the Kidneys, fortify the brain, boost the marrow and essence

Acupuncture treatment: KI-3, GB-39, BL-23, BL-52, GV-16, GV-20

Acupuncture modifications:
Steaming bone and tidal fever, red tongue, rapid pulse + GV-14, HT-6
Heart palpitations, fright/fear, vexation, agitation, restlessness + PC-7
Severely impaired memory and unclear speech + Si Shen Cong
Epileptiform symptoms + LR-3, LI-4, GV-14

Herbal treatment:
Zi Yin Da Bu Wan (Great Tonify the Yin Pill)
[Shu Di 60g, Nui Xi 45g, Shan Yao 45g, Shan Zhu Yu 30g, Du Zhong 30g, Fu Ling 30g, Ba Ji Tian 30g, Wu Wei Zi 30g, Xiao Hui Xiang 30g, Rou Cong Rong 30g, Yuan Zhi 30g, Shi Chang Pu 20g, Gou Qi Zi 20g]

Modifications:
Steaming bone and tidal fever, red tongue, rapid pulse + Di Gu Pi 9g, Zhi Mu 9g, Huang Bai 9g
Heart palpitations, fright/fear, vexation, agitation, restlessness + Suan Zao Ren 12g, Long Gu 12g, Mu Li 12g
Piercing headache due to stagnant Blood + Hong Hua 9g, Tao Ren 9g, Jiang Can 9g, Quan Xie 6g

Empirical Formulas for Post-Concussion Syndrome

Xiao Yi Tang (Disperse Sequelae Decoction)

> ***Functions***: Settles the Heart and quiets the spirit, upbears the pure while downbearing the turbid, quickens the Blood and transforms stasis, rectifies the Qi and courses the Liver, supplements the Kidneys and boosts the Spleen
> [Dang Shen 15–30g, Bai Shao 15g, Gou Qi Zi 15g, Ci Shi 15g, Long Chi 15g, Da Fu Pi 12g, Sang Bai Pi 12g, Tao Ren 12g, Chi Shao 9g, Jing Jie 6g, Chai Hu 6g, Xiang Fu 6g, Hu Po 3g, Zhu Sha 3g]

San Bian Di Huang Tang (Scatter the Inclined Rehmannia Decoction)

> ***Functions***: Quickens the Blood and transforms stasis, courses the Liver and boosts the Spleen, enriches the Kidneys and boosts essence
> [Shu Di 15–30g, Bai Shao 15–30g, Shan Zhu Yu 10–30g, Chuan Xiong 15–20g, Shan Yao 10–15g, Bai Zhi 6–12g, Xiang Fu 6–12g, Bai Jie Zi 6–12g, Mu Dan Pi 6–12g, Gan Cao 3–10g]

> ***Modifications***:
> Severe headache + Hong Hua, Dan Shen, Chi Shao
> Dizziness + Tian Ma 9g, Gou Teng 9g, Ju Hua 9g
> Insomnia + Suan Zao Ren 15, He Huan Pi 9g, Fu Shen 9g, Hu Po 3g
> Concomitant Qi and Blood deficiency + Tai Zi Ren 15g, Huang Qi 15g, Dang Gui 9g
> Severe Liver–Kidney deficiency + Gou Qi Zi 9g, Hu Tao Ren 9g, Du Zhong 9g, Lu Jiao Jiao 9g, Gui Ban Jiao 9g

Chapter 14

Treatment of Acute Brain Injury with Chinese Medicine

Due to the acute stage of a brain injury being a critical period, Chinese medical physicians will usually suggest combined management with modern Western medical methods if they are involved in treatment during this acute stage. Most practitioners will not see these cases, and many of the traditional formulas contain either substances which contain toxicity or are derived from endangered animal sources. For this reason, caution should be taken in applying these methods. While herbal substitutes can be made with similar actions, often these effects will be to a significantly lessened degree, requiring higher doses. However, for the sake of completeness of this text, it would be remiss not to include these treatment approaches.

Blockage of Qi

Primary symptoms: Unresponsiveness, severe confusion, agitation, delirium, restlessness, flushed face, twitching, and increased breath rate

Secondary symptoms: Fever, flushed faces, agitation

Tongue: Pale, flaccid

Pulse: Rapid, weak

Treatment principles: Remove the pathogenic factors blocking the aperture of the Heart

Acupuncture treatment: GV-20, GV-26, KI-1, LU-11, HT-9, SI-1, PC-9, LI-1, LR-3, ST-40, PC-8

Herbal treatment:

An Gong Niu Huang Wan (Calm the Palace Pill with Cattle Gallstone)
[Niu Huang 30g, She Xiang 7.5g, Xi Jiao 30g, Huang Lian 30g, Zhi Zi 30g, Bing Pian 7.5g, Yu Jin 30g, Zhu Sha 30g, Zhen Zhu 15g, Xiong Huang 30g, Jin Bo (Gold Foil)]

Note: Zhu Sha and Xiong Huang are potentially toxic heavy metals and Xi Jiao and She Xiang are derived from endangered animals. Today they are generally substituted with other substances with similar actions.

Zi Xue Dan (Purple Snow Pill)
[Xi Jiao 15g, Shi Gao 150g, Han Shui Shi 150g, Hua Shi 150g, Xuan Shen 50g, Sheng Ma 50g, She Xiang 0.15g, Mu Xiang 15g, Ding Xiang 3g, Chen Xiang 15g, Ling Yang Jiao 15g, Zhu Sha 9g, Ci Shi 150g, Po Xiao 500g, Xiao Shi 9.6g, Huang Jin 300g, Zhi Gan Cao 24g]

Note: Zhu Sha is a potentially toxic heavy metal and Ling Yang Jiao, Xi Jiao, and She Xiang are derived from endangered animals. Today they are generally substituted with other substances with similar actions.

Zhi Bao Dan (Greatest Treasure Special Pill)
[She Xiang 0.3g, Bing Pian 0.3g, An Xi Xiang 45g, Xi Jiao 30g, Niu Huang 0.3g, Dai Mao 30g, Jin Bo (Gold Foil), Yin Bo (Silver Foil), Zhu Sha 30g, Hu Po 30g, Xiong Huang 30g]

Note: Zhu Sha and Xiong Huang are potentially toxic heavy metals and Xi Jiao and She Xiang are derived from endangered animals. Today they are generally substituted with other substances with similar actions.

Notes

These medications are also used for coma or severe agitation due to other etiologies such as stroke, high fever, meningitis, or encephalitis. An Gong Niu Huang Wan is the pill most commonly prescribed. Its extracts for intravenous injection, named Xing Nao Jing, are available in China. Several preliminary controlled studies have shown the effectiveness of the intravenous application of Xing Nao Jing to treat the comatose state.

One of the major contents of An Gong Niu Huang Wan, Niu Huang (Bos Calculus), is bovine gallbladder, a mixture of bilirubin metabolites and endogenous bile acids. After traumatic brain injury and stroke, massive bleeding can produce significant iron-mediated oxidative stress, programmed cell death (apoptosis), and neurodegeneration. Bilirubin metabolites were found to be potent endogenous antioxidants with neuroprotective effects. One of the major endogenous bile acids, tauroursodeoxycholic acid, was found to have the ability to modulate cell death by interrupting classic pathways of apoptosis and has wide-ranging neuroprotective effects after brain injury. However, because this formulation contains small amounts of arsine and mercury, the patient should be closely monitored and prolonged use of An Gong Niu Huang Wan is not recommended.

Qi Exhaustion

Qi exhaustion by severe traumatic brain injury is a very serious and critical condition.

Primary symptoms: Deep coma with unresponsiveness, loss of jaw control with spontaneous mouth opening, heavy perspiration, loss of bladder control, and distal limb cooling

Tongue: White coat

Pulse: Weak

Treatment principles: Consolidation of vital energy

Acupuncture treatment: CV-4, CV-6, CV-8 (moxa on all)

Herbal treatment:
Shen Fu Tang + San Qi Powder (Ginseng and Prepared Aconite Decoction)
[Ren Shen 9g, Pao Fu Zi 6g, San Qi 3-9g]

Chapter 15

Treatment of Chronic Brain Injury with Chinese Medicine

Subacute TBI Management with Oriental Medicine

Following the acute stages of a brain injury a number of residual symptoms and symptom patterns may present and persist. Many clinical presentations have similarities to cases of post-stroke sequelae. For this reason, the treatment approaches as well tend to be similar. In this chapter emphasis is placed on those patterns along with Chinese medical treatment approaches, pharmacological actions of formulas, and notes of relevant research as etiology, pathogenesis, and additional recommendations are explored specifically in other chapters of this text.

Stasis of Blood

Primary symptoms: Persistent sharp/stabbing headache usually in a fixed location, cognitive deficiency

Tongue: Purple or purple spots on tongue body

Pulse: Wiry (bowstring), choppy

Treatment principles: Remove stasis, move Qi and Blood, relieve pain, nourish the brain

Acupuncture treatment: SP-10, BL-17, LR-3, GV-20, GV-16

Herbal treatment:
Xue Fu Zhu Yu Tang (Drive Out Stasis in the Mansion of Blood Decoction)

[Tao Ren 12g, Hong Hua 9g, Di Huang 9g, Dang Gui 9g, Chi Shao 6g, Chuan Xiong 4.5g, Chai Hu 3g, Zhi Qiao 6g, Jie Geng 4.5g, Chuan Nui Xi 9g, Gan Cao 6g]

Pharmacological effects: Antiplatelet, anticoagulant, reduced blood pressure, regulatory effect on blood vessels (vasoconstriction or vasodilation), antihyperlipidemic

Shu Jing Huo Xie Tang (Relax the Channels and Invigorate the Blood Decoction) [Dang Gui 3.6g, Bai Shao 4.5g, Di Huang 3g, Tao Ren 3g, Fu Ling 2.1g, Cang Zhu 3g, Chen Pi 3g, Qiang Huo 1.8g, Bai Zhi 1.8g, Wei Ling Xian 3g, Fang Ji 1.8g, Fang Feng 1.8g, Long Dan Cao 1.8g, Chuan Xiong 3g, Gan Cao 1.2g]

Pharmacological effects: Analgesic, anti-inflammatory

Note: Recent research has confirmed the beneficial effects of these groups of Chinese medicines on neural regeneration. It was reported that after the extracts of Shu Jing Huo Xie Tang were added in a culture medium of neural cells, the neurite outgrowth induced by nerve growth factor (NGF) increased approximately 30-fold compared to NGF alone.[1]

Deficiency of Qi and Stagnancy of Blood

Primary symptoms: Fatigue, dull headache worse with fatigue, tired appearance, low voice

Secondary symptoms: Lassitude, lack of strength, anorexia, palpitations, shortness of breath, aversion to cold, cool limbs

Tongue: Thin white coat

Pulse: Thready, weak

Treatment approaches: Boost Qi, move Blood, stop pain, nourish the brain

Acupuncture treatment: ST-36, SP-6, LI-10, CV-4, CV-6, GV-16, GV-20

Herbal treatment:
Bu Yang Huan Wu Tang (Tonify the Yang to Restore Five Decoction)
[Huang Qi 100g, Dang Gui Wei 6g, Chuan Xiong 3g, Chi Shao 4.5g, Hong Hua 3g, Tao Ren 3g, Di Long 3g]

Pharmacological effects: Brain blood vessel dilation and increased blood perfusion to brain, antiplatelet, anticoagulant, thrombolytic, antihyperlipidemic
Tao Hong Si Wu Tang (Four Substance Decoction with Safflower and Peach Pit)

---

1   Shinichiro Takaguchi, Tsutomu Nohno, Yoshio Kano, *et al*. Chinese medicine induces neurite outgrowth in PC12 mutant cells incapable of differentiation. *American Journal of Chinese Medicine*. 2002; 30: 287.

[Shu Di Huang 15g, Dang Gui 12g, Bai Shao 10g, Chuan Xiong 8g, Tao Ren 6g, Hong Hua 4g]

Pharmacological effects: Dilates coronary arteries and increases blood perfusion to cardiac muscle, antihyperlipidemic (total cholesterol and triglycerides), anti-inflammatory

Notes: Most TBI cases with hypopituitarism fall into this pattern. Bu Yang Huan Wu Tang has been reported to show benefits on disturbances of the hypothalamus–pituitary–thyroid axis after brain ischemic injury.[2] Animal studies have found that Bu Yang Huan Wu Tang may protect brain neurons from apoptosis after cerebral ischemia. It has been postulated that the mechanism for this action could be attributed to its effects on the improvement of cerebral energy metabolism, regulation of nitric oxide synthesis, and antagonism of toxic excitatory amino acids.[3] The Tao Hong Si Wu Tang Decoction is effective in hydroxyl radical scavenging and is effective in inhibiting lipid peroxidation.[4]

Kidney Yin Deficiency

Primary symptoms: Constant dull headache with a feeling of emptiness often worsening with exercise

Secondary symptoms: Lassitude, debility, aching, weakness of the lower back and legs, forgetfulness, decreased intelligence, dizziness, tinnitus, dry mouth, flushed cheeks, and a hot sensation in the palms and soles

Tongue: Red, scanty, or no coat

Pulse: Deep, thready, and weak

Treatment principles: Nourish Kidney Yin, boost Qi, reduce deficiency fire, stop pain, nourish the brain

Acupuncture treatment: KI-3, KI-6, SP-6, BL-23, GV-20, GV-16

Herbal treatment:
Liu Wei Di Huang Wan (Six-Ingredient Pill with Rehmannia)

---

2   Mu, Q., Liu, P., Hu, X., Gao, H., Zheng, X., and Huang, H. Neuroprotective effects of Buyang Huanwu Decoction on cerebral ischemia-induced neuronal damage. *Neural Regeneration Research*. 2014; 9(17): 1621–1627. doi:10.4103/1673-5374.141791

3   Sun, K., Fan, J., and Han, J. Ameliorating effects of traditional Chinese medicine preparation, Chinese materia medica and active compounds on ischemia/reperfusion-induced cerebral microcirculatory disturbances and neuron damage. *Acta Pharmaceutica Sinica B*. 2015; 5(1): 8–24. doi:10.1016/j.apsb.2014.11.002

4   Hsieh, M-T., Cheng, S-J., Lin, L-W., Wang, W-H., and Wu, C-R. The ameliorating effects of acute and chronic administration of Liuwei Dihuang Wang on learning performance in rodents. *Biological and Pharmaceutical Bulletin*. 2003 Feb; 26(2): 156–161. https://doi.org/10.1248/bpb.26.156

[Shu Di Huang 24g, Shan Zhu Yu 12g, Shan Yao 12g, Ze Xie 9g, Mu Dan Pi 9g, Fu Ling 9g]

Pharmacological effects: Lowered plasma cholesterol and triglyceride levels, lowered plasma glucose levels, immunostimulant (increased white blood cell count and activity), adaptogenic, hepatoprotective, nephroprotective, antiarrhythmic, hypotensive, increased sperm count, increased weight of sex organs

Modifications: With Liver Yang Rising + Zhen Gan Xi Feng Wan
[Niu Xi 30g, Zhe Shi 30g, Long Gu 15g, Mu Li 15g, Gui Ban 15g, Xuan Shen 15g, Tian Dong 15g, Bai Shao 15g, Yin Chen Hao 6g, Chuan Lian Zi 6g, Mai Ya 6g, Gan Cao 4.5g]

Note: Animal studies have shown Liu Wei Di Huang Wan to possess memory-enhancing properties and anti-amnesia effects.[5] It was suggested that the formula corrects the abnormal expressions of hippocampal genes in dementia animals.[6] Traditionally, Kidney tonic Chinese medications containing Liu Wei Di Huang Wan are used widely for general health condition improvement. These medications are able to improve immune function by regulating the ratio of T and B cells and control over-expression of cytokine genes from activated mononuclear cells.[7]

Kidney Yang Deficiency

Primary symptoms: Constant dull headache with a feeling of emptiness often worsening with exercise

Secondary symptoms: Lassitude, debility, aching, weakness of the lower back and legs, forgetfulness, decreased intelligence, impotence, aversion to cold, cold limbs, nocturia, and pale complexion

Tongue: Pale, thick white coat

Pulse: Deep, thready, and weak

Treatment principles: Nourish Kidney Yin, boost Qi, reduce deficiency fire, stop pain, nourish the brain

Acupuncture treatment: KI-3, KI-7, SP-6, BL-23, GV-4, GV-20, GV-16

5   Hsieh, M-T., Cheng, S-J., Lin, L-W., Wang, W-H., and Wu, C-R. The ameliorating effects of acute and chronic administration of Liuwei Dihuang Wang on learning performance in rodents. *Biological and Pharmaceutical Bulletin.* 2003 Feb; 26(2): 156–161. https://doi.org/10.1248/bpb.26.156

6   Zhang, M-H., Ji-ping Liu, J-P., Liang Feng, L., *et al.* Neuroprotective effect of Liuwei Dihuang Decoction on cognition deficits of diabetic encephalopathy in streptozotocin-induced diabetic rat. *Journal of Ethnopharmacology.* 2013; 150(1): 371–381. http://dx.doi.org/10.1016/j.jep.2013.09.003

7   Yang, S., Zhang, Y.X., and Lu, X.D. [Study on immunomodulating mechanism of the active fraction of Liuwei Dihuang Decoction]. *Zhongguo Zhong Xi Yi Jie He Za Zhi.* 2001 Feb; 21(2): 119–122. Translated from Chinese.

Herbal treatment:
You Gui Wan (Restore the Right [Kidney] Pill)
[Rou Gui 6–12g, Fu Zi 16–18g, Shu Di Huang 24g, Shan Zhu Yu 9g, Shan Yao 12g, Gou Qi Zi 12g, Lu Jiao Jiao 12g, Tu Si Zi 12g, Du Zhong 12g, Dang Gui 9g]

Pharmacological effects: Immunostimulant (macrophage), adaptogenic, improved cognition/memory, antiplatelet, hepatoprotective

Jin Gui Shen Qi Wan (Kidney Qi Pill from The Golden Cabinet)
[Shu Di Huang 6g, Shan Zhu Yu 6g, Shan Yao 6g, Ze Xie 6g, Mu Dan Pi 6g, Fu Ling 6g, Fu Zi 9g, Rou Gui 3g, Chuan Niu Xi 6g, Che Qian Zi 6g]

Pharmacological effects: Antiaging, immunostimulant (lymphocytes), endocrine stimulant (gland weight), hypoglycemic, increased sperm count and motility

Liver Blood Deficiency with Liver Yang Rising

Primary symptoms: Headache characterized by cramping pain in the temple and vertex worse with anger, tremors

Secondary symptoms: Faintness, giddiness, dizziness, bitterness in the mouth, decreased self-control, irritability, restlessness and insomnia, twisting of the body, and localized or generalized convulsions

Tongue: Thin yellow coat

Pulse: Wiry (bowstring), rapid

Treatment principles: Subdue Liver heat, calm internal wind, stop pain, nourish the brain

Acupuncture treatment: LR-2, LR-3, LR-8, GB-20, GV-16, GV-20

Herbal treatment:
Tian Ma Gou Teng Yin (Gastrodia and Uncaria Decoction)
[Tian Ma 9g, Gou Teng 9g, Zhi Zi 12g, Huang Qin 9g, Shi Jue Ming 9g, Yi Mu Cao 18g, Chuan Niu Xi 9g, Du Zhong 12g, Sang Ji Sheng 9g, Shou Wu Teng 9g, Fu Shen 9g]

Pharmacological effects: Antihypertensive, regulatory effect

Dan Zhi Xiao Yao San (Augmented Rambling Powder)
[Chai Hu 9g, Dang Gui 9g, Bai Shao 9g, Bai Zhu 9g, Fu Ling 9g, Zhi Gan Cao 4.5g, Mu Dan Pi 9g, Zhi Zi 9g]

Pharmacological effects: Anxiolytic (neurosteroid synthesis → GABA(A)/benzodiazepine receptor stimulation)

Qi Deficiency

Primary symptoms: Dull headache worse with fatigue, lassitude

Secondary symptoms: Lack of strength, anorexia, palpitations, shortness of breath

Tongue: Thin white coat

Pulse: Thready, weak

Treatment principles: Boost Qi, nourish the Spleen and Stomach, stop pain, nourish the brain

Acupuncture treatment: ST-36, SP-6, BL-20, BL-21, LI-4, LI-10, GV-16, GV-20

Herbal treatment: Bu Zhong Yi Qi Tang (Supplement the Center and Boost the Qi Decoction)
[Huang Qi 9g, Ren Shen 12g, Bai Zhu 9g, Zhi Gan Cao 9g, Dang Gui 18g, Chen Pi 9g, Chai Hu 12g, Sheng Ma 9g]

Pharmacological effects: Gastrointestinal regulation (peristalsis), gastric acid production/release increase (large dose only), adaptogenic, antiaging (monoamine levels in brain), immunostimulant (T-lymphocyte, IFN, and IL-2 count), NK cell and macrophage activity, antiallergic, anticancer, radioprotective, antibiotic, antiviral, antidepressive, antinociceptive

Blood Deficiency

Primary symptoms: Headache, dizziness, palpitations, insomnia

Secondary symptoms: Dreamful sleep, blurred vision, numbness in the limbs

Tongue: Pale

Pulse: Thready

Treatment principles: Nourish Blood, stop pain, nourish the brain

Acupuncture treatment: SP-10, LR-8, BL-17, BL-18, GV-16, GV-20

Herbal treatment: Si Wu Tang (Four Substance Decoction)
[Shu Di Huang 12g, Dang Gui 9–12g, Bai Shao 9–12g, Chuan Xiong 6–9g]

Pharmacological effects: Hematopoietic, antiplatelet, radioprotective, memory/cognitive increases, antioxidant, antiaging, increased diastolic and mean blood pressure, antipruritic, anti-inflammatory, antitumor (preventative of endometrial carcinogenesis)

Other Formulas Showing Effectiveness in the Post-Acute Stage of Brain Injury

Kang Nao Shuai Dan (Anti-cerebral Fatigue Capsule)
[Ren Shen, He Shou Wu, Dan Shen, Fu Ling, Ju Hua, Long Gu, Shi Chang Pu, Yuan Zhi]

Nao Shang Ning (Brain Concussion Treatment)
[Ren Shen, Huang Qi, Lu Rong, Chuan Xiong, Tao Ren, Ce Bai Ye, Ju Hua, Chi Shao]

Dian Kuang Meng Xing Teng (From the Bad Dream of Psychosis Awakening Decoction)

Clinical signs: Typical indications are abnormal states of mind such as constant crying, laughing, singing, and swearing no matter who is present; dream-like confusion, aggression such as throwing of objects, etc.

Additional symptoms: Insomnia, lack of appetite, dark complexion

Tongue: Dark or purple tongue with protruding sublingual veins

Pulse: Deep, rough

Action: Dispels Blood stasis, moves stagnated Liver Qi, and transforms phlegm

[Tao Ren 32g, Chai Hu 12g, Xiang Fu 8g, Mu Tong 12g, Chi Shao 12g, Ban Xia 8g, Da Fu Pi 8g, Qing Pi 8g, Chen Pi 12g, Sang Bai Pi 12g, Su Zi 16g, Gan Cao 20g]

This formula is effective for cases of manic depressive psychosis with Blood stasis and Qi stagnation.

Modifications: Profuse phlegm + Wen Dan Tang (Gallbladder Warming Decoction)

Chapter 16

Headache/Migraine

According to the International Headache Society, a post-traumatic headache is defined as one which onsets within seven days of the injury or returning to a conscious state following TBI. It may spontaneously resolve over the next six months or it may become chronic. Fortunately, headaches often respond quite well to Chinese medical approaches. The ability to determine an effective treatment strategy based on proper pattern differentiation aids this effectiveness.

Post-traumatic headache diagnosis is more prevalent in cases of mild TBI (95% reporting pain) compared to moderate-to-severe TBI (22% reporting pain). Nearly one/third of soldiers returning from deployment who sustained a concussion met criteria for post-traumatic headache. Approximately 40–50 percent of patients with TBI report headache at 3, 6, and 12 months. A chronic headache is defined as one which occurs at least 15 days per month for at least three months. This must also not be linked to any type of medication overuse or withdrawal.

Looking at the neurological structure of the head and neck region, there are multiple peripheral receptors that may be affected. These receptors are located at the end of nerves that begin near the spinal cord and communicate with specific pain centers of the brain. This is termed peripheral nociception. The afferent nerves possibly involved in post-traumatic headache include:

- Cranial Nerve V (trigeminal)
- Cranial Nerve IX (glossopharyngeal)
- Cranial Nerve X (vagus)
- Greater Occipital Nerve (C2 root origin)
- Lesser Occipital Nerve (C3 root origin)

In assessing headaches, it is important to distinguish between a primary headache with no specific cause and secondary headaches which may have an identifiable cause.

Diagnostic Testing

- CBC (complete blood count)
- Chem screen
- ESR (erythrocyte sedimentation rate)
- Glucose
- Urinalysis
- CSF (cerebral spinal fluid) collection
- EENT
- X-ray
- MRI
- CT scan

Signs and Symptoms

- Determine frequency, duration, character, location, severity
- Malocclusion of teeth
- Palpate neck for stiffness/tightness
- Palpate head, mastoid processes, occiput
- Jaundice, herpes lesions on face
- Ophthalmoscopic, press on eyeballs

History Taking

- OPQRST
  - Rapidity of onset
  - Times of day
  - Location: unilateral not as commonly benign
  - Recent head trauma
- Hypertension
- Relationship to meals, foods
- Stress
- Eye strain, visual defects
- Fevers, sinusitis
- Occupation
- Toxic exposure
- Allergies
- Improper yoga, exercise
- Family history
- Try to determine what hurts—nerves, arteries, other tissues—intracranial vs. extracranial

Differential Diagnosis

- Common signs of systemic or intracranial infection, intracranial tumor, severe hypertension, cerebral hypoxia, EENT

- Most patients suffer from muscle tension, migraine, or idiopathic origins; headaches are a common final pathway for many

Headache Types: Non-Vascular Headaches

Tension Headache

Tension headaches are the most common form of primary headache. Related to brain trauma, one-year prevalence rates were 38.3 percent for episodic and 2.2 percent for chronic tension headaches. Stemming from muscle spasm or postural sprain, tension headaches are estimated to make up 70 percent of all non-vascular headaches. They tend to have a gradual onset as muscle tension builds with cyclical periods of tension and relaxation. It is common for the muscles of the neck and skull to be tender to palpation. The muscular strain causes inflammation and a release of noxious stimuli such as serotonin, bradykinin, histamine, and prostaglandins. These then interact with calcitonin gene-related peptide, substance P, and neurokinin A, bringing on the pain response. These substances further lower tissue pH and activate an arachidonic acid cascade. Tension headaches share common nociceptive pathways involved in many migraines. Craniomandibular and cervicogenic headaches make diagnostic differentiation through neurologic testing difficult. The muscles most commonly involved here are innervated by C1–C3 nerve roots, trigeminal nerves, and occipital nerves, which all converge into the trigeminal caudate nucleus.

Tension headaches are often felt bilaterally as a band-like tightness or pressure in the back of the head and upper neck. They may also be reported as a band of pressure encircling the head or feeling like a vice clamping across the head with the most intense pain over the eyebrows. Pain tends to remain generally mild (not disabling), allowing most people to be able to function despite the headache. Tension headaches are not associated with aura, nausea, vomiting, or sensitivity to light and sound. They tend to occur infrequently and without a pattern, but can occur frequently and even daily in some people. Physical activity does not tend to impact pain intensity. Most people are able to function despite their tension headaches.

Tension Headache Treatment Considerations

- NSAIDs and OTC pain medication—Aspirin, Ibuprofen (Motrin, Advil), Acetaminophen (Tylenol), Naproxen (Aleve)

- Antidepressants, anticonvulsants, Botox

- Massage, acupuncture, physiotherapy

- Therabands and resistive exercise systems
- Biofeedback, stress management

Cervicogenic Headache

This refers to head pain primarily being generated from the cervical spine. The C1–C2 segment will refer pain to the periorbital region and ear. C2–C3 will refer paint the parietal and frontal regions. C3–C4 will refer to the upper thoracic region and lateral cervical region. The Brain Injury Association of America states that no pharmaceutical interventions have been found efficacious for this type of headache. Manual therapies may be used. Nerve injections, freeing the nerves, or even ablation may be recommended in persistent cases.

Craniomandibular Headache

This refers to head pain associated with the temporo-mandibular joint. These may be very debilitating, causing difficulty with eating, talking, or other movements of the jaw and mouth. Pain may be near the mandibular condyles with mouth open or pain with palpation of the condyles. Physical examination may reveal crepitus. Bite blocks may be recommended, and in persistent cases surgery may be recommended.

Other Potential Non-Vascular Etiologies

Anxiety: Often bizarre pain, vice-like, vertex or general, emotional disturbance prominent

Post-traumatic: History of trauma, manifestations vary

EENT lesions: Eye strain, otitis, sinusitis, TMJ syndrome, manifestations vary

Brain tumor: Mild to severe, localized initially, then becomes generalized as tumor grows, intermittently persistent; slowly progressive weakness, convulsions, visual changes, aphasia, vomiting, mental changes; better or worse with postural changes

Brain abscess: History of EENT infection, lung abscess, rheumatic heart disease

Meningitis: Constant, severe, generalized; fever, vomiting; preceding upper respiratory infection

Subdural hematoma: Trauma, changes in consciousness

Headache Types: Vascular Headaches
Intracerebral Hemorrhage

The result of a rupture of an arteriosclerotic vessel from hypertension or thrombus. Headaches tend to onset abruptly and severely. Neurological deficits steadily increase over time.

Subarachnoid Hemorrhage

An intercranial aneurysm, usually congenital, ruptures, causing an abrupt, severe onset of headache. This may be accompanied by syncope, vomiting, dizziness, stiff neck, and a positive Kernig's, Brudzinski's, and Babinski's test.

Toxic states: Moderate, generalized, pulsating, constant; history of toxic exposure—infections, alcohol, uremia, lead, arsenic, etc.

Hypertension: Throbbing, paroxysmal, occipital, and vertex

Migraine Headaches

Migraines are considered a form of vascular headache caused by vasodilation of the large arteries of the brain. This dilation stretches the nerves that coil around the blood vessels, causing the nerves to release chemicals which cause inflammation, pain, and further vasodilation. This creates a feedback loop which magnifies the pain. Hoffman *et al.* showed migraines being reported more frequently than any other type of headache, contrary to the previously believed notion of tension headache being more common. Fifty-eight percent of returning soldiers who had post-traumatic headache experienced what were considered post-traumatic migraines.

Etiology

- Family history

- More frequent in women [~three-quarters of cases]

- Begins between the ages of 10 and 30

- Often subsides after age 50

- Vascular instability

- Prodrome may be due to vasoconstriction of cerebral blood vessels

- Headache from vasodilation

- Possible platelet abnormality—aggregation

Symptoms of Migraine Headaches

Described as an intense, throbbing, or pounding pain that involves one temple or behind one eye and spreading outward. (Sometimes the pain is located in the forehead, around the eye, or at the back of the head.) Application of heat, presence of bright lights, and excessive physical activity will tend to worsen symptoms. Migraines tend to be unilateral; however, about a third of instances present bilaterally. Unilateral headaches typically change sides from one attack to the next. Unilateral headaches that always occur on the same side should be referred to a primary care physician to consider a secondary headache.

In approximately 40–60 percent of cases the migraine may be preceded by prodrome that may include scintillating scotomas, visual field defects, paresthesias, dizziness, mood swings/irritability, sleepiness, fatigue, depression or euphoria, yawning, and craving sweet or salty foods. The individual may experience a short period of depression, irritability, restlessness, and anorexia. It is common for nausea, vomiting, diarrhea, facial pallor, cold and/or cyanotic hands or feet, and sensitivity to light and sound to accompany migraine headaches. Prominent scalp arteries may also be present. Due to photophobia, sufferers of migraines usually prefer to lie in a quiet, dark room during an attack. Each patient tends to follow a particular pattern of how the migraine manifests. A typical attack lasts between 4 and 72 hours.

Types of Migraine Headaches

Classic migraine: Patients experience an aura before their headaches; are usually much more severe than common migraines.

Common migraine: Accounts for 80 percent of migraines. There is no aura before a common migraine.

Migraine Aura

An estimated 20 percent of migraine headaches are associated with an aura. The most common auras are:

- Flashing, brightly colored lights in a zigzag pattern (referred to as fortification spectra), usually starting in the middle of the visual field and progressing outward

- A hole (scotoma) in the visual field, also known as a blind spot.

Some elderly migraine sufferers may experience only the visual aura without the headache. A less common aura consists of pins-and-needles sensations in the hand and the arm on one side of the body or pins-and-needles sensations around the mouth and the nose on the same side. Other auras include auditory (hearing) hallucinations and abnormal tastes and smells.

Migraine Headache Treatment

Self-care at home:

- Using a cold compress to the area of pain

- Resting with pillows comfortably supporting the head or neck

- Resting in a room with little or no sensory stimulation (light, sound, odors)

- Withdrawing from stressful surroundings

- Sleeping

- Drinking a moderate amount of caffeine

- Nonsteroidal anti-inflammatory drugs (NSAIDs)

- Acetaminophen (Tylenol)

- Combination medications: include Excedrin Migraine, which contains acetaminophen and aspirin combined with caffeine.

Biomedical Treatment of Migraine Headaches
Abortive:

- Eletriptan (Relpax)

- Triptans, which specifically target serotonin. They are all very similar in their action and chemical structure

- Sumatriptan (Imitrex)

- Zolmitriptan (Zomig)

- Combination of aspirin, acetaminophen, and caffeine

- Naratriptan (Amerge, Naramig)

- Rizatriptan (Maxalt)

- Frovatriptan (Frova)

- Almotriptan (Axert)

The following drugs are also specific in affecting serotonin, but they affect other brain chemicals. Occasionally, one of these drugs works when a triptan does not:

- Ergotamine tartrate (Cafergot)

- Dihydroergotamine (DHE 45 Injection, Migranal nasal spray)

- Acetaminophen-isometheptene-dichloralphenazone (Midrin)

The following drugs are mainly used for nausea, but they sometimes have an abortive or preventive effect on headaches:

- Prochlorperazine (Compazine)

- Promethazine (Phenergan)

Weak narcotics: used primarily as a "backup" for the occasions when a specific drug does not work:

- Butalbital compound (Fioricet, Fiorinal)

- Acetaminophen and codeine (Tylenol with codeine)

Preventive: considered if a patient has more than one migraine per week, the goal being to lessen the frequency and severity of the migraine attacks. Medications include the following:

- Antihypertensives:
  - Beta-blockers (propranolol [Inderal])
  - Calcium channel blockers (verapamil [Covera])
- Antidepressants:
  - Amitriptyline (Elavil)
  - Nortriptyline (Pamelor)
- Anticonvulsants:
  - Gabapentin (Neurontin)
  - Valproic acid (Depakote)
  - Topiramate (Topamax)
- Antihistamines and anti-allergy drugs
  - Diphenhydramine (Benadryl)
  - Cyproheptadine (Periactin)

Other therapies:

- Botulinum toxin (Botox) injection

Cluster Headaches

These are headaches which occur in groups (clusters) lasting weeks or months, separated by pain-free periods of months or years. Pain typically occurs once or twice daily, but some patients may experience pain more than twice daily. Each episode of pain generally lasts from 30 to 90 minutes with attacks that tend to occur at about the same time every day and often awaken the patient at night from a sound sleep.

The pain is typically excruciating and located around or behind one eye. Some patients describe the pain as feeling like a hot poker in the eye. The affected eye may become red, inflamed, and watery. The nose on the affected side may become congested and runny.

Unlike patients with migraine headaches, patients with cluster headaches tend to be restless. They often pace the floor, bang their heads against a wall, and can be driven to desperate measures. Cluster headaches are much more common in males than females.

Treatment:

- Inhalation of high concentrations of oxygen (though this will not work if the headache is well established)

- Injection of triptan medications

- Injection of lidocaine into the nostril

- Dihydroergotamine (DHE, Migranal), a vasoconstrictor

- Caffeine

Preventative cluster headache treatment considerations may include the following:

- Calcium channel blockers

  ° Verapamil (Calan, Verelan, Verelan PM, Isoptin, Covera-HS)

  ° Diltiazem (Cardizem, Dilacor, Tiazac)

- Prednisone (Deltasone, Liquid Pred)

Antidepressant medications:

- Lithium (Eskalith, Lithobid)

- Valproic acid, divalproex (Depakote, Depakote ER, Depakene, Depacon)

- Topiramate (Topamax) (often used for seizure control)

Secondary Headaches

The International Headache Society lists a number of categories of secondary headache. A few examples in each category are noted (this is not a complete list):

- Head and neck trauma

- Blood vessel problems in the head and neck

- Stroke or transient ischemic attack (TIA)

- Arteriovenous malformations (AVM)

- Carotid artery inflammation

- Temporal arteritis (inflammation of the temporal artery)

- Non-blood vessel problems of the brain

- Brain tumors

- Seizures

- Idiopathic intracranial hypertension (once named pseudotumor cerebri)

- Excessive cerebrospinal fluid pressure in the spinal canal

- Medications and drugs (including withdrawal from those drugs)

- Infection

- Meningitis

- Encephalitis

- HIV/AIDS

- Systemic infections

- Post-craniectomy (Syndrome of Trephined): headache, dizziness, cognitive changes, etc. Shrinking of the skin flap due to positional changes; treatment: cranioplasty to replace the bone flap

Problems of homeostasis:

- Hypertension

- Dehydration

- Hypothyroidism

- Renal dialysis

- Problems of the eyes, ears, nose, throat, teeth, and neck

- Psychiatric disorders

- Craniosacral fluid dynamics— excessive with increased intracranial pressure: shunt; or a deficiency involving greater than 10 percent to volume decrease

Chinese Medical Perspective: Tóu Tòng ("Head pain")

The head is considered the meeting point for the clear Yang Qi of the body; it is also the location of the "sea of marrow." Head trauma can disrupt Qi and Blood flow, leading to Blood stasis in the channels and collaterals. The resulting headache will occur in a fixed location. Even without a history of traumatic injury, Blood stasis can often complicate other patterns of chronic headaches based on the notion that "Enduring diseases lodge in the collaterals."

Exogenous pathogenic factors:

- Wind is the primary pathogenic factor. "When injured by Wind, the upper part of the body will be affected first." Wind, Yang in nature, has the ability to attack the meeting point of all Yang Qi. Wind then carries other pathogens into the body

- Wind-Cold can congeal Qi and Blood

- Wind-Heat can flare upwards, disturbing the flow of Qi and Blood

- Wind-Dampness can block the flow of Qi

Any of these processes can obstruct the flow of clear Yang Qi to/in the head, resulting in headache.

Internal organs dysfunction: The brain relies on Essence and Blood from the Liver and Kidney for nourishment. It also depends on the Spleen and Stomach to transform and transport water and food, and to distribute Qi and Blood upwards to the head. Therefore, dysfunction of the Liver, Kidney, and Spleen leads to malnourishment of the head. Phlegm can form as a secondary component of Spleen dysfuntion, causing the Yang Qi to not be capable of not rising upward to the head.

Exterior vs. Interior Pathogenesis

Exterior: Sudden severe onset with sharp, throbbing, burning, distending, heavy, and/or constant pain

Interior: Gradual mild onset with dull, empty, lingering, and/or intermittent pain that is worse with exertion

Location Identification by Channel

Taiyang: Back of head, occiput, into the neck

Yangming: Forehead, eyebrows, and maxilla

Shaoyang: Temporal and/or auricular region

Jueyin: Vertex and eyes

Shaoyin: Radiating to the cheeks and teeth

Quality Differentiation by Pattern

Blood stasis: Sharp, stabbing with fixed location, worse at night, history of head trauma

Phlegm turbidity: Accompanied by nausea and vomiting

Qi and Blood deficiency: Dull

Dampness/Phlegm: Heaviness

Liver Yang rising, Liver fire, wind-heat: Distending, throbbing

Wind-cold: Stiff

Kidney deficiency: "Empty" sensation

Other factors which may provoke or have a palliative effect on headache are provided in Table 16.1.

TABLE 16.1 Provocation and Palliation Tendencies

Activity/rest	Worse with activity, better with rest	Qi and Blood deficiency
	Better with light activity	Liver Yang rising
Time of day	Worse during daytime	Qi/Yang deficiency
	Worse in evening or at night	Blood or Yin deficiency, Blood stasis
Weather/ temperature	Worse with heat, better with cold	Liver Yang rising, Liver fire
	Worse with cold	Yang deficiency
	Worse with damp weather	Dampness or phlegm

Emotions	Worse with anger	Liver Yang rising, Liver fire
	Worse with relaxation	Liver Yang rising
Sexual activity	Worse after intercourse	Kidney deficiency
	Better after intercourse	Liver fire
Food	Worse after eating	Dampness, phlegm
	Better after eating	Qi and Blood deficiency
Menstruation	Worse before menses	Liver Yang rising, Liver Qi stagnation
	Worse during menses	Liver fire, Blood stasis
	Worse after menses	Blood deficiency
Pressure	Worse with pressure	Excess
	Better with pressure	Deficiency

TCM Pattern Differentiation/Treatment

Wind-Cold Invasion

Primary symptoms: Headache accompanied by stiffness of the neck and back

Additional symptoms: Aversion to cold, absence of thirst

Tongue: Thin, white coat

Pulse: Tight, floating, superficial

Treatment principles: Eliminate wind, scatter cold, relieve pain

Acupuncture treatment: GB-20, BL-12, LI-4, LU-7 + points for affected channel

Herbal treatment:
Chuan Xiong Cha Tiao San (Tea-Blended Ligusticum Powder)
[Chuan Xiong 9g, Jing Jie 9g, Bai Zhi 6g, Qiang Huo 6g, Xi Xin 3g, Fang Feng 6g, Gan Cao 6g, Bo He 9g]

Wind-Heat Invasion

Primary symptoms: Distending or "splitting" headache

Additional symptoms: Fever, aversion to wind, flushed face, thirst with desire for cold drinks, runny nose with yellow discharge, sore throat, swollen tonsils, red eyes, constipation, dark urine

Tongue: Red, dry, white, or yellow coat

Pulse: Rapid, floating

Treatment principles: Eliminate wind, clear heat, relieve pain

Acupuncture treatment: LI-4, LI-11, GB-20, GV-14, TW-5 + points for affected channel

Herbal treatment:
Ju Hua Cha Tiao San (Chrysanthemum Flower Powder to Be Taken with Green Tea)
[Chuan Xiong Cha Tiao San + Bai Jiang Can 6g, Ju Hua 12g]

Wind-Damp Invasion

Primary symptoms: Headache with sensation of heaviness, made worse by damp or cloudy weather

Additional symptoms: Heaviness of extremities, loss of appetite, sensation of chest and epigastric oppression, scanty urine, constipation, loss of appetite, fever

Tongue: White, greasy coating

Pulse: Soft

Treatment principles: Eliminate wind, resolve dampness, relieve pain

Acupuncture treatment: LI-4, LU-7, GB-20, ST-8, SP-9 + points for affected channel

Herbal treatment:
Qiang Huo Sheng Shi Tang (Notopterygium Dampness-Overcoming Decoction)
[Qiang Huo 6g, Du Huo 6g, Gao Ben 6g, Fang Feng 6g, Man Jing Zi 6g, Chuan Xiong 6g, Zhi Gan Cao 3g]

Liver Yang Rising

Primary symptoms: Throbbing or distending headache accompanied by dizziness and vertigo

Additional symptoms: Irritability, restlessness, restless sleep, costal pain, red eyes, flushed face, bitter taste in the mouth, tinnitus, hypochondriac pain and/or distension

Tongue: Red, thin yellow coating

Pulse: Wiry, forceful, thin, rapid

Treatment principles: Soothe Liver, descend Liver Yang, relieve pain

Acupuncture treatment: GB-20, GV-20, GB-5, GB-43, LR-2

Herbal treatment:

Tian Ma Gou Teng Yin (Gastrodia and Uncaria Beverage)
[Tian Ma 9g, Gou Teng 12g, Shi Jue Ming 18g, Shan Zhi Zi 9g, Huang Qin 9g, Chaun Niu Xi 12g, Du Zhong 9g, Yi Mu Cao 9g, Sang Ji Sheng 9g, Ye Jiao Teng 9g, Fu Shen 9g]

Kidney Essence/Yin Deficiency

Primary symptoms: Headache with a sensation of emptiness of the head with dizziness and vertigo

Additional symptoms: Weakness and aching of the low back and knees, fatigue, seminal emission, tinnitus, insomnia

Tongue: Red, scanty coating

Pulse: Thin, thready, forceless

Treatment principles: Strengthen the Kidney, supplement Essence, nourish Yin, relieve pain

Acupuncture treatment: BL-23, BL-18, KI-3, SP-6, GV-20, GV-23

Herbal treatment:

Da Bu Yuan Jian (Major Origin-Supplementing Brew)
[Shu Di Huang 24g, Shan Zhu Yu 12g, Shan Yao 12g, Gou Qi Zi 12g, Ren Shen 9g, Dang Gui 9g, Zhi Gan Cao 6g]

Kidney Yin Deficiency: Liu Wei Di Huang Wan (Six Flavor Pill with Rehmannia)
[Shu Di Huang 24g, Shan Zhu Yu 12g, Shan Yao 12g, Ze Xie 9g, Mu Dan Pi 9g, Fu Ling 9g]

Kidney Yang Deficiency

Primary symptoms: Headache accompanied by cold body

Additional symptoms: Pale complexion, cold extremities, sore low back and knees, tiredness, fatigue

Tongue: Pale

Pulse: Deep, slow, thready

Treatment principles: Warm and supplement Kidney Yang, relieve pain

Acupuncture treatment: BL-23, CV-4, KI-3, GV-4, GV-20, GV-23

Herbal treatment:

You Gui Wan (Right-Restoring Kidney Yang Pill)

[Shu Di Huang 24g, Shan Yao 12g, Shan Zhu Yu 9g, Gou Qi Zi 12g, Lu Jiao Jiao 12g, Tu Si Zi 12g, Du Zhong 12g, Dang Gui 9g, Rou Gui 6g, Zhi Fu Zi 6g]
Jin Gui Shen Qi Wan (Golden Coffer Kidney Qi Pill)
[Shu Di Huang 24g, Shan Zhu Yu 12g, Shan Yao 12g, Ze Xie 9g, Mu Dan Pi 9g, Fu Ling 9g, Rou Gui 3g, Pao Fu Zi 3g]

Qi Deficiency

Primary symptoms: Constant dull headache aggravated by over-exertion

Additional symptoms: Weakness, fatigue, loss of appetite

Tongue: Pale, thin white coating

Pulse: Weak

Treatment principles: Supplement Qi, relieve pain

Acupuncture treatment: CV-6, BL-20, ST-36, LI-4, GV-20, GV-23

Herbal treatment:
Bu Zhong Yi Qi Tang (Supplement the Center and Boost the Qi Decoction)
[Huang Qi 15g, Ren Shen 9g, Bai Zhu 9g, Dang Gui 9g, Chen Pi 6g, Sheng Ma 3g, Chai Hu 3g, Zhi Gan Cao 6g]

Blood Deficiency

Primary symptoms: Dull headache accompanied by dizziness and vertigo, symptoms aggravated by over-exertion

Additional symptoms: Pale and lusterless complexion, blurred vision, palpitation, tiredness, fatigue, difficulty falling asleep, possible history of bleeding

Tongue: Pale

Pulse: Weak, thready

Treatment principles: Nourish Blood, relieve pain

Acupuncture treatment: BL-18, BL-17, BL-20, SP-6, GV-23, ST-36

Herbal treatment:
Si Wu Tang (Four Gentlemen Decoction)
[Dang Gui 12g, Bai Shao Yao 12g, Shu Di Huang 12g, Chuan Xiong 9g, Ju Hua 9g, Man Jing Zi 9g, Huang Qin 3g, Gan Cao 6g]

Phlegm Turbidity

Primary symptoms: Headache accompanied by dizziness and heaviness of the head

Additional symptoms: Epigastric and chest fullness and stuffiness, nausea, vomiting phlegm and/or mucus

Tongue: White, greasy coating

Pulse: Slippery, wiry

Treatment principles: Transform Turbid Phlegm, descend rebellious Qi, relieve pain

Acupuncture treatment: CV-12, LI-4, ST-36, ST-40, GV-20, Yintang

Herbal treatment:
Ban Xia Bai Zhu Tian Ma Tang (Pinellia, Atractylodes, and Gastrodia Decoction) [Fa Ban Xia 9g, Tian Ma 6g, Fu Ling 6g, Ju Hong 6g, Bai Zhu 15g, Gan Cao 3g, Sheng Jiang 3g, Da Zao 2pc]

Blood Stasis

Primary symptoms: Persistent, fixed, stabbing headache

Additional symptoms: Possible history of trauma to head

Tongue: Dark, purplish

Pulse: Choppy, thready, wiry

Treatment principles: Quicken the Blood, resolve stasis, relieve pain

Acupuncture treatment: BL-18, BL-17, BL-20, SP-6, GV-23, ST-36

Herbal treatment:
Tong Qiao Huo Xue Tang (Orifice-Freeing Blood-Quickening Decoction) [Chi Shao 3g, Chuan Xiong 3g, Tao Ren 9g, Hong Hua 9g, Cong Bai 3g, Da Zao 5pc, She Xiang 0.1g, Huang Jiu (Yellow wine) 50cc]

Additional Acupuncture and Moxibustion Considerations

By location: Local and distal points

Frontal headache: ST-8, Yintang, GV-23, LI-4, ST-44

Vertex headache: GV-20, SI-3, BL-67, LR-3

Occipital headache: GB-20, BL-10, GV-19, BL-60, SI-3

Temporal headache: Taiyang, GB-8, TW-5, GB-41, GB-43

Guiding Herbs

Taiyang: Qiang Huo, Ge Gen

Yangming: Bai Zhi, Man Jing Zi

Jueyin: Wu Zhu Yu, Gao Ben, Chuan Xiong

Shaoyang: Chuan Xiong, Chai Hu, Tian Ma

Shaoyin: Xi Xin

Clinical Notes

- It is imperative to rule out serious underlying pathology before treating headache in the clinic. Severe headaches of recent onset that have not been evaluated require immediate referral, particularly if pain is increasing in severity.

- Pay specific attention to the duration of the headache, as well as to the pain characteristics and specific location of the pain.

- To treat stubborn headaches, incorporate herbs that move Blood and unblock the collaterals. In chronic headache, the pathology involves a deep obstruction in the collaterals. This complication of obstructed circulation of Qi and Blood in the small collaterals causes poor response to therapy requiring the addition of herbs such as Tao Ren, Hong Hua, Chi Shao, and Si Gua Luo, as well as "insect" medicinals such as Quan Xie, Wu Gong, and Di Long to root out the pathogen.

Other Treatment Considerations

- Cold compress coated in a combination of lavender and peppermint essential oils
- Liver/Kidney drainage if excess crystals present
- Treat underlying allergies
- Avoid cheese, chocolate, beer, and wine, and allergens such as wheat or dairy
- Consider environmental allergens

Orthomolecular Considerations

- Tryptophan
- 5-HTP
- Magnesium (Migraine)—400–800mg/day
- Vitamin B2 (Riboflavin) (Migraine)
- Quercetin—500mg 15 minutes before eating
- Omega 3 fatty acids
- Niacin 100–400mg at first onset of symptoms

Phytotherapeutic Considerations

- Feverfew

- Butterbur

- Rosemary

- Majoram herbal tea

- Partenelle

- Meadow-sweet

- German chamomile

Research Studies

- A three-armed, parallel, randomized exploratory study was carried out in three military treatment facilities in the Washington, DC metropolitan area of previously deployed service members (18–69 years old) with mild-to-moderate TBI and headaches. Mean Headache Impact Test scores decreased in auricular acupuncture and traditional Chinese medicine groups, while they increased slightly in the "usual care" only group from baseline to week 6. Both acupuncture groups had sizable decreases in Numerical Rating Scale (Pain Best), compared to usual care.[1]

- Clinical signs of chronic headache (CH) disappeared markedly after three months of treatment with acupuncture. The amount of interleukin (IL)-1β, IL-6, and tumor necrosis factor-α (TNF-α) in LPS culture supernatant was significantly increased in the patients with CH compared to the healthy control group. Those cytokines came down toward the levels of the healthy group after treatment with acupuncture, although the levels still remained elevated. Significantly reduced plasma (cytokine) levels of TNF-α were also observed. "These data suggest that acupuncture treatment has an inhibitory effect on pro-inflammatory cytokine production in patients with [chronic headache]."[2]

- Before acupuncture treatment, the migraine without aura patients had significantly decreased functional connectivity in certain brain regions within the frontal and temporal lobe when compared with the healthy controls. After acupuncture treatment, brain regions showing decreased functional connectivity revealed

---

1   Jonas, W., Bellanti, D., Paat, C., *et al.* A randomized exploratory study to evaluate two acupuncture methods for the treatment of headaches associated with traumatic brain injury. *Medical Acupuncture.* 2016 Jun; 28(3): 113–130. https://doi.org/10.1089/acu.2016.1183

2   Jeong, H-J., Hong, S-H., Nam, Y-C., *et al.* The effect of acupuncture on proinflammatory cytokine production in patients with chronic headache: a preliminary report. *The American Journal of Chinese Medicine.* 2003; 31(6): 945–954.

significant reduction in migraine patients compared to before acupuncture treatment. Conclusions: Acupuncture treatment could increase the functional connectivity of brain regions in the intrinsic decreased brain networks in migraines without aura.[3]

- A review of studies found acupuncture may positively influence not just dynamic but also static cerebral autoregulation during the interictal phase depending on the intervals between sessions of acupuncture as dose units. "Point-through-point" needling (at angles connecting acupoints) was found to possibly be clinically superior to standard acupuncture; thus needling angles may affect treatment effectiveness.[4]

---

3   Zhang, Y., Li, K-S., Liu, H-W., *et al.* Acupuncture treatment modulates the resting-state functional connectivity of brain regions in migraine patients without aura. *Chinese Journal of Integrative Medicine.* 2016 Apr; 22(4): 293–301.

4   Lo, M-Y., Lin, J-G., Wei, O-M., and Sun, W-Z. Cerebral hemodynamic responses to acupuncture in migraine patients: a systematic review. *Journal of Traditional Complementary Medicine.* 2013; 3: 213–220.

Chapter 17

Fatigue

Fatigue is among the most common post-concussion symptoms. It can span all levels of injury severity and persist for many years in those with moderate-to-severe injuries. No correlation has been drawn between self-reported fatigue and injury severity or overall cognitive impairment. Fatigue is defined as "The awareness of a decreased capacity for physical and/or mental activity due to an imbalance in the availability, utilization, and/or restoration of resources needed to perform activity."[1]

Many people who have sustained a brain injury experience a reduction in the speed of information processing and have difficulties with attention, memory, and executive function. This can make cognitively demanding tasks more daunting and draining. Studying may be difficult, and energy for social interactions and engagement in leisure activities may be affected. This can cause isolation and confinement at home, which may turn to depression, even further exacerbating fatigue. This may impact major life activities or employment.

As with headaches, fatigue can be primary or secondary in nature. Secondary fatigue may be a result of chronic pain, sleep disturbance, stress, or a poorer overall quality of life. Depression and anxiety are also strongly associated with self-reported fatigue. Primary fatigue can be the result of diffuse brain injury as well as injury to the brain centers controlling arousal, attention, and response speed. This may include the ascending reticulating activating system, limbic system, anterior cingulate, middle frontal lobe, and basal ganglia.

It has also been proposed that fatigue may be associated with neuroendocrine dysregulation resulting from the injury. Growth hormone deficiency is common following a brain injury, with studies showing as high as a 60 percent occurrence rate, and is believed to be associated with subsequent fatigue. Others have proposed a significant correlation between hypothalamic injury and fatigue following a brain injury. This argument is substantiated by lower levels of CSF hypocretin-I as a result of the loss of hypocretin neurons which promote wakefulness. This results in an increased daytime sleepiness.

---

1   Aaronson, L.S., Teel, C.S., Cassmeyer, V., *et al.* Defining and measuring fatigue. *Image—The Journal of Nursing Scholarship*. 1999; 31: 45–50.

Physiological Fatigue vs. Psychological Fatigue

Physiological fatigue may be caused by depletion of energy, hormones, neurotransmitters, and/or reduction in neural connections due to injury. Fatigue arising from the peripheral nervous system can be assessed using motor tasks such as testing grip strength, thumb pressing, or finger tapping speed as these are unlikely to be affected by injury to the central nervous system.

Psychological fatigue is a state relating to reduced motivation, prolonged mental activity, or boredom which may result from chronic stress, anxiety, and depression. As all of these factors may be in play after a brain injury, psychological fatigue is an important factor to consider.

Fatigue can be addressed using Chinese medicine by generally tonifying any found deficiencies. This can often relate to the Earth and Water phases. Addressing the stagnations present is also necessary. This chapter will look at treatment approaches for chronic fatigue to gauge therapeutic principles and the Chinese medical approach to the deficiency taxation.

Chronic Fatigue

Chronic fatigue syndrome, or chronic fatigue immune deficiency syndrome, is a constellation of neurological, neuromuscular, and immunological abnormalities combined with cognitive impairments, disabling fatigue, and recurrent bouts of flu-like symptoms.

Etiology and Symptoms

Unknown. Viral infection is strongly suspected, with 85 percent of sufferers experiencing an initial acute onset of flu-like symptoms such as:

- Mild fever
- Sore throat
- Tender lymph nodes

- Chills
- Fatigue with minimal exertion

This is then followed by such chronic manifestations as:

- Myalgia (muscle pains)
- Migrating arthralgias (joint pains)
- Sleep disorders
- Headaches
- Hyper- or hyposensitivities
- Cognitive disorders—spatial disorientation, short-term memory loss

- Disabling fatigue and malaise
- Depression, anxiety, irritability, and/or confusion
- Fluctuations in weight
- Abdominal pain
- Nausea and/or vomiting

Patients with this condition also often have a history of multiple allergies. Most patients are between 25 and 40 years of age.

Biomedical Diagnosis

There are no absolute clinical indicators or laboratory tests confirming this diagnosis. It is diagnosed primarily by presenting symptoms and history.

Differential Diagnosis

- Lupus

- Rheumatoid arthritis

- Fibromyalgia

Biomedical Treatment

There is no specific biomedical treatment for chronic fatigue. Its current treatment is based on the management of symptoms.

For sleep: Tricyclic depressants, serotonin reuptake inhibitors, benzodiazepine, clonazepam

For headache: NSAIDs (tension headache), calcium channel blockers (migraine)

For myalgias / arthralgias: Muscle relaxants, NSAIDs, clonazepam

For candidiasis: Ketoconazole (Nizoral), fluconazole (Diflucan)

For depression: Antidepressants

For fatigue: Buproprion (Wellbutrin) and intramuscular B12 injections

Chinese Medical Perspective: Deficiency Taxation (Xu Lao)[2]
Chinese Medical Etiology

- External invasion of pathogens
- Internal damage by the seven emotions
- Unregulated eating and drinking

- Iatrogenesis
- Aging

---

2 Damone, Bob. *Ye Tian-Shi on Vacuity Detriment: a model for a mode of inquiry in Chinese medicine*. www.chinesemedicinedoc. com/ye-tian-shi-on-vacuity-detriment. Web. 18 Oct. 2017.

Pattern Differentiation

Interior Deficiency–Exterior Excess

Acute onset of sore, swollen throat, fever, sweating or no sweating, muscle aches, fatigue, lack of strength, torpid intake.

Tongue: Pale, fat, teeth marks with yellow and white coat

Pulse: Floating, fine, wiry (bowstring), slightly rapid

Treatment principles: Dispel wind and clear heat, support the righteous Qi

Acupuncture treatment: LI-4, GV-14, BL-12, ST-36

Herbal treatment:
Xiao Chai Hu Tang Jia Wei (Minor Bupleurum Decoction Plus Modifications)
[Ban Lan Gen 15g, Xuan Shen 15g, Niu Bang Zi 9g, Huang Qin 9g, Chai Hu 9g, Dang Shen 9g, Ban Xia 9g, Gan Cao 6g, Sheng Jiang 6g, Da Zao 6g]

Modifications:
Marked lymph node swelling: + Zhi Bei Mu 15g, Xia Ku Cao 15g

Blood deficiency / one catches cold with each menses: + Shu Di Huang 12g, Dang Gui 9g, Bai Shao 9g, Chuan Xiong 9g

Nasal congestion: + Bai Zhi 9g, Bo He 9g

Marked joint pain: + Qiang Huo 9g, Fang Feng 9g, Ge Gen 15g

High fever and thirst: + Shi Gao 20g, Zhi Mu 12g

Taxation Malaria Pattern

Spleen Qi deficiency signs: Fatigue, especially after eating, abdominal bloating after eating, loose stool, cold hands and feet, lack of strength in the four extremities, dizziness when standing up, easily bruised, easily catches colds and flu

Liver Blood / Kidney Yin deficiency with heat signs: Night sweats, hot flashes, 5-palm heat, tinnitus, dizziness, thirst/dry mouth with little desire to drink, recurrent dry sore throat, malar tidal flush, stiff sinews, numbness/tingling of the extremities, matitudinal insomnia

Liver depression signs: Premenstrual or menstrual lower abdominal distension, lower abdominal cramping, premenstrual breast distension and pain, irritability, emotional depression

Tongue: Pale red or red tongue with red tip, scanty coat

Pulse: Fine, rapid, or possibly floating, surging

Treatment principles: Supplement deficiency, course the Liver, rectify the Qi

Acupuncture treatment: PC-5, GV-14, LI-4, ST-36, KI-7, BL-20, BL-21

Herbal treatment:

Bu Zhong Yi Qi Tang Jia Wei (Supplement the Center and Boost the Qi Decoction Plus Modifications)

[Huang Qi 15g, He Shou Wu 15g, Niu Xi 12g, Dang Shen 9g, Bai Zhu 9g, Zhi Mu 9g, Wu Mei 9g, Cao Guo 9g, Gan Cao 6g, Dang Gui 6g, Chen Pi 6g, Sheng Ma 4.5g, Chai Hu 1–3g]

Modifications:

Severe fatigue: Increase Dang Shen to 20g, Huang Qi to 30g

Fatigue or abdominal bloating after eating: + Shi Chang Pu 9g, Mu Xiang 9g

Night sweats: Huang Bai 9g, Di Gu Pi 9g

Matitudinal insomnia: + Suan Zao Ren 12g, He Huan Pi 12g, Bai Zi Ren 12g

Liver Qi depression signs: + Xiang Fu 9g, Chuan Xiong 9g, Bai Shao 9g

Stiffness in sinews/Numbness of the extremities: + Ji Xue Teng 20g

Heart Malnourishment with Liver Depression

Primary symptoms: Long period of extreme fatigue, wan affect, emotional depression, insomnia, impaired memory

Additional symptoms: Occasional desire to sigh, shortness of breath, a faint voice or disinclination to speak, heart palpitations or fluster, no thought of eating or drinking, lack of strength, flabby muscles, possible muscle/joint soreness or pain

Tongue: Fat pale red tongue; white coat

Pulse: Fine, wiry

Treatment principles: Supplement the Heart Qi and Blood by fortifying the Spleen and boosting the Qi, course the Liver and resolve depression, quiet the spirit

Acupuncture treatment: BL-15, CV-17, HT-7, ST-36, SP-6, LR-3

Herbal treatment:

Bu Gan Yi Qi Tang (Supplement the Liver and Boost the Qi Decoction)

[Huang Qi 30g, Xian He Cao 30g, Bai He 30g, Hong Shen 9g, Shan Zhu Yu 9g, Chai Hu 9g, Zhi Ke 9g, Chen Pi 9g, Dang Gui 9g, Bai Zhu 12g, Bai Shao 12g]

Modifications:

Tendency toward heat: + Huang Lian 3–6g, Huang Qin 3–6g

With Yang deficiency: + Yin Yang Huo 9g, Xian Mao 9g

With Yin deficiency: + Gou Qi Zi 10g, Nu Zhen Zi 10g, Wu Wei Zi 10g, and/or He Shou Wu 10g

Torpid intake: + Shen Qu 9g, Shan Zha 9g, Mai Ya 9g

Insomnia and heart palpitations: + Ku Shen 9g, Suan Zao Ren 12–15g

With Blood stasis: + Chi Shao 9g, Dan Shen 9g, Mu Dan Pi 9g, and/or Yi Mu Cao 9g

Hidden or deeply lying pathogens in the blood level: Zi Cao 9–15g, Jin Yin Hua 9–15g, Lian Qiao 9–15g, Pu Gong Ying 9–15g, and/or Ban Lan Gen 9–15g

Clinical Notes

- Regulating and maintaining sleep is a very important component to fatigue after a brain injury as the body needs plenty of rest to allow for the healing process

- Identify and remove causes of stress or learn to accept it if it can't be changed

Other Treatment Considerations

Dietary Considerations

- Stabilize glucose

- Eat frequent meals (every two to three hours) in the glycemic healthy range for the individual

- Eat a protein and healthy fatty acid rich breakfast

- Don't wait until hungry—eat regularly to maintain a regular nutritional intake

- Nuts/seeds/eggs/jerky (low sugar)

- Avoid fruit juice and carrot juice and junk food

- Vegetables, meat—high quality, grass fed, whole grains

Avoid concentrated simple sugars, caffeine, nicotine, alcohol, allergies, trans fats, omega 6 fatty acids (inhibit steroid synthesis and disrupt normal anti-inflammatory cytokines), and artificial sweeteners (block conversion of phenylalanine to tyrosine, affecting catecholamine synthesis in adrenal medulla).

Somatic and Mind-Body Considerations

- Stress reduction techniques

- Meditation

- Yoga

- Positive mental image

- Sedona technique

- Contract muscles and relax

- Exercise in aerobic range, no overtraining

Orthomolecular Considerations

- Omega 3 fatty acids
- B vitamins
- Sulfer amino acids, milk thistle: detox support
- Phosphatidyl serine (affects cortisol)
- Royal jelly
- Cordyceps

Phytotherapeutic Considerations

- Astragalus
- Ashwaghanda
- Rhodiola
- Licorice root
- Panax ginseng
- Maca
- Holy basil

Research Studies

- One hundred patients with chronic fatigue syndrome were randomly assigned to two groups of acupuncture in the Qi Huang point (eight acupuncture needles in a 0.5-inch radius around the navel at 45-degree angles forming a complete circle) and the control group with routine therapy of acupuncture. Both groups received acupuncture for 30 minutes once every three days, ten times for one course, treatments lasting for two courses. Fatigue scale 14 (FS-14) and the self-rating depression scale (SDS) were used to evaluate the patients before and after treatment. Scores after treatment were significantly lower than those before treatment in two groups. Acupuncture in the Qi Huang point of Chuang medicine was shown to have better effects on chronic fatigue symptoms than the control group.[3]

- Forty-seven cancer patients with moderate to severe fatigue were treated. Significant improvements were found with regards to general fatigue ($P < 0.001$), physical fatigue ($P = 0.016$), activity ($P = 0.004$), and motivation ($P = 0.024$). At the end of the intervention, there was a 36 percent improvement in fatigue levels in the acupuncture group, while the acupressure group improved by 19 percent and the sham acupressure group by 0.6 percent.[4]

---

3   Li, M-K., Mo, Q-L., He, X-F., *et al.* Effect of acupuncture in Qi Huang point of Chuang medicine on treatment of 48 cases of chronic fatigue syndrome. *Guangxi Medical Journal.* 2014; 12: 1722–1724.

4   Molassiotis, A., Sylt, P., and Diggins, H. The management of cancer-related fatigue after chemotherapy with acupuncture and acupressure: a randomised controlled trial. *Complementary Therapies in Medicine.* 2007; 15(4): 228–237. http://dx.doi.org/10.1016/j.ctim.2006.09.009

- One hundred and twenty-eight individuals with post-stroke fatigue were given either pharmaceuticals or electroacupuncture (EA) with cupping. Findings showed the effective rate of EA plus cupping group was "obviously higher than that of medication group" and that the acupuncture plus cupping over the lumbo-back "can effectively relieve fatigue of post-stroke patients, and its therapeutic effect is superior to medication."[5]

5   Zhou, Y., Zhou, G-Y., Li, S-K., and Jin, J-H. Clinical observation on the therapeutic effect of electroacupuncture combined with cupping on post-stroke fatigue. *Zhen Ci Yan Jiu* [Acupuncture Research]. 2010 Oct; 35(5): 380–383.

Chapter 18

Dizziness

Dizziness following a brain injury can be a common hindrance that may stem from changes or damage to the visual or vestibular system. Given the wide range of impact it can have, visual system concerns will be discussed in a separate chapter later in this text. Here we will explore vestibular system dysfunction.

A variety of vesibular conditions may occur following a brain injury. These include labyinthine concussion (unilateral vestibular hypofunction). This is typically the result of trauma and bleed into the labyrinth. Symptoms may include dizziness, balance loss, or oscillopsia (visual input seems to oscillate, blur, or periodically jump), with rotation of the head, unilateral nystagmus, and postural instability. Most cases (nearly 95%) improve from this condition within six months of injury.

> *Post-traumatic Meniere's disease*: This is often the result of areas of scarring and intermittent fluid build-up (which are known as hydrops) that impacts the pressure within the endolymphatic system. This can occur both shortly after or a while following an injury. Symptoms include low tone hearing loss with or without dizziness. Key in diagnosis here are intermittent bouts of dizziness. The membrane may rupture, worsening symptoms.

> *Vestibular migraine*: This may or may not be associated with a headache. Symptoms include episodic spinning dizziness lasting a few minutes and occurring multiple times within a month. Photophobia, hearing loss, and tinnitus may also be present.

> *Basilar skull fracture*: At the time of injury, bleeding or leakage of CSF into the ear can cause severe imbalance or dizziness. Medical observation or surgery are the commonly accepted medical treatments for this condition.

> *Perilymphatic fistula*: This is an instance of perilymph leakage which causes abnormal communication between the inner and middle ear. The individual may experience dizziness or loss of balance while blowing their nose with eyes closed,

a high tone hearing loss, and increased dizziness with exposure to loud sounds. Minor surgery is the primary form of treatment.

Benign paroxysmal positioning vertigo: This is the result of inner ear crystals in the semicircular canals being out of place or having debris attached to them. The person may experience the sensation of spinning with certain movements without hearing loss. This may include rolling in one direction, bending over, or changing positions while in bed. A Dix-Hallpike movement test is used to diagnose this condition, noting nystagmus or signs of dizziness with provoking positions. The repositioning maneuver can at times fully alleviate symptoms.

Bilateral vestibular hypofunction: This condition results in posture and gait abnormalities as well as difficulty focusing with movements of the head. Due to both sides of the vestibular system being affected, nausea or vertigo are rarely reported. Individuals affected may require assistive devices.

Central vertigo: This may be the result of trauma to the afferent (sensory) inputs in the cervical spine or due to a vertebrobasilar insufficiency. Dizziness will be persistent as well as possibly coupled with symptoms based on the brain regions injured and whether the central or peripheral nerves are affected, as stated in Table 18.1.

TABLE 18.1 Central vs Peripheral Nerve Involvement in Dizziness/Vertigo

Central nerves affected	Eye movements abnormal (saccades, smooth pursuits)
	Rare hearing loss (unless due to other trauma)
	Diplopia (double vision)
	Lateropulsion (tendency to fall to one side)
	Acute vertigo symptoms unable to be suppressed by visual fixation
	Pendular nystagmus with eyes equal
	Vertical nystagmus persists despite changes in position
Peripheral nerves affected	Normal eye movement screen
	Nystagmus with positional testing
	May experience tinnitus, fullness in ears, or insidious hearing loss that may recover
	Very intense acute vertigo in which visual fixation can help
	Jerk nystagmus present (both fast and slow phases)
	Spontaneous horizontal nystagmus (generally resolves in ~1 week or less)

Diagnostic Testing

A physiatrist may examine to determine the nature of vestibular dysfunction. Possible diagnostics include:

- Audiogram
- Video or electronystagmography (VNG/ENG)
- Electrocochleography (EcoG)
- Platform posturography
- MRI
- MRA/MRV
- CT
- Arteriography

Biomedical Approaches

- Meclizine hydrochloride (Antivert)
- Scopolamine transdermal patch (Transderm-Scop)
- Promethazine hydrochloride (Phenergan)
- Metoclopramide (Reglan)
- Odansetron (Zofran)
- Diazepam (Valium)
- Lorazepam (Ativan)
- Clonazepam (Klonopin)
- Prednisone (Deltasone, Liquid Pred, Sterapred)

Emerging Treatment Methods

Balance deficits can be very common following a TBI and can cause physical limitations that can be both difficult to deal with and frustrating. It has been estimated that almost all individuals admitted to an inpatient rehabilitation environment with a TBI have some form of balance impairment. An emerging evidence-based treatment for those with neurogenic balance impairment is the use of virtual reality systems that allow them to view a virtual environment and dynamically respond and interact with it in real time.

Chinese Medical Perspective: Dizziness and Vertigo (Xuan Yun)

Xuan means blurred vision or blackouts, while Yun refers to the subjective sensation that the body or the environment is spinning. Xuan Yun can range from mild lightheadedness that may only show changes in posture, to severe vertigo with loss of balance, nausea and vomiting, perspiration, and even fainting.

Relevant Biomedical Conditions

- Traumatic head injury
- Hypertension
- Hypotension
- Hypoglycemia

- Anemia
- Labyrinthiti
- Meniere's disease

Chinese Medical Etiology

Emotional stress:

- *Liver*: Depression, anger, frustration, or irritability can result in Qi stagnation which, in turn, can generate Heat. Pathological Heat can damage Liver and Kidney Yin, resulting in failure to nourish the Liver and dysregulation between Yin and Yang. This will cause Liver Yang to rise hyperactively, disturbing the clear orifices and causing dizziness and vertigo.

- *Spleen*: Excessive pensiveness can weaken the Spleen, causing failure to generate Qi and Blood and lack of nourishment to the Brain, resulting in dizziness and vertigo.

Improper diet, overwork, hemmorhage: improper diet and overwork can weaken the Spleen and Stomach, causing failure to generate Qi and Blood and lack of nourishment to the Brain, resulting in dizziness and vertigo. Spleen and Stomach deficiency also can result in an accumulation of Phlegm-Dampness. Turbid Phlegm prevents clear Yang Qi from rising to the Brain.

Chronic illness, aging, congenital deficiency, excessive sexual activity: the preceding factors result in Kidney Essence deficiency with inability to generate Marrow and failure to nourish the Brain.

Pattern Differentiation
Liver Yang Rising

Primary symptoms: Dizziness and vertigo often accompanied by a pounding or distending headache, symptoms worse with emotional stress/anger

Additional symptoms: Irritability, tinnitus, blurred vision, dream-disturbed sleep, insomnia, flushed face, red eyes, bitter taste in the mouth

Tongue: Red, scanty, yellow coating

Pulse: Wiry (bowstring), rapid

Treatment principles: Settle the Liver, subdue Yang, nourish and supplement the Liver and Kidney, relieve dizziness and vertigo

Acupuncture treatment: LR-2/LR-3, BL-18, BL-23, KI-3, SP-6, GB-20

Herbal treatment:
Tian Ma Gou Teng Yin (Gastrodia and Uncaria Beverage)
[Tian Ma 9g, Gou Teng 12g, Shi Jue Ming 12g, Shan Zhi Zi 9g, Huang Qin 9g, Chuan Niu Xi 12g, Du Zhong 9g, Yi Mu Cao 9g, Sang Ji Sheng 9g, Ye Jiao Teng 9g, Fu Shen 9g]

Phlegm-Damp in the Middle Jiao

Primary symptoms: Dizziness and vertigo, heaviness of the head, cloudy thinking and poor concentration

Additional symptoms: Nausea, poor appetite, sleepiness, oppressive feeling in the chest, obesity

Tongue: White, greasy coating

Pulse: Soggy, slippery, soft

Treatment principles: Strengthen the Spleen, harmonize the Stomach, dry dampness, resolve phlegm, relieve dizziness and vertigo

Acupuncture treatment: ST-8, ST-36, ST-40, CV-12, PC-6, GB-20, BL-20

Herbal treatment:
Ban Xia Bai Zhu Tian Ma Tang (Pinellia, Atractylodes, and Gastrodia Decoction)
[Fa Ban Xia 9g, Tian Ma 6g, Fu Ling 6g, Ju Hong 6g, Bai Zhu 15g, Gan Cao 4g, Sheng Jiang 3g, Da Zao 2pc]

Phlegm-Fire in the Middle Jiao

Primary symptoms: Dizziness and vertigo, heaviness of the head

Additional symptoms: Nausea, headache, irritability, red eyes that feel distended, bitter taste in the mouth, thirst without desire to drink, oppressive sensation in the chest

Tongue: Yellow, greasy coating

Pulse: Slippery, wiry (bowstring)

Treatment principles: Transform phlegm, drain heat, relieve dizziness and vertigo

Acupuncture treatment: ST-8, ST-40, LR-2, GB-20, PC-6, CV-12

Herbal treatment:
Wen Dan Tang (Gallbladder-Warming Decoction)
[Fa Ban Xia 6g, Zhu Ru 6g, Zhi Shi 6g, Chen Pi 6g, Gan Cao 6g, Fu Ling 9g,

Sheng Jiang 2pc, Da Zao 3pc]
Plus: Huang Lian 9g, Huang Qin 9g

Qi and Blood Deficiency

Primary symptoms: Positional dizziness and vertigo in mild cases. In severe cases fainting is possible

Additional symptoms: Pale complexion, nails, and lips, fatigue, shortness of breath, disinclination to speak, palpitations, poor memory, insomnia, loss of appetite, often occurs during recovery from severe illness or severe blood loss

Tongue: Pale

Pulse: Weak, thready

Treatment principles: Strengthen Spleen and Stomach, supplement Qi and Blood, relieve dizziness and vertigo

Acupuncture treatment: BL-17, BL-18, CV-6, CV-4, GV-20, SP-6, ST-36, GB-39, LR-8

Herbal treatment:
Gui Pi Tang (Spleen-Returning Decoction)
[Huang Qi 9g, Ren Shen 9g, Bai Zhu 9g, Fu Shen 9g, Long Yan Rou 9g, Suan Zao Ren 9g, Mu Xiang 6g, Dang Gui 6g, Yuan Zhi 3g, Zhi Gan Cao 6g, Shang Jiang 3g, Da Zao 5pc]

Kidney Essence and Yin Deficiency

Primary symptoms: Dizziness and vertigo that does not abate

Additional symptoms: Listlessness, insomnia and/or dream-disturbed sleep, poor memory, achy and weak low back and knees, seminal emission, tinnitus, five-centers heat, night sweating

Tongue: Red, scanty coating

Pulse: Thready, rapid, wiry

Treatment principles: Supplement the Kidney, nourish Yin, relieve dizziness and vertigo

Acupuncture treatment: KI-3, BL-18, BL-23, GV-20, ST-36, SP-6

Herbal treatment:
Zuo Gui Wan (Left-Restoring Kidney Yin Pill)
[Shu Di Huang 24g, Shan Yao 12g, Shan Zhu Yu 12g, Gou Qi Zi 12g, Chuan Niu Xi 9g, Tu Si Zi 12g, Lu Jiao Jiao 12g, Gui Ban Jiao 12g]

Kidney Essence and Yang Deficiency

Primary symptoms: Dizziness and vertigo that does not abate

Additional symptoms: Cold body and extremities, listlessness, poor memory, weak and aching low back and knees, impotence, tinnitus, seminal emissions, insomnia

Tongue: Pale, scanty, white coating

Pulse: Deep, weak

Treatment principles: Supplement the Kidneys, tonify Kidney Yang, relieve dizziness and vertigo

Acupuncture treatment: BL-17, BL-23, KI-6, GV-20, CV-4, GV-4

Herbal treatment:
You Gui Wan (Right-Restoring Kidney Yang Pill)
[Shu Di Huang 24g, Shan Yao 12g, Shan Zhu Yu 9g, Gou Qi Zi 12g, Lu Jiao Jiao 12g, Tu Si Zi 12g, Du Zhong 12g, Dang Gui 9g, Rou Gui 6g, Zhi Fu Zi 6g]

Other Acupuncture Considerations

Ear points: Shen Men, Kidney, Occiput, Inner Ear, Subcortex
Scalp points: Yun Ting Qu (vertigo and hearing region)

Clinical Notes

- In middle-aged and older patients, there is a distinct possibility that more severe cases of dizziness and vertigo, particularly caused by Liver Yang rising, may result in Wind-Stroke. Hence, prevention and prompt treatment of dizziness and vertigo in older patients are very important.

- Preventive measures include decreasing consumption of rich foods and alcohol, abstaining from hot, spicy foods, controlling the emotions, and engaging in appropriate physical exercise.

Research Studies

- Sixty recruited patients in an emergency room. A variation of the Visual Analog Scale demonstrated a significant decrease between two groups after two different durations: 30 minutes and seven days. Heart rate variability also showed a significant increase in high frequency (HF) in the acupuncture group. No adverse event was reported in this study. It was concluded that "Acupuncture demonstrates a significant immediate effect in reducing discomforts and VAS [Visual Analog

Scale] of both dizziness and vertigo. This study provides clinical evidence on the efficacy and safety of acupuncture to treat dizziness and vertigo in the emergency department."[1]

- A summary of the literature showed that acupuncture in the treatment of cervical vertigo acts to dilate blood vessels, diminish vessel resistance, and increase blood flow, hence to improve micro-circulation and oxygen supply to the brain.[2]

- The investigation at Jianghan University employed a combination of electroacupuncture and ultrasound for the treatment of vertigo, focusing on efficacy for the treatment of vertigo due to posterior circulation ischemia from dysfunction of the vertebrobasilar arterial system. This combination achieved a 94.29 percent total effective rate. As a standalone therapy, electroacupuncture achieved a 68.57 percent total effective rate. Using only ultrasound, the researchers achieved a 71.43 percent total effective rate. Based on the data, the researchers conclude that a combination of electroacupuncture and ultrasound therapies achieves superior patient outcomes over using either modality alone.[3]

1   Chiu, C-W., Lee, T-H., and Hsu, P-C. Efficacy and safety of acupuncture for dizziness and vertigo in emergency department: a pilot cohort study. *BMC Complementary and Alternative Medicine: The official journal of the International Society for Complementary Medicine Research (ISCMR)*. 2015; 15: 173. https://doi.org/10.1186/s12906-015-0704-6

2   Wang, Ai-ping. Research progress of acupuncture in treating cervical vertigo. *Journal of Acupuncture and Tuina Science*. 2004 Feb; 2(1): 57–60.

3   Huang, L-M., Wei, R-X., Chen, X-L., Yu, J-L., and Yang, Q-P. Curative efficacy of dynamic ultrasound combined with electric acupuncture for vertigo. *Chinese Journal of Rehabilitation*. 2014; 29(5).

Chapter 19

Tinnitus

Tinnitus is a ringing, buzzing, roaring, whistling, or hissing sound that seems to originate from within the ear or head. It is a commonly occurring symptom following a TBI. The noise may be constant or intermittent and vary in pitch from a low roar to a high squeal. It may be heard in one or both ears. It is not a single disease, but rather a symptom of an underlying condition. Heavy use of antibiotics or aspirin can also cause tinnitus to occur.

In many cases (though not all) tinnitus itself is not a serious problem, but rather a nuisance. Much of the literature on brain injury makes mention of it but does not tend to elaborate greatly. Statistics on experiencing some form of hearing loss have rates as high as 44 percent of persons whose injuries were not caused by a blast injury and 62 percent in cases of blast injuries.[1]

This can have an impact on one's means of communicating with others. Hearing loss can go unnoticed, however, and be attributed to confusion or deficits in attention and memory. An assessment by an audiologist may be needed to gauge the severity of hearing loss and possible causes.

Until fairly recently, most of the accounts of tinnitus in textbooks said it was exclusively due to ear damage which could not be fixed. More recent research, however, suggests that with the majority of cases of tinnitus there are no definable physical abnormalities within the ear. Researchers using positron emission tomography (PET scan) to view the brain activity of people with tinnitus have been able to show that these phantom auditory sensations originated somewhere in the brain, not within the ear. It seems, therefore, that tinnitus can be something akin to a phantom limb pain or focal dystonia, where symptoms result from aberrant neural activity in the brain.[2]

---

1   Lash, Marilyn. *The Essential Brain Injury Guide.* 5th ed. Vienna, VA: Academy of Certified Brain Injury Specialists, Brain Injury Association of America. 2016. Print.

2   University at Buffalo. Searching for the brain center responsible for tinnitus. *ScienceDaily*, 9 October 2007. www.sciencedaily.com/releases/2007/10/071005185125.htm

Etiology

- Traumatic (e.g. injury to head and neck)

- Atherosclerosis

- Occupational/noise-induced

- Toxic (e.g. aminoglycoside antibiotics, aspirin)

- Congenital (e.g. otosclerosis)

- Infectious (e.g. otitis media)

- Cardiovascular (also known as pulsatile tinnitus)

- Age-related (also known as presbycusis)

- Hypertension

- Turbulent blood flow

- Arteriovenous malformation

- Head and neck tumors

- Other (physical obstruction such as earwax, Meniere's disease, acoustic neuroma)

Biomedical Approaches

There are, as yet, no cures for tinnitus but there are several treatments currently used to produce relief:

- Acoustic therapy: The addition or enhancement of external sounds that can reduce the perception of tinnitus using any of the following:

  ◦ Sound generators that are worn in the ears

  ◦ Hearing aids

  ◦ Tapes, CDs, and bedside units that can help with sleep or concentration

  ◦ Pillows embedded with small speakers that can plug into any tape, CD, or sound generation machine

- Pharmaceutical: Tricyclic antidepressants such as amitriptyline, nortriptyline, gabapentin (Neurontin), and acamprosate (Campral)

- Surgical intervention

- Diet and lifestyle changes

- Counseling

- Tinnitus retraining therapy (TRT): A combination of low-level, broadband noise and counseling to achieve the habituation of tinnitus. That is, the individual becomes no longer aware of their tinnitus, except when they focus their attention on it, and even then tinnitus is not annoying or bothersome.[3]

Chinese Medical Perspective: Tinnitus and Deafness (Er Ming Er Long)

Er Ming: "Ear ringing" (e.g. cicadas, ocean tides)
Er Long: "Deafness; decline or loss of hearing"

Tinnitus and deafness may or may not present simultaneously clinically. While they have different manifestations, their pathogenesis in Chinese medical terms is essentially identical; this is the reason they are traditionally described together. Tinnitus can be one of the most difficult problems to treat. It can be categorized as either resistant or responsive tinnitus.

Resistant tinnitus is hearing nerve damage or damage to the inner ear due to tumor, acoustic trauma, surgery, otosclerosis, and cochlear and auditory nerve lesions. Responsive tinnitus is broken down by etiology: stress, fatigue, and idiopathic tinnitus, as well as local vs. central or medication induced.

Local problems are defined as ear wax blockage, Eustachian tube abnormality, severe ear infection, flow disturbances of the carotid artery or jugular vein, allergies, and cervical injury. Central problems include high or low blood pressure, lyme disease, diabetes, anemia, and side effects of medication (anti-inflammatories, sedatives, antidepressants, cancer treatment medication, aspirin, nicotine, antibiotics).

Chinese Medical Etiology

- Differentiate excess from deficiency

- Excess patterns are characterized by a sudden onset and loud, high-pitched ringing

- Deficiency patterns are characterized by a gradual onset and soft, low-pitched sounds

TCM Pattern Differentiation
Wind-Heat Invasion

Primary symptoms: Common wind-heat symptoms include sore throat, fever, aversion to cold, headache, and dry mouth

Additional symptoms: Distension and obstruction within the ears with possible earache leading to tinnitus and impairment of hearing

---

3 Jastreboff, P. and Jastreboff, M. Tinnitus retraining therapy: an update. *Audiologyonline.com*. 23 October 2000. www.audiologyonline.com/articles/tinnitus-retraining-therapy-an-update-1286

Tongue: Possible red tongue tip, thin, yellow tongue coating

Pulse: Floating and rapid

Treatment principles: Disperse wind, clear heat, open the orifices

Acupuncture treatment: [TW-3, TW-17, TW-21, SI-19, GB-2, GB-43] + TW-5, LI-4, LI-11

Herbal treatment:
Yin Qiao San (Honeysuckle and Forsynthia Powder)
[Jin Yin Hua 10–30g, Lian Qiao 10–30g, Dan Dou Chi 10g, Niu Bang Zi 10g, Bo He 10g, Jing Jie 10g, Jie Geng 5g, Lu Gen 10g, Gan Cao 3g]

Liver and Gallbladder Fire

Primary symptoms: Sudden onset of loud tinnitus or deafness with the tinnitus resembling ocean waves or claps of thunder; onset of symptoms or increase in severity of symptoms with anger or frustration

Additional symptoms: Headache, dizziness and vertigo, epistaxis, earache, distending sensation of the ears, flushed complexion, red eyes, dry mouth, bitter taste in mouth, irritability, irascibility, restlessness, insomnia, distension and pain of the chest and hypochondrium, constipation, dark urine

Tongue: Red with yellow coating

Pulse: Rapid, wiry, forceful

Treatment principles: Drain Liver and Gallbladder Fire, open the orifices

Acupuncture treatment: [TW-3, TW-17, TW-21, SI-19, GB-2, GB-43] + LR-2, LR-3, GB-34, GB-41

Herbal treatment:
Long Dan Xie Gan Tang (Gentiana Decoction to Drain the Liver)
[Long Dan Cao 10–15g, Huang Qin 10g, Shan Zhi Zi 10g, Ze Xie 10g, Mu Tong 6g, Dang Gui 10g, Che Qian Zi 10g, Sheng Di Huang 10g, Chai Hu 6g, Gan Cao 6g]

Herbal treatment for Liver Depression transforming to Heat (less pronounced Fire):
Jia Wei Xiao Yao San (Augmented Rambling Powder)
[Chai Hu 10g, Bai Shao 10g, Dang Gui 10g, Bai Zu 10g, Fu Ling 10g, Zhi Gan Cao 6g, Pao Jiang 6g, Bo He 6g, Zhi Zi 10g, Mu Dan Pi 10g]

Binding Depression of Phlegm-Fire

Primary symptoms: Tinnitus and deafness accompanied by dizzy spells, sensation of heaviness of the head

Additional symptoms: Oppression in the chest, profuse phlegm, bitter taste in the mouth, irregularity of urination and bowel movements

Tongue: Red with greasy, yellow coating

Pulse: Slippery, wiry, or rapid

Treatment principles: Drain fire, transform phlegm, open the orifices

Acupuncture treatment: [TW-3, TW-17, TW-21, SI-19, GB-2, GB-43] + ST-40, PC-8

Herbal treatment:
Huang Lian Wen Dan Tang Jia Wei (Coptis Decoction to Warm the Gallbladder Plus Additions)
[Zhu Ru 10g, Zhi Shi 10g, Ban Xia 10g, Chen Pi 6g, Fu Ling 10g, Huang Lian 5g, Gan Cao 6g, Sheng Jiang 3pc]

Blood Stasis

Primary symptoms: Persistent tinnitus and/or hearing loss, possibly associated with black discharge from the ear or dark matter mixed with ear wax; possible earache

Additional symptoms: Dark complexion, possible headache

Tongue: Purple or purple spots with thin coat

Pulse: Wiry or choppy and thready

Treatment principles: Quicken the Blood, eliminate stasis, open the orifice

Acupuncture treatment: [TW-3, TW-17, TW-21, SI-19, GB-2, GB-43] + LR-3, LI-4, SP-10, SP-6, BL-17

Herbal treatment:
When stasis is confined to head: Tong Qiao Huo Xue Tang (Open the Portals and Quicken the Blood Decoction)
[Tao Ren 10g, Hong Hua 10g, Chi Shao Yao 10g, Chuan Xiong 9g, She Xiang 0.15g, Cong Bai 3g, Sheng Jiang 3pc, Da Zao 7pc]

When Blood stasis is more systemic: Xue Fu Zhu Yu Tang (Drive Out Stasis in the Mansion of Blood Decoction)
[Tao Ren 12g, Hong Hua 10g, Chuan Niu Xi 10g, Dang Gui 10g, Chi Shao Yao 6g, Chuan Xiong 6g, Zhi Ke 6g, Jie Geng 6g, Chai Hu 6g, Gan Cao 3g]

Note: This pattern usually follows after some trauma to the head or injury to the ear, including exposure to loud noise or sudden pressure changes. It can also complicate other chronic patterns of tinnitus or hearing loss.

Kidney Essence Depletion

Primary symptoms: Gradual onset of tinnitus or hearing loss/deafness associated with aging or chronic illness; tinnitus resembles the buzzing of cicadas, may be intermittent, and is often worse at night

Additional symptoms: Dizziness and vertigo, insomnia, weak, aching low back and knees, seminal emission

Tongue: Red with scanty coating

Pulse: Thin or rapid

Treatment principles: Supplement the Kidneys, secure the Essence

Acupuncture treatment: [TW-3, TW-17, TW-21, SI-19, GB-2] + BL-23, KI-3, SP-6, CV-4, GV-4

Herbal treatment:
Er Long Zuo Ci Wan (Pill for Deafness that is Kind to the Left [Kidney])
[Shu Di Huang 24g, Shan Zhu Yu 12g, Shan Yao 12g, Mu Dan Pi 9g, Ze Xie 9g, Fu Ling 9g, Shi Chang Pu 6g, Wu Wei Zi 6g, Ci Shi 30g]

Spleen and Stomach Qi Deficiency

Primary symptoms: Tinnitus and deafness aggravated by overwork, sensation of emptiness and coolness within the ears

Additional symptoms: Accompanied by tiredness, fatigue, poor appetite, loose stools, epigastric distension after eating and a sallow, withered complexion, pale tongue with white coating, weak pulse

Treatment principles: Strengthen the Spleen and Stomach, boost Qi

Acupuncture treatment: [TW-3, TW-17, TW-21, SI-19, GB-2] + BL-20, BL-21, ST-36, SP-6, CV-6

Herbal treatment:
Bu Zhong Yi Qi Tang (Supplement the Center and Boost the Qi Decoction)
[Huang Qi 10–60g, Dang Shen 10g, Bai Zhu 10g, Dang Gui 10g, Chen Pi 10g, Sheng Ma 5–15g, Chai Hu 5g, Zhi Gan Cao 3g]

Auricular acupuncture:

Subcortex, Endocrine, Liver, Kidney, Inner Ear, Shen Men

Occiput, Inner Ear, (Outer) Ear, Kidney

Scalp and electroacupuncture treatment of tinnitus and deafness: Insert three needles along Jiao Auditory Line (a 4cm horizontal line, with the midpoint 1.5cm directly above the apex of the ear; at about GB-8). Needle the two end points and the middle point obliquely downward, angled towards the apex.

Clinical Notes

- The pitch or loudness of tinnitus should not be taken as a sure indicator of excess; always corroborate these signs with the individual's other symptoms to determine the pathology and pattern.

- Children are less likely to complain of tinnitus or loss of hearing, but will complain of earache.

- Chronic tinnitus, especially of gradual onset, can be very recalcitrant to treatment by acupuncture alone, especially when Kidney Xu (Deficiency) is an important etiologic factor.

- Consider distal points on Gall Bladder, Triple Warmer, and/or Small Intestine channels if onset of the tinnitus followed an incident of physical trauma to such areas which may have left residual Xue Yu (Blood Stasis) and subsequently affected the channel(s) in its relationship to the ear.

- TW-17 and GB-20 can be a potent combination and can release the musculature in the occipital region, so much so that stimulation with the lift–thrust technique or twisting the needle can sometimes bring the volume of ringing down in real time almost like a volume knob on a stereo. Taking time to find the proper angle and position can at times provide significant relief to the individual.

Herbs Specific for Ear Disorders

- Ci Shi
- Dong Chong Xia Cao
- Ge Gen
- He Shou Wu

- Long Dan Cao
- Mu Li
- Nu Zhen Zi
- Shan Zhu Yu

Other Treatment Considerations
Orthomolecular Considerations

- Oral magnesium (aspartate)—low levels of magnesium (~200mg) are associated with noise-induced hearing loss; supplementation with magnesium has been shown to prevent noise-induced hearing loss.[4]

- Cobalamin (B12)—individuals with tinnitus and noise-induced hearing loss have demonstrated significant vitamin B12 deficiency. Determination of vitamin B12 status in individuals with tinnitus and noise-induced hearing loss is warranted. If low, supplement with 2000 mcg daily for one month, followed by 1000 mcg daily thereafter (sublingual methylcobalamin is preferred form). Take with folic acid.[5]

Phytotherapeutic Considerations

- Oats: Nerve tonic

- Prickly ash: Circulatory stimulant

- Ginkgo biloba (standardized extract): 40mg, three times a day. It may take three months or more of continued use

- Goldenseal: Catarrhal deafness and tinnitus

- St. John's wort: Internally; oil, locally in the ear canal

- Catsfoot: Tinnitus aurium

- Mullein

- Periwinkle[6, 7]

- Black cohosh: Vertigo from auditory tinnitus

Dietary Considerations

Eating principles:

- Low fat diet, low sugar, high complex carbohydrates

- Protein 12–15 percent of diet

- Low cholesterol foods

- Vegetarian cleansing diet or short fasts

---

4   Attias, J., Weisz, G., Almog, S., *et al.* Oral magnesium intake reduces permanent hearing loss induced by noise exposure. *American Journal of Otolaryngology.* 1994; 15: 26–32.

5   Shemesh, Z., Attias, J., Ornan, M., Shapira, N., and Shahar, A. Vitamin B12 deficiency in patients with chronic-tinnitus and noise-induced hearing loss. *American Journal of Otolaryngology.* 1993; 14(2): 94–99. http://dx.doi.org/10.1016/0196-0709(93)90046-A

6   Patyar, S., Prakash, A., Modi, M., and Medhi, B. Role of vinpocetine in cerebrovascular diseases. *Pharmacological Reports.* 2011; 63(3): 618–628. https://doi.org/10.1016/S1734-1140(11)70574-6

7   Hahn, A., Radkova, L., Achiemere, G., Klement, V., Alpini, D., and Strouhal, J. Multimodal therapy for chronic tinnitus. *International Tinnitus Journal.* 2008; 14(1): 69–72.

Chronic:

- Elimination/rotation diet, rotation diet, rotation diet expanded

Kidney (Deficiency) type:

- Foods that tonify the Kidney, Yang, and foods that tonify the Yin: black sesame seeds, black beans, celery, oyster shells, pearl barley, adzuki beans, black jujube, yams, lotus seed, chestnuts, grapes

- Avoid stimulating foods, hot, spicy foods, rich foods, coffee, alcohol

Liver Fire type:

- Heat-clearing foods, soothe the Liver foods, tonify the Liver foods

- Liver-cleansing foods: beets, carrots, artichokes, lemons, parsnips, dandelion greens, watercress, burdock root, chrysanthemum flowers and tea

- Avoid: stimulating foods, hot, spicy foods, rich foods, coffee, alcohol

Research Studies

- Two separate groups were tested with the acupuncture point prescriptions. Both groups had an acupuncture needle retention time of 30 minutes. Acupuncture was conducted once per day for a grand total of 18 acupuncture treatments. The first set of acupuncture points outperformed the second set by 30 percent with a total effective rate of 80 percent. A total of 64.17 percent of patients fully recovered, 14.71 percent had significant improvements, 11.76 percent had slight improvements, and 8.82 percent had no improvements. The total effective rate was 91.18 percent. The researchers concluded that acupuncture combined with ginger moxibustion is effective for the treatment of intractable tinnitus. The researchers note that widespread adoption of this clinical treatment protocol is warranted based on the significant rate of positive patient outcomes.[8]

- Fifty patients (46 males, 4 females) suffering from tinnitus were randomly assigned to three groups: a manual acupuncture group (MA), an electrical acupuncture group (EA), and a placebo group (PL). The frequency of tinnitus occurrence, tinnitus intensity, and reduction of life quality were recorded before treatment (Baseline), after six treatments (After-Treatment), and one month after the completion of treatment (1-Month-After). Standard audiometric tests were conducted on each patient at Baseline and After-Treatment. Six treatments were performed at weekly intervals. The frequency of tinnitus occurrence and the tinnitus loudness were

---

8   Song, Y., Li, S., Xiao, Y., and Wu, J. Efficacy observation of acupuncture combined with ginger moxibustion to treatment of 34 cases of intractable tinnitus. *Zhongyi Zhongyao* [Traditional Chinese Medicine and Herbs]. 2013 Aug: 277–278.

significantly decreased After-Treatment compared with Baseline in the EA group. Life quality was improved After-Treatment and at 1-Month-After compared with Baseline in both MA and EA groups. However, no significant differences were detected among the three groups, with the audiogram not showing any significant changes after treatment in either group (P > 0.091). The overall subjective evaluation indicated significant improvements After-Treatment compared with Baseline in both MA and EA groups. After-Treatment subjective evaluation was significantly better in the EA group compared with either the MA or PL group.[9]

- Ninety cases of nervous tinnitus were randomly divided evenly into three groups, 30 cases in each group. The acupuncture group were treated with acupuncture at cervical Jiaji (EX-B 2), 20 minutes each session, once a day, with ten sessions constituting one course. The Chinese herbs group was treated with modified Buzhong Yiqi Decoction (decocted in water), one dose each day, with ten doses constituting one course; the Western medicine group with bandazol, Dextran 40, Danshen tablet, and vitamin B12, with ten days constituting one course. After three courses, the therapeutic effects were evaluated, finding the effective rates in the three groups, which were 73.3 percent, 40.0 percent, and 33.3 percent, respectively, with significant differences among the three groups. It was concluded that "Acupuncture has obvious therapeutic effect on nervous tinnitus, and acupuncture at cervical Jiaji (EX-B 2) is an effective therapy for nervous tinnitus, and its therapeutic effect is better than those of Chinese herbs and Western medicine."[10]

9   Wang, K., Bugge, J., and Bugge, S. A randomised, placebo-controlled trial of manual and electrical acupuncture for the treatment of tinnitus. *Complementary Therapies in Medicine*. 2010; 18(6): 249–255. http://dx.doi.org/10.1016/j.ctim.2010.09.005

10   Tan, K-Q., Zhang, C., Liu, M-X., and Qiu, L. [Comparative study on therapeutic effects of acupuncture, Chinese herbs, and Western medicine on nervous tinnitus]. *Zhongguo Zhenjiu* [Chinese Acupuncture and Moxibustion]. 2007 Apr; 27(4): 249–251.

Chapter 20

Nausea and Vomiting

Nausea can frequently occur following a brain injury. This is particularly true initially following a mild TBI. In cases where other symptoms are present or become chronic such as headaches, migraines, dizziness/vertigo, dysphagia, visual disturbances, and seizures, nausea may accompany them as a secondary concern. Because nausea generally accompanies these other conditions, it is rarely addressed or studied on its own. This results in a lack of occurrence statistics within the literature. Because at times nausea and/or vomiting can become severe enough to warrant specific treatment, it is worth including treatment methods as found in the Chinese medical literature.

Vomiting (emesis) is the actual oral expulsion of gastrointestinal contents resulting in contractions of the gut and the thoracoabdominal wall musculature. This contrasts with regurgitation, which is the effortless passage of gastric contents into the mouth. Retching is the term used to describe the muscular events of vomiting without expulsion of vomitus (i.e. "dry heaves"). The term nausea refers to a subjective feeling of the need to vomit. The nauseated patient does not necessarily vomit or retch. Nausea should be distinguished from dyspepsia (upset stomach), which encompasses epigastric burning, gnawing discomfort, bloating, or pain. It is not uncommon for nausea to accompany dyspepsia, but they are distinct events.

The vomiting center lies in the medulla oblongata and comprises the reticular formation and the nucleus of the tractus solitarius. When activated, motor pathways descend from this center and trigger vomiting. These efferent pathways travel within the 5th, 7th, 9th, 10th, and 12th cranial nerves to the upper gastrointestinal tract, the lower tract signaling traveling within vagal and sympathetic nerves. Signals within spinal nerves travel to the diaphragm and abdominal muscles. The vomiting center can be activated directly by irritants or indirectly following input from four principal areas: the gastrointestinal tract, cerebral cortex and thalamus, vestibular region, and the chemoreceptor trigger zone (CRTZ). The CRTZ is closest in proximity, lying between the medulla and the floor of the fourth ventricle. Unlike other brain centers, it is not protected by the blood–brain barrier. This is to say that the endothelium of its capillaries is not tightly joined or surrounded by glial cells and is easily permeated by irritants regardless of their lipid solubility or molecular size.[1] Before vomiting occurs, there may be a period of antiperistalsis, in which rhythmic contractions occur up the digestive tract instead of downward. This may commence as far down as the ileum, with the antiperistaltic wave pushing contents of the lower small intestine upward into the duodenum and stomach within a few minutes. Distension within these upper portions of the gastrointestinal tract then generates afferent impulses to the vomiting center, where the actual act of vomiting is initiated. For this reason, an empty stomach does not preclude the expulsion of vomitus. At the onset of vomiting, intrinsic contractions occur in both the duodenum and the stomach, the lower esophageal sphincter relaxes, and vomitus moves from the stomach into the esophagus. Next, the inspiratory and abdominal muscles contract and expel the vomitus upward.

Biomedical Approaches

Antiemetic Drugs

Those that block acetylcholine and histamine appear most useful when vestibular triggers are suspected. Dopamine blockade targets the emetogenic influence of opioids in the vomiting center and CRTZ. Unfortunately, their ability to also block dopamine transmission in the basal ganglia can result in so-called extrapyramidal syndromes (EPSs) that include akathisia (restlessness), parkinsonian symptoms, and tardive dyskinesia. The serotonin antagonists act not only in the vomiting center but within the GI tract, where surgical manipulation or many of the chemotherapeutic agents generate a noxious influence. Anxiolytic medications are useful in cases where anticipatory anxiety is high.

Dopamine Antagonists

- Promethazine (Phenergan)—a commonly used antiemetic
- Prochlorperazine (Compazine)—another commonly used antiemetic
- Metoclopramide (Reglan)—has a prokinetic action on the upper digestive tract
- Droperidol—may trigger tachyarrhythmia

5-HT3 (Serotonin) Blockers

The 5-HT3 (serotonin) antagonists were introduced initially to combat radiation and chemotherapy-induced nausea and vomiting. This was due to chemotherapeutic agents triggering serotonin release within the gastrointestinal wall.

- Ondansetron (Zofran)

---

1   Becker, D. Nausea, vomiting, and hiccups: a review of mechanisms and treatment. *Anesthesia Progress.* 2010; 57(4): 150–157. PMC. Web. 17 Oct. 2017.

Novel Agents

Drugs that block the neurokinin 1 (NK1) receptor have proven efficacy in chemotherapy-induced nausea and vomiting. They are most effective in preventing delayed nausea and generally are used in conjunction with 5-HT3 antagonists for this reason.

- Aprepitant (Emend)

- Cannabinols such as tetrahydrocannabinol found in marijuana and dronabinol (Marinol), a synthetic derivative, have proven effective for chemotherapy-induced nausea and vomiting

- Glucocorticoids

- Dexamethasone: mechanism unknown but may suppress production of inflammatory autacoids that may somehow potentiate known vomiting pathways within the vomiting center. Benefit is limited to prophylactic regimens

Chinese Medical Perspective: Nausea (Ě Xīn) and Vomiting (Ǒu Tù)

Vomiting results from disharmony of the Stomach and rebellion of Stomach Qi. Nausea shares the same etiology and pathology as vomiting in TCM, so the two are discussed together.

Classically, Chinese medicine distinguished between heaving (ǒu = vomiting accompanied by sound), disgorgement (tù = vomiting without any sound), and retching (gān ǒu = involuntary effort to vomit accompanied by sound but without actual emesis). Despite these classical distinctions, today vomiting is looked upon as one disorder (ǒu tù).

Relevant Biomedical Diseases

- Acute or chronic gastritis
- Acute hepatitis
- Acute pancreatitis
- Acute cholecystitis
- Acute appendicitis
- Meniere's disease
- Morning sickness
- Viral or bacterial infection
- Esophageal obstruction
- Pyloric obstruction
- Head trauma (concussion)
- Peptic ulcer
- Renal failure
- Medication induced

Chinese Medical Etiology

The pathology of nausea and vomiting ultimately involves rebellion of Stomach Qi regardless of the pattern.

- Invasion of wind, cold, damp, or summer-heat pathogens may lead to rebellious Stomach Qi

- Improper diet (excessive consumption of raw, cold, greasy food or consumption of contaminated food or excessive antibiotic use) may lead to injury of the Spleen/Stomach, creating food stagnation or phlegm-fluids and ultimately rebellious Stomach Qi

- Rumination or excessive worry may lead to Qi stagnation in the Stomach or impairment of transformation and transportation of the Spleen, creating phlegm-fluids and rebellious Stomach Qi

- Anger and frustration may lead to stagnation of Liver Qi to where Liver Qi overacts onto the Stomach or Liver Qi overacting on Spleen, causing an impairment of transformation and transportation of the Spleen, creating phlegm-fluids and rebellious Stomach Qi

- Chronic disease, congenital deficiency, taxation fatigue, chronic poor diet, or chronic emotional distress may lead to Spleen/Stomach deficiency which may cause cold rebellious Stomach Qi

- Chronic disease, congenital deficiency, taxation fatigue, febrile disease, chronic poor diet, or chronic emotional distress may lead to Stomach Yin deficiency and ultimately rebellious Stomach Qi

Differential Diagnosis

Acid reflux (tūn suān): The swallowing of upwelling stomach acid; nausea and vomiting uncommon

Hiccup (è ni): Involuntary contraction of the diaphragm causing sudden, audible inspiration that is checked by a spasmodic closure of the glottis; nausea and vomiting uncommon

Stomach reflux (fǎn wèi): Vomiting of undigested food that was ingested many hours before

Dysphagia-occlusion (yē gé): Yē means difficulty swallowing; gé means blockage that prevents the downward passage of food and liquids after swallowing; dysphagia may occur alone but often leads to occlusion

Sudden turmoil disorder (huò luàn): A disease characterized by simultaneous vomiting and diarrhea usually followed by severe cramps; overlaps with cholera and acute gastroenteritis in biomedicine

Accompanying Signs and Symptoms

- Headache and fever: Exogenous pathogen

- Acute with cramping abdominal pain: Exogenous pathogen, Liver Qi stagnation

- With epigastric distension, belching, and bad breath: Stagnation of food in the Stomach

- Symptoms aggravated by emotional stress: Liver Qi attacking the Stomach

Type of Vomitus

- Scanty vomitus or dry retching: Stomach Yin deficiency

- Watery vomitus: Phlegm-Fluids or Spleen/Stomach deficiency cold

TCM Pattern Differentiation
Exogenous Pathogen Attacking the Stomach

Primary symptoms: Sudden onset of vomiting with a history of contraction of EPI

Additional symptoms, tongue, and pulse:

- Accompanied by fever, chills, headache, no sweating, thin, white tongue coating, and floating tight pulse if caused by pathogenic Wind-Cold

- Accompanied by fever, sweating, dysphoria, thirst, red tongue with yellow greasy coating, and moderate rapid pulse if caused by Summer-Heat and Dampness

- Accompanied by fever, aversion to wind, headache, spontaneous sweating, red tongue with thin yellow coating, and floating rapid pulse if caused by pathogenic Wind-Heat

Treatment principles: Dispel exogenous pathogenic factors, transform turbidity with aromatic herbs to harmonize the Stomach and descend Stomach Qi

Acupuncture treatment: [CV-12, ST-36, SP-4, PC-6] + LI-4, GB-20

Herbal treatment:
Huo Xiang Zheng Qi San (Agastache/Patchouli Qi Righting Powder)
[Huo Xiang 12g, Zi Su Ye 6g, Bai Zhi 6g, Chen Pi 9g, Da Fu Pi 9g, Hou Po 9g,

Bai Zhu 12g, Fu Ling 9g, Jie Geng 9g, Sheng Jiang 6g, Da Zao 2pc, Zhi Gan Cao 3g]

Modifications:
Heat type: Use Yin Qiao San
Summer-Heat type: Use Xiang Jia Xiang Ru Yin
If abnormal sweating: Also consider Gui Zhi Tang (if scratchy throat + Jie Geng)

Food Stagnation in the Stomach

Primary symptoms: Vomiting of acidic, foul-smelling vomitus, aggravated by eating and relieved after vomiting

Additional symptoms: Fullness and distension in the epigastrium and abdomen, bad breath, abdominal pain relieved after vomiting, anorexia, foul-smelling loose or dry stools

Tongue: Thick, greasy coating

Pulse: Slippery

Treatment principle: Disperse food, eliminate stagnation, and relieve vomiting

Acupuncture treatment: [CV-12, ST-36, SP-4, PC-6] + CV-10, CV-21

Herbal treatment:
Bao He Wan (Harmony Preserving Pill)
[Ban Xia 10g, Chen Pi 10g, Zhi Gan Cao 10g, Shan Zha 10g, Shen Qu 10g, Lai Fu Zi 10g, Lian Qiao 10g]

Accumulation of Phlegm-Fluids in the Stomach

Primary symptoms: Vomiting of clear liquid and mucus

Additional symptoms: Distension in the chest and epigastrium, poor appetite, dizziness, palpitation

Tongue: White, greasy coating

Pulse: Slippery

Treatment principle: Warm and transform Phlegm-Fluids, harmonize the Stomach, relieve vomiting

Acupuncture treatment: [CV-12, ST-36, SP-4, PC-6] + CV-17, ST-40

Herbal treatment:
Xiao Ban Xia Tang + Ling Gui Zhu Gan Tang (Minor Pinellia Decoction + Poria, Cinnamon, Atractylodes, and Licorice Decoction)

[Ban Xia 10g, Sheng Jiang 10g, Fu Ling 10g, Gui Zhi 5g, Bai Zhu 10g, Zhi Gan Cao 3g]

Liver Qi Attacking the Stomach

Primary symptoms: Vomiting accompanied by acid regurgitation and frequent eructation that temporarily relieves nausea, symptoms aggravated by emotional stress

Additional symptoms: Fullness and pain in the chest and hypochondrium

Tongue: Normal color or slightly red on the sides, thin, greasy coating

Pulse: Wiry (bowstring)

Treatment principle: Soothe the Liver, harmonize the Stomach to descend Qi and relieve vomiting

Acupuncture treatment: [CV-12, ST-36, SP-4, PC-6] + LR-3, LR-24, GB-24

Herbal treatment:
Ban Xia Hou Po Tang (Pinellia and Magnolia Bark Decoction) + Zuo Jin Wan (Left Gold Pill)
[Ban Xia 9–12g, Hou Po 9g, Fu Ling 12g, Sheng Jiang 15g, Zi Su Ye 6g + Huang Lian 3g, Wu Zhu Yu 0.5g]

Spleen and Stomach Deficiency Cold

Primary symptoms: Chronic, intermittent vomiting, often induced by a slight increase in food intake

Additional symptoms: Poor appetite, indigestion, epigastric fullness, lusterless face, lassitude, preference for warmth and aversion to cold, cold extremities, loose stools, possible dry mouth without desire to drink

Tongue: Pale with thin white coating

Pulse: Thin, weak

Treatment principle: Warm the middle Jiao, strengthen the Spleen, harmonize the Stomach and descend rebellious Qi

Acupuncture treatment: [CV-12, ST-36, SP-4, PC-6] + BL-20, BL-21

Herbal treatment:
Li Zhong Tang (Center Rectifying Decoction)
[Ren Shen 10g, Bai Zhu 10g, Gan Jiang 6g, Zhi Gan Cao 6g]

Stomach Yin Deficiency

Primary symptoms: Chronic, recurrent vomiting with scant vomitus or simply dry heaves

Additional symptoms: Dry mouth and throat, hunger without desire to eat, dull epigastric pain or discomfort, dry stool

Tongue: Dry and red with scanty coating

Pulse: Thin, rapid

Treatment principle: Nourish Stomach Yin, descend rebellious Qi, stop vomiting

Acupuncture treatment: [CV-12, ST-36, SP-4, PC-6] + SP-6, KI-3

Herbal treatment:
Mai Men Dong Tang (Ophiopogon Tuber Decoction)
[Mai Men Dong 15–18g, Ban Xia 15–18g, Ren Shen 6g, Jing Mi 15–30g, Da Zao 3–4pc, Gan Cao 6g]

Clinical Notes

- Referral to an acute-care medical facility is strongly recommended if dehydration due to severe vomiting is evident. Referral is also necessary if there is projectile vomiting with blood in the vomit, high fever, severe headache, irritability, lethargy, or unconsciousness.

- It may be difficult for a patient who is nauseated or vomiting to take a herbal decoction. Therefore, it may be helpful to administer the daily dose of the decoction in smaller quantities at more frequent intervals.

- Patients with persistent nausea may benefit from placement of intradermal needles over one of the primary acupuncture points. Palpation and holding points for five to ten seconds to gauge which elicits the greatest relief may guide which point(s) to utilize.

- "Sea Bands" or similar products that apply pressure over PC-6 may be a useful and accessible option for some.

Other Treatment Considerations
Potential Contributing Factors

- Variations in blood calcium levels
- Potassium excess

- Zinc toxicity

- Biotin toxicity

- Manganese excess

- Niacin toxicity

- Iodine toxicity

- Selenium excess

Dietary Recommendations

- Avoid spicy meals, alcohol, and fats

- Ginger (Gan Jiang) can often be effective for nausea

- Peppermint

Research Studies

Stimulation of point PC-6 has been studied and been found to be significantly effective in cases of postoperative nausea and vomiting (PONV). Acupuncture may reduce nausea and vomiting via endogenous beta-endorphin release in the cerebrospinal fluid or a change in serotonin transmission via activation of serotonergic and noradrenergic fibers. The exact mechanisms have yet to be established. Electroacupuncture at this point is also effective for postoperative nausea. "Stimulation of P6 has been shown to be as effective as pharmacological treatment for PONV with ondansetron in both adults and children."[2]

---

2   Chernyak, Grigory V. and Sessler, Daniel I. Perioperative acupuncture and related techniques. *Anesthesiology*. 2005; 102(5): 1031–1078.

Chapter 21

Dysphagia

Dysphagia is a disturbance in ability to swallow. It can occur for many reasons including motor control impairment, weakness of facial, masticatory, pharyngeal, or laryngo-esophageal muscles, a loss of coordination between breathing and muscle function, and changes in sensory processing. The gastrointestinal system involves regulation from the hypothalamus via the parasympathetic and sympathetic nervous systems. The gastrointestinal tract and the higher brain structures also regulate nutritional intake. Either sensory or motor neural deficits can lead to oropharyngeal dysphagia. Isolated cranial nerve deficits can include the facial nerve (CN VII), glossopharyngeal nerve (CN IX), vagus nerve (CN X), and hypoglossal nerve (CN XII).

Diagnostic Testing

Diagnostically a modified barium swallow test will be done by a radiologist or physiatrist and speech language pathologist.

- The Videofluoroscopic Swallowing Study (VFSS) is a barium-swallowing examination employing real-time X-rays for the visualization of bolus flow and structural movements in the aerodigestive tract. The VFSS is particularly helpful in determining improvements for swallowing food and developing strategies toward restoring oral nutrient intake.

- The water-swallowing test (WST) is a functional exam that detects aspiration and is useful in developing strategies to prevent pneumonia. The WST assesses drinking and its relation to successful swallows, swallowing speed, time to swallow, coughing, choking, or otherwise having to stop ingestion of water.

- The Swallowing Quality of Life Questionnaire (SWAL-QOL) evaluates 44 items and ten quality of life components to determine patient satisfaction and the quality of therapeutic care.

Following a brain injury an individual may require being intubated for a period of time. A feeding tube will provide both hydration and calories via the tube being surgically implanted into either the stomach (gastrostomy) or the small intestine (jejunostomy). These require nurses, trained staff, or family to assure proper administration to prevent risks of aspiration or over-distension. There are four levels of diet abilities in dysphagia. The level of lowest functionality is dysphagia pureed, followed by dysphagia mechanically altered, dysphagia advanced, and finally regular diet, with each level allowing for consumption of more complex foods. This information is found in Table 21.1.

TABLE 21.1 Diet Ability Levels in Dysphagia

Level	Dysphagia Severity	Description
Level 1 Dysphagia pureed	Moderate to severe	Consists of pureed, homogenous, and cohesive foods with a consistency akin to pudding. Foods requiring bolus formation, controlled manipulation, and chewing are not allowed
Level 2 Dysphagia mechanically altered	Mild to moderate and/ or pharyngeal dysphagia	All foods from level 1, plus foods that are moist, soft textured, and easily form a bolus. Food pieces no larger than 1/4 inch. Some chewing ability
Level 3 Dysphagia advanced	Mild	This level includes most textures except hard, sticky, or crunchy foods. It includes soft foods that require chewing ability
Level 4 Regular diet	N/A	All foods are tolerated

There are also four levels of liquid viscosity tolerated, as shown in Table 21.2.

TABLE 21.2 Liquid tolerance Levels in Dysphagia

Level	Description
Thin	No alteration
Nectar-like	Slightly thicker than water, the consistency of un-set gelatin
Honey-like	A liquid with the consistency of honey
Spoon-thick	A liquid with the consistency of pudding

Therapeutic Interventions

- Cold stimulation
- Practicing of swallowing
- Breath hold techniques
- Voicing exercises

- Throat contraction exercises
- Throat lifting exercises
- Face and lips muscle functional training

Other Possible Concerns

Gastrointestinal concerns following a brain injury include hyperphasia (excessive eating), coughing while eating, dehydration, anorexia (disinterest or loss of appetite), and gastroesophageal reflux disease (GERD).

Biomedical Approaches

Biomedical medications for GERD include Prilosec, Protonix, Zantac, Pepcid, and Reglan.

Though blocking acid production and reflux, these may increase the risk of cognitive changes or impairment.

The detrimental effects of dysphagia can have a significant impact. The metabolic needs of the individual increase significantly following a moderate-to-severe brain injury as the body requires these resources to heal the brain. This is required for the health of all cells, adequate cognitive function, and overall recovery. The Congress of Neurological Surgeons states that a person will need at least 40 percent more calories in the acute phase than prior to the injury. This increases in relation to the severity of the injury and the effects can at times persist indefinitely.

Chinese Medical Perspective: Dysphagia Occlusion (Ye Ge)

Dysphagia in Chinese medicine is referred to as dysphagia occlusion (Ye Ge), wind-stroke, or Yin Fei.

Chinese Medical Etiology

A deficiency of Kidney Yin, emptying of the sea of marrow, and obstruction of the meridians and collaterals by wind-phlegm and/or Blood stasis are possible etiological factors in dysphagia.[1] It is not explored in many sources as a separate condition, but rather the pattern differentiation of the previous chapter on nausea and vomiting applies. Acupuncture's efficacy as a treatment for dysphagia is linked to its ability to:

- Increase production of saliva
- Restore the swallowing reflex by stimulating local nerve sensory receptors

---

1   Flaws, Bob and Lake, James. *Chinese Medical Psychiatry: a textbook and clinical manual: including indications for referral to Western medical services.* Boulder, CO: Blue Poppy. 2003. Print.

- Inhibit the fibrosis process[2]

In this chapter we will list acupuncture points indicated for dysphagia or difficulty swallowing as well as some of the research that has been done.

Acupuncture Point Considerations

In addition to pattern differentiation there are a number of points indicated for either difficulty swallowing or dysphagia. Local points near the larynx or hyoid regions can aid in stimulating the smooth musculature of the esophagus and aid in swallowing. It is very important to perform shallow needling in these points so as to avoid puncturing the vasculature or the airway.

> *Local*: SI-17, CV-17, CV-22, CV-23, CV-24, ST-4, LI-18

> ***Distal points and their relevant clinical indications***:
> PC-8 "Inability to Swallow Food"
> GB-39 "Occlusion of the throat with oppressive feeling, difficulties in swallowing"
> TW-7 "Tongue paralyzed, cannot swallow (glosso-labio-pharyngeal paralysis)"
> BL-17 "Difficulty swallowing"
> BL-21 "Dysphagia"
> LI-11 "Dysphagia"
> Points correlating to potentially affected cranial nerves according to Yamamoto New Scalp[3]

Acupuncture may also be helpful, including:

- Facial nerve (CN VII)
- Vagus nerve (CN X)
- Glossopharyngeal nerve (CN IX)
- Hypoglossal nerve (CN XII)

Other Therapeutic Considerations
Phytotherapeutic Considerations

- Tan Xiang (White Sandalwood)
- Blackcurrant
- Fig
- Silver Linden

---

2   Chan, S-L., Or, K-H., Sun, W-Z., *et al.* Therapeutic effects of acupuncture for neurogenic dysphagia—a randomized controlled trial. *Journal of Traditional Chinese Medicine.* 2012; 32(1): 25–30. http://dx.doi.org/10.1016/S0254-6272(12)60027-2

3   Yamamoto, T. and Yamamoto, H. *Yamamoto New Scalp Acupuncture*: YNSA. Tokyo: Medical Tribune. 2003. Print.

Research Studies

- A meta-analysis of six enrolled trials showed that the acupuncture group had a better therapeutic effect on dysphagia after stroke than the control group, although quality of the studies was lacking.[4]

- Tongguan Liqiao acupuncture therapy has been shown to treat dysphagia effectively after stroke-based pseudobulbar paralysis. Sixty-four patients with dysphagia following brainstem infarction were divided into groups according to infarction location: medulla, midbrain, and pons, and a multiple cerebral infarction group according to MRI results. Acupuncture was done at PC-6, GV-26, SP-6, GB-20, GB-12, and TW-17 twice daily (30-minute retention time) for 28 days. The total efficacy rate was 92.2 percent after treatment, and was most obvious in patients with medulla oblongata infarction (95.9%). These findings suggest that Tongguan Liqiao acupuncture therapy can repair the connection of upper motor neurons to the medulla oblongata motor nucleus, promote the recovery of brainstem infarction, and improve patients' swallowing ability and quality of life.[5]

- Another meta-analysis of the literature showed treatment duration averaging 24.8 minutes in length, with an average total effective rate of 91.2 percent. In these studies, CV-23, GB-20, GV-16, and TW-17 were the most commonly used acupoints from the regular meridians, while Jinjin (EX-HN 12) and Yuye (EX-HN 13) were the most commonly used acupoints from the extraordinary meridians.[6]

- A total of 90 dysphagia patients with craniocerebral injuries (CCIs) participated. A total of 43 patients were cases with cerebral infarction, 24 cases with cerebral hemorrhage, 13 cases with traumatic injury, and ten other cases of CCIs. They were randomly split into three groups of rehabilitation exercises only, rehabilitation exercises with additional neuromuscular electrical stimulation, and rehabilitation exercises with additional neuromuscular electrical stimulation and acupuncture. Acupuncture using points ST-7, ST-6, ST-4, HT-5, and LI-4 was shown to have a significant benefit.[7, 8]

4   Wang, L-P. and Xie, Y. [Systematic evaluation on acupuncture and moxibustion for treatment of dysphagia after stroke]. *Zhongguo Zhenjiu* [Chinese Acupuncture and Moxibustion]. 2006 Feb; 26(2): 141–146.

5   Zhang, Chun-hong, Jin-Ling Bian, Zhi-hong Meng, *et al.* Tongguan Liqiao acupuncture therapy improves dysphagia after brainstem stroke. *Neural Regeneration Research*. 2016; 11(2): 285–291.

6   Chan, S. Survey on acupuncture treatment of neurogenic dysphagia and analysis of regularity of acupoint selection. *Journal of Acupuncture and Tuina Science*. 2015; 13: 273. doi:10.1007/s11726-015-0866-2

7   Wang, H.M., Cai, C., and Zhang, Z.F. Clinical observation on neuromuscular electrical stimulation combined with acupuncture and rehabilitation exercise for relieving dysphagia in patients with craniocerebral injury. *Journal of Nanjing University of Traditional Chinese Medicine*. 2015; 31(2).

8   Wang, S.X., Wang, Q., An, X.L., *et al.* Effect of swallowing function training and acupuncture and neuromuscular electrical stimulation on dysphagia after cerebral apoplexy. *Hebei Medical Journal*. 2013; 35(20): 3175–3176.

Chapter 22

Seizures

A seizure is defined as a sudden, brief attack of altered consciousness, motor activity, sensory phenomena, and/or inappropriate behavior. It may be recurrent or paroxysmal and is thought to involve an excessive discharge of cerebral neurons when a brief, strong surge of electrical activity affects part or all of the brain. One in ten adults are estimated to have a seizure sometime during their life. Each year 200,000 new cases of epilepsy are diagnosed with higher incidences of seizure activity in those under the age of two and over 65. Seventy percent of these new cases have no apparent or known cause.

Seizures can last from a few seconds to a few minutes. They can have many symptoms, from convulsions and loss of consciousness to some that are not always overtly recognized as seizures by the person experiencing them or by healthcare professionals. These may include blank staring, lip smacking, or jerking movements of arms and legs.

Incidence of post-traumatic seizures varies with the amount of time since the injury, severity of the injury, and the age of the individual at the time of trauma. On account of this, statistics range from a 4 to 53 percent incidence in individuals with brain injury. Being a young adult and military injuries tend to have the greatest risk of development. Trauma is said to be responsible for 20 percent of cases of symptomatic epilepsy. Epilepsy is unique in that it can recur suddenly and unexpectedly, which can lead to setbacks, both physical and psychological, that can be detrimental to recovery. Greater injury severity, cortical damage, and hemorrhage are correlated with a higher risk of epilepsy. Five percent of individuals with a closed head injury have been shown to develop post-traumatic epilepsy, while those sustaining an open injury showed a 30–50 percent incidence.

Post-traumatic seizures and epilepsy can affect an individual's quality of life, employment ability, and ability to drive, as well as increasing the risk of physical injury. This includes subsequent head injury. Individuals with epilepsy are considered to have a fourfold risk of a psychiatric disorder. Depression is the most common, being estimated to affect 25–50 percent of individuals. The association between epilepsy and depression is considered to be bidirectional—depression may be a causal risk factor for developing epilepsy, while those with epilepsy may develop depression as a result of the disorder. Anxiety disorders are less frequent but may also affect quality of life. Postictal psychosis is a common and significant problem associated with temporal lobe epilepsy and believed to be the result of temporal–limbic dysfunction. This can occur immediately following a seizure or after a brief period referred to as a "lucid interval" that may last up to a week before further symptoms present. Suicide incidence is a serious concern as there is an associated risk of up to eight times greater among those with epilepsy compared to the general population.

Etiology

Closed head injuries may involve diffuse axonal injury and neuronal shearing, focal hemorrhage, and contusion. Penetrating injuries carry risk of bone or missile fragments making their way into the cranial cavity. Cicatrix (new tissue that forms a scar) on the cortical surface may also form. Early seizures may be due to metabolic changes such as edema, ischemia, or the release of toxic mediators such as cytokines and bioactive lipids in the damaged brain tissue. Late post-traumatic seizures have been correlated to an iron deposition in the cortical tissue as a result of hemoglobin breaking down and forming free radicals that cause peroxidation of lipid membranes. This disrupts cell walls, and causes cell death and subsequent gliosis. Nitric oxide synthase activity may be reduced as a result. Seizure activity may also occur as a result of increased excitatory neurotransmitters (e.g. glutamate), while inhibitory neurotransmitters such as GABA become decreased. Those who develop seizure disorders postinjury have been shown to have a statistically higher mortality rate.

Post-Traumatic Seizure Types

Immediate Post-Traumatic Convulsions (IPTC)

These occur within seconds of impact, involving a loss of consciousness and involuntary movements. It is hypothesized to be a brief traumatic functional decerebration (loss of cerebral brain function) that results from the loss of cortical inhibition. This may also involve a reflexive brainstem activation. It may be associated with suppression of cholinergic or dopaminergic systems or activation of serotinergic systems or other neurochemical alterations. These episodes are generally considered non-epileptic events and closer to a syncope. They may start with a short period of tonic posturing, followed by clonic or myoclonic jerks that last less than two to three minutes. Following the acute episode there may be a brief postictal period where the individual experiences an altered state of consciousness that tends to be associated with retrograde and anterograde amnesia. The majority of the literature on IPTC is derived from observation of sports injuries wherein the incidence rates were estimated to occur in 1 out of 70 concussions. There is thought to be a low risk of recurrent seizures in cases of IPTC and thus no necessary use of anticonvulsant medications for prevention of such.

Early Post-Traumatic Seizures (EPTS)

These seizures occur within the first seven days following an injury to the brain. Fifty percent of convulsive EPTS occurs within the first 24 hours of injury, with 25 percent of cases occurring within the first hour. These can be found in mild as well as more severe TBI and have been reported to have an incidence of 2–10 percent in brain injuries. Most reports involve convulsive seizures wherein there is abnormal motor behavior. While statistics on non-convulsive EPTS have not been gathered, the Brain Injury Association of America states that it may occur in as many as 5 percent of EPTS cases. This is relevant as there has been some evidence of hippocampal shrinkage associated with non-convulsive EPTS.

Late Post-Traumatic Seizures (LPTS)

These are seizures which occur more than one week following an injury. Onset generally happens within the first 18 to 24 months of the brain injury but have been reported many years later. The reported incidence of LPTS ranges anywhere from 1.9 to 50 percent. While an isolated seizure incidence is possible, most sources will use the term post-traumatic epilepsy interchangeably with LPTS as they carry a higher risk of epilepsy than other seizure types. The exact pathomechanism and neurological changes are not fully understood at this time. Changes such as gliosis, atrophy, transmitter alterations, and vascular changes as secondary processes following an injury are thought to play a role. Children were found to be less prone to LPTS, while those over 65 years of age seemed more at risk. The strongest risk factors for LPTS seem to be missile wounds, bilateral or multiple contusions, and multiple craniotomies. Military personnel exposed to missile or blast injuries have a higher reported incidence.

Status Epilepticus

This is a condition defined as greater than 30 minutes of continuous seizure activity or two or more events occurring without a full recovery of consciousness between episodes. This condition occurs in approximately 10 percent of individuals after an acute head injury. It is more commonly found in children. There is a high mortality risk associated with the emergence of status epilepticus. Confused states following a brain injury need to be distinguished from the possibility of non-convulsive status epilepticus (NCSE). NCSE can involve a confusional state as well as bizarre behavior, sedation, or stupor. Failing to recognize cases of NCSE can result in persistent confusion, kindling of epileptic foci, and possible superimposed injury leading to ongoing memory or other cognitive deficits.

Biomedical Approaches

Pharmaceutical interventions for prophylaxis or post-traumatic seizures are summarized in Table 22.1.

TABLE 22.1 Pharmaceutical Intervention in Seizure

Antiepileptic Drug	Beneficial Effects	Potentially Harmful Effects
Barbiturates: e.g. phenobarbital (Solfoton)	Anxiety, mood stabilization, sleep	Aggression, impaired cognition and attention, depression, irritability, impaired sexual function and desire
Carbamazepine (Tegretol)	Aggression, mania, mood stabilization	Irritability, impaired attention
Ethosuximide (Zarontin)	Data not available	Aggression, confusion, depression, insomnia
Gabapentin (Neurontin)	Anxiety, insomnia, social phobia, mood stabilization	Irritability/agitation (usually in children with disabilities)
Lamotrigine (Lamictal)	Depression, mood stabilization, mania	Insomnia, irritability (usually in children with disabilities)
Levetiracetam (Keppra)	Data not available	Anxiety, depression, irritability (all appear more common in children), highest rate of psychiatric side effects (more common in those with psychiatric history)
Phenytoin (Dilatin)	Mania	Depression, impaired attention
Tiagabine (Gabitril)	Mania, mood stabilization	Depression, irritability
Topiramate (Topamax)	Binge eating, mania, mood stabilization, ethanol dependence	Depression, impaired cognition (word finding, memory) and attention, irritability
Valproate (Depakote)	Agitation, aggression, irritability, mania, mood stabilization	Depression
Zonisamide (Zonegran)	Mania	Aggression, emotional lability, irritability

Other Possible Pharmaceuticals

- Clonazepam (Klonopin)
- Primidone (Mysoline)
- Lacosamide (Vimpat)
- Rufinamide (Banzel)

- Diazepam (Valium)
- Lorazepam (Ativan)
- Oxcarbazepine (Trileptal)
- Pregabalin (Lyrica)

Cognitive or sedative side effects need to be taken into careful consideration in those with a brain injury. Topiramate has the highest incidence of cognitive side effects, followed by phenytoin and oxcarbazepine. Lamotrigine has been noted to enhance cognitive functioning and quality of life. Antiperoxidants and free radical scavengers have shown prophylactic effects in experimental models, though have not been studied in a controlled manner.

- Status epilepticus
- Benzodiazepines
- Intravenous phenytoin or fosphenytoin

- Barbiturates
- Propofol
- Valproate

Other Possible Causes of Seizures

Symptomatic

High fever, CNS infections, metabolic disturbances (hypoglycemia), toxic, cerebral hypoxia, neoplasms, congenital brain defects, cerebral edema, cerebral trauma, anaphylaxis, cerebral infarct, or hemorrhage.

Idiopathic

- Seventy-five percent of all seizures occur in young adults
- Before age two—developmental defects, metabolic disturbances, birth injury
- After age 25—tumors, trauma
- Focal brain disease can cause seizures at any age

Classifications

Generalized Seizure

Affects both cerebral hemispheres from the beginning of the seizure. Involves loss of consciousness and motor function. See Table 22.2 for subcategories.

TABLE 22.2 Subcategories of Generalized Seizure

Absence (petit mal)	*Grand mal (tonic-clonic)*	*Atonic (astatic, akinetic)*
Generalized	Generalized	Brief, generalized
10–30-second loss of consciousness with eye or muscle flutterings	Occasional aura	Complete loss of muscle tone and consciousness
	Loss of consciousness	Head drops, loss of posture, or sudden collapse
Stops activity and then resumes it after attack is over	Tonic-clonic contractions of muscles of extremities, trunk, head	
	2–5 minutes	Because abrupt, individual may fall, causing injury to head/face. Protective headgear is sometimes used.
Often when sitting quietly	Postictal state—sleep, headache, muscle soreness	
Genetic		
Does not begin after age 20		Tends to resist drug treatment
Myoclonic	*Infantile spasms*	*Febrile*
Brief, quick jerks or clumsiness	Sudden flexion of arms and trunk with extension of legs	Three months to five years old
May be repetitive	Lasts a few seconds, several times daily	High fever
Occasionally involves only one arm or a foot	Only in first three years of life	In 4 percent of all children—2 percent of those develop epilepsy
No loss of consciousness	Associated with developmental abnormalities	

Partial Seizure

In partial seizures, the electrical disturbance is limited to a specific region within one cerebral hemisphere. Partial seizures may spread to cause a generalized seizure, in which case the classification category is partial seizures secondarily generalized. Partial seizures are the most common type of seizure experienced by people with epilepsy. Virtually any movement, sensory, or emotional symptom can occur as part of a partial seizure, including complex visual or auditory hallucinations.

Simple Partial (Focal)

- Specific sensory, motor, psychomotor phenomena without loss of consciousness—aura is one

- Jacksonian seizure

- Focal symptoms begin in hand or foot and march up extremity

- May be local or proceed to generalized seizure

Complex Partial (Psychomotor)

- One- to two-minute loss of contact with surroundings: purposeless movements, unintelligible sounds, staggering

- No understanding

- Structural pathology

Partial Seizure Manifestations

- *Frontal lobe*: Cephalic sensations, autonomic sensations, motor phenomena (focal or generalized), forced or obscure thoughts or actions

- *Frontal complex (orbital or mesial)*: Often occur nocturnally, strong effective expression—screaming or cursing, intense thrashing movements that appear bizarre, pelvic thrusting, complex automatisms (bicycling, boxing, etc.), irregular or desynchronized movements

- *Temporal lobe (mesial)*: Fear (via amygdala), sensation of somebody behind them (generally contralateral), deja vu, jamais vu, rising epigastric sensation, autonomic manifestations (flushing, tachycardia, hypertension, peristalsis, repisratory arrest, sweating, urinary incontinence, piloerection), vomiting (right lobe), illusions, visual hallucinations, olfactory hallucinations (foul odor via uncus or basal forebrain) depersonalization, derealization, ictal psychosis

- *Temporal lobe (lateral)*: Aphasia, vertigo, simple auditory hallucinations

- *Parietal lobe*: Simple or complex somatosensory phenomena, pain (rare)

- *Occipital lobe*: Simple or complex visual hallucinations (less experiential than temporal hallucinations), vomiting

Psychic Phenomena during Partial Seizures

- *Cognitive*: "Dreamy state," derealization, depersonalization, dissociation, mystical/religious experiences, forced thinking, altered speed of thoughts, distortion of time, distortion of body image

- *Dysphasic*: Speech arrest, nonfluent speech, paraphasias, comprehension deficit, repetitive utterances, dyslexia, agraphia

- *Dysmnesic*: Déjà vu, jamais vu, selective memory impairment, forced recollection

- *Affective*: Fear, depression, anger, pleasure, laughter, crying

- *Visual*: Illusions and hallucinations

Diagnosis Testing

Medical history: Family, trauma, infection, toxic exposure

Laboratory testing: Serum glucose, CBC, chemistry screen

Imaging: CT scan, MRI, EEG

Differential Diagnosis
Medical Disorders

Seizure disorders, cerebrovascular accident (CVA), myocardial infarction, transient ischemic attack (TIA)

Effects of substances:
Alcohol or illicit substance intoxication or withdrawal, side effects of medications

Psychiatric disorders:
Conversion disorder, anxiety disorders, disorders of impulse control, borderline personality disorder (BPD), histrionic personality disorder (HPD), schizophrenia and other psychotic disorders, major depressive episode, pseudoseizures

Factors Influencing the Decision to Treat

- Abnormal EEG
- Previous seizure
- Driver
- Other neurological impairment
- Elderly

Factors Influencing the Decision Not to Treat

- Single seizure
- No history
- Neurologically normal
- Young age
- Side effects

Potential Contributing Factors

- Aspartic acid excess
- Asparagine excess
- Taurine deficiency

Contraindicator of:

- Aspartic acid

- Asparagine

Biomedical Approaches

Vagus Nerve Stimulation

Vagus nerve stimulation therapy is another form of treatment that may be tried when medications fail to stop seizures. It is currently approved for use in adults and children over the age of 12 who have partial seizures that resist control by other methods. The therapy is designed to prevent seizures by sending regular small pulses of electrical energy to the brain via the vagus nerve.

Surgery

When antiepileptic drugs fail to control or substantially reduce seizures, surgery on the brain may be considered. Although some of the techniques are recent, surgical removal of seizure-producing areas of the brain has been an accepted form of treatment for more than 50 years. Most surgical patients are adults who have fought long and unsuccessful battles for seizure control. However, children with severe seizures are also being treated with surgery.

Ketogenic Diet

A ketogenic diet is used when pharmacotherapy fails to adequately control seizures. This forces a child's body to burn fat continuously throughout the day. Eighty percent of calories are derived from fat, while the rest come from carbohydrates and protein. The amounts of food and liquid at each meal must be carefully worked out and weighed for each person. Doctors don't know precisely why a diet that mimics starvation by burning fat for energy should prevent seizures, although this is being studied. Nor is it known why the same diet works for some children and not for others. Attempting such a diet on a child without medical guidance puts a child at risk of serious consequences. Every step of the ketogenic diet process must be managed by an experienced treatment team, usually based at a specialized medical center.

A child on the diet usually continues to take anti-seizure medicine, but may be able to take less of it later on. If a child does very well, the doctor may slowly taper the medication with the goal of discontinuing it altogether. About a third of children who try the ketogenic diet become seizure free, or almost seizure free. Another third improve but still have some seizures. The rest either do not respond at all or find it too hard to continue with the diet, either because of side effects or because they can't tolerate the food.

Chinese Medical Approach: Epilepsy Patterns/Xián Zhèng

The symptoms of epilepsy are understood in Chinese medicine to result from Liver wind triggering latent phlegm, which mists the clear orifices and obstructs the channels. Conditions can be divided into pre-heaven (prenatal) or post-heaven (postnatal).

Prenatally, if the mother experiences trauma or a significant fright during pregnancy, it can affect or damage the child's Jing (essence) and deplete the Kidney system. Kidney Yin may then fail to control Liver Yang, allowing it to become hyperactive, and wind may be stirred. This internal wind can cause involuntary movements and seizures. Flaws cites the pre-heaven factor as a key etiological part of this disease.[1]

Post-natal mechanisms include an affliction or imbalance of the seven emotions which, if unregulated, will cause a counterflow of the Qi mechanism, which becomes chaotic. If this occurs the internal organ systems will not remain harmonious. Phlegm, fire stagnation, and wind may then develop. This is particularly true in cases of great fear or fright. Trauma, in particular a brain injury, can be another factor leading to the disease. Phlegm obstructing is the key pathologic factor. The injury directly damages the brain Shen and leads to stagnation.

Relevant Biomedical Diagnoses

These are generalized epilepsy, severe hysterical attacks, brain injury, poison, tumors or vascular disease, and metabolic or endocrine system diseases.

Prognosis

Recurrent attacks can damage brain Shen and create the severe consequences of Shen disturbances or extreme weakness. Generally, the prognosis depends on the severity of injury to the brain. Today more information can be gained by referring to Western medical exams.

Identifying Organ Involvement during the Interictal Stage

Good history taking during periods of remission is essential to identify patterns of organ involvement, such as Spleen Qi Deficiency with excessive Phlegm, and Liver and Kidney Yin Deficiency.

Differential Diagnosis

Four disorders in TCM share the common symptom of loss of consciousness; they can be differentiated as follows:

---

1   Flaws, Bob and Lake, James. *Chinese Medical Psychiatry: a textbook and clinical manual: including indications for referral to Western medical services.* Boulder, CO: Blue Poppy. 2003. Print.

Epilepsy: During the seizure, the subject may fall with a loud cry. Additional manifestations include convulsions and drooling of white froth; subject recovers within seconds or minutes; sequelae are absent during remission.

Wind stroke: Characterized by a sudden, silent fall accompanied by facial paralysis, hemiplegia, and weakness or numbness on the affected side of the body with a slow recovery of consciousness; various degrees of sequelae are common after restoration of consciousness.

Syncope: Additional manifestations often include pale complexion and frigid extremities; convulsions are not present.

Hypertonicity disorder: Nuchal rigidity is the primary symptom, marked by tonic contractions of voluntary muscles or, in severe cases, opisthotonos with high fever, a prolonged period of unconsciousness, and difficult recovery.

Treatment Principles

Given the paroxysmal, transient, yet recurrent nature of epilepsy, a treatment strategy should be developed based on the stage of the disease in the pattern presenting at that time:

Ictal stage (during or immediately following): Focus on the branch by extinguishing wind, eliminating phlegm, opening the orifices, and arresting contractions

Interictal stage: Focus on the root by strengthening the Spleen, transforming phlegm, nourishing the Liver and Kidney, and nourishing the Heart in calming the Spirit

TCM Pattern Differentiation: Acute Stage
Blood Vessel Stasis and Obstruction

Primary symptoms: Sudden onset, falling down (fainting), contraction of limbs, habitual headache which is fixed in place, either pounding or piercing in nature, worse at night

Additional symptoms: Bluish face or extremities, cyanosis of lips and fingers, can be triggered by anger or strong emotion stimulation, possible history of injury to the head

Tongue: Purplish tongue with static macules on edges of tongue, white coat

Pulse: Choppy or small, wiry (bowstring)

Treatment principles: Quicken the Blood and dispel stasis, open the orifices and extinguish wind

Acupuncture treatment: SP-10, LR-3, LI-4, GB-8, GB-20, GB-41, BL-10, BL-17, GV-20, Yin Tang, Draining technique

Herbal treatment:
Tong Qiao Huo Xue Tang He Zhi Jing San Jia Jian (Open the Portals and Quicken the Blood Decoction Plus Modifications)
[Tao Ren 10g, Hong Hua 3–10g, Chi Shao 10–15g, Chuan Xiong 6–12g, Dan Pi 10–12g, Yu Jin 10g, Quan Xie 1–1.5g, Wu Gong 1–1.5g]

Modifications:
Severe headache: + Wu Ling Zhi, Pu Huang, Di Long
Simultaneous Qi deficiency: + Huang Qi, Dang Shen
Simultaneous Blood deficiency: + Dang Gui, Sheng Di

Profusion of Phlegm-Fire

Primary symptoms:
Mild presentation: Stopping activities abruptly; dropping objects suddenly, forward bending of the neck, staring upward; after consciousness returns, patient does not recall incident
Severe presentation: Falling down suddenly, sometimes preceded by a scream, loss of consciousness, convulsions, frothing mouth; after consciousness returns, patient feels fatigue, may have headache, and does not recall incident

Additional symptoms: Constipation, agitated emotional state, irritability, insomnia, dry mouth, bitter taste

Tongue: Red, yellow greasy coat

Pulse: Rapid, wiry (bowstring), slippery

Treatment principles: Clear the Liver, drain fire, resolve phlegm, open orifices, stabilize epilepsy

Acupuncture treatment: (GB-20, GV-8, Yao Qi, CV-15, LR-3, ST-40, PC-5, GV2–6, ST-6) + LI-4, CV-12, ST-36

Herbal treatment:
Long Dan Xie Gan Tang + Di Tan Tang (Gentiana Decoction to Drain the Liver + Scour Phlegm Decoction)
[Long Dan Cao 6g, Huang Qin 9g, Shan Zhi Zi 9g, Ze Xie 12g, Mu Tong 9g, Dang Gui 3g, Che Qian Zi 9g, Sheng Di Huang 9g, Chai Hu 6g, Gan Cao 6g] + [Fa Ban Xia 9g, Zhi Tian Nan Xing 6g, Chen Pi 9g, Zhi Shi 9g, Fu Ling 12g, Ren Shen 6g, Shi Chang Pu 9g, Zhu Ru 9g, Sheng Jiang 6g, Gan Cao 3g]

Modifications:
Headache with profuse phlegm + Shi Jue Ming, Gou Teng, Zhu Li, Di Long
Phlegm fire congestion, constipation + ST-36, ST-25

Obstruction by Wind-Phlegm

Primary symptoms:
Mild presentation: Stopping activities abruptly, dropping objects suddenly, forward bending of the neck, staring upward; after consciousness returns, patient does not recall incident
Severe presentation: Falling down suddenly, sometimes preceded by a scream, loss of consciousness, convulsions, frothing mouth; after consciousness returns, patient feels fatigue, may have headache, and does not recall incident

Additional symptoms: Dizziness and vertigo, sensation of chest oppression, and sudden weakness may precede loss of consciousness; incontinence, frequent and recurrent numbness of limbs, coughing or vomiting phlegm, nausea, swelling of the body, heavy head or body

Tongue: Pale swollen tongue; white, greasy coating

Pulse: Wiry (bowstring), slippery

Treatment principles: Expel phlegm, extinguish wind, open orifices, stabilize epilepsy

Acupuncture treatment: (GB-20, GV-8, Yao Qi, CV-15, LR-3, ST-40, PC-5, GV-26, ST-6) + GB-34, LI-4, CV-12, ST-36, SP-9, SP-6

Herbal treatment:
Ding Xian Wan (Epilepsy-Stabilizing Pill)
[Tian Ma 30g, Chuan Bei Mu 30g, Fa Ban Xia 30g, Fu Ling 30g, Fu Shen 30g, Dan Xing 15g, Shi Chang Pu 15g, Quan Xie 15g, Bai Jiang Can 15g, Hu Po 15g, Deng Xin Cao 15g, Chen Pi 20g, Yuan Zhi 20g, Dan Shen 60g, Mai Men Dong 60g, Gan Cao 12g, Zhu Li (Dried Bamboo Sap) 100ml, Jiang Zhi (Ginger Juice) 50ml]

Interictal Stage
Liver and Kidney Yin Deficiency

Primary symptoms: Chronic epilepsy accompanied by dizziness and vertigo

Additional symptoms: Insomnia, poor memory and concentration, weak and achy low back and knees, dry stools/constipation, irritability, tinnitus, dry eyes and mouth, thirst especially at night, possible hot flashes

Tongue: Red, scanty coating

Pulse: Rapid, fine, thready

Treatment principles: Nourish and supplement Liver and Kidney Yin, subdue Yang, quiet the Spirit

Acupuncture treatment: (Yao Qi, CV-15) + KI-3, KI-6, LR-3, LR-8, SP-6, BL-18, BL-23, HT-7, GV-20

Herbal treatment:
Zuo Gui Wan (Left-Restoring Kidney Yin Pill)
[Shu Di Huang 24g, Shan Yao 12g, Shan Zhu Yu 12g, Gou Qi Zi 12g, Chuan Niu Xi 9g, Tu Si Zi 12g, Lu Jiao Jiao 12g, Gui Ban Jiao 12g]

Modifications:
Severe Yin deficiency/Yang hyperactivity: + Mu Li, Bie Jia
Heart spirit restlessness: + Bai Zi Ren, Ci Shi
Severe phlegm fire: + Bei Mu, Tian Zhu Huag, Zhu Ru
Vexatious heart heat: + Zhi Zi, Lian Zi Xin; + PC-5
Dry stools: + Xuan Shen, Huo Ma Ren; + BL-25, ST-25
Lassitude of spirit, somber complexion, enduring condition: + He Che Da Zao Wan; + BL-20, ST-36

Spleen and Stomach Qi Deficiency

Primary symptoms: Chronic epilepsy, fatigue and tiredness, occasional dizziness and vertigo, poor appetite, lusterless complexion, loose stools

Additional symptoms: Nausea, vomiting (white or clear phlegm), bloating and distension of chest and epigastrium, heavy head or limbs, cold hands and feet

Tongue: Pale, white, greasy coating

Pulse: Soft/soggy, weak

Treatment principles: Strengthen the Spleen, boost Qi, calm the Stomach, transform turbid phlegm

Acupuncture treatment: (Yao Qi, CV-15) + BL-20, CV-6, CV-12, ST-36, ST-40, SP-6, SP-9, LR-13, GV-20

Herbal treatment:
Liu Jun Zi Tang (Six Gentlemen Decoction)
[Ren Shen 9g, Bai Zhu 9g, Fu Ling 9g, Jiang Ban Xia 6g, Chen Pi 6g, Zhi Gan Cao 6g]

Modifications:

Severe vomiting: + Zhu Ru, Zhi Ke

Phlegm harassing heart spirit with restlessness: + Shi Chang Pu, Yuan Zhi, Tian Nan Xing, Jiang Can

Nausea and vomiting: + PC-6

Heart Blood Deficiency, Shen Losing Nourishment

Primary symptoms: Palpitations, weak body or limbs, insomnia, nightmares, wake up in the early morning or sleep lightly, frequently feels anxious

Additional symptoms: Dreams a lot during sleep, easily startled, may sleep walk, and may have low Shen clarity, poor concentration and memory, pale or sallow complexion, Shen weakness, dizziness, vertigo, and headache

Tongue: Pale tongue, thin coat

Pulse: Weak, deep

Acupuncture treatment: BL-15, BL-17, BL-20, HT-7, ST-36, SP-10, CV-14, GV-11, GV-20

Herbal treatment:

Modified Tian Wang Bu Xin Dan (Heavenly Emperor Tonifying the Heart Pill)

[Suan Zao Ren 30g, Bai Zi Ren 30g, Mai Dong 30g, Sheng Di 120g, Fu Ling 15g, Dan Shen 15g, Yuan Zhi 15g, Wu Wei Zi 30g, Lian Zi Xin 15g, Zhi Gan Cao 10g]

Ear acupuncture: Shen Men, Kidney, Stomach, Heart, Subcortex, Occiput, Brain

Clinical Notes

Chronic epilepsy patterns are often complicated by Qi stagnation and Blood stasis; therefore, treatments often include methods to rectify the Qi, quicken the Blood, and eliminate stagnation. The addition of entomological medicinals such as Quan Xie and Wu Gong have been found to be effective at extinguishing wind and relieving spasms, thus increasing the therapeutic effect for all epilepsy patterns. These are generally administered in powdered form at a dose of 1g bid; if administered together the dosage of each is reduced to 0.5g bid.

Other Treatment Considerations

Dietary Recommendations

- Food complements: Kelp. Take 4–5g of seaweed at mealtime once a day (powder in capsules or tablets)

- Orthomolecular treatment:

- Glucosamine: may dampen brain hyperexcitability[2]

- Taurine

- Alanine

- GABA

Research Studies

- Electroacupuncture was tested to determine the effects of low-frequency (10 Hz) stimulation of acupoint GB-20 (Fengchi) on epilepsy. Electroencephalogram (EEG) results demonstrate that electroacupuncture significantly suppresses brain epileptiform discharges and simultaneously improves sleep patterns. The researchers note that low frequency stimulation of GB-20 suppresses epilepsy and "blocks sleep disruption." The investigators cite research showing that opioid peptides and their receptors mediate the therapeutic effects of acupuncture.[3] Han *et al.* demonstrate that 2 Hz electroacupuncture stimulates an increase of met-enkephalin but not dynorphin. However, 100 Hz electroacupuncture increases dynorphin release and not met-enkephalin.[4,5]

- Sixty patients with epilepsy were randomly divided into a control group and an acupuncture group. The control group received only the pharmaceutical medication sodium valproate. The acupuncture group received both scalp acupuncture and body acupuncture plus sodium valproate. The acupuncture group demonstrated significantly superior patient outcomes over the medication-only group.
    Scalp acupuncture: chest area, Epilepsy-control area, chorea-tremor area.
    Body acupuncture: GB-20, GV-20, Si Shen Cong, Yintang, GV-26, PC-6, LI-4, ST-36, ST-40, SP-6, LR-3.

2   Stewart, L., Khan, A., Kai Wang, K. *et al.* Acute increases in protein O-GlcNAcylation dampen epileptiform activity in hippocampus. *The Journal of Neuroscience.* 2017; 37 (34): 8207. doi:10.1523/JNEUROSCI.0173-16.2017

3   Yi, P-L., Lu, C-Y., Jou, S-B., and Chang, F-C. Low-frequency electroacupuncture suppresses focal epilepsy and improves epilepsy-induced sleep disruptions. *Journal of Biomedical Science.* 2015; 22(1): 1–12.

4   Han JS. Acupuncture anesthesia versus Acupuncture-assisted anesthesia. Acupuncture Research. 1997;22 (1): 97–102.

5   Cheng, L-L., Ding, M-X., Xiong, C., Zhou, M-Y., Qiu, Z-Y., and Wang, Q. Effects of electroacupuncture of different frequencies on the release profile of endogenous opioid peptides in the central nerve system of goats. *Evidence-Based Complementary and Alternative Medicine: eCAM.* 2012; 2012: 476457. doi:10.1155/2012/476457=

Needles were retained for 30 minutes. A total of ten days comprised one course of care. There was a two-day break following each course of care. The treatment period was three months. Following the completion of acupuncture therapy, 12 acupuncture patients showed no epilepsy-related symptoms for at least one year. A total of nine patients showed excellent improvement, and six patients showed moderate improvement. The overall effective rate for the acupuncture group was 90 percent compared with 73.33 percent for the medication control group. The researchers conclude that acupuncture combined with sodium valproate has a synergistic clinical effect leading to improved patient outcomes.[6]

- Auricular acupuncture and body-style electroacupuncture reduced neuron overexcitation while simultaneously stopping epileptic seizures. Acupuncture's ability to regulate the TRPA1 ion (active in acute pain and neurogenic inflammation) signaling channel located on the plasma membrane of cells was quantified. Auricular and electroacupuncture demonstrate the ability to halt inflammation related to epileptic seizures while simultaneously downregulating TRPA1 in the hippocampus. Results were confirmed by western blot analysis, EEG, and electromyogram (EMG) techniques. The auricular acupuncture group received 2 Hz electroacupuncture stimulation from the ear apex to the ear lobe for 20 minutes on the left ear and ten minutes on the right ear per session. The body-style electroacupuncture group received 2 Hz electroacupuncture from acupoints ST-36 to ST-37. Both groups received acupuncture at a rate of three days per week for a total of six weeks. Auricular and body-style acupuncture were effective in providing relief from epileptic seizures, and both types of acupuncture regulated the TRPA1 signaling pathway and additional signaling pathways: PKC, pERK1/2.[7]

---

6   Niu, Xuexia. Clinical observations on treating 30 cases of epilepsy by head and body acupuncture. *Clinical Journal of Medicine.* 6.4 (2014): 65–67.

7   Lin, Y-W. and Hsieh, C-L. Auricular electroacupuncture reduced inflammation-related epilepsy accompanied by altered TRPA1, pPKCα, pPKCε, and pERK1/2 signaling pathways in kainic acid-treated rats. *Mediators of Inflammation.* 2014; 9 pages. Article ID 493480. doi:10.1155/2014/493480

Chapter 23

Chronic Pain

The most common pain conditions following a brain injury tend to be headaches, a topic specifically addressed in Chapter 16. This chapter will focus on other forms of body pain that may develop. Some more common conditions that are reported include head/neck pain, back pain, complex regional pain syndrome (CRPS), and fibromyalgia, among others. Pain can be due to tissue damage, spasticity or contracture, falls, heterotropic ossification, etc. within the general population. Service members run the additional risk of exposure to blast injuries with possible burns, traumatic amputation, high temperature gas inhalation, and physical displacement injuries. In order for pain to be considered chronic it must have persisted for six months or greater and may or may not be directly associated with any obvious tissue damage or pathological process.

There is an increasing amount of evidence demonstrating that in chronic postinjury pain, or other conditions, persistent pain may be correlated with an increased peripheral sensitization or "central sensitization." In this case, the pain relay system becomes hyperresponsive over time or will spontaneously discharge without direct stimulation. This sensitization of the peripheral afferent nerves can bombard the nociceptive impulses and result in further sensitization of second or third order neurons within the central nervous system. This sensitization has been correlated with dysfunctional functioning of the anterior cingulate cortex.

Post-traumatic stress conditions have also shown an association with the development of chronic pain. In some individuals there has been no physical trauma at all. Rather the onset, maintenance, severity, and exacerbation of pain is associated with psychological factors. Even with physical trauma present, psychosocial stressors can exacerbate pain conditions. In cases of brain injury it has been found that complaints of pain conditions were more than twice as frequent in those who sustained a mild brain trauma compared to a more severe injury. By the same token, chronic pain can and often does produce an impairment or exacerbation of cognitive functioning. This is particularly true in the realms of attentional capacity, processing speed, memory, and executive functions. Chronic pain has been further associated with mood change or emotional distress, somatic preoccupation, pain "catastrophization," sleep disturbance, fatigue, and chronic stress regarding the interference of daily activities.

The neuroanatomy of pain is a complex system which still remains not completely understood. Nociceptive receptors occur in the cutaneous, muscular, and visceral structure of the body. Afferent sensory neurons that are primary in this process include A delta fibers and C fibers. Delta fibers are small mylenated neurons that relay the responses of localized, sharp, fast, and well-defined pain patterns. C fibers are generally smaller, slower, unmylenated fibers that relay what tends to be slow, diffuse, poorly localized pain that feels more like a burning, throbbing, or gnawing sensation. Chronic pain has been associated with decreased density of the prefrontal and thalamic gray matter, as well as stress-induced hypothalamic–pituitary-axis dysfunction, serotonin deficiency, depressed somatomedic C levels, and increased norepinephrine levels.

Pain may also be distinguished as affecting either the lateral or medial pain systems. While there is a significant overlap between the two systems (which creates a unitary experience of pain in the individual), Table 23.1 lists distinctions that have been observed.

TABLE 23.1 Lateral vs. Medial Pain Systems

Lateral Pain System	Medial Pain System
Primarily mediates sensory-discriminatory components of pain	Primarily mediates emotional–motivational components of pain
Associated more with acute pain	Associated more closely with chronic pain
Inputs to thalamus and somatosensory cortex	Projections of medial–thalamic nuclei: projections to the anterior cingulate (area 24) and forebrain regions
	Supraspinal sensitization with limbic structures seem to mediate pain response

Brain Regions and Pain

Subcortical lesions (especially of the thalamus, less often with destruction of the anterior cingulate) can cause a loss of sensation or an inability to react to pain. At the neocortical level, although pain responsiveness may be diminished or absent following damage to these tissues, elementary sensation remains intact and the ability to differentiate is retained. For example, one is still able to differentiate between dull and sharp. This deficit is usually bilateral.

Cortical Regions and Their Role in Sensation

Somatosensory areas 1 and 2: Pain, touch, temperature sense, pressure sense, position sense, vibration sense, sensation of movement

Prefrontal area: Pain, executive function, creativity, planning, empathy, action, emotional balance, intuition

Anterior cingulate: Pain, emotional self-control, sympathetic control, conflict detection, problem solving

Posterior parietal lobe: Pain, sensory, visual, auditory perception, mirror neurons, internal location of stimuli, location of external space

Supplementary motor zone: Pain, planned movement, mirror neurons

Amygdala: Pain, emotion, emotional memory, emotional response, pleasure, sight, smell, emotional extremes

Insula: Pain, quiets the amygdala, temperature, itch, empathy, emotional self-awareness, sensual touch, connects emotion with bodily sensation, mirror neurons, disgust

Posterior cingulate: Pain, visuospatial cognition, autobiographical memory retrieval

Hippocampus: Helps to store pain memories

Orbital frontal cortex: Pain, evaluates whether something is pleasant vs. unpleasant, empathy, understanding, emotional attunement

Diagnostic Assessment
Self-Report

- Visual Analog Scale
- Numerical Rating Scale
- Onset, palliative, quality, radiation, severity, timing
- Intake of preinjury pain levels, pain vulnerabilities, relevant family history, etc.

Psychological Assessment

- Nociception Coma Scale (for those with disorders of consciousness)

Biomedical Approach

Biomedical approaches to treating chronic pain can vary greatly depending on symptom patterns. A summary of standard approaches is listed in Table 23.2.

TABLE 23.2 Treatment Approaches for Pain

Analgesics	Antidepressants	Anticonvulsants
Acetaminophen	Amitriptyline	Carbamazepine
Tramadol	Desipramine	Valproic acid
Steroids	Nortriptyline	Phenytoin
Prednisone	Fluoxetine	Clonazepam
Dexamethasone	Paroxetine	Gabapentin
	Duloxetin	Levetiracetam
		Lamotrigine
		Oxcarbazepine
		Pregabalin
Opioids	**Local Anesthetics**	**Topical Anesthetics**
Morphine	Lidocaine	Capsaicin
Hydromorphone	Mexiletine	"Speed Gel"
Codeine	Flecainide	
Hydrocordone		
Oxycodone		
Meperidine		
Fentanyl		
Physical Modalities	**Behavioral Treatments**	
Hot/cold packs	Patient education	
Heat lamps	Biofeedback	
Parrafin baths	Relaxation training	
Laser therapy	Operant treatment	
Cryotherapy	Cognitive–behavioral treatment	
Hydrotherapy	Social and assertive skills training	
Ultrasound	Imagery	
Phonopheresis	Hypnosis	
Diathermy	Habit reversal	
Transcutaneous nerve stimulations (TENS)	Body mechanics and ergonomics training	
Iontophoresis		
Cranial electrotherapy stimulation (CES)		
Traction		
Injections—prolotherapy, trigger point, plasma		
Epidural		
Sympathetic blocks		
Vestibular stimulation		

Chinese Medical Perspective
Painful Obstructive Syndrome (Bi Zheng)

Painful obstructive syndrome, Bi-syndrome, or Bi Zheng is caused by an invasion of exterior pathogenic factors such as wind, cold, dampness, and heat. These then obstruct the channels and collaterals, disturbing the blood circulation and Qi flow. The syndrome is characterized by localized discomforts in the muscles, joints, and tendons. Bì Zheng may affect the muscles, tendons, bones, and joints.

It is important to note that not all pain conditions fall into the category of Bi Zheng and that there are a number of very effective approaches to treating pain using various systems including local/ashi points, Master Tung's system, Dr. Tan's balancing approach, M-Test, and various microsystems (scalp, auricular, hand, reflexology, etc.), to name just a few.

Relevant Western Diseases

Rheumatoid arthritis, rheumatic arthritis, degenerative arthritis, osteoarthritis, gout, sciatica, subacromial bursitis, olecranal bursitis, carpal tunnel syndrome, fibromyalgia

Chinese Medical Etiology

Deficient Zheng Qi is the underlying etiology of painful obstructive syndrome.

- Unconsolidated interstitial layers between the muscles and skin allow for invasion of exogenous wind, cold, dampness, or heat.

- These pathogens obstruct the flow of Qi and Blood in the channels and collaterals, causing pain and restricted movement.

Invasion of exogenous pathogenic factors:

- Exogenous wind, cold, and dampness invade, causing obstruction of the channels and collaterals, muscles, and joints. This can result from one's living or working environment or from sudden exposure to cold or rainy weather.

- Exogenous heat invades, usually in combination with wind and dampness, causing wind-damp-heat bì. Heat bì can also form when wind-cold-damp invades a body that has pre-existing heat, either through Yang excess or Yin deficiency. Qi stagnation itself can potentially generate heat, and in individuals with pre-existing heat this process is greatly facilitated.

Distinguishing Pathogens

Wind/Wandering Bì: Characterized by pain that migrates from joint to joint; pain tends to be sore and aching

Cold/Painful Bì: Characterized by severe, excruciating pain in the affected joints with limited range of motion

Damp/Fixed Bì: Characterized by heavy aching with possible swelling and numbness in the joints and limbs

Heat Bì: Characterized by red, swollen, painful joints that are warm to the touch

Complicating Factors

The following complications are usually seen in chronic cases:

- Phlegm accumulation and Blood stasis

- Qi and Blood deficiency

- Liver and Kidney deficiency with Blood and Essence deficiency

Differential Diagnosis

Atrophy Syndrome (Wei Zheng)

Pattern Differentiation
Wind Bì

Primary symptoms: Soreness and pain that migrates from joint to joint, pain in indeterminate location, difficulty in flexion/extension of joints

Additional symptoms: Aversion to cold, fever in some cases, aversion to wind, limited range of movement

Tongue: Thin, white coat

Pulse: Floating, possibly wiry (bowstring)

Treatment principles: Expel wind, scatter cold, eliminate dampness, unblock collaterals, relieve pain

Acupuncture treatment: BL-12, BL-17, SP-10, GB-31, LI-4

Auxiliary points: For general pain over the entire body: + SI-3, BL-62, SP-21, LI-15, LI-11, LI-4, TW-4, GB-30, GB-34, GB-39, ST-41

Herbal treatment:
Fang Feng Tang (Siler Decoction)
[Fang Feng 12g, Qin Jiao 9g, Fu Ling 9g, Qiang Huo 6g, Gui Zhi 3g, Ma Huang 3g, Ge Gen 9g, Dang Gui 9g, Xing Ren 6g, Huang Qin 3g, Sheng Jiang 3g, Dao Zao 3pc, Gan Cao 4g]

Modifications:

Mainly affecting the upper extremities: + Qiang Huo 9g, Bai Zhi 6g, Jiang Huang 9g, Chuan Xiong 6g, Wei Ling Xian 9g

Mainly affecting the lower limbs: + Du Huo 9g, Niu Xi 9g, Mu Gua 6g, Fang Ji 6g, Bai Xie 6g

Mainly affecting the lower back or spine: + Du Zhong 12g, Sang Ji Sheng 12g, Ba Ji Tian 9g, Xu Duan 9g, Yin Yang Huo 9g

Swollen painful joints, dry sore throat, and a thin yellow tongue coat: Use Gui Zhi Shao Yao Zhi Mu Tang (Cinnamon Twig, Peony, and Anemarrhena Decoction)

Cold Bì

Primary symptoms: Excruciating pain in the affected joints and limbs. Pain is localized and aggravated by cold, pain decreases with heat, difficulty moving the affected parts

Additional symptoms: Stiffness of the joints with difficulty in movement, possible external pathogen invasion symptoms

Tongue: Thin white or moist white coating

Pulse: Floating and tight, slippery or slow, often wiry

Treatment principles: Scatter cold, warm the channels, dispel wind and eliminate dampness, relieve pain

Acupuncture: Moxa is primary reducing method with deep insertion and long retention time, BL-23, CV-4, GV-4

Herbal treatment:

Wu Tou Tang (Aconite Decoction)
[Zhi Chuan Wu Tou 6g, Ma Huang 6g, Huang Qi 12g, Bai Shao 9g, Gan Cao 6g, Feng Mi]

Modifications:

Complicated by constitutional Yang deficiency causing stubborn cold: + Rou Gui, Xi Xin

Pain of the elbow or shoulder joints is predominant: + Qiang Huo 9g, Wei Ling Xian 9g, Jiang Huang 9g

Pain of the knee and ankle joints is predominant: + Niu Xi 9g, Du Huo 9g, Mu Gua 9g

Pain in the lumbar region is predominant: + Du Zhong 12g, Sang Ji Sheng 12g, Xu Duan 9g

To enforce invigorating the blood and opening the collaterals: + Ji Xue Teng 12g, Dang Gui 9g, Luo Shi Teng 6g

Damp Bì

Primary symptoms: Swollen heavy, painful joints and numbness of the affected limbs, distension and swelling in some cases, pain in fixed location, limited range of motion, worse with cloudy or rainy weather

Additional symptoms: General soreness and heaviness, fatigue and lack of strength with difficult movement, possible external pathogen invasion symptoms

Tongue: White, greasy coating

Pulse: Soft and decelerating, slippery

Treatment principles: Eliminate dampness, unblock obstruction in the channels, dispel wind-cold, relieve pain

Acupuncture treatment: ST-36, BL-20, SP-5, SP-9

Herbal treatment:
Yi Yi Ren Tang (Coix Seed Decoction)
[Yi Yi Ren 30g, Cang Zhu 6g, Qiang Huo 9g, Du Huo 9g, Fang Feng 6g, Zhi Chuan Wu Tou 3g, Ma Huang 6g, Gui Zhi 6g, Dang Gui 9g, Chuan Xiong 9g, Sheng Jiang 6g, Gan Cao 6g]

Modifications:
Significant swelling in the joints: + Bi Xie 9g, Mu Tong 6g, Mu Gua 6g,
Fang Ji 6g, Jiang Huang 9g
Significant numbness: + Hai Tong 9g, Xi Xian Cao 9g, Ji Xue Teng 12g
Predominance of wind, cold, or dampness is not apparent: Use Juan Bi Tang
(Remove Painful Obstruction Decoction)

Heat Bì

Primary symptoms: Redness, swelling, and burning pain in joints that are warm to the touch, pain aggravated by pressure, preference for cold, limited range of motion

Additional symptoms: Aversion to wind/heat, fever, sweating, thirst, irritability and restlessness, sore throat, dark scanty urine

Tongue: Red tongue with yellow, dry, or possibly greasy coat

Pulse: Slippery, rapid

Treatment principles: Clear heat and unblock the collaterals, dispel wind, eliminate dampness, relieve pain

Acupuncture treatment: GV-14, LI-11

Herbal treatment:
Bai Hu Jia Gui Zhi Tang (White Tiger Decoction Plus Cinnamon Twig)
[Shi Gao 30g, Jing Mi 15g, Zhi Mu 9g, Gui Zhi 6g, Zhi Gan Cao 6g]

Modifications:
Clearing more heat and relieving toxicity: + Ren Dong Teng 12g, Lian
Qiao 12g, Huang Bai 9g, Jin Yin Hua 15g
Enhance invigorating the Blood, unblocking the collaterals, dispelling wind, and
eliminating dampness: + Hai Tong Pi 9g, Jiang Huang 9g, Wei Ling Xian 6g, Fang
Ji 9g, Sang Zhi 15g
Damp-heat descending to lower burner: Use San Miao Wan (Three Marvel Pill)

Phlegm Accumulation and Blood Stasis

Primary symptoms: Swollen joints with intermittent pain, possible deformity,
stiffness, difficulty in movement, subcutaneous nodules

Tongue: Purple or dark tongue with white, greasy coat

Pulse: Thready, choppy, deep-rough, or deep-slippery

Treatment principles: Transform phlegm, move Blood, expel stasis, unblock
channels, and stop pain

Acupuncture treatment: ST-40, SP-9, SP-6, CV-12, CV-9, BL-20, SP-10, BL-17,
BL-11

Herbal treatment:
Sheng Tong Zhu Yu Tang (Drive out Blood Stasis from a Painful Body Decoction)
[Tao Ren 9g, Hong Hua 9g, Dang Gui 9g, Chuan Xiong 6g, Mo Yao 6g, Wu Ling
Zhi 6g, Nui Xi 9g, Di Long 6g, Qin Jiao 3g, Qiang Huo 3g, Xiang Fu 3g, Gan
Cao 6g]
Tao Hong Yin (Peach Kernel and Safflower Decoction)
[Tao Ren 9g, Hong Hua 9g, Chuan Xiong 9g, Dang Gui Wei 9g, Wei Ling Xian
12g]

Modifications:
Strengthen transforming phlegm and dissipating nodules effect: + Bai Jie Zi
9g, Dan Nan Xing 4.5g
To enhance effects of invigorating the Blood, expelling stasis, and unblocking the
collaterals: + Chuan Shan Jia 9g, Di Long 9g, Zhe Chong 9g
Reinforce gathering wind and unblocking the collaterals effects: + Quan Xie 4.5g,
Wu Shao She 9g

Qi and Blood Deficiency

Primary symptoms: Chronic, aching pain in joints that is worse at night and better with light movement, difficult movement with limited range of motion, possible numbness or loss of sensation in affected areas

Additional symptoms: Fatigue, pale complexion, shortness of breath, palpitations, spontaneous sweating

Tongue: Pale with thin, white coat

Pulse: Thin, weak

Treatment principles: Boost Qi, nourish Blood, expel wind, eliminate dampness, scatter cold, stop pain

Acupuncture treatment: ST-36, SP-6, KI-3, LI-10, CV-4, CV-6, BL-17, BL-20, BL-23

Herbal treatment:
Huang Qi Gui Zhi Wu Wu Tang (From Ingredient Astragalus and Cinnamon Twig Decoction)
[Huang Qi 12g, Bai Shao 9g, Gui Zhi 9g, Sheng Jiang 12g, Da Zao 12pc]

Qi and Blood Deficiency (Liver and Kidney)

Primary symptoms: Intermittent joint pain with difficult movement, numbness of limbs

Additional symptoms: Soreness and weakness of the lower back, cold intolerance, prefers warmth, fatigue, lassitude, shortness of breath

Tongue: Pale tongue, white coat

Pulse: Thready, weak

Treatment principles: Expel wind-dampness, unblock the obstruction to alleviate pain, tonify Qi and Blood, nourish the Liver and Kidney

Acupuncture treatment: SP-6, LR-3, KI-3, BL-18, BL-20, BL-23

Herbal treatment:
Du Huo Ji Sheng Tang (Angelica-Loranthus Decoction)
[Du Huo 9g, Xi Xin 6g, Fang Feng 6g, Qin Jiao 6g, Rou Gui 6g, Ren Shen 12g, Fu Ling 6g, Dang Gui 6g, Chuan Xiong 6g, Sheng Di Huang 6g, Bai Shao 6g, Du Zhong 6g, Huai Niu Xi 6g, Sang Ji Sheng 6g, Zhi Gan Cao 6g]
San Bi Tang (Three Painful Obstruction Decoction)
[Xu Duan 30g, Du Zhong 30g, Fang Feng 30g, Rou Gui 30g, Xi Xin 30g, Ren Shen 30g, Fu Ling 30g, Dang Gui 30g, Bai Shao 30g, Gan Cao 30g, Qin

Jiao 15g, Sheng Di Huang 15g, Chuan Xiong 15g, Du Huo 15g, Huang Qi 30g, Chuan Niu Xi 30g, Sheng Jiang 6g, Da Zao 6g]

Modifications:
Significant pain + Zhi Chuan Wu, Di Long, Hong Hua, Bai Hua She
Preponderance of cold + Fu Zi
Preponderance of dampness + Fang Ji

Heart Bì

Primary symptoms: Palpitations, shortness of breath aggravated by exertion, oppression of the chest

Additional symptoms: Edema, pale or purplish complexion, nails, and lips

Tongue: Pale or purplish tongue

Pulse: Intermittent, knotted, or rapid forceless intermittent

Treatment principles: Augment the Qi, nourish the Heart, warm the Yang, and restore the regular pulse

Acupuncture treatment: Address palpitations and fatigue

Herbal treatment:
Zhi Gan Cao Tang (Honey Prepared Licorice Root Decoction)
[Zhi Gan Cao 12g, Ren Shen 6g, Gui Zhi 9g, Sheng Di Huang 24g, Mai Men Dong 9g, E Jiao 6g, Huo Ma Ren 9g, Sheng Jiang 9g, Da Zao 5pc]

Modifications:
Strengthen nourishing the Heart and calming the Shen effects + Yuan Zhi, Wu Wei Zi
Significant palpitations and dyspnea + Huang Qi, Bai Zhu
Accompanied by chest congestion and chest pain + Dan Shen, Yu Jin

Further Herbal Modification According to Affected Limbs

Shoulders, elbows, or upper extremity joints: + Qiang Huo, Bai Zhi, Gao Ben, Sang Zhi, Jiang Huang, Chuan Xiong, Wei Ling Xian

Knees, ankles, or lower extremity joints: + Du Huo, Niu Xi, Fang Ji, Mu Gua

Lower back or lumbar intervertebral joints: + Du Zhong, Sang Ji Sheng, Yin Yang Huo, Ba Ji Tian, Xu Duan

Red, swollen, and painful joints that are warm to the touch: + Ren Dong Teng, Shi Gao, Zhi Mu, Lian Qiao, Qin Jiao

In chronic cases of Bi patterns that manifest spasmodic pain and spastic contraction of limbs, entomological medicines such as Quan Xie 2.5g and Wu Gong 1–3g are used to free the collaterals and relieve pain.

Local Acupuncture Points (Based on the Location of Pain)

Shoulder: LI-15, TW-14, SI-10, SI-9, Jian Qian

Elbow: LI-11, LU-5, PC-3, HT-3, LI-10, TW-10, SI-8

Wrist: LI-5, TW-4, PC-7, LI-4, TW-5

Fingers: Ba Xie, LI-4, LI-3, TW-3, Si Feng

Hip: GB-30, GB-29, GB-34, ST-31, Huan Zhong

Sacrum: BL-32, BL-27, BL-28

Low back: BL-23, BL-27, BL-28

Knee: ST-35, Nei Xi Yan, ST-34, BL-40, GB-33, LV-8, GB-34, SP-9, KI-10, SP-10, He Ding

Ankle: BL-60, KI-3, ST-41, GB-40, SP-5, KI-6

Toes: Ba Feng, ST-44, SP-3

Spine: GV-14, GV-12, GV-3, Hua Tuo Jia Ji

Neck: GB-20, BL-10, BL-11, Hua Tuo Jia Ji

Auricular acupuncture: Points corresponding to affected parts, Sympathetic, Shen Men

Plum blossom: Used where swelling and distension are significant

External Chinese Formulas

Muscle and Tendon Bi, Wind-Cold-Damp, especially when acute: Chuan Wu, Cao Wu, Sheng Nan Xing, Fu Zi, Pao Jiang, Chi Shao, Rou Guo, Bai Zhi, Xi Xin

Muscle and Tendon Bi, cold and damp blood stagnation: Wheat Bran, Cang Zhu, Mu Xiang, Ru Xiang, Mo Yao

Boney Bi: Ru Xiang, Mo Yao, Hong Hua, Tu Bie Chong, San Qi, Chuan Wu, Cao Wu, Dang Gui, Du Zhong, Xu Duan, Tou Gu Cao

Wind-Damp-Heat, arthritis/gout, vessel Bi, sprain: Hong Hua, Chi Shao, Bai Zhi, Zhi Zi, Tao Ren, Ru Xiang, Mo Yao, Da Huang

Boney Bi, scars after surgery: Ru Xiang, Mo Yao, Bai Shao, Chuan Wu, Tao Ren, Xing Ren, Gu Sui Bu, Jiu Cai Zi

Damp-Heat Bi with swelling, good for scar tissue, more lower extremity, gout: Huang Bai, Sheng Ban Xia, Wu Bei Zi

Other Treatment Considerations

Orthomolecular Considerations

- Bromelain
- Gaba-linoleic acid
- Vitamin C
- Vitamin D
- SAMe
- Omega 3 fatty acids
- Probiotics

Phytotherapeutic Considerations

- Turmeric/curcumin
- Capsaicin
- Arnica
- Boswellia
- Willow bark
- Devil's claw
- Clove oil
- Ginger
- Fennel
- Feverfew
- Green tea
- Licorice root

Chapter 24

Neuralgia and Numbness

Neuralgia is pain that follows the path of a specific peripheral nerve tract. A summary of spinal-level nerve tracts and their associated muscle innervations is provided in Table 24.1, while organ innervations are included in Table 24.2. The causes of neuralgia can vary greatly. Trauma, chemical irritation, inflammation, compression of nerves by nearby structures (for instance, vertebral subluxations), and infections may all lead to neuralgia.

Trigeminal neuralgia is the most common form of neuralgia and is a result of inflammation or compression of the trigeminal nerve which runs along the side of the face. A related but rather uncommon neuralgia affects the glossopharyngeal nerve, which provides sensation to the throat. Symptoms of this neuralgia are short, shock-like episodes of pain located in the throat. The occipital nerve can also be affected, causing occipital neuralgia in the back of the neck and scalp. In cases where partial or full paralysis occurs or there is a loss of sensation to an area nerve, pain can occur along a nerve trajectory.

Neurogenic pain or discomfort may actually increase temporarily as feeling and/or range of motion increases with treatment. This is similar to a body part that has "fallen asleep," and discomfort can occur as it "wakes up" until full neural signaling is reestablished.

Biomedical Approaches

- Gabapentin (Neurontin)
- SSRIs
  - Fluoxetine (Prozac)
  - Citalopram (Celexa)
  - Paroxetine (Paxil)
  - Bupropion (Wellbutrin)

- Sedatives
  - Clonazepam (Klonopin)
- Anticonvulsants
  - Carbamazepine (Tegretol)
  - Oxcarbazepine (Trileptal)
  - Lamotrigine (Lamictal)
  - Phentoin (Dilantin)
- Anti-spasmotics
  - Baclofen (Gablofen)
- Botox injections
- Glycerol injections
- Microvascular decompression surgery
- Nerve blocks
- Nerve ablation

Differential Diagnosis

- Diabetic neuropathy
- Nerve compression
- Herpes zoster (shingles)
- Post-herpetic neuralgia
- Renal insufficiency
- Polyphyria
- Drug use

TABLE 24.1 Muscle Innervations

Spinal Exiting Nerve	Muscle Innervation
C1	None
C2	Longus colli, sternocleidomastoid (SCM), rectus capitis
C3	Trapezius, splenius capitis
C4	Trapezius, levator scapulae
C5	Supraspinatus, infraspinatus, deltoid, biceps
C6	Biceps, supinator, wrist extensors
C7	Triceps, wrist flexors

C8	Ulnar deviations, thumb extensors, thumb adductors
T1–T2	Minor innervations of intrinsic muscles of the hand, elbow, forearm, shoulder, scapulae, upper back, and neck
T3–T12	Innervations of the upper torso, as well as posterior and anterior aspects
L1	None
L2	Psoas, hip adductors
L3	Psoas, quadriceps, thigh atrophy
L4	Tibialis anterior, extensor hallucis
L5	Extensor hallucis, peroneals, gluteus medius, dorsiflexors, hamstrings, and calf atrophy
S1	Calf and hamstring, wasting of gluteals, peroneals, plantar flexors
S2	Calf and hamstring, wasting of gluteals, plantar flexors
S3	None
S4	Bladder, rectum

TABLE 24.2 Organ Innervation by Spinal Segment

Spinal Segment	Organ
T2–T4 (C3/C4)	Lung
T1–T5	Heart
T6–T10	Diaphragm
T6–T10	Stomach
T7–T10	Spleen
T7–T10	Pancreas
T7–T9	Liver and gallbladder
T9–T10	Small intestines
T11–L1 (to splenic flexure) L1–L2 (splenic flexure to rectum)	Large intestines
T10–L2	Kidneys
T11–L2	Bladder
T10–S3	Reproductive organs
S2–S4	Parasympathetic pathways of genital sex organs
T11–L2	Sympathetic pathways of genital sex organs
T1–T12	Ovaries

Spinal Segment	Organ
T11–L1	Fallopian tubes
T11–T12	Uterus
S2–S4	Vagina
L2–L1	Testicles
T12–L2	Prostate
L1–L2	Penis

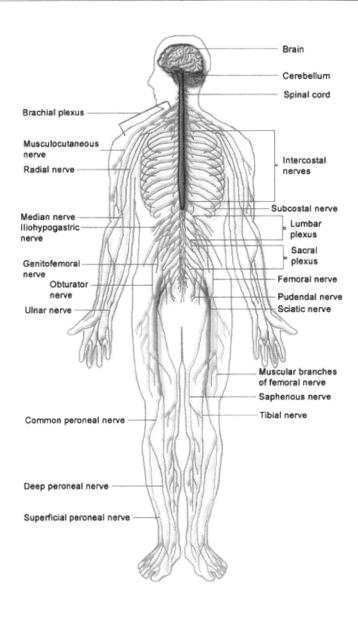

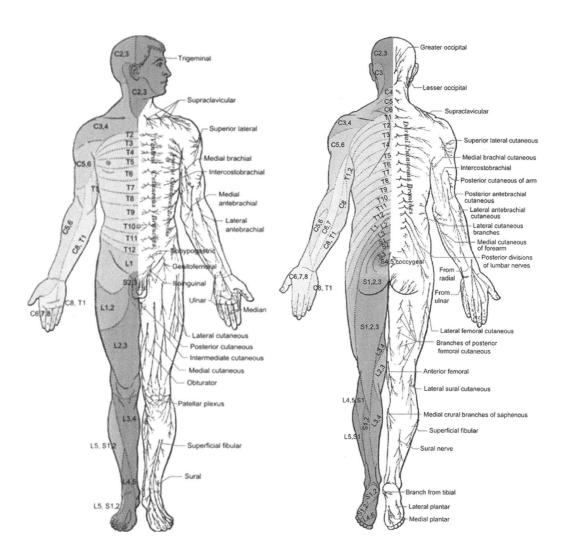

Chinese Medical Etiology

A common etiology in neuralgia consists of Blood stasis with associated Yin deficiency and/or Qi and Blood deficiency. Phlegm accumulation in the collaterals can also occur, causing numbness or tingling.

Pattern Differentiation
Wind-Heat Invasion

> *Primary symptoms*: Nerve pain, itchiness, headache, possible skin irritation

> *Additional symptoms*: Fever and chills, sore throat, runny nose with yellow discharge

> *Tongue*: Thin white or yellow coat, sides slightly red

Pulse: Floating, rapid

Treatment principles: Reduce pain, expel wind-heat, boost Lungs

Acupuncture treatment: LI-4, LU-3, LU-7, LU-11, BL-11

Herbal treatment:
Bai Hu Jia Gui Zhi Tang (White Tiger Decoction Plus Cinnamon Twig)
[Shi Gao 30g, Jing Mi 15g, Zhi Mu 9g, Gui Zhi 6g, Zhi Gan Cao 6g]

Modifications:
Clearing more heat and relieving toxicity: + Ren Dong Teng 12g, Lian
Qiao 12g, Huang Bai 9g, Jin Yin Hua 15g
Enhance invigorating the Blood, unblocking the collaterals, dispelling wind, and
eliminating dampness: + Hai Tong Pi 9g, Jiang Huang 9g, Wei Ling Xian 6g, Fang
Ji 9g, Sang Zhi 15g

Wind-Cold Invasion

Primary symptoms: Nerve pain, body ache, lack of sweat, possible headache

Additional symptoms: Fever and chills (chills predominant), stuffy nose with runny
mucus, sneezing, scratchy throat

Tongue: Thin white coat

Pulse: Floating, possibly slightly tight

Treatment principles: Reduce pain, expel wind, boost Lungs

Acupuncture treatment: LI-4, LI-20, TW-5, SI-10, BL-12

Herbal treatment:
Wu Tou Tang (Aconite Decoction)
[Zhi Chuan Wu Tou 6g, Ma Huang 6g, Huang Qi 12g, Bai Shao 9g, Gan Cao 6g,
Feng Mi]

Lung Phlegm-Cold

Primary symptoms: Intense stabbing pain, numbness/tingling, headache, mental
confusion

Additional symptoms: Chronic cough, profuse white sputum that is easily
expectorated, chest fullness, possible asthma

Tongue: Thin white coat

Pulse: Floating, possibly slightly tight

Treatment principles: Reduce pain, transform phlegm, boost Lungs, and course the channels

Acupuncture treatment: LI-4, LR-3, LU-7, KI-26, ST-40, SP-3, SP-9

Herbal treatment:
Bu Fei Tang (Restore the Lung Decoction)
[Dang Shen 10g, Huang Qi 10–15g, Shu Di 12g, Wu Wei Zi 10g, Zi Wan 10g, Bai Zhu 10g, Chen Pi 3g, Gan Cao 3–6g]

Blood Stasis

Primary symptoms: Intense stabbing pain, numbness/tingling, headache

Additional symptoms: Dry skin, dizziness, irregular menses

Tongue: Dark with sublingual vein distension, possible petechiae

Pulse: Choppy or tight

Treatment principles: Reduce pain, move Blood, and course the channels

Acupuncture treatment: BL-17, SP-10, LR-8, LR-3

Herbal treatment:
Shu Jing Huo Xue Wan Jia Jian (Sinew Soothing Blood-Quickening Decoction Plus Modifications)
[Du Huo 9g, Qiang Huo 9g, Fang Feng 9g, Jing Jie 6g, Dang Gui 12g, Xu Duan 12g, Qing Pi 6g, Huai Niu Xi 9g, Wu Jia Pi 9g, Du Zhong 9g, Hong Hua 6g, Zhi Ke 6g, Jiang Huang 6g, Yan Hu Suo 9g]
Shen Tong Zhu Yu Tang (Drive out Stasis from a Painful Body Decoction)
[Tao Ren 9g, Hong Hua 6–9g, Dang Gui 9g, Chuan Xiong 6g, Qiang Huo 3g, Qin Jiao 3–6g, Di Long 6g, Mo Yao 6g, Xiang Fu 3g, Chuan Niu Xi 9g, Gan Cao 6g, Wu Ling Zhi 6g]

Point Recommendations Based on Pain Location

Upper extremities: PC-6, LI-11, ST-12, LU-9, CV-17

Lower extremities: KI-1, LR-4, SP-6, KI-6, GB-34

Additional Dermal Treatments

- Regular massage
- Liniments (Zheng Gu Shui, liquid magnesium, etc.)
- Herbal compresses
- Plum blossom along affected nerve tract(s)

Clinical Notes

- Needling along the affected nerve tract(s) acts to initiate a healing cascade that can aid in reducing inflammation along the nerve. Acupuncture points have been shown to be located in areas where there is an abundance or terminance of superficial C nerve fibers and this may act as a method through which the therapeutic effect takes place.

- Determining any points of potential compression upon a nerve, if they exist, is imperative to treating neuralgia as local points and distal points both can be used to address this issue. If a structural realignment is necessary, make the appropriate referral to have this addressed, as only so much can be done if this is not properly addressed.

- Microsystem approaches such as scalp or auricular acupuncture may be helpful as a distal method of reducing pain.

Other Treatment Considerations
Orthomolecular Considerations

- Magnesium
- N-Acetylcysteine (NAC)
- Vitamin C
- Vitamins B1 (thiamine), B6, B9 (folic acid), B12
- Vitamin D
- Vitamin E
- Biotin

- 5-HTP
- GABA
- Omega 6 fatty acids
- CoQ10
- Alpha lipoic acid
- Acetyl L-carnitine
- L-Glutamine
- Taurine

Phytotherapeutic Considerations

- Angelica
- Capsaicin
- Cayenne
- Curcumin/turmeric
- Kava kava

- Evening primrose oil
- Skullcap
- Feverfew
- Oats
- Colloidal silver

Dietary Considerations

Eat food which contains a good source of vitamin B1, such as yeast, wheat germ, egg yolks, carrots, wholewheat bread, parsley, spinach, and rosemary.

Chapter 25

Paralysis/Muscular Atrophy

Paralysis and muscular atrophy can develop as a result of direct parietal lobe damage of the sensorimotor cortex. Lesions or tumors to the right lobe seem to be particularly impactful, affecting the contralateral-associated region of the body. If there is a loss of sensation, an individual may lose a sense of their body within space, which in turn can generate motor disturbances such as paresis with hypotonia or a reduction in the ability ("will") to initiate movement. Peripheral nerve injuries that no longer allow for full conduction of nerve impulses to the appendages, as well as progressive inflammation and cytotoxicity from diffuse axonal injury, may also cause paralysis. Unilateral spasticity (hemiplegia) of a limb or side of the body can frequently occur when the appropriate cortical regions are implicated.

Chinese Medical Perspective: Wei (Atrophy) Syndrome

This refers to a group of disorders whose symptoms range from flaccidity and weakness in the sinews and muscles to diminished muscle mass. Muscular atrophy may be localized or systemic. Atrophy syndrome is often considered to be caused by injuries to the internal organs, especially insufficient Essence and Blood or Yin deficiency with excessive fire. For this reason, symptoms pertaining to heat or deficiency are common.

Relevant Biomedical Disorders

- Myasthenia gravis
- Multiple sclerosis
- Polyneuritis or Guillain-Barre disease
- Acute myelitis (inflammation of the spinal cord)
- Sequela of infectious diseases of the CNS including poliomyelitis

Chinese Medical Etiology

The main pathomechanism of atrophy syndrome/Wĕi Zhèng is a lack of nourishment and moistening of the sinews (muscles, tendons, and vessels). External and internal pathogens can both cause this condition and can mutually affect each other.

- *External heat or prolonged febrile disease*: This can cause Lung heat which injures fluids and impairs the dispersing and descending functions of the Lung. Moisture and nourishment are not disseminated to the sinews and muscles; the extremities are affected, becoming weak and flaccid with decreased motor control.

- *Exposure to dampness or irregular diet*: Both of these can result in an accumulation of dampness in the sinews and muscles that transforms into damp-heat, obstructing the flow of Qi and Blood and consuming body fluids. The sinews and muscles lose nourishment, become weak and flaccid, lose mass, and atrophy.

- *Weak constitution, chronic disease, unhealthy lifestyle, aging, excessive sexual activity*: Results in Spleen/Stomach deficiency: inefficient rotting and ripening and transforming and transporting results in Qi, Blood, body fluids, and essence deficiency. Qi deficiency causes impaired circulation of Blood and body fluids. A deficiency in Blood and body fluids fails to nourish and moisten the sinews, muscles, and bones, causing atrophy.

- *Liver and Kidney deficiency*: The Liver governs the sinews and stores the Blood to nourish sinews, while the Kidney governs the bones and stores the essence that produces marrow to nourish the bones. If the Liver and Kidney are deficient, there will be flaccidity and weakness of the sinews and bones.

Deficiency vs. Excess

The majority of patterns for Wĕi Zhèng present as deficiency rather than excess and heat rather than cold, although patterns of temporary excess or mixed deficiency and excess are possible. Excess patterns are characterized by acute onset and rapid progression so that immobility and loss of muscle mass occur in a relatively short period of time. Deficient patterns are characterized by a gradual onset and slow progression, with the lower extremities being more often affected.

Pattern Differentiation
Lung Heat with Fluid Injury

> ***Primary symptoms***: Rapidly developing flaccidity and immobility of the extremities with muscular atrophy

Additional symptoms: Fever during the initial stage of the illness, or a fever followed by weakness, dry skin, irritability, thirst, cough, scanty sputum, scanty urine, and dry stool

Tongue: Red tongue, yellow coat

Pulse: Thin, rapid (thready)

Treatment principles: Clear heat, moisten dryness, nourish the Lung, and generate the fluid

Acupuncture treatment: BL-13, LU-5, LU-7

Herbal treatment:
Qing Zao Jiu Fei Tang (Eliminate Dryness and Rescue the Lungs)
[Sang Ye 9g, Shi Gao 7.5g, Mai Men Dong 3g, E Jiao 3g, Hei Zhi Ma 3g, Xing Ren 2g, Pi Pa Ye 3g, Ren Shen 2g, Gan Cao 3g]

Modifications:
High fever, thirst, and sweating: Ren Shen, E Jiao; + Zhi Mu, Jin Yin Hua, Lian Qiao, Bei Sha Shen, increase Shi Gao
Dry cough with scanty sputum or copious phlegm: + Bei Mu, Gua Lou
Fever abated, with loss of appetite and severe dry mouth and throat, indicating injury to the Lung as well as the Stomach Yin: Use Yi Wei Tang (Benefit the Stomach Decoction)

Damp-Heat Accumulation

Primary symptoms: Heaviness of the limbs, weak and flaccid extremities with occasional numbness, and slight swelling in the affected extremities; most often affects the lower extremities

Additional symptoms: Possibly fever, stifling sensation in the chest and epigastrium, and dark, scanty, painful, and difficult urination

Tongue: Red tongue, yellow greasy coat

Pulse: Soft, rapid, possibly slippery

Treatment principles: Clear heat and drain dampness

Acupuncture treatment: BL-20, SP-9, LI-11, CV-7

Herbal treatment:
Jia Wei Er Miao San (Supplemented Mysterious Two Powder)
[Huang Bai 9g, Cang Zhu 9g, Huai Niu Xi 9g, Fen Fang Ji 9g, Bi Xie 9g, Dang Gui 6g, Gui Ban 6g]

Si Miao Wan (Four Marvel Pill)
[Huang Bai 24g, Cang Zhu 12g, Niu Xi 12g, Yi Yi Ren 24g]

Modifications:
Strengthen the effect of draining damp-heat via urination: + Mu Tong, Fang Ji, Bi Xie
Predominance of dampness presenting white slimy tongue coat: + Hou Po, Fu Ling, Hua Shi
To disinhibit dampness and free the connections: Dang Gui, Gui Ban; + Yi Yi Ren, Mu Tong, Can Sha, Mu Gua
Excessive heat injuring the Yin: Cang Zhu + Sheng Di Huang, Gui Ban, Mai Men Dong, Tian Hua Fen
Numbness of the limbs, limited range of motion, purple tongue, and thready, choppy pulse: + Chi Shao, Dan Shen, Tao Ren, Hong Hua
During rainy summer weather: + Huo Xiang, Pei Lan

Spleen and Stomach Deficiency

Primary symptoms: Gradual onset of flaccidity and weakness of the extremities aggravated by exertion, gradual loss of muscle mass, fatigue, lassitude, and shortness of breath

Additional symptoms: Poor appetite, loose stool, sallow complexion, abdominal distension, facial puffiness

Tongue: Pale tongue, thin white coat

Pulse: Thin, forceless, thready

Treatment principles: Strengthen the Spleen and Stomach; augment the Qi

Acupuncture treatment: CV-4, CV-6, SP-6, ST-36, BL-20, BL-21

Herbal treatment:
Shen Ling Bai Zhu San (Ginseng, Poria, and Atractylodes Powder)
[Ren Shen 10g, Bai Zhu 10g, Fu Ling 10g, Zhi Gan Cao 10g, Shan Yao 10g, Bai Bian Dou 7.5g, Lian Zi 5g, Yi Yi Ren 5g, Sha Ren 5g, Jie Geng 5g]

Modifications:
Accompanied by food stasis: + Gu Ya, Mai Ya, Shan Zha, Shen Qu
Chills and cold extremities: + Zhi Fu Zi, Gan Jiang
With Qi and Blood deficiency: + Huang Qi, Dang Gui
Obesity with excessive phlegm: Use Liu Jun Zi Tang (Six Gentlemen Decoction)
Significant Qi deficiency or Qi sinking: Use Bu Zhong Yi Qi Tang (Tonify the Middle and Augment the Qi Decoction)

Liver and Kidney Deficiency

Primary symptoms: Slow and gradual onset, weak and flaccid lower limbs, soreness and weakness of the lower back and spine, the inability to stand for a long time. Total loss of mobility and severe loss of muscle mass can result with exacerbation

Additional symptoms: Dizziness, vertigo, hair loss, dry throat, tinnitus, fatigue, nocturnal emmision, enuresis, and irregular menstruation

Tongue: Red tongue, scanty coat

Pulse: Thready and rapid

Treatment principles: Tonify the Liver and Kidney, nourish the Yin, and clear heat

Acupuncture treatment: BL-18, BL-23, SP-6, CV-4, KI-3, LR-3

Herbal treatment:
Hu Qian Wan (Hidden Tiger Pill)
[Shu Di Huang 24g, Zhi Mu 12g, Gui Ban 30g, Huang Bai 9g, Bai Shao 9g, Gu Hu 6g, Chen Pi 6g, Suo Yang 6g, Gan Jiang 3g]

Modifications:
Enhance the effects of nourishing the Liver and Kidney, strengthening the sinews and bones: + Zhu Gu Sui, Niu Xi
Sallow complexion, palpitations, pink tongue, and weak, thready pulse: + Huang Qi, Dang Shen, Dang Gui, Ji Xue Teng
Strong heat: Suo Yang, Gan Jiang, or use Zhi Bai Di Huang Wan
Prolonged illness with injury of Yin that led to injury of Yang with physical cold, cold extremities, copious clear urine, impotence, pale tongue, and deep, thready, forceless pulse: Huang Bai, Zhi Mu; + Lu Jiao Jiao, Bu Gu Zhi, Ba Ji Tian, Rou Gui

Blood Stasis

Primary symptoms: Chronic flaccidity and weakness of the limbs with muscular atrophy; numbness of the limbs

Additional symptoms: Dark-colored skin, possible muscular pain, blood vessels may be visible on the skin surface

Tongue: Purple with thin, white coating

Pulse: Choppy

Treatment principles: Move Qi, quicken the Blood, eliminate stasis, open the channels and collaterals

Acupuncture treatment: CV-6, SP-6, SP-10, BL-40

Herbal treatment:

Sheng Yu Tang Jia Jian (Sage-like Healing Decoction Plus Modifications)
[Dang Gui 9g, Shu Di Huang 9g, Bai Shao 9g, Chuan Xiong 9g, Ren Shen 9g, Huang Qi 9g, Tao Ren 9g, Hong Hua 9g, Huai Niu Xi 9g]

Acupuncture prescription based on the affected limbs:

Upper limbs: LI-15, LI-11, LI-4, TW-5, Hua Tuo Jia Ji, Yang Ming channel Pai Ci
Lower limbs: ST-31, ST-34, ST-35, ST-41, GB-39, [GB-34], GB-30, [SP-10], Hua Tuo Jia Ji, Yang Ming channel Pai Ci
Korean Sa-Am protocol: Lung tonification LU-9(+), SP-3(+), LU-10(−), HT-8(−)

Clinical Notes

To treat Wĕi Zhèng, strategies addressing the Yang Ming channels and organs should be adopted. The Spleen and Stomach meridians generate Qi, Blood, Essence, and body fluids. Located in the Middle Burner, they send vital substances to the Lung for dissemination to the entire body. They also supply the Liver and Kidney with Blood and Essence to nourish the sinews and bones. The Spleen governs the muscles and provides them with nourishment. Strengthening the Spleen and Stomach ensures the proper function and adequate supply of vital substances.

- A strategy of "harmonizing Yin and Yang" by treating the Du Mai and Ren Mai can be used in which there is superficial threading along the Du Mai and Ren Mai with long needles, alternating between the two channels from treatment to treatment.

- Often Japanese Sotai techniques can be used as a gentle movement modality to assist in range-of-motion improvement in cases where muscle and tendon spasticity or contracture is present.

- Bai Shao Gan Cao Wan, a simple two herb formula, can be added to other herbal prescriptions or as a standalone prescription in cases of spasticity, contracture, and paralysis.

- Plum blossom needling along the Du Mai and Ren Mai, alternating between the two channels from treatment to treatment, may be considered.

- Moxa along the Du Mai and Ren Mai, alternating between the two channels from treatment to treatment, may be considered.

- Needling the major points along the Du Mai and Ren Mai (GV-3/4/14/16/20/26; CV-3/4/6/12/17/23/24), alternating between the two channels from treatment to treatment, may be considered.

Other Therapeutic Considerations
Somatic Considerations

- Sotai
- Massage

- Qigong
- Tai Ji Quan

Orthomolecular Considerations

- Magnesium (oral or topical)
- L-Dopa (in cases of low dopamine levels)

Dietary Considerations

- Foods which help nourish the Blood and Sinews

Chapter 26

Neuroendocrine Dysfunction

It has been recorded that up to two-thirds of individuals who sustain a brain injury experience single or multiple pituitary-target hormone disruptions. Twenty percent of those affected have a combination of two or more deficiencies, many being transient in nature. Hypopituitarism is considered a common sequela of brain injury, and it has been suggested that pituitary cells are particularly vulnerable to trauma, this being especially true for somatotrophs and gonadotrophs. This dysregulation more commonly affects the gonadal or growth hormone (15%) channels of the endocrine system, though a wide array of channels and regulatory functions can be affected. Common endocrine disturbances are listed in Table 26.1.

TABLE 26.1 Common Endocrine Disturbances Following a Brain Injury

Hypo/hyperthyroidism
Impaired growth hormone release
Impaired adrenal cortical function
Hypopituitarism
Hypothalamic hypogonadism
Precocious puberty
Hyperphagia
Hyperprolactinemia
Temperature dysregulation
Syndrome of inappropriate diuretic hormone
Diabetes insipidus
Menstrual irregularities
Changes in sexual function

Some of these concerns will be specifically addressed in the following chapters. The mechanisms of these effects have been identified as the result of a direct mechanical injury, cytotoxic processes, or both. This occurs to the central nervous system components of the hypothalamic–pituitary–organ axes. Infarction of the pituitary lobe can also result from compression or occlusion of the hypophysial blood vessels stemming from brain swelling and edema.

Thyroid Dysfunction: Hypothyroidism
Diagnosis

- Myxedema

- Thyroid hormone deficiency

Etiology

Primary:

- Autoimmune

- Hashimoto's thyroiditis

- Chronic influence of thyroid with lymphocytic infiltration caused by autoimmune factors

- In women, 8:1 more

- Often family history of thyroid disorders

Post-therapeutic:

- Surgery

- Drugs for hyperthyroidism

- Iodine deficiency—goiter

Secondary:

- Decrease in thyroid stimulating hormone from hypothalamus

- Decrease in thyroid stimulating hormone from pituitary

Signs and Symptoms of Hypothyroidism

- Insidious onset

- Fatigue

- Dull facies with periorbital edema

- Hoarse voice, slow speech

- Cold intolerance, hypothermia

- Coarse, dry, thin hair

- Coarse, dry, scaly, thick skin

- Weight gain

- Memory and intellectual impairment

- Constipation

- Paresthesias

- Anemia

- Macroglossia

- Bradycardia

- Pericardial, pleural effusion

- Carotenodermia (orange skin on palms and soles)

- Menorrhagia

- Brisk contraction, slow relaxation of reflexes

- Thyroid may be enlarged, tender or non-tender, smooth or nodular, firm or rubbery—if nodular, refer for evaluation

Diagnostic Testing

- Decreased serum T4 (thyroxine) [normal: 0.5–5.0; some suggest higher than 2.5 is troublesome]

- Decreased T3 uptake (triiodothyronine)

- Elevated or decreased TSH (thyroid stimulating hormone)

Biomedical Approaches

- Replacement therapy: desiccated thyroid [contains T1, T2, T3, T4], L-thyroxine (synthroid, levoxyl) [only T4]

- Iodine 4mg/day, tyrosin

- Vitamin D helps T3 bind to receptors

Chinese Medical Perspective

Acupuncture treatment protocol: CV-6, GV-20, Yintang, LI-10, LI-11, SP-6, KI-7, 8 points equidistant around 0.5 cun from the center of the navel plus pattern-specific points.[1]

Heart Yang Deficiency

Primary symptoms: Fatigue, palpitations, spontaneous sweating, cold limbs

Additional symptoms: Feeling of cold, pale face

Tongue: Pale, wet, swollen

Pulse: Empty

---

1   Abbate, Skya. The early diagnosis and treatment of hypothyroidism. *Acupuncture Today*. 2001 Jul; 2(7). Web. www.acupuncturetoday.com/mpacms/at/article.php?id=27779

Treatment principles: Nourish the Heart, raise Yang, boost Qi

Acupuncture treatment: [CV-6, GV-20, Yintang, LI-10, LI-11, SP-6, KI-7] + BL-15, HT-7, KI-1

Herbal treatment:
Bao Yuan Tang (Protect the Source Decoction)
[Huang Qi 20g, Ren Shen 20g, Rou Gui 8g, Gan Cao 5g]

Spleen Qi Deficiency

Primary symptoms: Poor appetite, distension after eating, weakness of the four limbs, fatigue, loose stools

Tongue: Pale and swollen with teeth marks

Pulse: Wiry (bowstring), slippery

Treatment principles: Boost Qi, nourish the Spleen

Acupuncture treatment: [CV-6, GV-20, Yintang, LI-10, LI-11, SP-6, KI-7] + SP-3, ST-36, BL-20

Herbal treatment:
Bu Zhong Yi Qi Tang Jia Jian (Supplement the Center and Boost the Qi Decoction Plus Modifications)
[Huang Qi 9g, Ren Shen 12g, Bai Zhu 9g, Kun Bu 9g, Hai Zao 9g, Zhi Gan Cao 9g, Dang Gui 18g, Chen Pi 9g, Chai Hu 12g, Sheng Ma 9g]

Spleen Yang Deficiency

Primary symptoms: Cold limbs, chilliness, edema, fatigue

Additional symptoms: Poor appetite, distension after eating, weakness of the four limbs, loose stools

Tongue: Pale, wet, and swollen with teeth marks

Pulse: Deep

Treatment principles: Tonify the Yang, boost Qi, nourish the Spleen, warm the middle

Acupuncture treatment: CV-6, GV-20, Yintang, LI-10, LI-11, SP-6, KI-7, SP-3, ST-36, BL-20, CV-4, CV-8 moxa

Herbal treatment:
Fu Zi Li Zhong Wan (Prepared Aconite Pill to Regulate the Middle)
[Gan Jiang 3–12g, Ren Shen 12g, Bai Zhu 9g, Zhi Fu Zi 6g, Zhi Gan Cao 5g]

Kidney Qi Deficiency

Primary symptoms: Fatigue, shortness of breath, cold limbs, weak back and knees, copious clear urine, incontinence, nocturia

Tongue: Pale

Pulse: Deep, weak, possibly tight

Treatment principles: Boost the Qi, nourish the Kidney

Acupuncture treatment: [CV-6, GV-20, Yintang, LI-10, LI-11, SP-6, KI-7] + KI-3, BL-23

Herbal treatment:
Zuo Gui Wan Jia Jian (Left-Restoring Kidney Yin Pill Plus Modifications)
[Shu Di Huang 24g, Shan Yao 12g, Shan Zhu Yu 12g, Gou Qi Zi 12g, Kun Bu 9g, Hai Zao 9g, Chuan Niu 9g, Tu Si Zi 12g, Lu Jiao Jiao 12g, Gui Ban Jiao 12g]

Kidney Yang Deficiency

Primary symptoms: Fatigue, pale complexion, cold extremities, sore low back and knees, tiredness

Tongue: Pale

Pulse: Deep, slow, thready

Treatment principles: Raise Yang, tonify the Kidney

Acupuncture treatment: [CV-6, GV-20, Yintang, LI-10, LI-11, SP-6, KI-7] + KI-3, GV-4, BL-23

Herbal treatment:
Jin Gui Shen Qi Wan Jia Wei (Kidney Qi Pill from The Golden Cabinet Plus Modifications)
[Shu Di Huang 6–10g, Shan Zhu Yu 6–10g, Shan Yao 6–10g, Fu Ling 6–10g, Ze Xie 6–10g, Dan Pi 3–6g, Fu Zi 3–6g, Rou Gui 3–6g, Yi Zhi Ren 6–10g, Shi Chang Pu 6–10g]
You Gui Wan Jia Wei (Restore the Right [Kidney] Pill Plus Modifications)
[Rou Gui 6–12g, Fu Zi 16–18g, Shu Di Huang 24g, Shan Zhu Yu 9g, Shan Yao 12g, Kun Bu 9g, Hai Zao 9g, Gou Qi Zi 12g, Lu Jiao Jiao 12g, Tu Si Zi 12g, Du Zhong 12g, Dang Gui 9g]

Thyroid Dysfunction: Hyperthyroidism
Thyrotoxicosis: Graves' Disease
Etiology
Unknown, but probably immunologic

Signs and Symptoms of Hyperthyroidism

- Nervousness, increased activity
- Increased perspiration, heat intolerance
- Fatigue, weakness
- Increased appetite, weight loss
- Insomnia

- Frequent bowel movements
- Goiter
- Tachycardia, atrial fibrillation
- Warm, moist skin
- Tremor
- Stare

In Graves' disease

- Exophthalmos
- Ocular muscle weakness

- Pretibial edema
- Non-pitting, pruritic edema

Diagnostic Testing

- Decreased TSH
- Elevated free T4

- Elevated T3 uptake
- Elevated T3

Biomedical Treatment

- Anti-thyroid agents— Propylthiouracil, Methimazole (Tapazole)

- Radioactive iodine
- Surgery

Chinese Medical Perspective
Chinese Medical Etiology

- Internal damage of the seven emotions
- Unregulated eating and drinking
- Aging
- Enduring disease

Pattern Differentiation
Qi Stagnation and Phlegm Congealing

Primary symptoms: Goiter swelling in the front of the neck that is soft and not painful, possible exophthalmia

Additional symptoms: Emotional depression, frequent suspicion, irritability, easy anger

Tongue: Pale red and thin, slimy coat

Pulse: Wiry (bowstring), slippery

Treatment principles: Course the Liver, rectify Qi, transform phlegm, scatter nodulation

Acupuncture treatment: LR-3, ST-40, TW-13, SI-16, LI-17, SI-17, CV-22

Herbal treatment:
Xiao Chai Hu Tang + Xiao Yao San (Minor Bupleurum Decoction + Rambling Powder)
[Xia Ku Cao 15g, Mu Li 12g, Zhe Bei Mu 12g, Fu Ling 12g, Chai Hu 9g, Dang Shen 9g, Bai Zhu 9g, Dang Gui 9g, Bai Shao 9g, Kun Bu 9g, Ban Xia 9g, Chen Pi 6g, Gan Cao 6g, Da Zao 3pc, Sheng Jiang 3 slices]

Modifications:
Depressive heat + Xuan Shen 15g, Huang Qin 12g
Increased appetite + Shi Gao 15g, Zhi Mu 9g
Hand or finger tremors + Jiang Can 15g, Chan Tui 15g

Liver Fire Flaring Upward

Primary symptoms: Marked goiter that is soft and not painful, possible exophthalmia

Additional symptoms: Emotional tension, irritability, impetuosity, red face, headache, dizziness, tinnitus, hand and tongue trembling, palpitations, insomnia, thirst, profuse drinking, bitter taste

Tongue: Red tongue, yellow coat

Pulse: Wiry (bowstring), rapid

Treatment principles: Clear the Liver and drain fire, transform phlegm, scatter nodulation

Acupuncture treatment: LR-2, GB-34, TW-13, SI-16, LI-17, SI-17, CV-22

Herbal treatment:

Long Dan Xie Gan Tang Jia Jian (Gentiana Drain the Liver Decoction Plus Modifications)

[Xia Ku Cao 15g, Xuan Shen 15g, Sheng Di 12g, Mu Li 12g, Long Gu 12g, Ban Xia 12g, Fu Ling 12g, Zhe Bei Mu 12g, Chai Hu 9g, Huang Qin 9g, Zhi Zi 9g, Dang Gui 9g, Hai Zao 9g, Kun Bu 9g, Chen Pi 6g, Gan Cao 6g]

Modifications:

Hand or finger tremors + Shi Jue Ming 15g, Gou Teng 9g, Bai Shao 9g

Fatigue + Huang Qi 20g

Oral thirst, profuse drinking + Mai Men Dong 12g, Tian Hua Fen 12g

Pain and distension in the eyes + Bai Zhi 15g, Gou Qi Zi 15g, Shi Chang Pu 9g, Ci Ji Li 9g

Yin Deficiency, Yang Excess

Primary symptoms: Goiter, possible exophthalmia, possible nodulations

Additional symptoms: 5-palm heat, insomnia, profuse dreams, dizziness, blurred vision, palpitations, restlessness, easy sweating, hot flashes, malar flush, shaking hands, tinnitus, increased food intake but emaciation, lack of strength

Tongue: Red tongue, scanty coat

Pulse: Wiry (bowstring), fine, rapid

Treatment principles: Enrich Yin, subdue Yang, transform phlegm, scatter nodulation

Acupuncture treatment: LR-3, HT-7, KI-7, TW-13, SI-16, LI-17, SI-17, ST-9

Herbal treatment:

Tian Wan Bu Xin Dan + Yi Guan Jian (Heavenly Emperor Supplement the Heart Elixir + One Link Decoction)

[Sheng Di 15g, Xuan Shen 15g, Huang Yaso Zi 15g, Mai Men Dong 12g, Tian Men Dong 12g, Gou Qi Zi 12g, Suan Zao Ren 12g, Long Gu 12g, Mu Li 12g, Fu Ling 12g, Chuan Lian Zi 9g, Yuan Zhi 9g, Wu Weri Zi 9g, Bai Zi Ren 9g, Ban Xia 9g, Hai Zao 9g, Kun Bu 9g, Chen Pi 6g, Huang Lian 3g]

Modifications:

Severe Yin deficiency: + Gui Ban 12g, He Shou Wu 12g, Nu Zhen Zi 12g

Severe deficiency fire: + Huang Bai 9g

Sudden Liver fire engendering wind: + Gou Teng 15g, Jiang Can 9g

Leukopenia: + Hu Zhang 12g, Gui Ban 12g

Qi and Yin Dual Deficiency

Primary symptoms: Spirit lassitude and fatigue, shortness of breath, dizziness, tinnitus, palpitations, emaciation, lack of strength

Additional symptoms: Dry rough eyes, pale lusterless complexion with possible malar flush, restlessness, insomnia, impaired memory, dry mouth and throat, possible tremors of hand and tongue

Tongue: Red tongue, thin or peeling coat

Pulse: Vacuous, rapid

Treatment principles: Boost the Qi, nourish Yin

Acupuncture treatment: BL-15, BL-18, BL-20, BL-23, TW-13, SI-16, SI-17, LI-17

Herbal treatment:
Jia Kang Zhing Fang (Heavy Hyperthyroid Formula)
[Huang Qi 30–45g, Xia Ku Cao 30g, He Shou Wu 20g, Sheng Di 15g, Bai Shao 12g, Xiang Fu 12g]

Modifications:
Bulging, distending eyes + Gou Qi Zi 15g, Bai Jie Zi 9g, Ze Xie 9g, Lai Fu Zi 9g, Di Gu Pi 9g, Ci Ji Li 9g
Severe palpitations, shortness of breath + Sheng Mai San
Yin deficiency with stirring of wind + Gui Ban 15g, Bie Jia 15g, Zhen Zhu Mu 15g

Visceral Agitation (Zang Zao)

Visceral agitation is a paroxysmal mental disease that primarily affects the Heart organ as a result of hormonal disruption. The agitation refers to agitation of the Blood that has resulted from damaged Yin and the rashness, impetuosity, and impatience that characterize this condition. The Chinese literature traditionally states that this condition is more common in adolescent females. It may, however, also be used to describe severe premenstrual tension, and is noted to often be seen in perimenopausal women. Visceral agitation often begins as melancholy, depression, and emotional lability but then progresses to alternating laughing and crying for no reason, sighing for no apparent reason, and vexation and agitation. When addressing these symptoms as a sequela of brain trauma and hormonal dysregulation, however, site and severity of the injury plays more of a role in determining the condition than does gender, age, or other factors.

Relevant Western Diseases

Psychoneurosis, depression, stress reactive types, and hormonal psychosis

Differential Diagnosis
Medical Disorders

- CNS disorders, including mass lesions, seizure disorders, etc.

- History of head trauma

- Effects of substances: Alcohol or illicit substance intoxication or withdrawal; side effects of medications

Psychiatric Disorders

- Histrionic Personality Disorder

- Other Personality Disorders

- Major Depressive Disorder

- Bipolar Affective Disorder (BAD)

- Premenstrual Dysphoric Disorder (PMDD)

Chinese Medical Etiology

Visceral agitation develops primarily from a lack of nourishment to the Heart Shen and harassment of the Shen by some sort of pathogenic heat. Lack of nourishment to the Heart may be the result of a Heart-Spleen dual deficiency. Pathogenic heat may be depressive heat, phlegm heat, or deficiency heat. Clinically, Liver depression is nearly always a present factor in visceral agitation. This is generally Liver depression with a Spleen deficiency which acts as mechanisms for Heart-Spleen deficiency with the development of both depressive and phlegm heat.

Chronic or severe depressive heat damages and consumes Yin and Blood, which may then give rise to Yin-deficient effulgent fire or Yin deficiency with Yang hyperactivity. Most cases of visceral agitation present with at least four simultaneous disease mechanisms (Liver depression, depressive heat, Spleen deficiency, and Heart Blood deficiency). In most cases, this disease is considered to be caused by stress, overexertion, poor diet, pregnancy and postpartum difficulty, and constitutional factors; however, as noted above, trauma may also be a pathomechanism.

Pattern Differentiation
Qi and Blood Deficiency

Primary symptoms: Cries frequently and does not talk, or not clear why they feel such sadness, may be crying and laughing inappropriately

Additional symptoms: Sensitive, Shen is very weak, moody, upset, depressed, easily angered, low appetite and energy, insomnia

Tongue: Pale tongue, thin white coat

Pulse: Weak, thready

Acupuncture treatment: PC-6, HT-3, HT-7, GV-20, SP-6, KI-9, Yintang

Herbal treatment:
Gan Mai Da Zao Tang (Licorice, Wheat, and Jujube Decoction)
[Gan Cao 9g, Fu Xiao Mai 9g, Da Zao 10pc]

Modifications:
Heart Blood deficiency: + Shu Di Huang, Long Yan Rou
Heart Yin deficiency: + Bai Zi Ren, Bai He
Heart Qi deficiency: + Ren Shen, Dang Shen
Heart Fire: + Sheng Di Huang, Gan Cao Shao
Heart Shen sedating: + Zhen Zhu Mu, Ci Shi

Heart Shen Not Being Nourished

Primary symptoms: Devitalized essence spirit, abstraction, sorrowfulness without apparent cause and abnormal laughing and crying, susceptibility to fright

Additional symptoms: Heart vexation, insomnia, profuse dreams, heart palpitations, lassitude of the spirit

Tongue: Tender and red

Pulse: Fine, wiry (bowstring)

Treatment principles: Enrich the Heart and supplement the Spleen, nourish the Blood and quiet the spirit

Acupuncture treatment: GV-26, GV-20, PC-6, HT-7

Acupuncture modifications:
During hysterical crisis: Use GV-26, PC-8, KI-1
Pronounced chest oppression: + CV-17
Plum pit Qi: + ST-40, CV-23, HT-5
Heart spirit lack of nourishment: + BL-15, BL-17, SP-6
Abnormal laughing and weeping: + SI-3
Essence spirit abstraction: + BL-15, BL-47

Herbal treatment:
Symptoms of Yin and Blood deficiency more pronounced: Gan Mai Da Zao Tang Jia Wei (Licorice, Wheat, and Jujube Decoction Plus Modifications)
[Suan Zao Ren 12g, Sheng Di 12g, Bai He 12g, Gan Cao 10–15g, Huai Xiao Mai 15–30g, Da Zao 5–15pc]

Symptoms of Liver depression more pronounced: Xiao Yao San He Gan Mai Da Zao Tang Jia Wei (Rambling Powder with Licorice, Wheat, and Jujube Decoction Plus Modifications)
[Chai Hu 6g, Bo He 3–6g, Bai Shao 10g, Dang Gui 10g, Bai Zhu 10g,

Fu Shen 12g, Gan Cao 10g, Huai Xiao Mai 15–30g, Suan Zao Ren 12–15g, Ye Jiao Teng 10–15g, Da Zao 5pc]

If complicated by phlegm heat: Wen Dan Tang He Gan Mai Da Zao Tang Jia Jian (Warm the Gallbladder Decoction with Licorice, Wheat, and Jujube Decoction Plus Modifications)
[Ban Xia 10g, Fu Ling 10g, Chen Pi 6g, Zhi Ke 6g, Zhu Ru 6–10g, Gan Cao 6g, Chai Hu 6–10g, Bai Shao 10g, Xiang Fu 10g, Dan Pi 10g, Zhi Zi 6g, Huai Xiao Mai 15–30g, Da Zao 5pc]

Symptoms of Heart–Spleen dual deficiency more pronounced: Gui Pi Tang He Gan Mai Da Zao Tang Jia Wei (Restore the Spleen Decoction with Licorice, Wheat, and Jujube Decoction)
[Huang Qi 10–15g, Dang Shen 10g, Bai Zhu 10g, Fu Shen 12g, Dang Gui 6–10g, Long Yan Rou 10g, Mu Xiang 6g, Yuan Zhi 6–10g, Suan Zao Ren 12g, Huai Xiao Mai 15–30g, Da Zao 5pc, Shi Chang Pu 6g, Gan Cao 10g]

Modifications:
Plum pit Qi: + Ban Xia, Hou Po
Even more pronounced Qi stagnation: + Fo Shou, He Huan Pi
Liver depression transformed into heat: + Dan Pi, Zhi Zi, Huang Qin

Heart–Liver Fire

Primary symptoms: Heart vexation, easy anger, lack of tranquility when sitting or lying down, crying and laughing without constancy, profuse dreams, susceptibility to fright

Tongue: Red tongue, thin yellow coat

Pulse: Fine, wiry (bowstring), rapid

Treatment principles: Clear the Liver and resolve depression, tranquilize the Heart and quiet the spirit

Acupuncture treatment: LR-3, SP-6, GV-16, HT-8

Acupuncture modifications:
Severe agitation + KI-1
Pronounced Liver depression + LR-3, TW-6
Liver depression transforming into fire + LR-2, GB-43
Chest oppression + CV-17
Accompanying phlegm or plum pit Qi + ST-40
Accompanying Blood stasis + SP-10

Herbal treatment:
Dan Zhi Xiao Yao San Jia Wei (Augmented Rambling Powder Plus Modifications)

[Zhi Shi Ying 15g, Long Gu 12g, Mu Li 12g, He Huan Pi 12g, Chai Hu 9g, Bai Zhu 9g, Fu Ling 12g, Dang Gui 9g, Bai Shao 9g, Dan Pi 9g, Shan Zhi 9g, Gan Cao 6g]

Modifications:
Severe heart vexation and insomnia: + Ci Shi, Mia Dong, Wu Wei Zi
Chest and rib-side distension and oppression with dry mouth and bitter taste: + Huang Qin, Sheng Di, Qing Pi
Headaches and dizziness: + Shi Hue Ming, Ju Hua, Sang Ye

Liver–Kidney Deficiency

Primary symptoms: Heart vexation, irritability, insomnia, heart palpitations, susceptibility to fright

Additional symptoms: Dry mouth, dry stools, 5-palm heat, dizziness, tinnitus, low back and knee soreness and limpness

Tongue: Red tongue and scanty, possibly dry, possibly yellow coat

Pulse: Fine, wiry (bowstring), and rapid or surging

Treatment principles: Enrich the Kidneys and clear the Liver, nourish the Heart and quiet the Shen

Acupuncture treatment: HT-7, PC-6, KI-3, SP-6, CV-4, GV-20, GV-26

Herbal treatment:
Yin deficiency or deficient heat: Bai He Di Huang Tang He Zi Shui Qing Gan Yin (Lily Bulb and Rehmannia Decoction with Enrich Water and Clear the Liver Decoction)
[Bai He 10g, Sheng Di 12g, Shu Di 12g, Shan Yao 10g, Shan Zhu Yu 10g, Dan Pi 6–10g, Fu Ling 10g, Zi Xie 6–10g, Chai Hu 3–6g, Bai Shao 10g, Zhi Zi 6–10g, Suan Zao Ren 12–15g, Dang Gui 10g]

Yin deficiency and Yang hyperactivity: Tian Ma Gou Teng Yin He Gan Mai Da Zao Tang Jia Wei (Gastrodia and Uncaria Decoction with Licorice, Wheat, and Jujube Decoction Plus Modifications)
[Tian Ma 10g, Gou Teng 10g, Du Zhong 10g, Niu Xi 10g, Shi Jue Ming 12g, Sheng Di 12g, Zhi Zi 6–10g, Huang Qin 10g, Chai Hu 6–9g, Fu Shen 12g, Ye Jiao Teng 10–15g, Huai Xiao Mai 10–15g, Gan Cao 6–10g, Da Za 5pc]

Yin deficiency with phlegm fire: Wen Dan Tang Jia Wei (Warm the Gallbladder Decoction Plus Modifications)
[Ban Xia 12g, Fu Ling 9g, Chen Pi 9g, Zhi Shi 6g, Zhu Ru 9g, Dan Nan Xing 9g, Ting Ling Zi 9g, Zhi Mu 9g, Mai Dong 12g, Ye Jiao Teng 12g, Gan Cao 6g, Da Zao 5pc]

Chapter 27

Incontinence and Bowel Disorders

Due to the brain housing the regulatory system for bowel and bladder function, a brain injury can disturb control over these functions and result in urinary or fecal incontinence.

Urinary incontinence is generally associated with bilateral central lesions as well as poor functional status. The individual will often experience an altered bladder sensation, lowered capacity, increased sense of urgency, and greater frequency. Damage to the spinal cord, pudendal nerve, or sacral nerve roots can also result in urinary incontinence. Urinary tract infection (UTI) can occur both early after injury as well as long after the initial incident. Interventions for urinary incontinence include maintaining adequate hydration, minimizing intake of caffeine and caramel-colored drinks, timed voiding, use of cranberry tablets or D-Mannose, and early detection and treatment of UTI. If incontinence persists even after time-voiding training, there may be a bladder study performed and a referral to a urologist familiar with brain injury-related bladder concerns. The urologist may recommend medications, generally anti-cholinergics, or an external portable collection device; adult disposable briefs may be considered.

Fecal incontinence does not occur as frequently, though it has been associated with similar cortical and spinal pathways to those that regulate bladder function. Diarrhea, constipation, impaction, or bowel obstruction may result from changes in mobility, tube feedings, food consistency and intake status, fluid intake, and medication. The impact of narcotics on bowel regularity, as used for acute and chronic pain management, is a challenge for many individuals and is of particular concern. Good bowel hygiene, including a routine that promotes emptying at least two or three times weekly, is necessary for the establishment of bowel continence and regularity. Additionally, ensuring dietary and fluid intakes include enough bulk, roughage, and fluid is important to aid in regularity. Medications used to restore and maintain bowel emptying include stool softeners, irritant cathartics that promote bowel regularity, bulk laxatives, suppositories, or low-volume enemas.

Individuals should be assessed for signs of constipation or impaction, including abdominal distension, nausea, and decreased appetite. Other signs of autonomic dysregulation such as high blood pressure and sweating may also indicate impaction. While constipation itself is not a critical disorder, the complications that can accompany constipation are clinically significant. Continued constipation can result in an auto-intoxication via resorption of toxins that remain in the intestines. Symptoms of auto-intoxication include dizziness, headache, loss of appetite, irritability, insomnia, acne, and dry, cracking, or peeling skin. Chronic constipation can also lead to stubborn perianal disorders that do not respond well to treatment, including hemorrhoids, perianal fissures and fistulas, and perianal abscesses. It is also possible for constipation to provoke a medical crisis; for example, cerebrovascular accident due to hemorrhage and myocardial infarction may be induced by forcing and straining during defecation.

If cognitive functioning is affected, the brain-injured individual may be a poor reporter of bowel emptying, which can be an issue for caregivers.

Brain Injury in Conjunction with Spinal Cord Injury

If an individual has a concomitant brain injury and spinal cord injury, they may not be able to feel or control their bowels. When this is the case, proper and routine bowel care becomes necessary to prevent further complications such as constipation or, in severe cases, toxic mega colon. This consists of a bowel program as well as assistance for the individual in eating properly: a high-fiber diet, drinking adequate fluids to ensure proper hydration, and being active through exercise. In cases where the individual requires a wheelchair, this means getting up from the chair at regular intervals.

Bladder control is also a concern here. Renal disease was recently the leading cause of morbidity in individuals with spinal cord injury. Necessary focus includes preventing UTI, maintaining low-pressure urine storage, and (if able) voiding without urinary leakage or over-distension of the urinary bladder. Depending on the level of the spinal cord injury, the bladder may be either reflexic or areflexic. Management usually entails an indwelling catheter, an intermittent catheter, or, in cases of men with a reflexic bladder, an external collector. Intermittent cathetization has a reduced risk of infection and is generally preferred despite associated risks of urethral trauma, strictures, and hematuria. An individual with memory problems may have difficulty remembering to maintain the 4–6-hour schedule of an intermittent catheter.

Chinese Medical Approaches: Urinary Incontinence
Relevant Chinese Medical Diseases

> Frequent urination (Xiǎo Biàn Pín Shuò), urinary incontinence (Xiǎo Biàn Bù Jìn), and nocturnal enuresis (Yí Niào)

The mechanisms of frequent urination, urinary incontinence, and nocturnal enuresis are essentially the same. Frequent urination refers to an obvious increase in the need to urinate over a period of time. Incontinence refers to a lack of control over urination. Leakage of varying amounts of urine may occur without warning or immediately on perceiving the urge to urinate. The latter is termed urge incontinence. Leakage which occurs as a result of increased intra-abdominal pressure caused by sneezing, coughing, or jumping is called stress incontinence. Nocturnal enuresis is urinary incontinence during sleep and is seen primarily in children.

Relevant Biomedical Diseases/Conditions

- Urinary tract infection (UTI)
- Prostatitis
- Diabetes mellitus/insipidus
- Post-menopausal atrophic changes in the bladder and urethral wall

- Hypothyroidism
- Multiple sclerosis
- Benign prostatitic hyperplasia (BPH)
- Interstitial cystitis

Chinese Medical Etiology

- Exogenous Damp-Heat
- Diet of greasy, spicy foods and alcohol can generate Damp-Heat
- Childbirth
- Constitutional deficiency

- Aging
- Excessive sexual activity
- Chronic cough
- Imbalance of any of the seven emotions

In most cases the pathology of frequent urination, urinary incontinence, and nocturnal enuresis is characterized by deficiency. Excess patterns, when they occur, tend to be more common in children.

Pattern Differentiation
Damp-Heat in the Bladder

Primary symptoms: Frequent urination, urinary incontinence, or nocturnal enuresis with dark scanty urine, burning sensation during micturition, distension in the lower abdomen

Additional symptoms: Bitter and sticky taste in the mouth, thirst with little desire to drink; constipation with incomplete defecation in some cases

Tongue: Red with yellow, greasy coating

Pulse: Slippery, rapid

Treatment principles: Clear heat, drain dampness

Acupuncture treatment: CV-3, SP-6, SP-9, TW-5, ST-28, BL-28

Herbal treatment:
Ba Zheng San (Eight Corrections Powder)
[Chuan Mu Tang 3–6g, Hua Shi 12–30g, Che Qian Zi 9–15g, Qu Mai 6–12g, Bian Xu 6–12g, Zhi Zi 3–9g, Jiu Da Huang 6–9g, Deng Xin Cao 3–6g, Gan Cao 3–9g]

Liver Qi Stagnation

Primary symptoms: Frequent urination, urinary incontinence, or nocturnal enuresis accompanied by emotional stress, anger/irritability, or depression

Additional symptoms: Distension and pain in the chest and hypochondriac regions

Tongue: Normal or dusky

Pulse: Wiry (bowstring)

Treatment principles: Soothe the Liver, regulate Qi

Acupuncture treatment: LR-1, LR-3, LR-8, LR-14

Herbal treatment:
Xiao Yao San Jia Wei (Augmented Rambling Powder)
[Chai Hu 9g, Dang Gui 9g, Bai Shao 9g, Bai Zhu 9g, Fu Ling 9g, Pao Jiang 6g, Zhi Gan Cao 6g, Bo He 3g, Wu Yao 6g]

Kidney and Heart Deficiency

Primary symptoms: Frequent urination, urinary incontinence, or particularly nocturnal enuresis accompanied by nervousness

Additional symptoms: Palpitations, insomnia, dream-disturbed sleep, disorientation, forgetfulness

Tongue: Pale with white coating

Pulse: Thin, slow, weak

Treatment principles: Boost Qi, supplement the Heart and Kidney, astringe fluids

Acupuncture treatment: HT-7, KI-3, BL-15, BL-23

Herbal treatment:
Sang Piao Xiao San (Mantis Egg Case Powder)

[Sang Piao Xiao 9g, Duan Long Gu 12g, Fu Ling 9g, Yuan Zhi 9g, Shi Chang Pu 9g, Ren Shen 12g, Dang Gui 9g, Zhi Gui Ban 15g]

Lung and Spleen Qi Deficiency

Primary symptoms: Frequent urination, urinary incontinence, or nocturnal enuresis which is worse with fatigue or exertion or when coughing or sneezing

Additional symptoms: Fatigue, weakness, shortness of breath, spontaneous perspiration, weak voice, poor appetite, chronic loose stools or diarrhea

Tongue: Pale with thin, white coating

Pulse: Weak and thready

Treatment principles: Supplement the Lung and Spleen, boost Qi, ascend the clear Yang Qi

Acupuncture treatment: SP-3, BL-20, CV-6, ST-36, LU-9, BL-13, LU-7, GV-20

Herbal treatment:
Bu Zhong Yi Qi Tang (Supplement the Center and Boost the Qi Decoction) [Huang Qi 15g, Dang Shen 10g, Bai Zhu 10g, Zhi Gan Cao 6g, Chen Pi 6g, Dang Gui 6g, Chai Hu 3g, Sheng Ma 3–4.5g]

Kidney Yang Deficiency

Primary symptoms: Frequent urination with copious or scanty clear urine, urinary incontinence, or nocturnal enuresis; worse with exposure to cold and after prolonged lifting or standing

Additional symptoms: Sore, weak low back and knees, cold limbs and body, pale complexion, fatigue

Tongue: Pale and moist with white coating

Pulse: Deep, weak, and thready, particularly in the chi position

Treatment principles: Warm and supplement Kidney Yang

Acupuncture treatment: KI-3, GV-4, GV-20, BL-23, CV-4 + moxa

Herbal treatment:
Jin Gui Shen Qi Wan (Golden Coffer Kidney Qi Pill)
[Shu Di Huang 6g, Shan Zhu Yu 6g, Shan Yao 6g, Ze Xie 6g, Mu Dan Pi 6g, Fu Ling 6g, Fu Zi 9g, Rou Gui 3g, Chuan Niu Xi 6g, Che Qian Zi 6g]

Kidney Yin Deficiency

Primary symptoms: Frequent urination with scanty dark urine and possible irritation or sensation of heat, urinary incontinence, nocturnal enuresis, dribbling of urine

Additional symptoms: Sore, weak low back and knees, dizziness, insomnia, dry throat, night sweats, tinnitus

Tongue: Red with little coating

Pulse: Thready and rapid

Treatment principles: Supplement the Kidney, nourish Yin, clear deficient heat

Acupuncture treatment: KI-3, KI- 6, KI-2, BL-23, CV-4

Herbal treatment:
Zhi Bai Di Huang Wan (Anemarrhena, Phellodendron, and Rehmannia Decoction) [Shu Di Huang 24g, Shan Yao 12g, Shan Zhu Yu 12g, Zhi Mu 9g, Huang Bai 9g, Fu Shen 9g, Bai Zi Ren 9g, Zhi Gan Cao 6g, Ci Shi 6g, Hu Po 6g, Suan Zao Ren 9g, Yuan Zhi 9g]

Clinical Notes

- In cases of brain injury causing incontinence, acupuncture points which have a direct effect on the brain/marrow should be considered. In cases of spinal cord injury, local acupuncture near the affected vertebrae/nerve tract is an important component. This may include relevant points along the Du meridian, Hua Tuo Jia points, or inner Bladder line meridian points.

- Stress incontinence can be treated with regular Kegel exercises, outlined below. These exercises help strengthen the muscles that control the bladder and can be done anywhere, at any time. It may take 3 to 6 months to see an improvement, so patients must be persistent and patient.

Other Considerations
Kegel Exercises

- To locate the right muscles, try stopping or slowing your urine flow without using your stomach, leg, or buttock muscles. When you're able to slow or stop the stream of urine, you've located the right muscles.

- Squeeze your muscles. Hold for a count of ten. Relax for a count of ten.

- Repeat 10 to 20 times, three times a day.

- You may need to start slower, perhaps squeezing and relaxing your muscles for four seconds each and doing this ten times, twice a day. Work your way up from there.

Bladder Training for Urge Incontinence

Some people who have urge incontinence can learn to lengthen the time between urges to go to the bathroom. Start by urinating at set intervals, such as every 30 minutes to two hours (whether you feel the need to go or not). Then gradually lengthen the time between urinating (for example, by 30 minutes) until it is every three to four hours. Relaxation techniques can be practiced when the urge to urinate is felt before it is time to go to the bathroom. Breathe slowly and deeply.

Think about the breath until the urge goes away. Kegel exercises can also be done if they help control urgency. After the urge passes, wait five minutes and then go to the bathroom even if there is no feeling of needing to urinate. When it's easy to wait five minutes after an urge, begin waiting ten minutes. Bladder training may take 3 to 12 weeks.

Bowel Incontinence

Etiology

Osmotic: Non-absorbable, water-soluble solutes in bowel—lactose, simple carbohydrates

Secretory: Secrete electrolytes and water—bacterial toxins, viruses

Exudative: Mucosal inflammation and ulceration

Decreased intestinal transit time: Not enough exposure to absorptive surface for a sufficient amount of time—18 to 30 hours is pretty average

Potential Contributing Factors

- Dysbiosis
- Magnesium excess
- Potassium excess
- Potential secondary eEffects
- Hypokalemia

Parasitic Infections

- Entameba histolytica

- Giardia lamblia

- Enterobius vermicularis/(pinworm)

- Diagnosis by Ovum and Parasite exam

Biomedical Approaches

- Find and treat underlying disorder

- Rehydration (water alone is not best—electrolytes, etc.)

- Avoid simple carbohydrates

- Charcoal

- Rice water

- Psyllium seed (Fiberall, Metamucil)

- Difenoxin (Motofen)

- Diphenoxylate (Lomotil, Lonox)

- Acidophilus

- Hydrastis (Goldenseal)

10–12 bowel movements a day may be an infection of candida.

Chinese Medical Approach: Diarrhea (Xie Xie)

Characterized by changes in the frequency and quality of bowel movement—frequent passage of unformed, loose/soft or watery stool that may or may not contain undigested food. These can occur in all seasons, but tend to be more common in summer and fall.

Relevant Biomedical Diseases

- Traumatic brain injury

- "Stomach flu"

- Acute gastritis

- Acute or chronic enteritis

- Acute or chronic colitis

- Malabsorption syndrome

- IBS

- Food poisoning

- IBD

- Intestinal tumor

Chinese Medical Etiology

- Attack of Spleen by exogenous dampness leading to damp accumulation

- Improper diet (poor food choices or excessive or irregular food intake) leads to food stagnation

- Intensive or persistent emotional stress leading to Liver attacking the Spleen (Liver/Spleen disharmony)

- Overexertion or pensiveness creates Spleen Qi deficiency with failure of the Spleen in transforming and transporting

- A weak constitution, prolonged disease, aging leads to Kidney and Spleen Yang deficiency

Table 27.1 provides a summary of stool characteristics and their associated imbalance.

TABLE 27.1 Identification of Pathology by Stool Characteristics

Damp-heat	Yellow sticky or pasty stool with a strong foul odor and burning sensation of the anus
Cold-damp	Bluish-gray or bluish-black stool with a clear and thin or watery consistency without significant odor
Food stagnation	Pasty stool containing undigested food with a foul odor like rotten eggs and a sensation of incomplete defecation
Liver–Spleen disharmony	Paroxysmal loose stool or diarrhea triggered or aggravated by emotional stress
Spleen deficiency	Loose stool or diarrhea aggravated by overexertion or rich foods
Yang deficiency	Watery stool or diarrhea containing undigested food with abdominal pain occurring in the early AM hours

Distinguishing Deficiency Patterns from Excess Patterns

- Deficiency patterns are characterized by a short course with an acute onset. Bowel frequency increases with possible abdominal pain that is aggravated by pressure and relieved by defecation.

- Excess patterns are characterized by a chronic and prolonged course of intermittent episodes of diarrhea. Abdominal pain is relieved by pressure and aggravated by defecation.

Distinguishing Cold Patterns from Heat Patterns

- Cold patterns result in a loose or watery stool that may contain undigested food and severe abdominal pain that is accompanied by loud borborygmus and relieved by warmth. The individual will tend to have no thirst or a desire for warm beverages. Urination will tend to be clear and profuse. The pulse will be deep and tight with a moist white tongue coat.

- Heat patterns result in sticky yellow stool with a foul smell. There will be a sense of urgency and often a burning sensation of the anus. There may be a burning abdominal pain and an intense thirst with a preference for cold beverages. Urination will tend to be dark and scanty. The pulse will be slippery and rapid with a red tongue and yellow coat.

Other Diagnostic Tips for Diarrhea

- *Exuberance of dampness:* Acute diarrhea with a short course

- *Spleen deficiency:* Chronic diarrhea with a long course and often induced by eating or overexertion

- *Decline of Mingmen/Yang deficiency:* Early AM diarrhea with coldness in the loins

- *Diarrhea with normal appetite:* Mild condition with good prognosis

- *Severe diarrhea with weight loss:* Severe condition with poor prognosis

TCM Pattern Differentiation
Attack by External Cold-Damp

Primary symptoms: Diarrhea with loose or watery stool, borborygmus, abdominal pain

Additional symptoms: Preference for warmth, fullness and distension in the epigastrum, poor appetite, no thirst, possible simultaneous chills and fever, headache, nasal congestion, general aching

Tongue: White, greasy coating

Pulse: Soggy and moderate

Treatment principles: Scatter cold to release the exterior, resolve dampness with aromatic medicinals, and stop diarrhea

Acupuncture treatment: ST-25, ST-36, CV-12, CV-6, SP-9

Herbal treatment:
Huo Xiang Zheng Qi San (Patchouli Qi Righting Powder)
[Huo Xiang 12g, Zi Su Ye 6g, Bai Zhi 6g, Chen Pi 9g, Da Fu Pi 9g, Hou Po 9g, Bai Zhu 12g, Fu Ling 9g, Jie Geng 9g, Sheng Jiang 6g, Da Zao 2pc, Zhi Gan Cao 3g]

Damp-Heat in the Middle Jiao

Primary symptoms: Urgent, foul-smelling, yellow/pasty, and explosive diarrhea with abdominal pain or sensation of incomplete defecation

Additional symptoms: Burning sensation in the anus during bowel movement, traditionally seen in the summer and fall, persistent fever, thirst with a desire for little drink, scanty yellow urine

Tongue: Yellow, greasy coating

Pulse: Slippery, rapid, or soggy

Treatment principles: Clear heat and eliminate dampness, stop diarrhea

Acupuncture treatment: ST-25, ST-36, ST-44, SP-9, LI-11, ST-37

Herbal treatment:
Ge Gen Qin Lian Tang (Pueraria, Scutellaria, and Coptis Decoction)
[Ge Gen 10g, Huang Qin 10g, Huang Lian 10g, Zhi Gan Cao 5g]

Food Stagnation in the Stomach and Intestines

Primary symptoms: Diarrhea or loose stool with the smell of rotten eggs that may contain undigested food; distending abdominal pain relieved after diarrhea

Additional symptoms: Borborygmus, fullness in the epigastrium and abdomen, belching with foul-smelling, acid regurgitation, foul breath, no appetite/anorexia

Tongue: Thick, greasy coating

Pulse: Slippery

Treatment Principles: Clear food, more stagnation, stop diarrhea

Acupuncture treatment: ST-25, ST-36, Inner Neiting, CV-10

Herbal treatment:
Bao He Wan (Harmony Preserving Pill)
[Ban Xia 10g, Chen Pi 10g, Zhi Gan Cao 10g, Shan Zha 10g, Shen Qu 10g, Lai Fu Zi 10g, Lian Qiao 10g]

Liver/Spleen Disharmony

Primary symptoms: Recurrent, painful diarrhea and borborygmus induced by anger or emotional strain; abdominal pain is somewhat relieved after diarrhea

Additional symptoms: Stuffiness or distension in the chest and hypochondrium, depression, anger/irritability, moodiness, belching, poor appetite, gas

Tongue: Thin, white coat

Pulse: Wiry (bowstring)

Treatment principles: Soothe the Liver, regulate Qi, strengthen the Spleen, stop diarrhea

Acupuncture treatment: ST-25, ST-36, BL-18, LR-3, LR-13, CV-12

Herbal treatment:
Tong Xie Yao Fang (Pain and Diarrhea Formula)
[Bai Zhu 15g, Bai Shao Yao 12g, Chen Pi 6g, Fang Feng 6g]

Spleen Qi Deficiency

Primary symptoms: Loose or watery stools that may contain undigested food; increased frequency of bowel movement after exertion or after eating rich and greasy foods

Additional symptoms: Epigastric and abdominal fullness and distension (particularly after eating), poor appetite, sallow complexion, lassitude, fatigue

Tongue: Pale with white coating

Pulse: Thin, weak

Treatment principles: Strengthen the Spleen, benefit the Stomach, resolve dampness, stop diarrhea

Acupuncture treatment: ST-25, ST-36, CV-12, BL-20, SP-3, GV-20

Herbal treatment:
Shen Ling Bai Zhu San (Ginseng, Poria, and Atractylodes Powder)
[Dang Shen 15g, Bai Zhu 12g, Fu Ling 12g, Shan Yao 12g, Bai Bian Dou 9g, Yi Yi Ren 6g, Lian Zi 6g, Sha Ren 6g, Jie Geng 6g, Zhi Gan Cao 12g]

Diarrhea Manifesting as Spleen and Kidney Yang Deficiency

Primary symptoms: Watery diarrhea with undigested food that occurs at dawn; bowel movement preceded by cold abdominal pain that is relieved after diarrhea

Additional symptoms: Aversion to cold, cold limbs, sore, cold, and weak lower back and knees

Tongue: Pale with a white coating

Pulse: Deep, fine, weak

Treatment principles: Strengthen the Spleen, boost Kidney Yang, warm the middle Jiao, stop diarrhea

Acupuncture treatment: ST-25, ST-36, CV-4, GV-4, BL-23, KI-3, BL-20

Herbal treatment:
Si Shen Wan (Four Spirits Pill)
[Bu Gu Zhi 10g, Wu Zhu Yu 3g, Wu Wei Zi 6g, Rou Dou Kou 10g]

Clinical Notes

- In cases of brain injury causing incontinence, points which have a direct effect on the brain/marrow should be considered. In spinal cord injuries, local acupuncture near the affected vertebrae/nerve tract is an important component. This may include relevant points along the Du meridian, Hua Tuo Jia points, or inner Bladder line meridian points.

- Excessive Dampness and Spleen deficiency are the two major proximal causes of diarrhea and have a tendency to influence each other. Damp accumulation can hinder the function of the Spleen, causing diarrhea; the treatment principle in such a case emphasizes the action of expelling pathogenic factors. Therefore, bitter, warm, and aromatic herbs should be used to dry dampness. A deficient Spleen may generate internal dampness, causing diarrhea. The treatment principle in this case focuses on supporting Upright Qi; sweet, warm herbs should be used for strengthening the Spleen to stop diarrhea.

- The underlying cause of diarrhea in each case should be taken into consideration when forming the treatment plan. In acute onset diarrhea, the method of binding and astringing is not recommended as a strategy as this may retain pathogenic factors. In cases of chronic diarrhea, apply the strategy of astringing and binding, and consider raising Yang Qi.

- With proper treatment, most cases of diarrhea resolve in a few days; however, inappropriate treatment can prolong recovery and lead to chronic diarrhea. Pathological crisis related to diarrhea is rare. Severe, excessive, and unremitting diarrhea, however, will lead to severe loss of Yin and body fluids, eventually depleting Yin and devastating Yang. Clinical manifestations of this type of crisis include intense thirst with desire to drink, profuse bleeding and cold extremities, pale complexion, and minute pulse. Biomedically, this is termed a fluid and electrolyte imbalance.

Other Therapeutic Considerations
Orthomolecular Considerations

- Sodium
- Potassium
- Charcoal
- Chlorine (persistent)
- Active Lactobacillus

Phytotherapeutic Considerations

- Vinca minor (periwinkle)

Dietary Considerations

- Remove all simple carbohydrates

Constipation

Signs and Symptoms

- Three to five stools per week
- More than three days without stool
- Stool weight less than 35g

Etiology

- Obstruction
- Drugs
- Tumors
- Functional disorders
- IBS, hypothyroidism
- Psychological

Potential Contributing Factors

- Variations in blood calcium levels
- Arginine deficiency

Potential Complications

- Hemorrhoids
- Diverticulosis
- Colon cancer

Biomedical Approaches

- Hydration, fiber, allergies, exercise
- Psyllium (Fiberall, Metamucil)
- Lactulose (Constulose, Enulose, Generlac, Kristalose)
- Polyethylene glycol (Colyte, GoLYTELY, Gycolax, Miralax, NuLYTELY, Trylite)
- Abdominal massage
- Magnesium, vitamin C

Chinese Medical Perspective: Constipation (Bìan Bì)

Constipation entails difficult and/or infrequent defecation which includes conditions where the stool is hard and dry, or where stool quality is normal and there is a desire to defecate but evacuation is difficult and requires significant straining. It may also manifest with sluggish or incomplete bowel movements.

Constipation primarily involves the impairment of the Large Intestine's ability to transport and guide turbidity downwards. However, dysfunction of the Spleen, Stomach, Lung, Liver, and Kidney can also lead to constipation.

Relevant Biomedical Diseases

- Habitual constipation
- Atonic constipation
- Spastic constipation
- Intestinal neurosis
- Irritable bowel syndrome
- Bowel obstruction
- Intestinal tumor
- Perianal perforation and infection (fissure or fistula)
- Hemorrhoids
- Side effect of medication
- Chronic laxative use

Chinese Medical Etiology

In Chinese medicine constipation essentially comes down to two factors: either a "lack of water to float the boat," indicating a deficiency of body fluids, Blood, or Yin; or a "lack of force to move the boat," which indicates a Qi or Yang Qi deficiency.

Accumulated heat consuming body fluids in the stomach and intestines (pathology) is caused by:

- Diet: excessive consumption of alcohol, spicy foods
- Pungent and hot drugs/herbs
- Constitutional Yang excess
- Febrile diseases creating heat shifting downward to the intestines
- Qi stagnation leading to heat in the Stomach and Large Intestine
- Heat in the Stomach channel leads to intestinal heat (the Large Intestine channel is functionally related to the Stomach via the Six Channel schema)

Qi stagnation (pathology) is caused by:

- Emotional stress (sorrow, sadness, pensiveness, depression, anger) leading to a deficiency or stagnation of Qi

- Physical inactivity creates stagnation of Qi in the intestines

- Failure of Lung Qi to descend

- Causes Qi to become stuck and unable to move; this causes impairment of body fluids due to depressive heat or fire

Deficiency of Qi, Blood, Yin, and Essence (pathology) is caused by:

- Childbirth and loss of blood

- Overwork

- Aging

- Chronic illness (constipation with medium stool)

Results in insufficient body fluids to moisten the Large Intestine, leading to dryness and difficult passage of stool.

Yang deficiency with cold stagnation (pathology) is caused by:

- Excessive consumption of raw and cold food

- Bitter and cold drugs/herbs

- Constitutional Yang deficiency

- Aging

- Chronic illness leading to impaired flow of body fluids in intestines due to cold stagnation (via Qi stagnation)

- Direct attack of pathogenic cold: cold "congeals" Yang Qi, leading to poor fluid distribution and difficulty in the Large Intestine's ability to transmit stool

Identification of Types of Constipation

Table 27.2 provides a summary of various constipation patterns.

TABLE 27.2 Identification of Types of Constipation

Heat	Dry, hard stool, infrequent and difficult defecation, accompanied by a red face, fever, bad breath, mouth sores, dark scanty urine, dry yellow tongue coating, and a forceful slippery pulse
Qi stagnation	No significant alteration in the quality of stool (though it can be hard if Qi stagnation has generated Heat), stool sometimes can be thinner than normal, incomplete or sluggish defecation, belching, distension in the chest and hypochondrium, distending abdominal pain, a thin, greasy tongue coating, and a wiry pulse

Qi deficiency	Normal desire for defecation, ineffective straining to force bowel movements, great effort and prolonged time required for defecation, stools generally not dry or hard, a pale complexion, fatigue, spontaneous sweating and shortness of breath, thin tongue coating, vacuous pulse
Blood deficiency	Dry pebble-like stool that is difficult to evacuate, pale complexion, palpitations, dizziness, a pale tongue, and a thin or choppy pulse
Yin deficiency	Dry pebble-like stool that is difficult to evacuate, malar flush, dizziness, vertigo, thirst with desire for sips of water, night sweats, palpitations, soreness and weakness of the lower back and knees, emaciation, red tongue with little or no coat, fine and rapid pulse
Yang deficiency	Stools generally neither dry nor hard, difficult and sluggish defecation requiring great effort, cold limbs and/or general cold intolerance, copious clear urine, a moist white tongue coating, and a deep, slow pulse

Pattern Differentiation

Heat Accumulating in the Large Intestine and Stomach

Primary symptoms: Dry stool with difficult, infrequent defecation, dark scanty urine (urinary frequency with Stomach heat)

Additional symptoms: Abdominal distension or pain that increases with pressure, red complexion, sensation of heat, dry mouth, halitosis, or even ulcerations in the mouth

Tongue: Red with a dry yellow coating

Pulse: Slippery, rapid

Treatment principles: Clear heat, moisten the intestines, and promote bowel movement

Acupuncture treatment: [ST-25, BL-25, SP-15, TW-6, KI-6] + LI-11, LI-4, ST-44

Herbal treatment:
Ma Zi Ren Wan (Hemp Seed Formula)
[Ma Zi Ren 20g, Da Huang 10g, Xing Ren 10g, Bai Shao 10g, Zhi Shi 10g, Hou Po 10g]

Qi Stagnation

Primary symptoms: Constipation with a desire for defecation, well-formed stool (not necessarily dry) which is hesitant and difficult to push out

Additional symptoms: Frequent sighing, fullness and distension in the chest and hypochondrium, distension and pain in the abdomen, irritability

Tongue: Thin, greasy coating

Pulse: Wiry

Treatment principles: Course the Liver, regulate Qi, eliminate stagnation

Acupuncture treatment: [ST-25, BL-25, SP-15, TW-6, KI-6] + CV-12, LR-3, CV-6

Herbal treatment:
Liu Mo Tang (Six Ground-Herbs Decoction) **or** Xiao Chai Hu Tang/Da Chai Hu Tang (Minor Bupleurum Decoction/Great Bupleurum Decoction)
[Mu Xiang 10g, Wu Yao 10g, Chen Xiang 3g, Da Huang 10g, Bing Lang 10g, Zhi Shi 10g]

Qi Deficiency

Primary symptoms: Difficult defecation despite the need to move the bowels, stools are neither particularly hard nor dry, possible feeling of fatigue after bowel movement

Additional symptoms: Bright-white or pale complexion, spirit fatigue/listlessness, disinclination to speak, shortness of breath, spontaneous perspiration

Tongue: Pale and tender with a thin white coating

Pulse: Weak

Treatment principles: Boost Qi, promote bowel movement

Acupuncture treatment: [ST-25, BL-25, SP-15, TW-6, KI-6] + ST-36, SP-6, CV-4, BL-20

Herbal treatment:
Huang Qi Tang (Astragalus Decoction)
[Huang Qi 20g, Huo Ma Ren 15g, Feng Mi 12g, Chen Pi 12g]

Modifications:
Hypertension with concerns about Huang Qi's ascendant quality: + Huang Qin, Xia Ku Cao, Zhi Shi, Zhi Ke, Niu Xi

Blood Deficiency

Primary symptoms: Constipation with small, dry, and round stools

Additional symptoms: Pale and sallow complexion, palpitations, anemia, dizziness, vertigo, blurred vision, tingling of the limbs, pale lips, possibly following labor/surgery

Tongue: Pale

Pulse: Fine

Treatment principles: Nourish Blood, moisten the intestines, promote bowel movement

Acupuncture treatment: [ST-25, BL-25, SP-15, TW-6, KI-6] + SP-6, ST-36, BL-17, BL-20, CV-4

Herbal treatment:
Run Chang Wan (Moisten the Intestines Pill) **or** Ba Zhen Tang (Eight Treasures Decoction)
[Sheng Di Huang 20g, Dang Gui 15g, Tao Ren 10g, Huo Ma Ren 10g, Zhi Ke 6g]

Yin/Fluid Deficiency

Primary symptoms: Constipation with dry, hard stool

Additional symptoms: Malar flush, dizziness, vertigo, thirst with desire for sips of water, night sweats, palpitations, soreness and weakness of the lower back and knees, emaciation

Tongue: Red with little or no coat

Pulse: Fine and rapid

Treatment principles: Nourish Yin, supplement the Kidney, moisten the intestines, promote bowel movement

Acupuncture treatment: [ST-25, BL-25, SP-15, TW-6, KI-6] + SP-6, KI-3, LU-7

Herbal treatment:
Zeng Ye Tang (Increasing Fluids Decoction)
[Xuan Shen 30g, Sheng Di Huang 24g, Mai Men Dong 24g]

Kidney Yang Deficiency

Primary symptoms: Difficult defecation, dry or moist (well-formed) stools, profuse clear urine

Additional symptoms: Abdominal coldness and pain, preference for warmth with aversion to cold, cold limbs, soreness and coldness of the lower back, bright-white or bluish complexion

Tongue: Pale with a white coat

Pulse: Deep, slow

Treatment principles: Warm the Yang, supplement the Kidney, and promote bowel movement

Acupuncture treatment: [ST-25, BL-25, SP-15, TW-6, KI-6] + CV-8, CV-6, BL-23, GV-4 + moxa

Herbal treatment:

Ji Chuan Jian (Float the Boat Decoction) **or** Zhen Wu Tang (True Warrior Decoction)
[Rou Cong Rong 12g, Dang Gui 10g, Huai Niu Xi 10g, Ze Xie 5g, Zhi Ke 3g, Sheng Ma 5g] + Tu Si Zi

Auricular: Stomach, Large Intestine

Clinical Notes

- In cases of brain injury causing incontinence, points which have a direct effect on the brain/marrow should be considered. In a spinal cord injury, local acupuncture near the affected vertebrae/nerve tract is an important component. This may include relevant points along the Du meridian, Hua Tuo Jia points, or inner Bladder line meridian points.

- Discontinue bitter and cold herbs that drain downwards once the desired effect has been achieved. The most common method for treating constipation is draining heat and unblocking intestinal obstruction. This strategy incorporates herbs that are very cold and bitter. As a result, they have a tendency to injure the Spleen/Stomach and should be discontinued once the therapeutic effect has been achieved.

- Support Upright Qi to restore normal bowel movements. In the late stages of a warm-febrile disease, constipation is a common symptom. This is the result of decreased food and water intake during the acute stage. Treatment to promote bowel movement might not be necessary in such a case. Instead, nourish Stomach Yin and strengthen Stomach Qi. Once the Upright Qi recovers and normal food and fluid intake resumes, bowel movements will be restored.

Other Therapeutic Considerations

- Abdominal massage can help to regulate or initiate peristalsis
- Consider allergies, particularly milk, if there is alternating constipation/diarrhea

Dietary Recommendations

- Drink two liters of water/day
- Eat vegetable fibers which are necessary for a healthy intestinal tract: green vegetables and fruit, bran (cholesterol must be lowered), muscilages

- Avoid spicy food

- Eat wholewheat organic bread (bran), cooked prunes, prune juice, green vegetables, fresh figs

- No pulses or bananas

Orthomolecular Considerations

- Magnesium 600–900mg/day

- Vitamin C 10g/day

- Glucomannan

- Fructo-oligosaccharides

- Vitamin B complex

Research Studies

In a controlled investigation, acupuncture plus topical herbal medicine had a higher total effective rate and a higher complete recovery rate than drug therapy for post-stroke constipation. In addition, acupuncture plus topical herbal medicine had a significantly lower failure rate than drug therapy.[1]

---

1   Xiong ZH et al. Therapeutic Observation of Abdominal Electroacupuncture plus Chinese Medicinal Application at Umbilicus for Poststroke Constipation [J]. Shanghai Journal of Acupuncture and Moxibustion, 2017, 36 (3): 265–268.

Chapter 28

Sexual Dysfunction

Given that the brain is involved in all aspects of hormonal regulation and sexual functioning, a brain injury can result in various changes in libido, arousal, and sexual performance. This includes everything from stimulus, ability to communicate in forming intimate relationships, and an awareness of excitement, to the physiological responses that happen at cognitive, neurological, and genital levels. Sexuality involves diverse brain regions including the frontal lobes, limbic structures, and the temporal lobes. Lesions to the right hemisphere in particular are of relevance. These alterations in functioning can be further compounded by hormonal changes and medication side effects.

Trauma to the pituitary gland can disrupt hormonal levels in the body, which can cause disruption of menstrual cycles in women or affect testosterone levels. Reproductive health can become a prominent concern as UTIs, dysmenorrhea, polycystic ovarian symptoms, and pre-menstrual mood dysphoria become possible along with accompanying depression, hormonally regulated migraines, osteoporosis, or endocrine disorders. Over the long term, risks of cardiovascular disease and cancer increase.

Women with a TBI may be limited in their use of oral contraceptives or estrogen replacement therapy as a result of deep vein thrombosis (DVT) or embolus postinjury. Medications can cause earlier onset of menopause. This is particularly true of anti-seizure medications. This can be compounded by the impact of seizures that do occur on the hypothalamic–pituitary axis.

Hygiene can also become a concern for some affected by a brain injury who may not be able to fully tend to their own hygiene. Routine gynecological, testicular, and prostate examinations, contraceptive counseling, and awareness of STD risk should be given consideration for individuals.

Hormonal treatment of progesterone or estrogen has been studied as an acute injury treatment approach. Progesterone modulates GABA and inhibits apoptosis, gliosis, and the production of inflammatory agents by which it may reduce brain edema. Estrogen is a powerful antioxidant with a vasoprotective action. In animal models administration of estrogen seemed to only show benefit in males, while administration to females was shown to be detrimental and associated with an increased injury-related mortality risk.

The American Brain Injury Association cites ten notable areas in which sexuality may be affected by a brain injury:

- *Difficulty with sexual energy, desire, or drive:* This may stem from the often felt general fatigue following a brain injury as well as the ability to manage sleep, stress, and health habits. Some individuals find that they have a reduced interest in all drives, including sexual. This may cause difficulty in maintaining romantic relationships despite being a neurobiological issue which does not act as a direct reflection of the feelings felt for another, the value placed on the relationship, or the perceived attractiveness of the individual.

- *Reduction/loss of sensation or orgasm:* An injury can affect the neural circuitry that carries signals of feeling pleasure that lead to orgasm. Additionally, many prescription medications can have this same effect.

- *Positioning, movement, and pain difficulties:* Due to pain or difficulties in movement following an injury, certain movements or sexual positions can be limited. These may be addressed through physical therapy, physiotherapies that reduce pain, and the possible use of adaptive positioning aids.

- *Altered body image, mood, and self-confidence:* Depression, a loss of confidence, or reduced self-esteem have been associated with brain injury in up to 50 percent of cases for both men and women. This may additionally stem from, or be compounded by, disability, unemployment, or changes in family or social roles.

- *Decreased ability to sexually satisfy one's partner:* Individuals may not be able to remember the proper exchanges or patterns of interaction involved in intimacy. Due to increased mental and physical expenditure, the individual may not be able to process these exchanges in the moment. When interacting with a partner after an injury, both parties may have to be patient in relearning one another. Couples counseling may be helpful in order to effectively communicate with one another and reestablish new foundations between them.

- *Disinhibition and hypersexuality:* Hypersexuality does not seem to occur as frequently as disinterest; however, it can cause a number of issues for those affected. In cases where the frontal lobe has been injured, it is possible that the inhibitory function on the base animalistic drives of the limbic system and lower brain centers may fail. This can result in uninhibited offensive comments, changes in character behaviors, and, seemingly, a loss of moral judgment and ability to gauge social appropriateness. This may include compulsive sexual pursuit, exhibitionism, touching themselves or others in public, masturbation in inappropriate situations, a disregard for the rights or space of others, and demonstrating little regard for cultural norms, situational contexts, and religious teachings or traditions. The individual may proposition caregivers, strangers, friends, or family. They may patronize sex workers (sometimes multiple times a day) and there is the possibility of developing violent sexual behavior that was unknown prior to injury. This can cause difficulty for the individual or among family members, caretakers, or medical practitioners. Severe cases may require inpatient care.

- *Incontinence and issues of adaptive equipment*: An individual who experiences bowel or bladder incontinence may avoid sexual activity due to embarrassment of these issues or out of fear that an accident may occur. Management of a voiding schedule may assist in this matter and may be addressed with their healthcare provider.

- *Diminished capacity for sexual ideation*: One's ability to think about or imagine sexual activity can be affected. This may further reduce one's drive and interest in sexual matters. Counseling and increased communication among partners may assist in this matter.

- *Greater sexual concerns among those with mild TBI*: An injury that is mild may recover quite well but have persistent symptoms. Because the individual is more consciously aware of any deficits or difficulties than those with severe brain injury, this can be of great concern and may exacerbate depression.

- *Sexual intimacy issues may predate TBI*: It is important to be aware of any intimacy concerns present prior to the onset of injury.

Primary Causes of Sexual Dysfunction

Neuroendocrine/hormonal changes: 40–62 percent of persons have shown pituitary damage; 42 percent showed hypothalamic lesions.

Secondary Causes of Sexual Dysfunction

- Physical changes
- Spasticity
- Hemiparesis
- Ataxia

- Balance
- Movement disorders
- Sensory deficits

Cognitive Impairments

- Attention and concentration
- Initiation (motivation to act)
- Social communication abilities

- Impaired awareness
- Memory loss
- Executive dysfunction

Emotional and Behavioral Changes

- Depression
- Child-like or dependency behaviors
- Disinhibition or trouble self-monitoring

- Apathy/decreased initiation
- Self-centeredness
- Low self-esteem or poor body image

Other Potential Factors

- Marital or family dysfunction
- Role changes
- Financial stress
- Parenting strain

- Decreased communication between partners
- Social isolation
- Medication side effects

Effects of Certain Pharmaceutical Classes on Sexual Functioning

A number of pharmaceutical medications can have an impact on sexual function and drive. Table 28.1 provides a summary of these potential effects.

TABLE 28.1 Effects of Certain Medication Classes on Sexual Functioning

Drug Category	Examples	Potential Benefits	Potential Effects on Sexual Functioning
Antidepressants	Prozac, Elavil, Norpramin	Control/improve mood	Delay orgasm, anorgasma (not Wellbutrin)
Antispasmodics	Probathine, Baclofen	Reduce/control spasms	Modify sensory experience of orgasm
Antipsychotics	Zyprexa, Seroquel, Haldol	Control/improve psychotic symptoms	Decrease sexual drive, increase fatigue, delay orgasm, especially older medications
Antihypertensives	Inderol, beta blockers	Control blood pressure	Decrease sexual drive, erectile dysfunction
Stimulants	Ritalin, Adderal	Improve attention, enhance cognition	Increase sexual drive, decrease fatigue

Antiseizure drugs	Dilantin, Tegretol, Depakote	Reduce/control seizures	Decrease sexual drive, increase fatigue, disinterest
Antihistamines	Actifed, Atarax, Claritin	Control allergy symptoms	Older medications decrease sexual drive and anorgasmic response, increase fatigue. New medications—no effects identified
Anti-inflammatories	Advil, Naprosyn	Control inflammation and reduce pain	Increase sexual drive, decrease menstrual pain, increase sexual response
Antibiotics	Cipro, Penicillin	Control infection	May increase vaginal itching and yeast infections
Antiemetics	Reglan, Compazine	Control nausea	Decrease sexual drive, decrease orgasmic response
Oral contraceptives	"The Pill"—various formulations	Prevent conception	Various types may either increase or decrease sexual drive
Androgen anabolic steroids	Winstrol, Anadrol	Minimize wasting syndromes	Increase sexual drive, absence of menstrual period, clitoral enlargement
Hormone replacement therapy	Estratest, Premarin	Adjusts hormone levels following menopause/ hysterectomy (risk)	Increases sexual drive, prevents vaginal atrophy

Differential Diagnosis

Frontal lobe: Sexual automatisms, such as sexual hypermotoric pelvic or truncal movements, are common in frontal lobe seizures

Temporal lobe: Discrete genital automatisms, like fondling and grabbing the genitals, are more common in seizures involving the temporal lobe

In most instances, "sexual" seizures are associated with being located in the right frontal lobe. However, patients may also become hyposexual, especially with left frontal injuries, and/or experience genital pain with left temporal seizures.

Chinese Medical Perspective: Decreased Sexual Desire (Yang Wei, Weak Yang)

This differs from impotence in that with impotence desire may exist but the ability to become physically aroused does not. With decreased sexual drive the individual does not have difficulty in physical arousal. In Chinese medicine, sexual desire is primarily a function of the Mingmen fire and Kidney Yang.[1]

Chinese Medical Etiology

Psychological causes: Emotional factors such as anger, sadness, fright, and worry can influence a patient's sexual response. Other factors such as environmental surroundings, financial difficulties, stress, or excessive workload can decrease desire to engage in intercourse. Previous relationship experiences or sexual traumas may also impact sexual drive.

Constitutional causes: Those with a weak constitution or who are experiencing chronic diseases may also have no sexual interest. Common conditions that could possibly affect a person's constitution include Addison's syndrome, hypothyroidism, diabetes, anemia, cerebral vascular diseases, neurological disorders, or chronic diseases of the Heart, Liver, or Kidneys. All of these can influence the endocrine system by reducing testosterone levels which, in turn, may diminish desire for sex.

Reproductive disorders: Disorders such as vulvitis; vaginitis; atrophy of the vagina; pelvic inflammatory disease; uterine prolapse; improper development of the uterus or ovaries; pituitary cancer; or polycystic syndrome can decrease sexual drive.

Drugs/medications: Excessive intake of alcohol or prolonged drug use produces an inhibitory effect on the central nervous system that can lead to a drop in sexual cravings. Diuretics may additionally decrease vaginal lubrication and influence sexual function.

Other:

Impotence can be the most significant and recognized condition leading to decreased sexual yearnings and activities.

Excessive taxation and fatigue—all forms of taxation eventually damage the Kidneys. Physical work, overthinking, pre-occupation, and worry all damage the Heart and Spleen. Over time these can develop into a Kidney deficiency

Spleen–Kidney dual deficiency—Spleen Qi deficiency leads to Kidney Yang deficiency

---

1   Sionneau, Philippe and Gang, Lu. *Treatment of Disease in TCM*. Vol. 6, Diseases of the Urogenital System and Proctology. Fletcher, NC: Blue Poppy Press. 1999. Print.

Liver Depression Qi stagnation—Emotional frustration creates Qi stagnation which prevents the free flow of Yang Qi to the genitals via the Liver meridian

Kidney Essence and Original Qi insufficiency—insufficient Kidney Yang Qi to stir desire

Diagnostic Keys

- Continuous lack of orgasm, even during erotic circumstances (more often with the same partner)

- Inability to produce or maintain vaginal lubrication during sexual activity

- A sudden drop of sexual desire following a stressful or emotional situation

- Age, either premenopausal/andropausal or postmenopausal/andropausal, which can play a role in diagnosing sexual activity

- Appropriate clinical lab testing, which can disclose underlying factors

Differential Diagnosis

A comprehensive personal and family history, and a thorough physical examination, are invaluable in determining the source of the disorder with other diagnoses.

Pattern Differentiation
Heart–Spleen–Kidney Deficiency

Primary symptoms: Weak sexual desire, possible impotence or incomplete erection

Additional symptoms: Fatigue, hypersomnia, lassitude of the spirit

Tongue: Pale, white coat

Pulse: Moderate, relaxed, forceless

Treatment principles: Nourish the Heart, fortify the Spleen, boost the Kidneys

Acupuncture treatment: BL-15, BL-20, BL-23, SP-6, CV-4, KI-7

Herbal treatment:
Fu Wei Qi Wan (Restore Weakness and Raise the Yang Pill)
[Ren Shen 6g, Shan Yao 9g, Yuan Zhi 9g, Suan Zao Ren 9g, Wu Wei Zi 9g, Gou Qi 9g, Yin Yang Huo 9g, Ron Cong Rong 9g, Dang Gui 9g]
Fu Tu Wan (Poria and Cuscuta Special Pill)
[Fu Ling 15g, Tu Si Zi 30g, Shi Lian Zi 9g, Wu Wei Zi 21g, Shan Yao 18g]

Kidney and Heart Disharmony Due to Fright

Primary symptoms: Decreased libido, emotional suppression, being easily frightened, dramatic emotional fluctuations in which the patient overacts easily

Additional symptoms: Insomnia; irritability; soreness and pain of the back and knees

Tongue: Red, scanty coating

Pulse: Deep, thready

Treatment principles: Nourish the Kidney and Liver, tranquilize the spirit

Acupuncture treatment: ST-36, SP-9, BL-23, LI-4, PC-6, SP-6, BL-15, KI-3, HT-7, ear Shenmen

Herbal treatment:
Zhi Bai Di Huang Wan (Anemarrhena, Phellodendron, and Rehmannia Decoction) [Shu Di Huang 24g, Shan Yao 12g, Shan Zhu Yu 12g, Zhi Mu 9g, Huang Bai 9g, Fu Shen 9g, Bai Zi Ren 9g, Zhi Gan Cao 6g, Ci Shi 6g, Hu Po 6g, Suan Zao Ren 9g, Yuan Zhi 9g]

Modifications:
Loose stool + Bai Zhu, Sha Ren
Yin deficiency heat with 5-palm heat and thready rapid pulse + Zhi Mu

Spleen–Kidney Dual Deficiency

Primary symptoms: Weak sexual desire, lassitude of the spirit

Additional symptoms: Fatigue, torpid intake, loose stools, possible spontaneous sweating, tinnitus, dizziness, nocturia, cold feet, low back and knee weakness

Tongue: Pale

Pulse: Deep, fine, forceless

Treatment principles: Fortify the Spleen, boost the Kidneys

Acupuncture treatment: CV-4, GV-4, BL-52, SP-6, ST-36

Herbal treatment:
Fu Zheng Yi Shen Wan (Restore the Righteous and Boost the Kidney Pill) [Ren Shen 6g, Huang Qi 15g, Fu Ling 9g, Ji Nei Jin 6g, Bai Zhu 9g, Dang Gui 6g, Shi Chang Pu 9g, Yuan Zhi 9g, Yin Yang Huo 9g, Xian Mao 9g, Ba Ji Tian 9g, Lu Rong 1g]

Liver Depression Qi Stagnation

Primary symptoms: Weak sexual desire that is worse with emotional upset, possible incomplete erection, irritability

Additional symptoms: Emotional depression, low spirits, vexation and agitation, chest oppression, rip side distension and pain, eructation, frequent sighing, irregular menstruation, dysmenorrhea, dark menstrual blood with clots, occasional pain in the lower abdomen and genital area during intercourse

Tongue: Normal or dark/red, thin coat

Pulse: Deep, wiry (bowstring), possibly slow, weak

Treatment principles: Course the Liver and boost the Kidney, resolve depression and quiet the emotions

Acupuncture treatment: LR-3, PC-5, HT-7, CV-4, SP-6, ST-36, Yintang, ear Shenmen

Herbal treatment:
Jie Yu Xing Yang Wan (Resolve Depression and Move Yang Pill)
[Chai Hu 6g, Yu Jin 9g, Xiang Fu 9g, Bai Shao 9g, Dang Gui 6g, Shi Chang Pu 9g, Yuan Zhi 6g, Yin Yang Huo 12g, Rou Cong Rong 6g, Ba Ji Tian 6g]
Jia Wei Xiao Yao San (Augmented Free and Easy Wanderer)
[Chai Hu 30g, Dang Gui 30g, Bai Shao 30g, Bai Zhu 30g, Fu Ling 30g, Gan Cao 15g, Sheng Jiang 30g, Bo He 3g, Mu Dan Pi 3g, Zhi Zi 3g]

Modifications:
Breast distension or pain + Qing Pi
Dysmenorrhea + Yan Hu Suo, Pu Huang, Wu Ling Zhi
Menstrual blood clots + Chuan Xiong, Hong Hua, Tao Ren, Gui Zhi

Kidney Essence and Original Qi Deficiency, Mingmen Fire Depleted

Primary symptoms: Weak sexual desire, impotence or incomplete erection, sterility

Additional symptoms: Low back and knee soreness and weakness, bowed head, weak constitution, fatigue, tinnitus, dizziness, listlessness of the essence spirit, loss of hair, loose teeth, cold limbs

Tongue: Pale, tender, scanty coat

Pulse: Fine, weak, forceless

Treatment principles: Supplement the Kidneys, foster essence, and invigorate the Mingmen fire of the Kidney

Acupuncture treatment: CV-6, CV-4, BL-23, ST-36, SP-6, SP-9, LI-4, GV-4, KI-2

Herbal treatment:

Yu Jing Wen Yang Wan (Boost the Essence and Warm Yang Pill)
[He Shou Wu 12g, Shu Di Huang 18g, Gou Qi 15g, Shan Zhu Yu 12g, Ba Ji Tian 9g, Rou Cong Rong 9g, Yin Yang Huo 9g, Lu Rong 1g]
Stronger focus on Mingmen—Zhan Yu Dan (Special Pill to Aid Fertility)
[Lu Jiao Shuang 9g, Du Zhong 9g, Tu Si Zi 9g, Dang Gui 9g, Fu Ling 9g, She Chuang Zi 7g, Bai Zhu 7g, Rou Cong Rong 9g, Shu Di Huang 9g, Jiu Cai Zi 9g, Ba Ji Tian 9g, Xian Mao 7g, Yin Yang Huo 15g, Rou Gui 9g, Fu Zi 7g]

Modifications:

Qi deficiency: + Ren Shen, Bai Zhu
Loose stool, diarrhea, or abdominal pain: + Ren Shen, Rou Dou Kou
Lower abdominal pain: + Wu Zhu Yu
Trickling vaginal discharge: + Bu Gu Zhi
Lower back and knee pain: + Dang Gui, Du Zhong

Note: Yu Jing Wen Yang Wan has a stronger focus on building the essence, while Zhan Yu Dan has a stronger effect on the Mingmen fire.

Qi and Blood Deficiency

Primary symptoms: Decreased libido, dizziness, blurry vision, shortness of breath, fatigue, pale and dull complexion

Additional symptoms: Poor appetite, dry mouth, light menstrual color (scanty amount)

Tongue: Pale, thin white coating

Pulse: Thready, rapid

Treatment principles: Tonify Qi and Blood

Acupuncture treatment: ST-36, SP-9, BL-23, LI-4, LR-8, SP-10, CV-4, CV-6, GV-4, PC-6

Herbal treatment:

Ba Zhen Tang (Eight Gentlemen Decoction)
[Ren Shen 3g, Bai Zhu 3g, Fu Ling 3g, Zhi Gan Cao 1.5g, Shu Di Huang 3g, Dang Gui 3g, Bai Shao 3g, Chuan Xiong 3g, Sheng Jiang 3g, Da Zao 3g]

Modifications:

Dizziness and blurry vision + Gou Qi, Nu Zhen Zi
Fatigue and shortness of breath + Ren Shen, Huang Qi, Ling Zhi
Poor appetite + Bian Dou, Bai Zhu, Fu Ling

Tina Chen's recommended formula for sexual arousal disorder: Zi Shi Ying Zhu Yang Fang

"This formula is best for people with low sex drive with no physical or mental abnormalities or symptoms."[2, 3]

[Yin Yang Huo 15g, Zi Shi Ying 30g, Xu Duan 15g, Hua Jiao 1.5g, Ba Ji Tian 10g, Hu Lu Ba 10g, Tu Si Zi 10g, Rou Gui 6g, Sang Piao Xiao 12g, Jiu Xiang Chong 10g]

Lifestyle Recommendations

Increase the intake of foods with warm properties such as lamb, onions, and chives. A balanced diet should go along with a balanced lifestyle that includes proper work hours, exercise, and play.

Hypersexuality/Disinhibition

As discussed above, Chinese medicine sexual desire is primarily a function of the Mingmen fire and Kidney Yang. The outward expression of one's sexuality is regulated by the Fire element and, in particular, the Heart and Pericardium organs.

Chinese Medical Etiology

- Heart Qi and Blood Deficiency

- Heart Fire

- Phlegm Fire Harassing the Pericardium

- Liver Qi Stagnation

- Kidney Yin or Essence Deficiency with Deficiency Heat

Pattern Differentiation
Heart Qi/Blood Deficiency

Primary symptoms: Hypersexuality, palpitations (may be more pronounced in the evening), insomnia

Additional symptoms: Fatigue, shortness of breath, spontaneous sweating, pale face, poor memory, anxiety, dream-disturbed sleep, easily startled, pale lips, dizziness

2   Chen, T. and Jang, M-C. Sexual arousal disorder: Western and Oriental medical perspectives. Part 1. *Acupuncture Today*. 2002; 3(8). www.acupuncturetoday.com/mpacms/at/article.php?id=28021. Web. 2017.

3   Chen, T. and Jang, M-C. Sexual arousal disorder: Western and Oriental medical perspectives. Part 2. *Acupuncture Today*. 2002; 3(10). www.acupuncturetoday.com/mpacms/at/article.php?id=28073. Web. 2017.

Tongue: Normal color or pale, slightly dry, possible midline crack and swollen sides

Pulse: Empty, choppy, or fine

Treatment principles: Tonify Heart Qi, tonify the Blood and Heart, soothe the Shen

Acupuncture treatment: HT-5, HT-7, PC-6, BL-15, BL-17, BL-20, CV-14, CV-15, CV-17, CV-4, CV-6

Herbal treatment:
Tian Wang Bu Xin Dan (Heavenly Emperor Tonifying the Heart Pill)
[Di Huang 120g, Xuan Shen 15g, Tian Men Dong 30g, Mai Men Dong 30g, Dan Shen 15g, Dang Gui 30g, Ren Shen 15g, Fu Ling 15g, Suan Zao Ren 30g, Wu Wei Zi 30g, Bai Zi Ren 30g, Yuan Zhi 15g, Jie Geng 15g]

Modifications:
Constipation + Zhi Shi, Hou Po
Severe palpitations, insomnia, restlessness + Long Yan Rou, Shou Wu Teng
Inability to concentrate, forgetfulness, or to enhance memory + Yuan Zhi, Shi Chang Pu, Yin Xing Ye
Dizziness and vertigo + Chuan Xiong, Bai Zhi
Excessive thinking and worrying + Xiao Yao San
Insomnia or restless sleep + Suan Zao Ren Tang

Heart Fire

Primary symptoms: Hypersexuality, palpitations, sexual and general impulsiveness

Additional symptoms: Mouth and tongue ulcers, mental restlessness, insomnia, dream-disturbed sleep, bitter taste in the mouth, blood in the urine or dark urine, thirst and sensation of heat
If accompanying Heart Yin deficiency: Poor memory, anxiety, low grade fever, malar flush, night sweats, 5-palm heat, dry mouth and throat

Tongue: Red with very red tip, swollen with petechiae, possible midline crack, yellow coat

Pulse: Rapid and full especially in the Heart position, possibly irregular

Treatment principles: Clear the Heart, nourish Kidney Yin, soothe the Shen

Acupuncture treatment: HT-9, HT-8, HT-7, CV-15, SP-6, KI-6
Accompanying Heart Yin deficiency: + PC-6, CV-14, CV-4
Night sweats + HT-6, KI-7

Herbal treatment:
Xie Xin Tang (Draining the Heart Decoction)
[Huang Qin 3g, Huang Lian 3g, Da Huang 6g]

Modifications:
Delirium + Shi Chang Pu, Yu Jin
Severe constipation + Mang Xiao, Zhi Shi, Hou Po
Bleeding due to heat in the Blood level + Mu Dan Pi, Di Huang

Phlegm Fire Harassing the Pericardium

Primary symptoms: Disinhibition, palpitations, rash behavior, mental confusion

Additional symptoms: Feeling of oppression in the chest, thirst, red face, bitter taste in the mouth, expectoration of phlegm, rattling sound in the throat, mental restlessness, insomnia, dream-disturbed sleep, agitation, incoherent speech, tendency to hit or scold people, uncontrolled laughter or crying, shouting, muttering to oneself, mental depression and dullness, manic behavior

Tongue: Red and swollen with yellow sticky coat; deep heart crack tip may be redder

Pulse: Full, rapid, slippery; or possibly full, rapid, wiry

Treatment principles: Drain Pericardium and Heart fire, resolve phlegm, open the mind's orifices, calm the mind

Acupuncture treatment: PC-5, HT-7, HT-8, PC-7, CV-15, BL-14, BL-15, ST-40, SP-6, LR-2, GV-20, GV-24, GB-13, GB-17

Herbal treatment:
Wen Dan Tang (Warming the Gallbladder Decoction)
[Ban Xia 6g, Zhu Ru 6g, Zhi Shi 6g, Chen Pi 9g, Fu Ling 4.5g, Zhi Gan Cao 3g]

Modifications:
Insomnia due to depression + Yue Ju Wan
Insomnia and palpitations due to fright + Suan Zao Ren
Epilepsy + Yu Jin, Shi Chang Pu
Epilepsy and convulsions + Dan Nan Xing, Gou Teng, Quan Xie
Dizziness and vertigo + Ju Hua, Huang Qin

Liver Qi Stagnation

Primary symptoms: Disinhibition, irritability, emotional lability

Additional symptoms: Rib side distension and pain, depression, moodiness, melancholy, plum pit Qi, nausea, vomiting, epigastric pain, diarrhea, irregular menstruation, PMS

Tongue: Normal tongue body, thin white coat

Pulse: Wiry (bowstring)

Treatment principles: Regulate sexual impulse, course the Liver, regulate Qi

Acupuncture treatment: LR-3, LR-5(−), GB-34, GB-40, LR-13, LR-14, TW-6, PC-6

Herbal treatment:

Jia Wei Xiao Yao San (Free and Easy Wander Plus Modifications)
[Chai Hu 30g, Dang Gui 30g, Bai Shao 30g, Bai Zhu 30g, Fu Ling 30g, Zhi Gan Cao 15g, Mu Dan Pi 30g, Zhi Zi 30g]

Liver Yang Rising

Primary symptoms: Disinhibition, headache (may be at temples, eyes, or lateral head), irritability, feeling "worked up," propensity to outbursts of anger

Additional symptoms: Dizziness, tinnitus, deafness, blurred vision, dry mouth and throat, insomnia, stiff neck

Tongue: May be pale or slightly red on sides without coat

Pulse: Wiry (bowstring)

Treatment principles: Subdue Liver Yang, nourish Yin and Blood

Acupuncture treatment: LR-3, LR-8, TW-5, PC-6, LI-4, GB-20, GB-38, GB-43, BL-2, SP-6, KI-3, KI-6

Herbal treatment:

Tian Ma Gou Teng Yin (Gastrodia–Uncaria Decoction)
[Tian Ma 9g, Gou Teng 12g, Zhi Zi 9g, Huang Qin 9g, Shi Jue Ming 18g, Yi Mu Cao 9g, Chuan Niu Xi 12g, Du Zong 9g, Sang Ji Sheng 9g, Shou Wu Teng 9g, Fu Shen 9g]

Modifications:

Post-stroke complications + Chi Shao, Tao Ren, Hong Hua
Thirst and phlegm accumulation + Bei Mu, Zhu Ru

Ling Jiao Gou Teng Tang (Antelopis–Uncaria Decoction)
[Ling Yang Jiao 4.5g, Gou Teng 9g, Sang Ye 6g, Ju Hua 9g, Bai Shao 9g, Di Huang 15g, Chuan Bei Mu 12g, Zhu Ru 15g, Fu Shen 9g, Gan Cao 2.4g]

Modifications:

Phlegm accumulation that alters consciousness + Tian Zhu Huang, Zhu Li

Kidney-Yin or Essence Deficiency with Deficiency Heat

Primary symptoms: Excessive sexual desire, mental restlessness, nocturnal emissions with dreams

Additional symptoms: Malar flush, insomnia, night sweating, low grade fever, 5-palm heat, dark urine, blood in the urine, dry throat especially at night, thirst with desire for small sips, dizziness, tinnitus, low back ache

Tongue: Red, cracked with a red tip, no coat

Pulse: Floating, empty, and rapid

Treatment principles: Nourish Kidney Yin, clear empty heat, calm the mind

Acupuncture treatment: KI-2, KI-3, KI-6, KI-9, KI-10, CV-4, SP-6, HT-5, HT-6, LU-7, LU-10, LI-11, GV-24

Herbal treatment:
Liu Wei Di Huang Wan Jia Wei (Six Ingredient Rehmannia Pill Plus Modifications) [Shu Di Huang 24g, Shan Zhu Yu 12g, Shan Yao 12g, Ze Xie 9g, Mu Dan Pi 9g, Fu Ling 9g, Di Gu Pi 9g, Zhi Mu 12g, Huang Bai 6g]

Modifications:
Insomnia, neurasthenia: + Suan Zao Ren, Bai Zi Ren
Irregular menstruation: + Xiang Fu, Ai Ye
Nocturnal emissions: + Jin Suo Gu Jing Wan

Individual Herbs for Sexual Dysfunction

Sexual dysfunction: Che Qian Zi, Dang Gui, Dong Chong Xia Cao, Ge Jiue, Guan Mu Tang, Hai Ma, Hai Shen, Long Gu, Ren Shen, Xiao Mao, Yin Yang Huo, Ze Xie

Deficiency

Decreased sexual drive / impotence: Yin Yang Huo, Hai Gou Shen, Dong Chong Xia Cao

Low sexual response (women): Rou Cong Rong, Lu Rong, Lu Jiao Jiao, Zi He Che, Shu Di, Ren Shen, Tu Si Zi

Excess

Sex drive increased abnormally: Zhi Mu

Easily aroused: Huang Bai

Chapter 29

Visual Disturbances

Visual problems are very common following a brain injury, with a number of different pathologies that may arise. Most commonly these are concerns that adversely affect versional and vergent oculomotor abnormalities, accommodative dysfunctions, dry eye, cataracts, and visual field defects. Other indirect pathologies such as orbital fractures, lid abnormalities, blepharitis, blepharoconjunctivitis, pupillary abnormalities, optic nerve abnormalities, and retinal defects may occur. In a sample study the most common of these included exophoric deviations (41.9%), oculomotor dysfunctions (39.7%), and visual field defects (32.5%). Functional vision abnormalities can negatively affect one's ability to perform daily activities such as reading, writing, walking, and driving, among others.

Refractive changes may cause constant blurred vision. Reduced best-corrected visual acuity can also occur due to damage along the primary visual pathway anywhere between the optic nerve head and the occipital cortex. Appropriate spectacles may help adjust for these afflictions.

A summary of common visual disturbances is provided in Table 29.1, while common deficits and their related symptomology are provided in Table 29.2.

TABLE 29.1 Visual Disturbances Common in Brain Injury

Spots (floaters)	A result of vitreous debris from the degeneration of the membranous attachment of the vitreous body to the optic nerve and retina early in life. Although potentially bothersome, they lack pathological significance
Retinal detachment	Usually from trauma to the head or eye, it is typically preceded by a shower of sparks in one quadrant of the visual field, followed by a sensation akin to a curtain falling over the the eye

Scotomas	A (−) scotoma is a blind spot in the visual field. It can often be unnoticed by the patient unless it occurs in the central vision. A (+) scotoma is described as a light spot or scintillating flash that occurs as a response to abnormal stimulation of some portion of the visual system (e.g. during a migraine prodrome)
Myopia (nearsightedness)	The visual image strikes in front of the retina due to an elongated eyeball or excessive refractive power. The individual can see near objects but not far ones
Hyperopia (farsightedness)	The visual image strikes behind the retina due to a shortened eyeball or weak refractive power. It is the most common refractive error. Presbyopia is a hyperopia that occurs with advancing age as the lens becomes less pliable
Astigmatism	Refraction of the eyeball is unequal in its different meridians
Anisometropia	A different refractive error in each eye
Strabismus	Deviation of one eye from parallel view. If the condition is congenital, there is no diplopia (double vision), as the vision in the deviated eye is suppressed by the brain. This suppression results in amblyopia, which is reduced visual acuity
Diplopia (double-vision)	This can occur for a variety of reasons. It is often seen in acute ophthalmoplegia and extraocular muscle palsies

TABLE 29.2 Deficits of the Visual System

Deficit	Symptoms	Treatment Approaches
Deficits of accommodation	Constant or intermittent blur, easy visual fatigue, inability to hold prolonged near vision, tearing, occasional headache	Separate pair of reading spectacles with or without concurrent oculomotor rehabilitation
Refractive changes	Constant blur at a particular viewing distance	Spectacles
Versional ocular motility deficits	Reading difficulty, slower reading speed and loss of place when reading, texts appears to "swim," misreading or rereading words, difficulty shifting gaze or tracking objects with ambulation	Oculomotor rehabilitation Differential diagnosis: vestibular defects
Vergent ocular motility deficits	Constant or intermittent diplopia, eliminated with covering one eye, easy visual fatigue, reading words may appear to "float," intermittent closing of one eye, may avoid eye contact to avoid diplopia	Fusional prisms, oculomotor rehabilitation (vision therapy), surgical intervention (vertical oculomotor deviations), visual occlusion (vertical oculomotor deviations)

Deficit	Symptoms	Treatment Approaches
Visual–vestibular disturbances	Disequilibrium, dizziness with increased sensitivity to visual motion in multiple visually stimulating environments (e.g. malls, supermarkets), accompanied by nausea and/or headache	Neurology/neurotology referral, vestibular rehabilitation (e.g. vestibulo-ocular reflex training), oculomotor rehabilitation
Photosensitivity	Elevated sensitivity to light (may be selective to fluorescent lights or general)	Tinted lenses, wearing brimmed hats
Visual field impairment	Missing a portion of one's visual field with or without inattention. Having relative defects scattered throughout field of vision	Laterally displaced prism spectacles, half-Fresnel prisms, mirrors

Anatomy and Visual Pathways

The eyes are more than just intimately connected to the brain, they are an actual external extension of the brain. They are the only part of the brain we are able to see. The eye is structurally made up of the cornea, conjunctiva, sclera, iris, aqueous humor, anterior and posterior chamber, crystalline lens, vitreous humor, retina, and choroid.

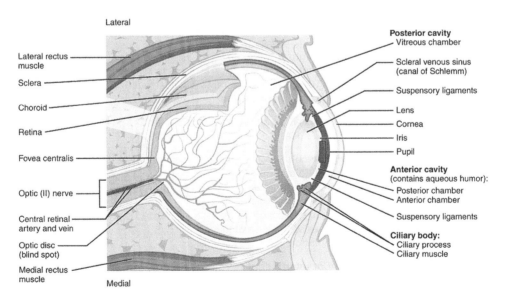

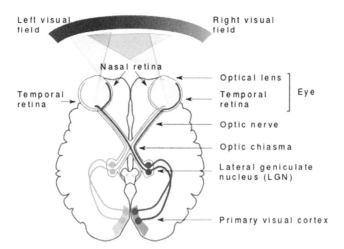

The primary visual pathway begins at the retina where two types of ganglion cell axons, magnocellular (transient cells) and parvocellular (sustained cells), exit at the optic nerve via the optic nerve head. These axons extend to the optic chiasma where partial decussation of nerve fibers of each eye occurs to ensure hemispheric visual information is kept separated. The visual signals then travel down the optic tract to the lateral geniculate body where they are combined with non-visual neural signals. From here, fibers travel to a few different locations:

- *Primary visual cortex (occipital cortex) via the optic radiations*: Early visual processing

- *Tectum*: To aid pupillary function

- *Superior colliculus*: Aids in eye movement and related multisensory integrative behaviors

The secondary visual pathway begins at the extrastriate portion of the visual cortex. From here the ventral visual pathway, primarily composed of parvocellular cells communicating with the inferior temporal area, is associated with visual identification and object recognition. The dorsal visual pathway, primarily composed of magnocellular cells which extend via the middle temporal area to the parietal cortex, gauges motion and spatial vision. Other cortical areas are also involved in oculomotor subsystems and can impact ocular motility if damaged, including the cerebellum, midbrain, frontal eye fields, superior colliculus, parietal cortex, and visual cortex.

Pathophysiology

Mechanisms of visual impairments and associated clinical findings are summarized in Table 29.3. Varying structural impairments will also tend to affect the visual system in different ways. These are as follows:

- *Soft tissue injuries*: Extraocular muscular avulsion, hemorrhage, and edema

- *Orbital fractures*: Floor, medial wall, lateral wall, roof

- *Cranial neuropathies*: Oculomotor nerve, trochlear nerve, abducens nerve, sphenocavernous syndrome, orbital apex syndrome

- *Intra-axial brainstem damage*: Internuclear ophthalmoplegia, horizontal gaze paresis, vertical gaze paresis, Perinaud's syndrome, skew deviation, abnormalities of convergence, accommodation and fusion, cerebellar lesions, vestibular system dysfunctions

- *Cerebral lesions*: Saccades, pursuit

TABLE 29.3 Visual Impairments, Mechanisms and Associated Manifestations

Deficit	Possible Mechanism	Clinical Manifestations
Blurred vision	Ocular injury to cornea, lens, and/or retina	Constant or intermittent blurred vision in one or both eyes
	Damage to the optic nerve or anywhere along the primary visual pathway	Fatigue or eye strain with sustained visual tasks
	Cranial nerve 3 damage	
	Midbrain injury	
	Refractive error	
	Amblyopia	
	Side effect of medications	
Binocular vision abnormalities	Diminished oculomotor control (cranial nerve 3, 4, or 6, palsy or paresis)	Constant or intermittent diplopia in some or all positions of gaze
	Midbrain injury affecting medial longitudinal fasciculus and/or the oculomotor nuclei	Reduced accuracy in depth perception
		Difficulty localizing objects in space
		Confusion with sustained visual activities
Nystagmus	Brainstem damage	Abnormal ocular oscillations resulting in oscillopsia, nausea, blurred vision, and visual confusion
	Cerebellar damage	
Deficits of pursuit	Lesion in either hemisphere with or without brainstem damage	Difficulty tracking in any plane
Deficits of saccades	Lesion in frontal eye field (area 8) and parietal area	Difficulty in rapid localization of objects in space
		Difficulty with reading

Chinese Medical Perspective

In Chinese medicine the eyes are considered "clear orifices" of the head which are nourished by Essence, Qi, Blood, and body fluids. Essence moistens and nourishes the eyes and has a close relationship to Shen. The "true Qi" or Yuan Qi which rises to the eyes is rooted in the Kidneys and ceaselessly rises, descends, exits, and enters, allowing for clarity of vision and pupil dilation. If the Qi is damaged then vision may become blurred. Blood nourishes the eyes as well, carrying Qi and fluids upward into the eyes, where it is said to turn to "jelly," which protects the pupils and preserves vision. The body fluids derive from the triple warmer to moisten the exterior of the eyes as well as form tears. If fluids become deficient, dry eyes may develop and cause further visual problems. The Shen is also said to be visible through an individual's eyes and is of common diagnostic note. If one's Shen seems unclear or they do not seem wholly present, then it may indicate visual problems or problems of a mental–emotional nature.

Roles of the Organ Systems as They Relate to Visual Disturbances

Heart: Generates Blood which nourishes the eyes. Houses the Shen which one's consciousness manifests through the eyes. Lateral and medial angles of the eyes correlate to the Heart, such as cracks in the skin, dandruff, scabs, pus, etc. in these areas.

Liver: Liver Blood and Qi moisten and nourish the eyes. The Liver stores Blood, while the Liver meridian flows through the eyes and is said to be in direct contact with the "connections of the eye," which is equivalent to the optic nerve and blood vessels behind the eyeball. The ability to distinguish colors is attributed to the Liver, as is the "dark of the eye" (area of the cornea and iris).

Spleen: In charge of tranformation and transportation of Qi, Blood, and body fluids; these then ascend to the eyes. The eyelids and the external eye muscles which provide structure and binding of the eyeball are governed by the Spleen.

Lung: Assists the Heart Qi in carrying Blood and assists the Spleen in carrying refined Qi to the eyes. In charge of the "white of the eye," including the sclera and conjunctiva, where visible vasculature, yellowing, or nodules may develop.

Kidney: Distribution, regulation, and harmonization of internal fluids of the eye. Corresponds to the pupil.

Gallbladder: Clear Yang Qi from the liquid of the Gallbladder rises up to form the vitreous fluid and moistens and nourishes the pupil.

Urinary Bladder: Stores liquids, transforms Qi, and moves water, which is dependent on the Kidney's ability to provide these materials. The meridian of the Bladder begins at the inner canthus and controls the surface of the whole body.

Triple Warmer: Moves the primal Qi (Yuan Qi) and refined Qi from food upward to the eyes.

The Five Wheels

Literature on Chinese medical ophthalmology describes five "wheels," each of which is associated with regions of the eye and organ system correlations. The five wheels are the muscle wheel, Blood wheel, Qi wheel, wind wheel, and water wheel. These are summarized in Table 29.4.

TABLE 29.4 The "Five Wheels" of the Eyes and Their Correlates

Wheel	Location	Organ System	Phase
Muscle wheel	Eyelids, tarsus, palpebral conjunctiva	Spleen	Earth
Blood wheel	Inner and outer canthus, lacrimal caruncle, plica semilunaris, lacrimal puncta	Heart	Fire
Qi wheel	Anterior sclera, bulbar conjunctiva	Lungs	Metal
Wind wheel	Cornea, iris	Liver	Wood
Water wheel	Pupil, aqueous humor, lens, vitreous body, choroid, retina, mascula, optic nerve, etc.	Kidneys	Water

Primary Pathogenic Environmental Contributing Factors

Heat/Fire: Swelling, inflammation, redness (common in acute eye disease), more in lacrimal sacs and eyelids, conjunctival hyperemia, keratitis with photosensitivity, abundant lacrimal fluid, yellow viscous secretion.

Cold: Slow onset, sharp pain (most cases of chronic degenerative vision loss)— keratitis, tense, dry, and aching eyes, dark purple edematous eyelids, painful spasms of blood vessels in head and eyes.

Wind: Sudden and rapid onset (common in acute eye disease)—itching, lacrimation, eyelid edema or paresis, facial nerve paralysis, paretic strabismus.

Dampness: Mucus, edema (local swelling), secretions, slow onset, heaviness, protracted keratitis, scleral ictitis.

Dryness: Dryness, itching, redness, low grade conjunctival hyperemia, punctate corneal lesions.

Summer Heat: Inflammation with mucus, hyperemia and edema of conjuctiva and eyelids, visual impairment.

Emotional causes of degenerative vision loss: Emotional states, particularly long-standing imbalances, are said to negatively impact the visual system over time and degrade the quality of one's vision.

Anger: Anger upsets the Liver and causes Qi (pathogenic heat) to rise, and the eyes become congested with excess. This heat can disturb the blood vessels and the physical structures of the eyes, causing severe tissue damage and reduced function. Prolonged anger and rage can cause severe visual impairment.

Fear: Fear causes the Qi to sink. When the energy of the body sinks, Qi, Blood, and body fluids are literally drained from the top of the body. The opposite action of anger, fear, results in too little nourishment reaching the eyes. Fear also drains the Kidney Yin (which controls the eyes).

Worry: Worry causes the Qi to knot and jam up. Worrying about the past and future creates stress. Actions that focus on helping others with their problems will usually minimize a person's own problems.

Chaos and overstimulation: Chaos, overstimulation, and overexcitement can disrupt the circulation of blood, the Heart Qi, and finally the Heart Yang. When the Heart grows weak, it slowly deprives the eyes of vital nourishment.

Fright: Fright scatters Qi and disrupts the normal flow pattern of Qi and Blood. This disruption will impair the circulation and nourishment to the eyes.

Grief/Depression: Grief and depression consume Qi. Energy consumption will reduce function and impair a person's capacity to regenerate. Grief and depression can also cause a congestion of the Lung Qi, which can lead to cataracts.

General Therapeutic Considerations Affecting the Visual System

Lifestyle Considerations

- Sufficient, regular sleep
- Regular, moderate exercise
- Ensuring proper breaks are taken during physical activity or mental work

Environmental Considerations

- Exposure to fluorescent lights
- Reading in poor (dim) lighting

- Environmental allergens
- Chlorine in swimming pools
- Air conditioning and forced hot air or baseboard heating

Somatic Therapies

- Vision therapy
- Eye exercises
- Qigong exercises for nourishing the eyes—pressure with thumb and index finger, intensifying when exhaling and decreasing when inhaling. Massage with circular movements both clockwise and counterclockwise: BL-1, BL-2, Yu Yao, TW-23, GB-1, ST-1, ST-2, LI-20, GB-14, Tai Yang, GB-20, LI-4

Orthomolecular Considerations

- Lutein
- Omega 3/6 fatty oils

Herbal Considerations

- Dusty Miller: Weak vision due to constitutional or acute conditions
- Eyebright: As a compress, relieves redness, swelling, and visual disturbance in acute and subacute inflammation and fresh eye injuries
- Bilberry fruit: Especially with diabetic retinopathy, macular degeneration, or retinal inflammation
- Chamomile
- Chrysanthemum
- Rue
- Black cohosh
- Seneca snakeroot

Nutrition

Therapeutic foods:

- Foods rich in vitamin A, C, B-complex
- Blueberries, blueberry jam, bilberry, burdock root, carrot, black beans, cod liver oil, huckleberries, endive

Specific remedies:

- Itchy eyes due to contacts: Vitamin B6

- Tired vision due to overuse and strain: Blueberries, fresh or in jam or extract

- Blurred vision: Longan fruit

Representative Chinese Formulas for Visual Conditions

- Sang Ju Yin: Acute Wind-heat

- Qi Ju Di Huang Wan: Liver Yin Deficiency with Kidney Yin Deficiency

- Jin Gui Shen Qi Wan: Kidney Yin Deficiency and Kidney Yang Deficiency

- Xiao Yao Wan: Liver Qi Stagnation

- Gui Pi Tang: Heart Blood Deficiency with Spleen Qi Deficiency

Acupuncture

Table 29.5 summarizes common points known for their effect on vision or the visual system.

TABLE 29.5 General Local Acupuncture Points with Significance to Eye Diseases

Point	Effect on Eye Diseases	Point	Effect on Eye Diseases
BL-1	Meeting point of Yin Qiao and Yang Qiao Mai—clears vision, disperses wind, clears heat, opens network vessels	GB-17	Meeting point with Yang Wei Mai—disperses wind
BL-2	Clears vision, disperses wind, opens the network vessels	GB-18	Meeting point with Yang Wei Mai—disperses wind and wind-heat, regulates Liver Qi
BL-3	Disperses wind	GB-20	Meeting point with Yang Wei Mai and Yang Qiao Mai—disperses wind, clears heat, clears vision
BL-6	Disperses wind, transforms dampness, eliminates "eye screens"	ST-1	Meeting point with Yang Qiao Mai and Ren Mai—disperses wind, leaches out wind-heat, clears vision
BL-7	Disperses wind, relaxes spasms, dissipates wind-dampness blockages	ST-2	Disperses wind, clears vision, regulates the Liver
BL-8	Strengthens and raises Liver Qi, disperses wind, opens the network vessels	ST-3	Meeting point with Yang Qiao Mai—disperses wind, leaches out wind-heat, supports Liver Qi, moves Blood

Point	Effect on Eye Diseases	Point	Effect on Eye Diseases
BL-10	Disperses wind, opens the network vessels, transforms dampness	ST-4	Meeting point with Yang Qiao Mai and Ren Mai—calms internal wind
SI-18	Disperses wind diseases	ST-8	Meeting point with Yang Wei Mai—disperses wind, supports and regulates Liver and Gallbladder
TW-17	Clears vision, disperses wind	GV-16	Meeting point with Yang Wei Mai—disperses wind, relaxes spasms
TW-20	Eliminates "eye screens" and spasms, leaches out wind-dampness	GV-17	Supports and regulates Liver and Spleen, disperses wind, leaches out damp-heat
TW-22	Supports the Qi, disperses wind, leaches out dampness	GV-19	Disperses wind, regulates Liver Qi
TW-23	Moves the Blood, regulates Qi, disperses wind	GV-20	Meeting point with all Yang and Liver meridians—opens orifices, supports and regulates Liver, disperses wind, directs Liver Yang downward, directs true Yang upward
GB-1	Connection to divergent channels of the Liver, clears vision, disperses wind and wind-heat	GV-21	Disperses wind, leaches out wind-heat
GB-3	Disperses wind, relaxes spasms	GV-23	Leaches out wind-heat
GB-5	Regulates Qi, disperses wind, clears heat	GV-24	Disperses wind, directs flaring Yang downward
GB-7	Apoplectic symptoms	Yintang	Disperses wind and heat, sedates
GB-8	Disperses phlegm blockages, leaches out wind and wind-dampness	Taiyang	Clears the eyes, leaches out wind and wind-heat, clears heat
GB-12	Regulates Liver Qi, leaches out wind and wind-heat	Yu Yao	Leaches out wind and wind-heat, clears vision
GB-14	Meeting point with Yang Wei Mai—clears vision, disperses wind	Qiu Hou	Dissipates internal blockages, clears vision
GB-15	Meeting point with Yang Wei Mai—disperses wind, supports and regulates Liver and Gallbladder	Yi Ming	Clears vision, calms the Shen
GB-16	Meeting point with Yang Wei Mai—disperses wind, regulates Liver and Gallbladder		

Eye Strain/Fatigue
Symptoms

- Dryness and discomfort of the eyes

- Distending pain

- Dizziness

- Vexation and nausea after extensive work at close distances (reading, computer work, etc.)

- Symptoms may resolve with rest

Pattern Differentiation
Liver and Kidney Deficiency

Primary symptoms: Blurred vision after extensive use of eyes, distending eye pain, possible refractive errors such as myopia, hyperopia, or presbytia

Additional symptoms: Dizziness, tinnitus, lower back and knee weakness/soreness

Pulse: Thready

Tongue: Pale, thin coat

Treatment principles: Nourish Kidney and Liver, enrich essence, brighten the eyes

Acupuncture treatment: [ST-1, BL-1, BL-2, GB-20, BL-2, LI-4, TW-23, Qiu Huo, Yu Yao, Tai Yang] + LR-3, KI-3, BL-18, BL-23

Herbal treatment:
Qi Ju Di Huang Wan Jia Jian (Rehmannia Pill with Lycium Berry and Chrysanthemum plus Modifications)
[Shu Di Huang 10g, Shan Zhu Yu 10g, Shan Yao 10g, Ze Xie 10g, Fu Ling 10g, Mu Dan Pi 10g, Gou Qi Zi 10g, Ju Hua 10g, Chai Hu 10g, Ge Gen 10g, Gan Cao 3g, Huang Qin 10g, Chi Shao 10g, Zhi Mu 10g, Bei Mu 10g]

Modifications:
Severe eye dryness + Bei Sha Shen 10g, Mai Men Dong 10g

Spleen Qi Deficiency

Primary symptoms: Eye pain or distending pain, heavy eyelids, blurred vision after extensive reading or screen use

Additional symptoms: Fatigue, pale complexion, reduced appetite, weak limbs, loose stools

Pulse: Thready

Tongue: Pale

Treatment principles: Benefit Qi and raise Yang, dispel wind, stop pain

Acupuncture treatment: [ST-1, BL-1, BL-2, GB-20, BL-2, LI-4, TW-23, Qiu Huo, Yu Yao, Tai Yang] + ST-36, SP-6, BL-20, CV-6

Herbal treatment:
Zhu Yang Huo Xue Tang (Yang Helping and Blood Activating Decoction Plus Modifications)
[Huang Qi 20g, Bai Zhi 10g, Fang Feng 10g, Dang Gui 10g, Sheng Ma 10g, Chai Hu 10g, Zhi Gan Cao 10g, Man Jing Zi 10g]

Modifications:
Light loose stool + Chao Bai Zhi 15g, Gan Cao 3g
Severe eye pain at night + Xia Ku Cao 10g

Qi and Blood Deficiency

Primary symptoms: Eyeball pain and supraorbital bone pain, inability to see for a long period of time

Additional symptoms: Pale complexion and lips, mental fatigue, lack of strength, profuse and forgetful dreams

Pulse: Thready and weak

Tongue: Pale white

Treatment principles: Benefit Qi and nourish the Blood, dispel wind, stop pain

Acupuncture treatment: [ST-1, BL-1, BL-2, GB-20, BL-2, LI-4, TW-23, Qiu Huo, Yu Yao, Tai Yang] + ST-36, SP-6, LR-8, BL-17, BL-20, CV-6

Herbal treatment:
Dang Gui Yang Rong Tang (Chinese Angelica Qi Nourishing Decoction)
[Dang Gui 10g, Chuan Xiong 6g, Bai Shao 10g, Shu Di Huang 10g, Qiang Huo 6g, Fang Feng 6g, Bai Zhi 6g, Dang Shen 15g]

Modifications:
Severe Qi deficiency + Zhi Huang Qi 20g
Severe Blood deficiency + He Shou Wu 10g, Long Yan Rou 10g
Severe supra-orbital bone pain + Mu Gua 10g, Gou Teng 10g

Liver Constraint and Blood Deficiency

Primary symptoms: Inability to read for an extensive period of time, blurred vision, distending eye pain after long periods of reading, heavy eyelids, sore and dry eyes

Additional symptoms: Headache, tightness sensation of forehead

Pulse: Thready and rapid or deep, weak, forceless

Tongue: Pale white coat

Treatment principles: Enrich Yin and nourish Blood, clear the Liver and harmonize

Acupuncture treatment: [ST-1, BL-1, BL-2, GB-20, LI-4, TW-23, Qiu Huo, Yu Yao, Tai Yang] + SP-6, LR-3, LR-8, BL-17, BL-18, BL-20

Herbal treatment:

Zi Yin Yang Xue He Jie Teng (Yin Enriching, Blood Nourishing, and Harmonizing Decoction)

[Shu Di Huang 30g, Gou Qi Zi 12g, Mai Men Dong 10g, Sha Shen 10g, Dang Gui 5g, Bai Shao 5g, Huang Qin 10g, Ban Xiao 10g, Chai Hu 10g, Jing Jie 10g, Fang Feng 10g, Xiang Fu 10g, Xia Ku Cao 15g, Gan Cao 3g]

Modifications:

With dry stool: + Fan Xie Ye 10g

Loose stool and acid swallowing: Shu Di Huang; + Bai Zhu 10g, Wu Zhu Yu 10g

Floaters

Floaters occur within the vitreous fluid of the eye behind the retina. They appear as black dots, strands, or squiggles in one's visual field. As the net-like structure of collagen fibers deteriorates over time, they may tangle or clump together to create fibrils. Floaters are the result of shadows on the retina from encountering irregularities in the gelatinous matrix that is the vitreous fluid. They may be especially visible when one is looking at a plain, well-lit background. A sudden vitreous shrinkage, as may occur with a drying and thickening vitreous later in life, can cause a pulling away from the retina and the appearance of substantial floaters. Floaters tend to occur more frequently in those with myopia or diabetes.

Symptoms

- Dryness and discomfort of the eyes
- Distending pain
- Dizziness

- Vexation and nausea after extensive work at close distances (reading, computer work, etc.)
- Symptoms may resolve with rest

Conventional Approaches

None. Virectomies are available for more severe cases.

Chinese Medical Perspective: Pattern Differentiation
Liver and Kidney Deficiency

Primary symptoms: Floaters

Additional symptoms: Breast, chest, abdominal, and rib-side distension and fullness especially during the premenstrum, dizziness, headache, moodiness, pale white facial complexion and pale nails, scanty, delayed, or blocked menstruation

Tongue: Pale tongue, thin coat

Pulse: Fine, wiry (bowstring)

Treatment principles: Course the Liver and rectify the Qi, nourish the Blood and benefit the eyes

Acupuncture treatment: BL-1, KI-6, LR-3, LR-14, LI-4, Taiyang

Herbal treatment:
Hu Qian Wan (Hidden Tiger Pill)
[Shu Di Huang 24g, Zhi Mu 12g, Gui Ban 30g, Huang Bai 9g, Bai Shao 9g, Gu Hu 6g, Chen Pi 6g, Suo Yang 6g, Gan Jiang 3g]

Liver Qi Stagnation and Blood Deficiency

Primary symptoms: Floaters

Additional symptoms: Headache, dizziness, irritability, rib-side discomfort, palpitations, insomnia, blurred vision, numbness in the limbs, pale complexion

Tongue: Pale

Pulse: Thready, wiry (bowstring)

Treatment principles: Move Liver Qi, nourish Blood, benefit the eyes

Acupuncture treatment: BL-1, KI-6, LR-3, LR-14, LI-4, Taiyang

Herbal treatment:
Xiao Yao San (Rambling Powder)
[Chai Hu 10g, Dang Gui 10g, Bao Shao 10g, Bai Zhu 10g, Fu Ling 10g, Gan Cao 6g, Bo He 3–6g, Sheng Jiang 3g, Da Zao 3pc, Long Gu 12g, Mu Li 12g]

Other Therapeutic Considerations
Orthomolecular Considerations

- Omega3 fatty acids
- Vitamin A
- Vitamin C—strengthens connective tissue of the eye, <1500mg daily to prevent malabsorption of other minerals

- Vitamin E

- Beta-carotene

- Selenium

- Chromium—deficiency increases risk eightfold

- Glucosamine sulfate—repairs and rebuilds vitreous connective tissues to prevent detachment

- Lutein

- Spirulina, chlorella, blue–green algae

Phytotherapeutic Considerations

- Ginkgo biloba

- Chysanthemum (tea or compress)

- Grapeseed extract

- Bilberry

Dietary Considerations

- Proteins: Emphasize fish, soy, almonds, sunflower seeds, sesame seeds

- Avoid: Red meat, poultry, dairy

- Brown rice with whole grains instead of processed grains such as white bread or pasta—lots of vegetables

- Avoid: Nightshade family (tomatoes, green peppers, eggplant)

- Steam or bake foods instead of frying

- Drink primarily water (eight glasses/day)

- Minimize salt

Amblyopia

The conventional definition of amblyopia is a reduced vision resulting in disuse of the eye. It is not a turned or wandering eye but may be the consequence of either of these problems. If a person's eye becomes misaligned (e.g. crossed in or turned out), the brain may selectively ignore the image coming from the turned eye. In time, the nervous pathways from the eye to the brain become underdeveloped and a lazy eye develops.

Amblyopia is not an optical problem but a problem involving the pathway from the eye to the visual cortex of the brain. Although amblyopia is commonly called "lazy eye," the eye in this condition is not really lazy; it simply has not received proper stimulation, for the following reasons:

- The eye has a prescription much different from the other eye. This inequality in sight and the discrepancy in size of the images in the two eyes make it hard for the visual cortex of the brain to integrate the two received images. If this happens before the age of six, visual development will not proceed normally. The result is the reduced visual acuity called amblyopia.

- One eye turns in, out, or up at all times and the problem begins before age six. When the two eyes are not able to align on a target, the child will initially experience double vision. As double vision is intolerable to the brain, one of the adaptations to help eliminate it is to reduce the visual acuity in the turned eye so that the brain will learn to ignore it.

Amblyopia generally does not develop once the visual system has matured (after age eight or nine) without some external trauma.

Biomedical Approaches

A patch is prescribed for the "good" or normal eye, requiring the "lazy" eye to be used. It is thus made stronger out of necessity. The extent and duration of the patching depends on the age of the individual, the severity of the condition, and the response to treatment. Dilating the pupil of the normal eye is used in occasional cases where patching cannot be done. Methods to correct the underlying abnormality that may also correct the lazy eye include eye muscle surgery, vision therapy, prescription glasses, or lid surgery.

Other Treatment Considerations

Eye exercises, Qigong eye exercises

Nutrients: Lutein, bilberry, multi-green formula

Pattern differentiation

Chinese Medical Perspective: Pattern Differentiation
Kidney Yin Deficiency or Kidney Jing Deficiency

Primary symptoms: Amblyopia

Additional symptoms: Fatigue, 5-palm heat, weak and sore lower back and knees, lack of concentration or intelligence, malar flush

Tongue: Red or pale tongue, red tip

Pulse: Fine, possibly deep

Treatment principles: Nourish the Liver, enrich the Kidneys, improve vision

Acupuncture treatment: GV-20, LI-4, SP-6, ST-36, LR-8, KI-3, KI-6

Herbal treatment:
Qi Ju Di Huang Wan Jia Wei (Lycium Fruit, Chrysanthemum, and Rehmannia Pill

Plus Modifications)
[Shu Di 12g, Shan Yao 10g, Shan Zhu Yu 10g, Ze Xie 6g, Dan Pi 10g, Gou Qi Zi 10–12g, Ju Hua 10g, Huang Bai 10g, Long Gu 12g]

Myopia (Near-Sightedness)

In myopia, objects at close distances are seen more clearly than objects at far distances. It is believed to occur secondarily to an excessive curvature of the cornea and/or a longer-than-normal eyeball. When light comes into the eye, it is first bent by the cornea, then by the lens. In myopia, instead of focusing on the retina in the area called the fovea, the light focuses in front of the retina. This results in the image appearing blurred for objects at a distance.

Myopia affects more than 80 million people in the United States. Less than 5 percent of people are born near-sighted, with symptoms appearing in the first five years of life. The majority of people who develop near-sightedness do so within the first 18 years of life. By age ten about 10 percent of people are near-sighted; by age 18 it increases to 40 percent of the population. The progression of near-sightedness stops for most people in their early 20s.

Genetic predisposition, malnutrition, various syndromes such as Down's syndrome, or ophthalmological diseases can be factors. Environmental factors can play a role as well—the increasing percentages above correspond very well to the increasing near work required in school. As an individual reads more or does more work on a computer or smart phone, the ciliary muscles of the eyes that control the focusing of the eye are called upon to work harder to focus at these near distances. As they do this for longer and longer periods of time, the muscles find it hard to relax into a position that allows focus at a distance.

The degree of near-sightedness can vary, as can the age of onset and rate of progression. Near-sightedness does not develop suddenly, but slowly over time. Most near-sighted individuals develop symptoms by the age of eight or nine and progress over the next ten years, stabilizing by the late teens or early 20s.

Symptoms

- Blurred sight at a distance

- Generally bilateral but one may be worse than the other

- Sight tends to be worse at night

- Early signs of myopia tend to occur in the child who has his or her face in a book for long periods of time without ever looking up. That child might experience some blurring at distance as he or she looks up and finds it takes longer to get far-away objects into focus

Conventional Approaches

- Glasses or contacts are prescribed to correct the refraction error—concave lenses

- Laser refractive surgery

Other Treatment Considerations: Orthomolecular Considerations

- Calcium

- Magnesium

- Phosphorus

- Zinc

- Lutein

- Bilberry

- Multi-green formula

Chinese Medical Perspective

In TCM, myopia can be caused by Liver and/or Kidney deficiency, Liver Blood deficiency, Heart Yang deficiency, and/or Heart Yin deficiency, or combinations of these patterns.

Pattern Differentiation
Heart Yang Insufficiency

Primary symptoms: Near-sightedness

Additional symptoms: Pale complexion, palpitations, mental exhaustion

Pulse: Weak

Tongue: Pale

Treatment principles: Support the Heart, augment the Qi, calm the Shen, benefit the eyes

Acupuncture treatment: [GB-20, GB-1, BL-2, ST-1, BL-1, TW-23, ST-2, LI-4] + BL-2, BL-15, HT-7, PC-6, Yiming

Herbal treatment:
Ding Zhi Wan Jia Jian (Settle the Emotions Pill Plus Modifications)
[Yuan Zhi 10g, Shi Chang Pu 10g, Dang Shen 10g, Dang Gui 9g, Sheng Di Huang 9g, Fu Shen 6g, Gan Cao 6g]

Modifications:
Eye distancing pain and fatigue + Mu Gua 10g, Bai Shao 10g

Heart Yin Deficiency

Primary symptoms: Near-sightedness

Additional symptoms: Palpitations, shortness of breath worse with physical activity, insomnia, vivid dreaming, fatigue, 5-palm heat, malar flush

Pulse: Floating or empty

Tongue: Pale, little to no coat

Treatment principles: Support the Heart Yin, augment the Qi, clear deficiency heat, calm the Shen, benefit the eyes

Acupuncture treatment: [GB-20, GB-1, BL-2, ST-1, BL-1, TW-23, ST-2, LI-4] + CV-14, CV-17, HT-7, SP-6, KI-6, BL-15, HT-3

Herbal treatment:
Tian Wang Bu Xin Dan (Emperor of Heaven Special Pill to Tonify the Heart)
[Di Huang 120g, Xuan Shen 15g, Tian Men Dong 30g, Mai Men Dong 30g, Dan Shen 15g, Dang Gui 30g, Ren Shen 15g, Fu Ling 15g, Suan Zao Ren 30g, Wu Wei Zi 30g, Bai Zi Ren 30g, Yuan Zhi 15g, Jie Geng 15g]

Kidney/Liver Yin Deficiency

Primary symptoms: Near-sightedness

Additional symptoms: Vertigo, tinnitus, restless sleep, frequent dreams, low back and knee weakness

Pulse: Thin

Tongue: Pale

Treatment principles: Moisten and tonify the Liver and Kidney, nourish Blood, support the essence, benefit the eyes

Acupuncture treatment: [GB-20, GB-1, BL-2, ST-1, BL-1, TW-23, ST-2, LI-4] + LR-3, LR-14, KI-3, BL-18, BL-23, SP-6

Herbal treatment:
Qi Ju Di Huang Tang (Brighten the Eyes Formula)
[Shu Di Huang 18g, Shan Yao 10g, Shan Zhu Yu 6g, Ze Xie 6g, Fu Ling 10g, Mu Dan Pi 6g, Gou Qi Zi 12g, Ju Hua 12g]
Zhu Jing Wan Jia Jian (Preserve Vistas Pill Plus Modifications)
[Che Qian Zi 9g, Gou Qi Zi 9g, Wu Wei Zi 3g, Dang Gui 9g, Shu Di Huang 9g, Hua Jiao 3g, Chu Shi Zi 3g, Tu Si Zi 12g]

Liver Blood Deficiency

Primary symptoms: Near-sightedness, blurred vision

Additional symptoms: Vertigo, tinnitus, insomnia, pale complexion, dry or cracking skin, pale/brittle nails, muscle weakness or spasm

Pulse: Thready or forceless

Tongue: Pale, dry

Treatment principles: Nourish Blood, tonify the Liver, benefit the eyes

Acupuncture treatment: [GB-20, GB-1, BL-2, ST-1, BL-1, TW-23, ST-2, LI-4] + GV-20, SP-6, ST-36, LR-3, LR-8

Herbal treatment:
Ming Mu Di Huang Tang (Brighten the Eyes Formula)
[Shu Di Huang 12g, Sheng Di Huang 6g, Shan Yao 6g, Shan Zhu Yu 6g, Ze Xie 6g, Mu Dan Pi 6g, Chai Hu 6g, Fu Shen 6g, Dang Gui 6g, Wu Wei Zi 6g]

Hyperopia (Far-Sightedness)

This refractive condition is due to either a smaller-than-normal length of the eye or a relatively flat curvature of the cornea. In hyperopia, objects at far distances are seen more clearly than those in close proximity. The amount of far-sightedness can vary with age. It can be overcome somewhat by strengthening the focusing power of the lens to help see near-objects clearly. Hyperopia is normal in newborn and young children and tends to lessen as children get older.

Symptoms

- Blurred vision
- Eye strain or headaches when looking at near-objects

Conventional Approaches

Glasses are prescribed to correct the refractive error.

Other Therapeutic Considerations

Nutrients: Lutein, bilberry, multi-green formula

Chinese Medical Approach

In Chinese medicine, moderate-to-severe hyperopia may be caused by Yin essence deficiency, Yin deficiency, or deficiency of Qi and Blood.

Pattern Differentiation
Yin Essence Deficiency

Primary symptoms: Hyperopia symptoms

Additional symptoms: Dizziness, tinnitus, vertigo, sore back, constipation, malar flush, night sweats, hot palms, hot feet and/or hot chest, hot flashes, insomnia, low libido, chronic dry throat, anxiety, easily startled

Pulse: Thin or fine, possibly weak or floating

Tongue: Possibly red, no coat

Treatment principles: Nourish the Liver, enrich the Kidneys, improve vision

Acupuncture treatment: [GB-1, GB-20, ST-1, TW-23, BL-1, LI-4] + CV-4, KI-6, SP-6, ST-36

Herbal treatment:
Ming Mu Di Huang Tang (Brighten the Eyes Decoction)
[Shu Di Huang 12g, Sheng Di Huang 6g, Shan Yao 6g, Shan Zhu Yu 6g, Ze Xie 6g, Mu Dan Pi 6g, Chai Hu 6g, Fu Shen 6g, Dang Gui 6g, Wu Wei Zi 6g]

Qi and Blood Deficiency

Primary symptoms: Hyperopia symptoms

Additional symptoms: Fatigue, loose stools, poor appetite, dizziness, pale complexion, weak voice, sweating with little exertion, pale or brittle nails

Pulse: Weak, thin

Tongue: Pale, thin white coat, possibly teethmarks

Treatment principles: Tonify and augment Qi and Blood

Acupuncture treatment: [GB-1, GB-20, ST-1, TW-23, BL-1, LI-4] + SP-6, ST-36, LR-8, BL-17, BL-20

Herbal treatment:
Ba Zhen Tang (Eight Treasure Decoction)
[Ren Shen 3g, Bai Zhu 3g, Fu Ling 3g, Zhi Gan Cao 1.5g, Shu Di Huang 3g, Dang Gui 3g, Bai Shao 3g, Chuan Xiong 3g, Sheng Jiang 3g, Da Zao 3g]

Astigmatism

Conventional theory is that astigmatism is caused by an irregularity in the shape of the cornea (and/or lens) of the eye whereby it becomes more oblong or "football shaped," rather than round. This distorts the light entering the eye and creates a blurred image on the retina. Astigmatism is quite common and frequently occurs along with near-sightedness and far-sightedness. It is generally bilateral but may occur unilaterally. Like other visual conditions, astigmatism is not necessarily a fixed entity. Keeping one's head held to the side for long periods of time (such as musicians) has shown changes in astigmatism due to the chronic straining of some eye muscles while relaxing others.

Symptoms

- Blurred, distorted vision at near, distance, or both, depending on the amount of astigmatism

- May involve symptoms of eye strain (such as headaches, dizziness, blurred vision, and eye redness and twitching)

- Straight lines may appear crooked; lines may be clearer in one direction than another direction

Conventional Approaches

- Glasses or contacts are prescribed if vision is impaired or eye strain present

- Refractive surgery

Other Therapeutic Considerations

Nutrients: Lutein, bilberry, multi-green formula

Chinese Medical Perspective

In TCM, astigmatism can be caused by Liver and/or Kidney deficiency, Liver Blood deficiency, Heart Yang deficiency, and/or Heart Yin deficiency, or combinations of these patterns.

Pattern Differentiation
Heart Yin Deficiency

Primary symptoms: Astigmatism symptoms

Additional symptoms: Palpitations, shortness of breath worse with physical activity, insomnia, vivid dreaming, fatigue, 5-palm heat, malar flush

Pulse: Floating or empty

Tongue: Pale, little to no coat

Treatment principles: Support the Heart Yin, augment the Qi, clear deficiency heat, calm the Shen, benefit the eyes

Acupuncture treatment: [GB-20, GB-1, BL-2, ST-1, BL-1, TW-23, ST-2, LI-4] + CV-14, CV-17, HT-7, SP-6, KI-6, BL-15, HT-3

Herbal treatment:
Tian Wang Bu Xin Dan (Emperor of Heaven Special Pill to Tonify the Heart) [Di Huang 120g, Xuan Shen 15g, Tian Men Dong 30g, Mai Men Dong 30g, Dan Shen 15g, Dang Gui 30g, Ren Shen 15g, Fu Ling 15g, Suan Zao Ren 30g, Wu Wei Zi 30g, Bai Zi Ren 30g, Yuan Zhi 15g, Jie Geng 15g]

Kidney/Liver Yin Deficiency

Primary symptoms: Near-sightedness

Additional symptoms: Vertigo, tinnitus, restless sleep, frequent dreams, low back and knee weakness

Pulse: Thin

Tongue: Pale

Treatment principles: Moisten and tonify the Liver and Kidney, nourish Blood, support the essence, benefit the eyes

Acupuncture treatment: [GB-20, GB-1, BL-2, ST-1, BL-1, TW-23, ST-2, LI-4] + LR-3, LR-14, KI-3, BL-18, BL-23, SP-6

Herbal treatment:
Qi Ju Di Huang Tang (Brighten the Eyes Formula) [Shu Di Huang 18g, Shan Yao 10g, Shan Zhu Yu 6g, Ze Xie 6g, Fu Ling 10g, Mu Dan Pi 6g, Gou Qi Zi 12g, Ju Hua 12g]
Zhu Jing Wan Jia Jian (Preserve Vistas Pill Plus Modifications) [Che Qian Zi 9g, Gou Qi Zi 9g, Wu Wei Zi 3g, Dang Gui 9g, Shu Di Huang 9g, Hua Jiao 3g, Chu Shi Zi 3g, Tu Si Zi 12g]

Liver Blood Deficiency

Primary symptoms: Near-sightedness, blurred vision

Additional symptoms: Vertigo, tinnitus, insomnia, pale complexion, dry or cracking skin, pale/brittle nails, muscle weakness or spasm

Pulse: Thready or forceless

Tongue: Pale, dry

Treatment principles: Nourish Blood, tonify the Liver, benefit the eyes

Acupuncture treatment: [GB-20, GB-1, BL-2, ST-1, BL-1, TW-23, ST-2, LI-4] + GV-20, SP-6, ST-36, LR-3, LR-8

Herbal treatment:
Ming Mu Di Huang Tang (Brighten the Eyes Formula)
[Shu Di Huang 12g, Sheng Di Huang 6g, Shan Yao 6g, Shan Zhu Yu 6g, Ze Xie 6g, Mu Dan Pi 6g, Chai Hu 6g, Fu Shen 6g, Dang Gui 6g, Wu Wei Zi 6g]

Strabismus

Two types:

- Paralytic (noncomitant)

- Nonparalytic (comitant or concomitant)

Symptoms

- Acute double vision

- Oculomotor nerve palsy: Ptosis, deviation of eye out and down, pupil may be involved

- Trochlear nerve palsy: Affected eye deviates up and out

- Abducens nerve palsy: Limited abduction of affected eye

- May occur unilaterally or bilaterally

- Compensatory head posturing

Etiology

- Paralytic: May follow defects in oculomotor nuclei, nerves, or muscles; may be caused by CNS, thyroid, muscle diseases, congenital abnormalities, trauma, neoplasm, infection

- Nonparalytic: Muscles function but do not properly converge; may follow vision problems, especially pediatric hyperopia

- Some physicians have noted mild strabismus associated with anxiety states in young people, particularly in anorexic/bulimic types

Conventional Approaches

- Ophthalmological treatment depending on clinical findings

- Conservative

- Surgical

Other Therapeutic Considerations
Somatic Considerations

- Eye exercises: Can include patching of strong eye

Chinese Medical Perspective
Chinese Medical Etiology

- Liver Blood deficiency not nourishing the eyes, which may generate wind that settles in the network vessels around the eyes, inhibiting movement

- Transforming ability of the Spleen becomes inhibited, generating accumulation of dampness and phlegm alongside wind. Wind-phlegm attacks the upper body and the eye orifice

- Kidney Yin deficiency fails to subdue Yang. Water no longer moistens wood, allowing Liver Yang to flare upward, generating wind

Pattern Differentiation
Liver Blood Deficiency

Primary symptoms: Rapid onset, diplopia in varying intensity, possibly involving eyelid

Additional symptoms: Pale, lusterless complexion, rotary vertigo, tinnitus, pale nails, possible limb numbness, tremor, hypomenorrhea

Tongue: Pale, white coat

Pulse: Thin

Treatment principles: Disperse wind, unblock the network vessels, nourish Liver, tonify Blood

Acupuncture treatment: ST-3, ST-4, ST-8, BL-2, BL-3, GB-20, LI-4, BL-17, BL-18, BL-62, TW-5, LR-3, Taiyang

Herbal treatment:
Yang Xue Dang Gui Di Huang Tang (Tangkuei and Rehmannia Decoction to Nourish Blood)
[Shu Di Huang 20g, Dang Gui 9g, Chuan Xiong 6g, Bai Shao 10g, Gao Ben 6g, Fang Feng 6g, Bai Zhi 6g, Xi Xin 3g, Qiang Huo 6g, Di Long 6g]

Dampness and Phlegm Accumulation

Primary symptoms: Rapid onset, diplopia in varying intensity, possibly involving eyelid

Additional symptoms: Headache, vertigo, lack of appetite, abdominal tension, fatigue, loose stool, abundant phlegm

Pulse: Wiry (bowstring) or slippery

Tongue: Thick sticky white coat

Treatment principles: Disperse wind, transform phlegm, unblock the network vessels, strengthen the Spleen and Stomach

Acupuncture treatment: LU-7, ST-36, ST-40, SP-6, LI-4, SI-4, BL-2, BL-10, TW-20, GB-1, GB-8, GB-20, Taiyang

Herbal treatment:
Qian Zheng San Jia Jian (Lead to Symmetry Powder Plus Modifications)
[Bai Fu Zi 3g, Chen Pi 6g, Ban Xia 6g, Mu Gua 6g, Xi Xin 3g, Da Zao 5g, Sheng Jiang 3g, Jiang Can 6g, Quan Xie 3g]

Liver and Kidney Yin Deficiency

Primary symptoms: Rapid onset, diplopia in varying intensity, possibly involving eyelid

Additional symptoms: Dizziness, vertigo, tinnitus, forgetfulness, sleep disturbances, frequent dreams, dry mouth, 5-palm heat, extreme thirst, polyuria, night sweats

Tongue: Red tongue, thin yellowish coat

Pulse: Thin and wiry (bowstring)

Treatment principles: Moisten and nourish the Liver and Kidney Yin, extinguish wind, eliminate phlegm

Acupuncture treatment: LI-4, SP-6, BL-2, BL-18, BL-23, BL-64, ST-2, LR-3, GB-1, GB-20, Taiyang

Herbal treatment:
Da Ding Feng Zhu (Major Arrest the Wind Pills)
[Sheng Di Huang 18g, Mu Li 25g, Bai Shao 10g, Huo Ma Ren 12g, Gou Teng 12g, Mai Men Dong 9g, Tian Ma 6g, E Jiao 6g, Wu Wei Zi 3g, Gan Cao 3g, egg yolk]

Yang Qiao Mai Excess and/or Yin Qiao Mai Deficiency

Acupuncture treatment: GB-20, TW-3, LI-4, ST-2, BL-1

Modifications:
Internal strabismus: Tai Yang, Qiu Hou
External strabismus: Jian Ming, Xia Jing Ming
Excess: BL-62, SI-3 to open Yang Qiao Mai
Deficiency: KI-6, LU-7 to open the Yin Qiao Mai

Chapter 30

Sleep Disturbances

According to surveys, approximately 30–70 percent of individuals who have experienced a brain injury have reported sleep disturbances following the event. These may include post-traumatic hypersomnia, narcolepsy, central and obstructive deep apnea, periodic limb movement disorder, and insomnia. Often this dysregulation of the body's daily cycles and lack of proper time to rest and rejuvenate its resources can exacerbate other symptoms such as pain, irritability, and cognitive or mood problems.

Multiple discrete centers in the brain for sleep production and wakefulness have been identified. The brainstem, basal forebrain, and hypothalamus regulate the normal sleep–wake cycle. The neurotransmitters serotonin and acetylcholine are intimately involved in this process, as are other endogenous products such as substance C and S, hypocretin, dopamine, and norepinephrine. The sleep–wake cycle is also regulated by the interactions of internal synchronizers, or "biological clocks," stemming from the suprachiasmic nucleus of the hypothalamus and the endogenous production of "process S." External synchronizers of the body are referred to as Zeitgebers, and include light–darkness changes, eating and social schedule, temperature, and relative humidity. Cognitive deficits and/or sensory deprivation may further impact disorders of sleep in individuals with brain injury.

A study of individuals with moderate-to-severe TBI showed low cerebrospinal fluid levels of hypocretin 1, a neuropeptide known to be low or absent in those with narcolepsy. These decreased levels were associated with a lower level of arousal. Individuals with TBI were also shown to have an increase in slow wave sleep and reduced REM sleep that resulted in frequent awakenings at night.

It has been suggested that sleep complaints may vary over time. Difficulty initiating and maintaining sleep tends to occur soon after injury, whereas excessive daytime somnolence occurs months or years after injury. Postinjury anxiety has been demonstrated to be the most consistent risk factor for worsening sleep status.

There are two distinct states of sleep. Rapid eye movement sleep, or REM sleep, occurs approximately every 90–100 minutes and lasts anywhere from 10 to 40 minutes. This state consists of increased brain and physiological activity similar to that of wakefulness.

Non-rapid eye movement sleep is a more restful, peaceful state with three stages. The states and stages are outlined in Tables 30.1 and 30.2.

TABLE 30.1 Sleep States

Rapid Eye Movement	Non-Rapid Eye Movement
• High level of brain activity • Physiological activity similar to wakefulness • Episodic bursts of rapid eye movement • Dreaming associated with vivid dream recall • Inability to regulate body heat (poikilothermia) • Absence of body movement but partial or full penile erection • Increase in pulse rate, blood pressure, and respiratory rate • Decreased ventilatory response to increased levels of carbon dioxide • Cortical electroencephalogram reveals low-voltage mixed-frequency waves	• Low level of brain activity • Physiological activity markedly reduced • No rapid eye movement activity • Three stages present, with arousal threshold lowest in stage 1 and highest in stage 3 • Hypothermia • Slight decrease in pulse rate, blood pressure, and respiratory rate • Decrease in blood flow through all tissues • Intermittent involuntary body movement • Cortical electroencephalogram reveals increased-voltage slowed-frequency waves

TABLE 30.2 Stages of Non-Rapid Eye Movement Sleep

Stage	General Characteristics	Electroencephalographic Findings
1	Light stage of sleep, lasts briefly Slow eye movement Occupies approximately 5 percent of sleep Hypnic jerks are common If aroused, feel they have been awake	3–7 cycles/second, low-voltage mixed-frequency waves Alpha waves disappear, theta waves appear
2	Occupies approximately 50 percent of sleep No eye movement Dreaming very rare Easily awakened	Spindle-shaped tracings at 12–14 cycles/second K complexes characterized by slow triphasic waves
3	Slow wave sleep Dreaming more common than other stages Stages most often involving parasomnias (e.g. sleepwalking, somniloquy, night terrors, sleep paralysis)	High-voltage delta waves at 0.5–2.0 cycles/second Occupies 20–50 percent of the tracing Delta waves dominant

Post-Traumatic Hypersomnia

This is a disorder in which there is hypersomnia as a result of a traumatic event involving the central nervous system. Key characteristics are excessive sleepiness and cognitive or physical fatigue. These may worsen over time as the individual gets farther out from the time of injury. Naps generally are not experienced as refreshing or effective in reducing sleepiness. No differences have been found between those experiencing hypersomnia and those without hypersomnic symptoms in terms of Glasgow Coma Scale score, length of coma, time since brain injury, nature of injury, gender, or medications. The Maintenance of Wakefulness Test (MWT) can be used to assess daytime sleepiness and predict dangerous driving in individuals.

Narcolepsy

While less common, narcolepsy can develop after a brain injury. This is typically characterized by:

- Catalepsy—sudden loss of bilateral muscle tone whereby one will suddenly collapse into sleep

- Hypnagogic hallucinations—vivid dream-like visual, auditory, or tactile sensations between waking and sleep states

- Repeated episodes of naps or lapses into sleep for short durations (10–20 minutes)

The individual will often begin to feel sleepy again after about 2 to 3 hours, repeating the cycle again. Generally, the individual's consciousness will remain clear, their respiration will be intact, and their memory will not be affected by cataleptic episodes which can last from a few seconds to several minutes.

Central and Deep Apnea

Obstructive sleep apnea syndrome is characterized by repetitive episodes of upper airway obstruction that occur during sleep. It is generally associated with a reduction in blood oxygen saturation. Loud snoring or brief gasps can often accompany this condition with silent periods of approximately 20–30 seconds. Cardiac arrhythmias commonly occur during sleep. Bradycardia can also occur during periods of apneic halting of breathing. Hypertension may also occur.

Central sleep apnea is a decreasing or stopping of breathing during sleep and is associated with lowered oxygen levels in the blood. It appears to be related to changes in the feedback loop between the lungs and the brain. An individual may appear restless as well as gasping, grunting, or choking during sleep.

Periodic Limb Movement Disorder

This entails periodic episodes of repetitive and highly stereotyped limb movements occurring during sleep. Most often this occurs in the legs, consisting of extension of the first toe and partial flexion of the ankle, knee, and sometimes hip. While less common, similar movements can occur in the upper limbs. They can occur when an individual is partially awake or waking up. They may not even be aware of these movements and rather simply describe frequently awakening throughout the night or unrestful sleep. Approaches to this condition can include proper hydration (as dehydration can be a factor), magnesium supplementation (internal or topical), or Bai Shao Gan Cao Wan—a simple formula consisting of white peony root and licorice root.

Insomnia

Insomnia is the most common sleep disturbance reported by those affected by brain injury. Literature suggests that more than 80 percent of those with a TBI complain of poor sleep and daytime sleepiness. Key components of insomnia include:

- Difficulty falling asleep

- Frequent awakenings with difficulty falling back asleep (over 30 minutes)

- Feeling of fatigue throughout the day

In order to meet the requirements for insomnia established in the DSM-5, the sleep disturbance must last for more than a month and occur greater than twice per week. It is suggested that in most cases this does not tend to subside over time following the injury. It has been shown that those who were found to have high anxiety scores had more trouble initiating sleep, while those with high depression scores had more difficulty maintaining sleep. Pain is also closely associated with insomnia in the general population.

Diagnosis

- Self-reporting
- Polysomnography (PSG)
- Multiple Sleep Latency Test (MSLT)
- Actigraphy

Biomedical Approaches
Benzodiazepine Hypnotics

- Lorazepam
- Temazepam
- Clonazepam (Klonopin)
- Triazolam

Nonbenzodiazepine Sedative-hypnotics

- Zolpidem (Ambien)
- Zaleplon (Sonata)
- Eszopiclone (Prosom)

Antidepressants

- Trazedone
- Amitriptyline

Antipsychotics

- Risperidone (insomnia and psychosis)
- Quetiapine (insomnia with paranoia or agitation)
- C-PAP or bi-level pressure oral appliances (sleep apnea)
- Modafinil (sleep apnea, narcolepsy)
- Melatonin
- Phototherapy
- Chronotherapy

Chinese Medical Perspective: Insomnia (Bu Mian)

Insomnia refers to the inability to experience normal sleep. In the *Nei Jing* this is also referred to as "inability to close one's eyes," or "inability to lie down."

In Chinese medicine, insomnia has a variety of meanings/presentations including difficulty falling asleep, frequent waking during the night, difficulty returning to sleep after wakening, restless sleep, shallow sleep, frequent nightmares or dream-disturbed sleep, and in severe cases complete inability to fall asleep. Headaches, dizziness, palpitations, fatigue, and forgetfulness frequently accompany insomnia.

Insomnia in biomedical terms is a symptom that may result from a variety of causes:

- Pain
- Depression, anxiety, bipolar disorder
- Sleep apnea
- Caffeine use
- Prescription medications and other drugs

Relevant Western Diseases

Insomnia can be found with depression, mania, schizophrenia, psychoneurosis, and reactive neurosis disorder as well as many physical situations.

Diagnosis

- *Mild*: Has difficulty falling sleep, but stays asleep once fallen asleep
- *Moderate*: Wakes easily or early, has disturbed sleep, tiredness in morning

- *Severe*: Has no sleep overnight at all and may feel exhausted in morning

- Accompanied by bodily symptoms like headache, dizziness, weakness, lack of concentration, palpitations, forgetfulness, etc.

- Frequent dreams during the sleep, nightmares, anxiousness, fearful and scary dreams, wake up with crying or expressing extreme emotion

- Insomnia that occurs three times or more in a week, continually over one month or more, requires treatment

- Nervous system and laboratory examinations may be negative or positive

Prognosis

Insomnia can be life-long; some patients suffer very severe insomnia if they have severe Shen disturbance. Today a high percentage of people regulate their sleep using medications or herbs.

Differential Diagnosis
Medical Disorders

- Degenerative neurologic diseases including Parkinson's disease, Huntington's disease, Alzheimer's disease, and other dementias

- Seizure disorders

- History of cerebrovascular accident (CVA)

- Sleep apnea (central or obstructive)

- Restless leg syndrome

Effects of Substances

- Alcohol or illicit substance intoxication or withdrawal

- Side effects of medications

Psychiatric Disorders

- Panic disorders

- Post-traumatic stress disorder

- Generalized anxiety disorder (GAD)

- Mood disorders

- Schizophrenia and other psychotic disorders

Chinese Medical Etiology

"In Chinese medicine, sleep is seen as the sinking of the clear Yang Qi of the heart spirit back down and into the interior of the body to be covered and enfolded by Yin."[1] The amount and quality of sleep is dependent on the state of the Shen, which is housed in the Heart and nourished by Heart Blood and Heart Yin. In general terms, insomnia is caused either by pathogenic factors agitating the Heart (excess) or by malnourishment of the Heart (deficiency).

The Ethereal Soul (Hun) also plays an important role in the physiology and pathology of sleep. It is said to control dreaming, and dream-disturbed sleep is often a result of this harmony.

Adequate Liver Blood or Liver Yin is necessary to root the Ethereal Soul (Hun). If Liver Blood or Liver Yin is deficient, sleep becomes restless and dreams may be excessively vivid and disturbing. The Ethereal Soul (Hun) is affected not only by a deficiency of the Liver but may also be affected by pathogenic factors such as heat/fire.

Emotional stress: Anger, frustration, irritability, or depression can injure the Liver and cause Liver Qi stagnation that, over time, may generate heat or fire that disturbs the Heart Shen.

Improper diet: Overeating or excessive consumption of greasy, spicy food can result in food stagnation and phlegm-heat in the Stomach, causing the Stomach Qi to rebel upwards and phlegm-heat to harass the Heart Shen.

Pensiveness: Excessive rumination or over-thinking injures the Spleen, leading to Qi and Blood deficiency which fails to nourish the Heart. Lack of Blood means the Shen has no residence, causing insomnia.

Congenital deficiency, aging, chronic illness, overwork, excessive sexual activity: Deficient Kidney Yin fails to nourish Heart Yin, causing Heart Yang to become hyperactive with empty fire agitating the Heart Shen.

Constitutional deficiency of both the Heart and Gallbladder can show in a personality that is timid, anxious, and indecisive. Sleep will be light with frequent waking during the night accompanied by panic, nightmares, and palpitations.

Spleen Qi deficiency may result in Blood deficiency with failure to nourish the Heart. Lack of Blood means the Shen has no residence; this causes insomnia.

Diagnostics

It is imperative to determine whether or not a patient's insomnia is secondary (caused by a known physical or mental condition) or primary. Do not diagnose insomnia when sleep is disturbed by other illnesses such as asthma, cough, pain, or itching from a

1   Flaws, Bob and Lake, James. *Chinese Medical Psychiatry: a textbook and clinical manual: including indications for referral to Western medical services.* Boulder, CO: Blue Poppy. 2003. Print.

dermatological condition. Primary insomnia is not caused by a sudden change in weather, drinking caffeinated beverages before bedtime, emotional distress or excitement, noise, or stimulation by bright light.

Difficulty falling asleep usually indicates Blood deficiency. Falling asleep easily but waking up frequently usually indicates deficient Yin. Waking up early in the morning or waking up with a startle indicates Heart and Gallbladder Qi deficiency.

A certain amount of dreaming is normal; however, nightmares, anxious dreams, angry dreams, or dreaming all night to the point where a person wakes feeling tired is considered abnormal in Chinese medicine.

Pattern Differentiation

Heart Qi and Blood Stagnation

Primary symptoms: Insomnia, may be recurrent type with palpitations, nightmares, headaches

Additional symptoms: May have chest tightness, heaviness, or painful sensations, easily startled, wakes up at night, worse at night, may be exacerbated by emotional changes, long-term history of stress or emotional problems, purplish complexion, especially lips

Tongue: Purplish tongue, white coat

Pulse: Wiry, choppy, irregular, and intermittent

Acupuncture treatment: [HT-7, SP-6, An Mian, KI-6, BL-62] + HT-5, CV-14, CV-17, LR-3, LR-14, BL-15, BL-17, BL-18, Taiyang, Yintang

Herbal treatment:
Xue Fu Zhu Yu Tang (Drive Out Stasis in the Mansion of Blood) [Tao Ren 9g, Hong Hua 9g, Shi Chang Pu 9g, Yuan Zhi 9g, Ban Xia 6g, Chuan Xiong 9g, Xiang Fu 6g, Gui Zi 6g, Jie Geng 6g, Zhi Qiao 6g, Chi Shao 12g, Chai Hu 12g, Chuan Niu Xi 9g]

Liver Depression Transforming into Fire

Primary symptoms: Insomnia, irritability, propensity toward angry outbursts, unpleasant dreams or nightmares

Additional symptoms: Red/bloodshot eyes, chest or rib-side distension, thirst, constipation, bitter taste in the mouth, dark urine

Tongue: Red tip with yellow coat

Pulse: Rapid, wiry (bowstring)

Treatment principles: Soothe the Liver, drain fire, calm the Spirit

Acupuncture treatment: [HT-7, SP-6, An Mian, KI-6, BL-62] + LR-2, LR-3, GB-44, GB-20, BL-18

Herbal treatment:
Long Dan Xie Gan Tang (Gentiana Long Dan Cao Decoction to Drain the Liver)
[Long Dan Cao 6g, Chai Hu 6g, Zhi Zi 9g, Huang Qin 9g, Dang Gui 3g, Sheng Di Huang 9g, Mu Tong 9g, Che Qian Zi 9g, Ze Xie 12g, Gan Cao 3g]

Modifications:
Tinnitus or red eyes: + Xia Ku Cao; + TW-17, TW-3 (tinnitus) or LI-5, Taiyang (red eyes)
Damp heat in lower burner: + Mu Tong, Ze Xie

An Mian Tang (Peaceful Sleep Decoction)
[Chai Hu 9g, Bai Shao Yao 9g, Chuan Xiong 9g, Fu Ling 9g, Chao Bai Zhu 12g, Huang Lian 6g, Chao Zhi Zi 9g, Sheng Di Huang 9g, Chao Suan Zao Ren 30g, Ye Jiao Teng 30g, Gan Cao 30g]

Phlegm-Fire Harassing the Interior

Primary symptoms: Insomnia, chest fullness with expectoration of copious phlegm, heaviness of the head

Additional symptoms: Aversion to eating, belching, acid regurgitation, nausea or vomiting, distension in the epigastrium, bitter taste in the mouth, irritability, dizziness, prefers spicy and junk food

Tongue: Red tip and yellow, greasy coat

Pulse: Rapid, slippery

Treatment principles: Clear heat, transform phlegm, harmonize the Stomach, calm the Shen

Acupuncture treatment: [HT-7, SP-6, An Mian, KI-6, BL-62] + ST-36, ST-40, ST-44, CV-12, LU-5, Yintang, GV-20

Herbal treatment:
Huang Lian Wen Dan Tang Jia Jian (Coptis Warm the Gallbladder Decoction Plus Modifications)
[Huang Lian 6g, Zhu Ru 6g, Zhi Shi 6g, Ban Xia 6g, Chen Pi 9g, Fu Ling 4.5g, Gan Cao 3g, Sheng Jiang 3–6g, Shi Chang Pu 10g, Yuan Zhi 10g, Suan Zao Ren 15g, Long Gu 15–20g, Mu Li 15–20g]

Modifications:
Constipation: + Gua Lou Ren, Da Huang
Food stagnation with stomach disharmony: − Ban Xia; + Ban Xia Qu, Shu Mi

Nausea or vomiting: + PC-6

Vertigo: + Dan Nan Xing, Tian Ma

Phlegm rheum with heat (dry throat, numb extremities, sudden startling, counterflow palpitations): Use Shi Wei Wen Dan Tang He Shu Mi Tang Jia Jian [Ren Shen 6g, Fu Ling 12g, Suan Zao Ren 12g, Zhi Mu 6–10g, Zhu Ru 6–10g, Ban Xia 10g, Shi Mu 15g]

Food Stagnation

Primary symptoms: Insomnia with distending, epigastric pain which is worse with pressure, belching, acid regurgitation, halitosis

Additional symptoms: Nausea, vomiting of undigested food, epigastric pain relieved after belching or vomiting, anorexia, incomplete evacuation of stool or loose, foul-smelling stool or constipation with dry stool, busy mind, prefers sweets and junk food

Tongue: Thick, greasy coating

Pulse: Slippery, wiry

Treatment principles: Disperse food, eliminate stagnation, relieve pain, calm the Spirit

Acupuncture treatment: [HT-7, SP-6, An Mian, KI-6, BL-62] + CV-6, CV-10, CV-12, ST-21, ST-25, Li Nei Ting, ST-44, LR-13, Yintang

Modifications:
Grain food stagnation: + ST-21
Meat food stagnation: + ST-24

Herbal treatment:
Bao He Wan Jia Jian (Harmony Preserving Pill Plus Modifications)
[Ban Xia 10g, Fu Ling 10g, Chen Pi 10g, Shan Zha 10g, Shen Qu 10g, Lai Fu Zi 10g, Lian Qiao 10g, Zhi Gan Cao 10g, Huo Po 10g, Zhi Shi 10g, Da Huang 3g]

Heart Yin Deficiency

Primary symptoms: Difficulty falling asleep, heart palpitations, deficiency vexation, impaired memory

Additional symptoms: Dream emission, profuse dreams, afternoon tidal heat, night sweats, 5-palm heat, sores in the mouth and on top of tongue, dry mouth and throat, dry stools

Tongue: Red tongue, scanty coat

Pulse: Fine, rapid

Treatment principles: Supplement the Heart and enrich Yin, nourish the Blood and quiet the Spirit

Acupuncture treatment: [HT-7, SP-6, An Mian, KI-6, BL-62] + HT-6, BL-15, KI-6

Herbal treatment:
Tian Wang Bu Xin Dan Jia Jian (Emperor of Heaven's Special Pill to Tonify the Heart Plus Modifications)
[Sheng Di 12g, Dang Shen 10g, Dan Shen 10g, Xuan Shen 10–15g, Fu Shen 12g, Wu Wei Zi 10g, Yua Zhi 10g, Dang Gui 10g, Tian Dong 12g, Ma Dong 12g, Bai Zi Ren 12g, Suan Zao Ren 12g]

Modifications:
Severe Heart palpitations: + Long Chi; + PC-6
Night sweats: + Long Gu, Bai Shao; + BL-43
Sores in mouth and tip of tongue: + Dan Zhu Ye, Huang Lian; + PC-8, CV-23
Impaired memory: + BL-52 with moxa

Yin Deficiency with Fire Affecting Shen

Primary symptoms: Insomnia, irritability, restlessness

Additional symptoms: Tossing and turning in bed, dizziness or tinnitus, hot feeling at night, 5-palm heat, night sweats, dream-disturbed sleep, excess dreams, low energy, lower back ache, sore legs and feet, emaciation, poor memory and concentration, yellow or scanty urination, constipation, scanty menses or amenorrhea, seminal emission

Tongue: Red with scanty or no coating

Pulse: Rapid, thin, or thready

Treatment principles: Nourish Kidney Yin, downbear Heart fire, calm the Shen, promote Heart/Kidney communication

Acupuncture treatment: [HT-7, SP-6, An Mian, KI-6, BL-62] + BL-15, BL-23, KI-3, PC-7, Yintang, KI-1 (can massage KI-1 before bed)

Modifications: If significant heat + KI-2

Herbal treatment:
Huang Lian E Jiao Tang Jia Jian (Coptis and Ass Hide Glue Decoction Plus Modifications)
[Huang Qin 6g, Huang Lian 12g, E Jiao 9g, Bai Shao 9g, Ji Zi Huang (egg yolk*), Fu Shen 12g, Suan Zao Ren 12g, Rou Gui 3g, Yuan Zhi 10g, He Shou Wu 9g]
*Stirred in while cooling

Modifications:
Severe insomnia + Zhu Sha, Hu Po
Severe deficient heat + Xuan Shen, Sheng Di; + ST-44
Dizziness + Zhen Zhu Mu, Long Gu; + GB-20
Tinnitus + Ci Shi; + SI-19
Seminal emission + Huang Bai, Zhi Mu; + BL-52
Tian Wang Bu Xin Dan (Emperor of Heaven's Special Pill to Tonify the Heart)
[Sheng Di Huang 120g, Fu Ling 15g, Dan Shen 15g, Ren Shen 15g, Dang Gui 30g, Bai Zi Ren 30g, Yuan Zhi 15g, Suan Zao Ren 30g, Tian Men Dong 30g, Mai Men Dong 30g, Wu Wei Zi 30g, Xuan Shen 15g, Jie Geng 15g, Zhu Sha 15g]

Liver/Heart Blood Deficiency with Empty Heat

Primary symptoms: Difficulty falling asleep; frequent, vivid dreams

Additional symptoms: Irritability, headache, chest or hypochondriac distension or pain, palpitations, night sweats, dry throat and mouth, dizziness

Tongue: Red tip, pale

Pulse: Wiry or thin, rapid

Treatment principles: Nourish Liver and Heart Blood, clear empty heat, calm the Shen

Acupuncture treatment: [HT-7, SP-6, An Mian, KI-6, BL-62] + BL-15, BL-18, BL-42, BL-47, LR-3

Herbal treatment:
Suan Zao Ren Tang Jia Jian (Zizyphus Seed Decoction)
[Suan Zao Ren 15g, Chuan Xiong 6g, Zhi Mu 10g, Fu Ling 10g, Gan Cao 3g, Huai Xiao Mai 15g]

Modifications:
Night sweats + Mu Li, Wu Wei
Severe deficient heat + Han Lian Cao, Nu Zhen Zi, Bai Shao

Heart and Spleen Deficiency

Primary symptoms: Difficulty falling asleep, light sleep, frequent and vivid dreams, palpitations, forgetfulness, difficulty concentrating

Additional symptoms: Dizziness, fatigue, pale complexion, lassitude of the spirit, shortness of breath, disinclination to talk, nervous and moody, sleepy in the daytime, prefers to lie down, poor appetite, weight loss, reduced food intake, loose stools

Tongue: Pale with thin coat

Pulse: Thin, weak, possibly thready

Treatment principles: Supplement the Heart and Spleen to promote the production of Qi and Blood, calm the Shen

Acupuncture treatment: [HT-7, SP-6, An Mian, KI-6, BL-62] + BL-15, BL-20, ST-36, SP-3, Si Shen Cong

Herbal treatment:
Gui Pi Tang (Spleen-Returning Decoction)
[Ren Shen 9g, Huang Qi 9g, Bai Zhu 9g, Fu Ling/Shen 9g, Dang Shen 10g, Suan Zao Ren 9g, Long Yao Rou 9g, Ye Jiao Teng 6g, Mu Xiang 6g, Zhi Gan Cao 6g, Dang Gui 6g, Zhi Yuan Zhi 3g, Sheng Jiang 3g/5 slices, Da Zao 5pc]

Modifications:
Severe insomnia:[2] + Bai Zi Ren
Impaired memory:[3] + Shi Chang Pu
Profuse dreams:[4] + Hu Po

Heart and Gallbladder Qi Deficiency

Primary symptoms: Insomnia with light sleep, frequent and vivid (sometimes disturbing) dreams, tendency to wake with a start

Additional symptoms: Timidity, palpitations, easily frightened or startled, shortness of breath, fatigue, copious, clear urine, plum pit Qi

Tongue: Pale

Pulse: Thin, wiry, weak, possibly slippery

Treatment principles: Supplement Qi, stop fright, calm the Spirit, stabilize the Mind

Acupuncture treatment: [HT-7, SP-6, An Mian, KI-6, BL-62] + HT-5, PC-7, GB-24, GB-40, BL-15, BL-19, BL-42

Herbal treatment:
An Shen Ding Zhi Wan Jia Jian (Spirit-Quieting Mind-Stabilizing Pill Plus Modifications)

---

2   Flaws, Bob and Lake, James. *Chinese Medical Psychiatry: a textbook and clinical manual: including indications for referral to Western medical services*. Boulder, CO: Blue Poppy. 2003. Print.

3   Flaws, Bob and Lake, James. *Chinese Medical Psychiatry: a textbook and clinical manual: including indications for referral to Western medical services*. Boulder, CO: Blue Poppy. 2003. Print.

4   Flaws, Bob and Lake, James. *Chinese Medical Psychiatry: a textbook and clinical manual: including indications for referral to Western medical services*. Boulder, CO: Blue Poppy. 2003. Print.

[Fu Ling 9g, Fu Shen 9g, Yuan Zhi 6g, Ren Shen 9g, Long Gu 30g, Shi Chang Pu 6g, Suan Zao Ren 12g, Hu Po 1g]

Ear points: Sub Cortex, Brain, Shen Men, Sympathetic, Heart, Spleen, Endocrine

Clinical Notes

- For insomnia due to deficient Qi, Blood, and Yin, focus the treatment on the use of herbs to supplement the Heart, Blood, Qi, and Yin and add a small quantity of herbs to anchor, settle, and calm the Spirit.

- For insomnia due to excess pathogenic factors that disturb the Shen, focus the treatment on the use of herbs that anchor, settle, and calm the Spirit, and add a small quantity of herbs to nourish the Heart and calm the Spirit.

- While the use of melatonin as a natural sleep aid can be beneficial, it is important to note that it is a hormone secreted by the pineal gland in response to fluctuations in light and darkness. Long-term and consistent supplementation of melatonin can establish an artificial external source of the hormone, making the body less likely to consistently produce it endogenously. Strong consideration should be given to utilizing melatonin either in the short term or in short periods followed by a brief break from supplementation. This may be taking it for two to three days, then taking a day off, or supplementing for a week, then taking two to three days off to allow the body to continue endogenous production.

- "Draining the South and tonifying the North" is a strategy appropriate for insomnia due to lack of communication between the Heart and Kidney. The Heart is representative of the South, while the Kidney represents the North. With Kidney Yin deficiency, water fails to nourish the Heart and empty fire flares; hyperactivity of Heart fire leads to insomnia, mental restlessness, irritability, and palpitations.

- Severe cases may give consideration to the following herbal combination: Suan Zao Ren 30g, Chen Pi 15g, Hu Po 15g.

Other Therapeutic Considerations
Somatic Therapies

- Aerobic exercise program
- Nourish breathing: Before bed
- Qigong
- Tai Qi Chuan

Just before bedtime, do the following exercise of contracting and then relaxing your muscles: While lying down, take five or six deep, slow breaths. Then tighten up the muscles of your face and neck into an ugly grimace for about two seconds. Then let go and relax. Then hunch your shoulders and tighten up the muscles of your arms. Let go and relax. Follow this pattern with the stomach muscles, legs, and then feet and toes. Then contract all the muscles of your body and relax. Repeat this whole sequence two or three more times, putting attention on deep breathing.

Orthomolecular Considerations

- Tryptophan
- 5-HTP
- Melatonin
- Phosphorus
- Lithium (anxious)

Phytotherapeutic Considerations

The following herbs used alone or in combination can help to induce quality sleep without producing the groggy, hard-to-awaken feeling the next morning that is common with sleeping pills:

- Chamomile
- Hops
- Passion flower
- Skullcap
- Valerian (which is a strong sedative)

If used as a tea, combine one tablespoon of herb per cup of boiling water. Steep for 20 minutes and drink half an hour before bedtime. If used as a tincture (liquid herbal extract), 30–60 drops of any combination are taken with a little water.

Dietary Considerations

Therapeutic foods:

- Increase foods that calm the Shen (Spirit), tonify the Heart, and harmonize the Stomach and Spleen
- Foods high in tryptophan: nuts, eggs, meat, fish, dairy

- If supplementing with tryptophan, give with cofactors (vitamins B3, B6, and C) and wholewheat toast, bananas, walnuts, and pineapples that are high in serotonin

- Increase foods high in vitamin C, vitamin B-complex

Avoid meat, alcohol, hot sauces, spicy foods, fried foods, fatty foods, rich foods, salty foods, coffee, caffeine, sweet foods, and sugar.

Nightmares/Night Terrors (Oppressive Ghost Dreams, Meng Yan)

Nightmares, or as Wiseman translates Meng Yan—"oppressive ghost dreams," occur during REM sleep. In contrast to night terrors, the disturbing dream content is remembered. Although nightmares typically cause awakening (also in contrast to night terrors), they are rarely correlated with an increase in heart or breath rate. They are usually relatively less disturbing than night terrors.

Chinese Medical Etiology

The Heart spirit becomes disquieted due to insufficient construction and nourishment or becomes harassed by an exogenous pathogen, namely heat and/or phlegm. Insufficient nourishment of the Heart may be caused by visceral deficiencies not engendering and transforming the Qi and Blood. The various organ deficiencies associated with nightmares include Heart–Liver Blood deficiency and Heart–Gallbladder Qi deficiency. Blood stasis may also result in blood deficiency as static blood hinders the generation of new or fresh blood.

Differential Diagnosis

Medical disorders:

- Narcolepsy

- Epilepsy

- Seizure disorders

Psychiatric disorders:

- Anxiety disorders

- Schizophrenia and other psychotic disorders

- Post-traumatic stress disorder (PTSD)

TCM Pattern Differentiation
Liver–Gallbladder Depressive Heat

Primary symptoms: Nightmares/profuse dreams, irritability

Additional symptoms: Bitter taste on arising, chest/breast/rib-side/abdominal distension and pain, menstrual irregularity, PMS, or dysmenorrhea, possible headaches, red eyes, dry mouth/throat

Tongue: Red tongue, dry and/or yellow coat

Pulse: Wiry (bowstring), rapid

Treatment principles: Course the Liver and rectify the Qi, clear heat, quiet the Shen

Acupuncture treatment: LR-3, SP-10, LI-4, HT-7, PC-6, ST-36, BL-15, BL-17

Herbal treatment:
Simple Liver–Gallbladder excess: Long Dan Xie Gan Tan Jia Jian (Gentiana Drain the Liver Decoction Plus Modifications)
[Long Dan Cao 6g, Huang Qin 10g, Zhi Zi 6–10g, Chai Hu 6–10g, Bai Shao 10–12g, Dang Gui 10g, Zhen Zhu Mu 12g, Hu Po 1g, Gan Cao 3–6g]

Liver depression creating heat with Spleen deficiency: Dan Zhi Xiao Yao San Jia Jian (Augmented Rambling Powder)
[Chai Hu 6–10g, Dang Gui 10g, Bai Shao 10–12g, Bai Zhu 10g, Fu Shen 12g, Zhi Zi 6–10g, Gan Cao 6g, Da Zao 3–5pc, Mu Li 12g, Hu Po 1g]

Liver Yang Rising

Primary symptoms: Nightmares, insomnia, dizziness, and vertigo

Additional symptoms: Tinnitus, headache, red eyes, distended/heavy head with simultaneous feeling of weakness or lack of grounding in the lower limbs, irritability, irascibility

Tongue: Red tongue, dry and/or yellow coat

Pulse: Fine, wiry (bowstring), rapid

Treatment principles: Drain the Liver, subdue Yang, quiet the Shen

Acupuncture treatment: LR-2, GB-20, GB-44, HT-7, PC-6

Herbal treatment:
Tian Ma Gou Teng Yin He Suan Zao Ren Tang Jia Jian (Gastrodia and Uncaria Drink Plus Modifications)
[Tian Ma 10g, Gou Teng 10g, Shi Jue Ming 15g, Zhi Zi 6–10g, Huang

Qin 6–10g, Niu Xi 10g, Du Zhong 10g, Sang Ji Sheng 12g, Ye Jiao Teng 12–15g, Fu Shen 12g, Suan Zao Ren 12g, Chuan Xiong 6–15g]

Phlegm Fire Harassing Above

Primary symptoms: Nightmares/profuse dreams, insomnia, irritability, vexation and agitation, profuse phlegm

Additional symptoms: Chest/abdominal oppression and fullness, palpitations, dizziness, possible nausea and vomiting

Tongue: Red tongue, thick, slimy, yellow coat

Pulse: Slippery, wiry (bowstring), rapid

Treatment principles: Clear heat and transform phlegm, open the orifices, quiet the Shen

Acupuncture treatment: LI-11, ST-40, ST-44, HT-7, PC-5

Herbal treatment:
With constipation: Meng Shi Gun Tan Wan (Mica Roll Phlegm Pills)
[Da Huang 3–6g, Huang Qin 10g, Huang Lia 3–6g, Meng Shi 3g, Chen Xiang 1g, Ban Xia 10g, Shi Chang Pu 6g]

No constipation: Huang Lian Wen Dan Tang Jia Wei (Coptis Warm the Gallbladder Decoction Plus Modifications)
[Huang Lian 3–6g, Huang Qin 10g, Ban Xia 10g, Zhu Ru 6g, Zhi Shi 6g, Chen Pi 6–10g, Fu Shen 12g, Dan Nan Xing 3–6g, Gan Cao 3–6g, Da Zao 3–5pc]

Heart–Liver Blood Deficiency

Primary symptoms: Frequent nightmares occurring soon after falling asleep, palpitations, tinnitus, impaired memory

Additional symptoms: Pale white facial complexion, pale lips and nails, blurred vision, night blindness, brittle nails, possible numbness of the extremities, scanty/delayed/blocked menstruation

Tongue: Pale body; white, possibly dry coat

Pulse: Fine, weak, possibly wiry (bowstring)

Treatment principles: Supplement the Heart, nourish the Liver, supplement the Blood, quiet the Shen

Acupuncture treatment: HT-7, SP-5, BL-15, BL-17, BL-18. Tonifying technique

Herbal treatment:

Zhen Zhu Mu Wan Jia Jian (Mother of Pearl Pill)
[Zhen Zhu Mu 15g, Dang Gui 10g, Suan Zao Ren 12–15g, Bai Zi Ren 12–15g, Shu Di 12g, Fu Shen 12g, Ye Jiao Teng 12–15g, Chen Xiang 1g, Hu Po 1g, Long Chi 15g]

Heart–Spleen Dual Deficiency

Primary symptoms: Profuse dreams, insomnia, impaired memory

Additional symptoms: Reduced food intake, somber white complexion, abdominal distension, loose stools, short of breath, disinclination to talk, fatigue, lack of strength

Tongue: Pale

Pulse: Soggy, fine

Treatment principles: Fortify the Spleen and boost the Qi, nourish the Heart, supplement the Blood

Acupuncture treatment: HT-7, BL-15, ST-36, SP-6, SP-1

Herbal treatment:

Gui Pi Tang Jia Jian (Restore the Spleen Decoction Plus Modifications)
[Huang Qi 15g, Dang Shen 10g, Bai Zhu 10g, Fu Shen 12g, Long Yan Rou 15g, Suan Zao Ren 12g, Mu Xiang 6g, Dang Gui 10g, Yuan Zhi 10g, Shi Chang Pu 6g, Hu Po 1g, Long Chi 12g, Gan Cao 6g]

Modifications:

Complicated by phlegm-heat: Use Yi Qi An Shen Tang (Boost the Qi and Calm the Spirit Decoction)
[Dang Gui 10g, Fu She 12g, Sheng Di 12g, Mai Men Dong 12g, Suan Zao Ren 12–15g, Yuan Zhi 6–10g, Ren Shen 3–6g, Huang Qi 15–18g, Dan Nan Xing 3–6g, Zhu Ye 10g, Huang Lian 3–6g, Gan Cao 3–6g]

Heart–Gallbladder Qi Deficiency

Primary symptoms: Nightmares/profuse dreams, waking from sleep with a fright, profuse dreams, insomnia, susceptibility to fright, timidity, impaired memory

Additional symptoms: Paranoia, palpitations, chest oppression, possible profuse phlegm or plum pit Qi

Tongue: Slightly dark or pale tongue; white, possibly slimy coat

Pulse: Fine, wiry (bowstring), possibly slippery

Treatment principles: Supplement the Heart and Gallbladder, boost the Qi, settle fright, quiet the Shen

Acupuncture treatment: HT-7, PC-7, GB-44, SP-5, BL-15, BL-18, BL-42, CV-8

Herbal treatment:

Da Ding Xin Tang Jia Jian (Major Arrest the Heart Formula Plus Modifications)
[Ren Shen 5g, Fu Ling 10g, Fu Shen 10–12g, Yuan Zhi 6–10g, Long Gu 15g, Rou Gui 3g, Gan Jiang 3g, Dang Gui 10g, Bai Zhu 10g, Bai Shao 10–12g, Hu Po 1g, Suan Zao Ren 12–15g, Ye Jiao Teng 15g]

Shi Wei Wen Dan Tang Jia Jian (Ten-Ingredient Formula to Warm the Gallbladder Decoction Plus Modifications)
[Ban Xia 10g, Zhi Shi 6g, Fu Shen 12g, Suan Zao Ren 12g, Yuan Zhi 10g, Wu Wei Zi 10g, Shu Di Huang 12g, Dang Shen 10g, Gan Cao 6g, Long Chi 12g, Ci Shi 12g]

Modifications:

More obvious Liver depression: + Chai Hu, Chuan Lian Zi

More obvious phlegm: + Shi Chang Pu, Zhu Ru

Depressive heat: + Huang Lian, Zhi Zi

Heart and Kidney Not Communicating

Primary symptoms: Profuse dreams, insomnia, heart vexation, palpitations

Additional symptoms: Low back and knee soreness and limpness, tidal heat, night sweats, seminal emission

Tongue: Red tongue; scanty or no coat

Pulse: Fine, rapid

Treatment principles: Nourish Yin and downbear fire, promote Heart and Kidney communication

Acupuncture treatment: HT-6, ST-41, KI-3, KI-1. Massage KI-1 strongly before sleep

Herbal treatment:

Huang Lian E Jiao Tang Jia Jian (Coptis and Ass Hide Gelatin Decoction Plus Modifications)
[Huang Lian 3–6g, Huang Qin 10g, Bai Shao 10g, E Jiao 6g, Yuan Zhi 10g, Fu Shen 12g, Tian Men Dong 12g, Ji Zi Huang 1pc]

Blood Stasis Obstructing Internally

Primary symptoms: Frequent nightmares, piercing lancinating headache which is fixed in location

Additional symptoms: Purplish-green lips and nails, dusky complexion, palpitations, chest/abdominal pain, all symptoms worse in evening, possible menstrual pain

Tongue: Dark purplish tongue; static spots or macules

Pulse: Fine, wiry (bowstring), possibly choppy

Treatment principles: Quicken the Blood and transform stasis, open the orifices, quiet the Shen

Acupuncture treatment: GV-14, GV-20, GV-24, SP-10, LI-4, SP-6, SP-1 (bleed). Draining technique

Herbal treatment:
Tong Qiao Huo Xue Tang (Open the Portals and Quicken the Blood Decoction) [Chi Shao 10g, Chuan Xiong 10–15g, Tao Ren 10g, Hong Hua 10g, Di Long 6g, Shi Chang Pu 6g, Yu Jin 10g, Dang Gui 10g]

Ear points: Shenmen, Sympathetic

Also consider treatment for "Internal Dragons" or "External Dragons":
External Dragons: GV-20, UB-11, UB-23, UB-61
Internal Dragons: Master point quarter inch below CV-15, ST-25, ST-32, ST-41

Other Therapeutic Considerations
Phytotherapeutic Considerations

- Lavender
- Passion flower
- Skullcap
- Peony seed (powdered)

- Pasque flower
- Swamp verbena
- Hops (use as small stuffed pillow)
- Mugwort (under pillow—folk remedy)

Dietary Considerations
Therapeutic foods:

- Increase foods that calm the Shen, tonify the Heart, and harmonize the Stomach and Spleen

Avoid:

- Meat, alcohol, hot sauces, spicy foods, fried foods, fatty foods, rich foods, salty foods, coffee, caffeine, sweet foods and sugar, processed foods
- Refined carbohydrate, food allergens

Somnolence/Hypersomnia

Etiology

- Lowering of basal metabolic rate accompanying hypothyroidism

- Central nervous system lesions affecting the hypothalamus or brainstem disrupt normal functioning of brain circuits that permit normal sleep

- Chronic abuse of marijuana, heroin, and other CNS depressants

- Psychopharmacological agents including many antidepressants and some OTC medications have significant sedating effects

- Dysregulation of serotonin, norepinephrine, or other neurotransmitters in depression

Excessive tiredness is generally due to either insufficient Yang Qi to nourish the Heart spirit or some external influence confounding the Heart. The primary external factors are phlegm and dampness. Damp depression, generally stemming from Spleen deficiency, hinders and obstructs the clear Yang from rising by its failing to transport and transform fluids. Phlegm heat may also confound the Heart and Shen.

Differential Diagnosis

Medical disorders:

- Hypothyroidism
- Hypothalamic lesions

- Seizure disorders
- Diffuse axonal injury

Effects of substances:

- Alcohol or illicit substance intoxication or withdrawal

- Side effects of medications

Psychiatric disorders:

- Depression

- Bipolar disorder, depressive phase

Pattern Differentiation

Spleen Qi Deficiency

Primary symptoms: Somnolence, lassitude of the spirit, pale complexion

Additional symptoms: Shortness of breath, disinclination to talk, poor appetite, diarrhea or loose stools

Tongue: Pale, tender, slimy coat

Pulse: Fine, weak

Acupuncture treatment: GV-20, GB-20, ST-36, SP-6

Herbal treatment:
Bu Zhong Yi Qi Tang (Supplement the Center and Boost the Qi Decoction)
[Huang Qi 15g, Dang Shen 10g, Bai Zhu 10g, Zhi Gan Cao 6g, Chen Pi 6g, Dang Gui 6g, Chai Hu 3g, Sheng Ma 3–4.5g]

Modifications:
Phlegm misting the mind: + Ban Xia, Fu Ling, Yuan Zhi, Dan Nan Xing
Food stagnation with fatigue somnolence especially after eating: Use Er Chen Tang Jia Wei (Two Cured Decoction Plus Modifications)
[Ban Xia 12g, Fu Ling 10g, Chen Pi 10g, Bai Zhu 15g, Dang Shen 15g, Mai Ya 10g, Shan Zha 6g, Gan Cao 3–6g]

Spleen–Kidney Yang Deficiency

Primary symptoms: Somnolence, sleeping with limbs huddled, lassitude of the spirit, disinclination to talk, decreased libido

Additional symptoms: Fear of cold, cold hands and feet, spontaneous sweating, dizziness, lower back pain and knee soreness, nocturia, long clear urination, possibly clear watery vaginal discharge

Tongue: Pale, white coat

Pulse: Fine, weak

Treatment principles: Fortify the Spleen and boost Qi, warm Yang and supplement the Kidneys

Acupuncture treatment: Tai Yang, BL-62, CV-4, CV-6, CV-8

Herbal treatment:
Fu Zi Li Zhing Wan He Shen Qi Wan Jia Jian (Aconite Rectify the Center Pills Plus Kidney Qi Pills Plus Modifications)
[Dang Shen 10g, Fu Zi 6g, Gan Jiang 6g, Bai Zhu 10g, Zhi Gan Cao 6g, Shu Di 12g, Shan Zhu Yu 10g, Shan Yao 10g, Fu Ling 10g, Ze Xie 6g, Mu Dan Pi 6–10g, Yi Zhi Ren 3g]

Modifications:
Phlegm confounding the spirit + Ban Xia, Yuan Zhi, Dan Nan Xing

Heart–Spleen Dual Deficiency

Primary symptoms: Somnolence, fatigue, reduced food intake, heart palpitations, lack of strength

Additional symptoms: Sallow or pale complexion, dizziness, impaired memory, abdominal distension, loose stools

Tongue: Pale, enlarged body, thin white fur

Pulse: Fine, weak

Treatment principles: Fortify the Spleen and boost Qi, nourish the Heart and supplement the Blood

Acupuncture treatment: BL-15, BL-20, ST-36, SP-6, BL-62

Herbal treatment:
Gui Pi Tang Jia Jian (Restore the Spleen Decoction Plus Modifications)
[Bai Zhu 12g, Huang Qi 15g, Long Yan Rou 10g, Suan Zao Ren 12g, Yuan Zhi 6–10g, Dang Gui 10g, Dang Shen 10g, Mu Xiang 6g, Shi Chang Pu 6g]

Kidney Essence Deficiency

Primary symptoms: Somnolence, fatigue, impaired memory, difficulty thinking

Additional symptoms: Tinnitus, deafness, dull effect, tendency to lower the head, low back and knee soreness and weakness

Tongue: Pale

Pulse: Fine, weak

Treatment principles: Enrich the Kidneys and foster essence, supplement the marrow and strengthen the brain

Acupuncture treatment: GV-20, ST-36, SP-6, KI-3, KI-6, BL-62

Herbal treatment:
He Che Da Zao Wan Jia Jian (Placenta Great Construction Pills with Modifications)
[Zi He Che 1g, Mai Men Dong 12g, Shu Di 12g, Niu Xi 12g, Du Zhong 10g, Gou Qi Zi 10g, Gui Ban Jian 10g, Lu Jiao Jiao 9g, Fu Ling 10g, Sha Ren 3g]

Spleen Encumbered

Primary symptoms: Somnolence, lassitude of the spirit, sensation of having a bag over, or hand wrapped tightly around, one's head, heavy encumbered limbs

Additional symptoms: Chest oppression and abdominal distension, poor appetite, loose stool

Tongue: Slimy white coat

Pulse: Soggy, slippery

Treatment principles: Eliminate dampness and arouse the Spleen

Acupuncture treatment: ST-36, SP-6, SP-9, Yintang, LI-2, LR-3

Herbal treatment:
Ping Wei San Jia Jian (Level the Stomach Powder with Modifications)
[Zi He Che 1g, Mai Men Dong 12g, Shu Di 12g, Niu Xi 12g, Du Zhong 10g,
Gou Qi Zi 10g, Gui Ban Jian 10g, Lu Jiao Jiao 9g, Fu Ling 10g, Sha Ren 3g]

Phlegm Heat Clouding and Sinking

Primary symptoms: Somnolence, difficulty thinking, heavy-headedness, profuse
yellow phlegm, irritability

Additional symptoms: Plum-pit Qi, heart vexation, chest and abdominal fullness,
possible nausea and vomiting, red facial complexion and red eyes, taciturnity
alternating with talkativeness, possible deranged speech, possible heart palpitations

Tongue: Red tongue, slimy yellow fur

Pulse: Slippery, wiry (bowstring), rapid

Treatment principles: Clear heat and transform phlegm, open the orifices and arouse
the spirit

Acupuncture treatment: ST-36, ST-40, ST-41, PC-5, CV-12, CV-17

Modifications:
Plum-pit Qi + HT-5, CV-23
Pronounced Spleen deficiency + BL-20, BL-21

Herbal treatment:
Huang Lian Wen Dan Tang Jia Jian (Coptis Warm the Gallbladder Decoction with
Modifications)
[Ban Xia 12g, Zhu Ru 12g, Shi Chang Pu 12g, Fu Ling 10g, Chen Pi 10g, Zhi Shi
10g, Huang Lian 6g, Gan Cao 3g]

Modifications:
With Spleen deficiency + Dang Shen, Cang Zhu

Clinical Notes

Spleen Qi deficiency somnolence typically responds well to relatively large doses of Huang
Qi and Dang Shen.

Chapter 31

Impaired Attention/ Concentration

Impairment in attention is a very prevalent occurrence following a brain injury at all levels of severity. Common symptoms include mental slowing, trouble following conversation, loss of train of thought, and difficulty in attending to more than one thing at once. The extent of changes following a brain injury reflects multiple factors, including severity of diffuse axonal injury, the length of amnesia, extent of atrophy, and the location and depth of the injury. Age, pre-existing morbidities, genetic factors, and any additional extracranial or systemic injuries such as hypoxia or hypotension can also be factors.

The early phases of recovery and post-traumatic amnesia can show signs of impaired awareness and wandering attention. Even mild injury can become restrictive of other processes such as learning new information due to the ability to maintain attention underpinning all aspects of cognition. The concept of attention can be subdivided into categories of selective, sustained, and divided attention. Information processing speed and supervisory (or executive) aspects of attention are also considered.

The brainstem reticular formation supports overall tone of attention and degree of responsiveness to stimuli. The right hemisphere has been postulated to have a greater role in sustained attention, while the left hemisphere may be more closely linked to selective and focused attention. Selective attention has also been attributed to the functioning of the posterior parietal, dorsolateral frontal, and cingulate regions of the brain, working in conjunction with the thalamus, basal ganglia, and midbrain.

Individuals who have sustained a brain injury frequently show a proportional slowing of reaction time relative to complexity of the task being performed. This is particularly true when needing to decide between several choices. Slowed cerebral processing time has been theorized to be responsible for many concerns of attention. Limitations on executive, or supervisory, control in attention has been hypothesized to govern lower-level attentional processes, including allocation of attention resources, target selection, interference control, shifting between tasks, monitoring, etc. This is thought of as a limited-capacity component involved in the processing of novel or non-routine tasks rather than those which are processed automatically. Subtypes of attention are described in Table 31.1.

TABLE 31.1 Attention Subtypes

Focused	Perceive and respond to internal and external stimuli. The selection of one source of information while withholding responses to irrelevant stimuli
Sustained	Maintain attention to complete a task accurately and efficiently over a period of time
Selective	Maintain attention in the presence of competing distractions
Alternating	Shift focus between tasks that demand different behavioral or cognitive skills
Divided	Respond simultaneously in multiple task demands while maintaining speed and accuracy

Other domains of cognitive functioning that may be affected by brain injury:

- *Categorization*: Ability to identify objects based on experiential or perceptual attributes (e.g. color, shape, construction, size, texture, detail, function)

- *Memory*: Consolidation, storage, and recall of information

- *Processing speed*: Speed at which information is processed

- *Executive functions*: Planning, reasoning, judgment, initiation and abstract thinking, problem solving, decision making

- *Metacognition*: Self-awareness and knowledge of one's strengths and weaknesses

Biomedical Approaches
Cholinergic Agents

- Physostigmine

- Cytidine-5-diphosphocholine

- Cholinesterase inhibitors (donepezil, rivastigmine, galantamine)

Catecholaminergic Agents

- Bromocriptine

- Amantadine

- Selegiline

- Psychostimulants (methylphenidate, dextroamphetamine)

- Levodopa

Other Agents

- Tricyclic antidepressants
- Memantine
- Atomoxetine (SNRI)
- Dopamine receptor agonists— pergolide, pramipexole, ropinirole
- Guanfacine
- Lamotrigine
- Other antidepressants—SSRIs, SNRIs, bupropion

Attention Processing Training (APT)—tasks are organized by increasing difficulty, and progression to a higher skill level occurs when the easier task is mastered. Repetition of a task results in a reduction in the amount of effort and attention control required.

Differential Diagnosis
Medical Disorders

- Seizure disorders
- Diseases of the CNS
- Toxic exposure
- Metabolic diseases

Effects of Substances

- Alcohol or illicit substance intoxication or withdrawal
- Side effects of medications (e.g. bronchodilators)

Psychiatric Disorders

- Attention deficit hyperactivity disorder (ADHD)
- Generalized anxiety disorder (GAD)
- Separation anxiety
- Oppositional–defiant disorder
- Conduct disorder
- Learning disorders
- Perceptual or cognitive processing deficits

Chinese Medical Perspective
Relevant TCM Diseases

Irritability (Yi Nu, Duo Nu), Insomnia (Bu Mian), Profuse Dreams (Duo Meng), Oppressive Ghost Dreams (Meng Yan), Vexation and Agitation (Fan Zao), Impaired Memory (Jian Wang)

Chinese Medical Etiology

In Chinese medicine, impaired attention and concentration has mainly to do with the Shen of the Heart. If the Shen is healthy, then it will be calm. If the Shen is calm, the mind is not agitated and the body will not become restless. Therefore, according to Chinese medicine, there are three basic mechanisms which may result in attention difficulties: the Shen may not be nourished sufficiently; some sort of external pathogen such as heat or wind harasses the heart Shen; or some sort of internal pathogen such as phlegm turbidity or Blood stasis blocks the orifices of the Heart.

Pattern Differentiation
Static Blood Obstructing Internally

Primary symptoms: Poor concentration, difficulty studying, easily angered over nothing, excessive movement and restlessness

Additional symptoms: Dry withered hair, scaly skin, prominent veins, possible history of birth trauma or traumatic brain injury with intracranial hemorrhage, blue green/dull dark complexion

Tongue: Dark and/or purple tongue, static spots or macules, engorged tortuous sublingual veins

Pulse: Deep, choppy, fine or bound, regularly intermittent

Treatment principles: Quicken the blood, transform stasis, nourish blood, engender essence, calm spirit, boost intelligence

Acupuncture treatment: Drain: SP-10, LI-4, BL-15; Tonify: BL-17, BL-23

Acupuncture modifications:
Scattered concentration: + GV-20, Si Shen Cong, PC-7
Hyperactive stirring: + BL-15, Ding Shen, An Mian
Labile emotions with vexation and agitation: + GV-24, CV-17, KI-6
Essence spirit lassitude, fatigue, shortness of breath, palpitations: + ST-36, SP-3, BL-20

Herbal treatment:
Huo Xue An Shen Tang (Move the Blood and Calm the Spirit Decoction)
[Tao Ren 6–10g, Hong Hua 6–10g, Chuan Xiong 3–6g, Chi Shao 3–6g, Shi Chang Pu 6–10g, Yi Zhi Ren 6–10g, Shan Zu Yu 6–10g, Shu Di Huang 6–12g, Huang Jing 6–10g]

Modifications:
Excessive movement and restless fidgeting: + Long Gu, Mu Li
Essence spirit lassitude, fatigue, shortness of breath, palpitations: + Huang Qi, Dang Gui

Torpid intake, sallow complexion, weak limbs: + Dang Shen, Bai Zhu, Fu Ling, Shan Yao

5-palm heat, insomnia, profuse dreams, emaciation, and red tongue: + Gui Ban, Sheng Di Huang, Zhi Mu, Huang Bai

Spleen Deficiency, Liver Hyperactivity

Primary symptoms: Difficulty maintaining attention, uncontrollable fidgeting, emotional tension, easy anger

Additional symptoms: Poor sleep, fatigue, diminished appetite, diarrhea due to stress

Tongue: Thin white coat

Pulse: Wiry (bowstring)

Treatment principles: Fortify the Spleen and harmonize the Liver

Acupuncture treatment: LR-3, LI-4, ST-36, HT-7

Acupuncture modifications: Same as above pattern

Herbal treatment:
Yi Gan San (Restrain the Liver Powder)
[Chai Hu 3–10g, Gou Teng 6–12g, Dang Gui 4–10g, Chuan Xiong 6–12g, Bai Zhu 6–10g, Fu Ling 6–12g, Gan Cao 3–10g]

Modifications:
Pronounced disquieted spirit: + He Huan Pi, Ye Jiao Teng; or Long Gu, Mu Li
Depressive heat: + Huang Qin and/or Huang Lian
Pronounced fatigue due to Spleen deficiency: + Dang Shen
Phlegm turbidity: + Ban Xia, Shi Chang Pu, Chen Pi

Heart–Spleen Dual Deficiency

Primary symptoms: Difficulty concentrating, sallow yellow or somber white facial complexion, pale nails and lips, fatigue, insomnia, profuse dreams, heart palpitations

Additional symptoms: Shortness of breath, poor appetite, tendency to loose stool, impaired memory

Tongue: Fat pale tongue with teeth marks, thin white coat

Pulse: Fine, weak

Treatment principles: Fortify the Spleen and supplement the Heart, boost the Qi and nourish the Blood

Acupuncture treatment: BL-15, BL-17, BL-47, BL-20, SP-3, HT-7

Acupuncture modifications: Same as first pattern

Herbal treatment:

Gui Pi Tang He Gan Mai Da Zao Tang Jia Jian (Restore the Spleen Decoction Plus Licorice, Wheat and Jujube Plus Modifications)
[Tai Zi Shen 6–10g. Bai Zhu 6–10g, Fu Shen 6–12g, Huang Qi 6–12g, Gan Cao 3–10g, Dang Gui 4.5–10g, Suan Zao Ren 6–12g, Yuan Zhi 4.5–10g, Shi Chang Pu 3–10g, Wu Wei Zi 6–10g, Da Zao 2–5pc, Huai Xiao Mai 12–25g]

Yin Deficiency–Yang Excess

Primary symptoms: Thin body type, poor concentration, insomnia, heart palpitations, easy agitation, easy anger, excessive movement and speech

Additional symptoms: Dizziness, tinnitus, possible low back pain, possible enuresis, flushed cheeks, dry mouth and throat, night sweats

Tongue: Red tongue, red tip, scanty coat

Pulse: Fine, rapid

Treatment principles: Enrich and nourish Kidney Yin, level the Liver and subdue Yang, calm the Heart and boost intelligence

Acupuncture treatment: Tonify: KI-3, SP-6; Drain: PC-6, GV-14, LI-11

Acupuncture modifications: Same as first pattern

Herbal treatment:

Zuo Gui Yin Jia Wei (Restore the Left [Kidney] Pill with Modifications)
[Shu Di Huang 6–12g, Shan Zhu Yu 6–10g, Gou Qi Zi 6–10g, Fu Ling 6–10g, Shan Yao 6–10g, Gan Cao 3–6g, Zhi Mu 6–10g, Huang Bai 6–10g, Gui Ban 10–15g, Nu Zhen Zi 6–10g, Long Gu 10–15g, Mu Li 10–15g, Shi Chang Pu 6–10g, Yuan Zhi 6–10g, He Shou Wu 6–10g]

Modifications:

Scattered concentration, poor memory + Yi Zhi Ren, Wu Yao
Disquieted sleep with spasms and contractions of hands and feet + Suan Zao Ren, Ye Jiao Teng, Gou Teng, Bai Shao

Phlegm Heat Harassing Internally

Primary symptoms: Lack of attention, excessive movement and speech, difficulty controlling oneself, lack of concentration, easy anger, pronounced irritability, vexation and agitation

Additional symptoms: Possible nausea, profuse phlegm, chest and abdominal fullness and oppression, torpid intake, possible bad breath, bitter taste in mouth, yellow-red urination

Tongue: Red tongue edges, slimy yellow coat

Pulse: Slippery, rapid, wiry (bowstring)

Treatment principles: Clear heat and disinhibit dampness, transform phlegm and calm the Heart

Acupuncture treatment: ST-40, CV-12, PC-6, GV-14, LI-11

Acupuncture modifications: Same as first pattern

Herbal treatment:
Huang Lian Wen Dan Tang Jia Jian (Coptis Decoction to Warm the Gallbladder Plus Modifications)
[Ban Xia 6–10g, Chen Pi 6–10g, Fu Ling 6–10g, Huo Po 6–10g, Yu Jin 6–10g, Shi Chang Pu 6–10g, Hua Shi 6–10g, Zhi Ke 6–10g, Lian Qiao 6–10g, Huang Lian 1.5–6g, Gan Cao 1.5–3g]

Modifications:
With Yin deficiency: + Shu Di Huang, Bai He, Shi Hu
Constipation due to heat: + Da Huang, Huang Qin, Zhi Zi
Severe phlegm and chest oppression: + Meng Shi, Chen Xiang

Yang Qi Deficiency

Primary symptoms: Poor concentration, excessive movement but not overexcitement

Additional symptoms: Lassitude of the spirit, somber white complexion, torpid intake, loose stools, low back and knee soreness and limpness, cold body and chilled limbs

Tongue: Pale tongue, moist coat

Pulse: Deep, weak

Treatment principles: Supplement the Kidneys and boost the Qi, strengthen the will (or mind) and quiet the spirit

Acupuncture treatment: BL-23, KI-7, GV-4, BL-51, CV-4, ST-36. Moxa

Herbal treatment: Jin Gui Shen Qi Wan Jia Wei (Kidney Qi Pill from The Golden Cabinet Plus Modifications)
[Shu Di Huang 6–10g, Shan Zhu Yu 6–10g, Shan Yao 6–10g, Fu Ling 6–10g, Ze Xie 6–10g, Dan Pi 3–6g, Fu Zi 3–6g, Rou Gui 3–6g, Yi Zhi Ren 6–10g, Shi Chang Pu 6–10g]

Other Therapeutic Considerations
Somatic Therapy Considerations

- Gentle exercise
- Eurhythmy

- Yoga
- Qigong

Phytotherapeutic Considerations

- Black cohosh
- Chamomile
- Wild oat
- California poppy
- Evening primrose
- Siberian ginseng
- Hops

- Oatstraw
- St. John's wort
- Lavender
- Melissa
- Passion flower
- Skullcap
- Valerian

Dietary Considerations

Diet can at times have a significant impact on attentional concerns, particularly if a food allergy or sensitivity is present.

Therapeutic foods:

- Whole-foods diet, high in protein and complex carbohydrates; reduce sugar and simple carbohydrates
- Increase foods that calm the Shen (Spirit), tonify the Heart, and harmonize the Stomach and Spleen
- Increase foods rich in vitamin B-complex
- Longan, oyster, rice, rosemary, wheat, wheat germ, mushroom (maitake, shiitake, reishi)

Also:

- *Avoid food additive sensitivities*: Eliminate processed foods that contain artificial colors, flavors, sweeteners, and preservatives, commonly listed as benzoates, nitrates, and sulfites. Common food additives also include calcium silicate, BHT, BHA, benzoyl peroxide, emulsifiers, thickeners, stabilizers, vegetable gums, and food starch
- *Minimize food sensitivities*: Eliminate or reduce the intake of cow's milk, soy, eggs, wheat, citrus, and other potential allergenic foods

- *Minimize sugars and simple carbohydrates to reduce risk of hypoglycemic reactions*: Avoid meat, alcohol, hot sauces, spicy foods, fried foods, fatty foods, rich foods, salty foods, coffee, caffeine, sweet foods, and sugar

Chinese Nutritional Approach

- *Heart Blood deficiency, Spleen Qi deficiency, Yin deficiency, and Yang hyperactivity*: Nourishing, cooked, warm, clear, bland diet, with slightly increased animal protein to help manufacture sufficient blood, for example soups with black beans, chicken or beef broth, and plentiful root and leafy green vegetables

- *Phlegm obstructing the Heart orifices*: Avoid sweet, cold, and damp foods which either weaken the Spleen, such as chilled, cold, raw foods or sugar and sweets, or foods which cause dampness and phlegm, such as sugar and sweets, dairy foods, and fatty, greasy, fried foods

- *Heat excess*: Eliminate all food additives, colorings, and flavorings; avoid oranges, sugar, and red meat, as well as hot foods such as hot spices, shellfish, and curries

- *Heat and phlegm*: Eliminate phlegm-producing foods such as dairy and peanut butter and high frequency of gluten intolerance which causes green phlegm and nasal congestion; avoid sweet and damp foods

- *Middle Jiao deficiency, including Spleen Qi deficiency*: Limit sweets and fruit juices, especially restricting cold food and drinks; no ice

- *Kidney Qi deficiency*: Limit sweets and cold food; no ice

Chapter 32

Memory Impairment

Memory dysfunction is considered a flagship feature following a brain injury. During the acute recovery phase, retrograde amnesia and post-traumatic amnesia can certainly have a distinct impact. Subjective memory complaints in the post-acute phase can often persist as well. In cases of mild TBI most symptoms tend to resolve within one to three weeks following the injury. In moderate-to-severe injuries, symptoms may chronically persist. A brain injury can affect anywhere along the process of memory functioning—encoding, storage, or retrieval of information may all be impacted. The transferring of information from short-term to long-term memory, a process known as consolidation, can also be influenced. In order for information to become encoded, it must be present and attended to, allowing for storage. The information must be stored in order to be later retrieved. As such, a dysfunction anywhere in this process will cause impairments in memory.

Individuals with brain injuries have generally been found to test more poorly in memory tasks, such as recalling a list of 15 words presented to them (either visually or aurally), than those who had not sustained such an injury.

The various types of memory are as follows:

Sensory memory: Holds a memory of sensory input for a matter of a few seconds after the stimulus. This allows the screening of large amounts of information and can be vulnerable to "washout." The five forms of sensory memory correlating to the five senses are echoic (auditory), iconic (visual), olfactory (smell), haptic (touch), and gustatory (taste).

Short-term memory: Information recall lasts for a few minutes to hours. Information is passively held. Some cognitive psychologists hold that short-term memory and working memory are interchangeable terms; others consider them separate functions.

Working memory: Active, rather than passive, this is a temporary storage of information in order to accomplish a task.

Long-term memory: Permanent consolidation and storage of information within long-term retention systems that may remain for a lifetime. Long-term memory can be further divided into either explicit, which can be consciously declared, or implicit, which is an unconscious procedural process.

- Examples of explicit memory—semantic memory (general knowledge/facts about the world), episodic memory (personal recollection of experiences)

- Examples of implicit memory—procedural memory (e.g. "muscle memory," tying shoes, riding a bike), cognitive skill memory (e.g. memory of procedures needed to solve a problem or win a game), classical conditioning

Aspects of Memory Relating to Executive Function

- *Working memory*: As defined above

- *Strategic memory*: Active organizing and elaborative strategies to enhance encoding and retrieval

- *Source memory*: Context in which episodic memory is formed—where and when, temporal order, recentness of presentation

- *Prospective memory*: Remembering to perform a task in the future at a certain time or following a specific event

- *Metamemory*: Awareness and knowledge of one's memory abilities

Episodic memory impairment is a hallmark feature of a TBI and generally corresponds to the severity of the injury. Working memory can also often be affected, in which the function of processing and manipulating information has been linked to the dorsolateral prefrontal region. This also corresponds to updating stored information, inhibiting unwanted thoughts, and the alteration between maintenance systems of verbal and visuospatial information. Spontaneous organizing strategies during learning tasks such as semantic categorization (e.g. "vegetables," "cars") has often been shown as being impaired. Prospective memory may also show deterioration. Individuals may fail to effectively gauge the degree of their memory impairment, believing they perform better than the actual results show. This demonstrates a deficit in self-awareness of one's abilities (metamemory). A traumatic brain injury tends to affect the brain's control/manipulation processes more than the passive storage/rehearsal aspects. Recognition memory tends to remain intact, as does implicit memory.

MRI findings have consistently demonstrated hippocampal atrophy following injury. This, coupled with a marked sensitivity of this structure to injury, strongly implicates the entorhinal cortex and hippocampus as the crucial structures in dysfunctions of explicit memory following a brain injury. Bilateral destruction of the anterior hippocampus results in profound disturbances involving memory and new learning (i.e. anterograde amnesia). The hippocampus is thus assumed to protect memory and the encoding of new information during the storage and consolidation phase by gating of afferent streams of information and the filtering/exclusion/dampening of irrelevant and interfering information. When the hippocampus is damaged, input overload may result as the neuroaxis is overwhelmed by neural noise. This disrupts the consolidation phase of memory to the degree that relevant information is not properly stored or even attended to. Consequently, the ability to form associations or alter preexisting schemas is negatively affected. Diencephalic and basal forebrain structures are also postulated to be strong potential candidates given their substantial role in episodic memory. Mnemonic functioning may be affected by injury to the frontal lobes.

Frontal–subcortical and memory-specific temporal networks have also been implicated in attention and executive function memory impairments. Inferior temporal neurons are involved in encoding, storage, and recall, and interact with the amygdala and hippocampus via the entorhinal cortex in regard to learning, memory, and recognition. These inferior neurons are involved in short-term emotional, as well as non-emotional, visual and cognitive processing and memory storage. Neurons in the inferior temporal gyrus convey information concerning current versus previous stimulus patterns and their behavioral context. As seen with a lesion of the inferior temporal lobe, visual and verbal memory functions may suffer. "Middle temporal firing patterns may contribute to the reactivation of neocortical circuits encoding a particular stimulus-context gestalt,"[1] which in turn makes recognition and retrieval possible. Electrical stimulation of the inferior and medial temporal lobe has produced exceedingly vivid personal memories which include snapshots of such things as complex scenes from early childhood, hearing conversations, seeing faces, or experiencing somesthetic sensations and related events. Diffuse axonal injury has also been suggested to affect the wider memory networks.

Damage or seizures of the left inferior temporal lobe can moderately disrupt immediate and severely impair delayed memory of verbal passages, and the recall of verbal associations, consonant trigrams, word lists, and number sequences. Electrical stimulation of the anterior and posterior temporal regions has shown severe anterograde and retrograde memory loss for verbal material. Right temporal lesions, on the other hand, significantly impair recognition memory for tactile and recurring visual stimuli such as faces and meaningless designs, and object positioning/orientation and visual–pictorial stimuli. Electrical stimulation of the right anterior and posterior temporal lobe also causes, respectively, severe anterograde and retrograde memory loss for designs, geometric stimuli, and faces. The anterior temporal region is more involved in the initial consolidation storage phase of memory, while the posterior temporal region is involved more with memory retrieval and recall. The temporal lobes directly interact with the frontal lobes in this process of memorization and remembering. The greater degree of activation in the frontal and temporal lobes (and associated tissues), the greater the likelihood individuals will remember, whereas reduced activity is associated with forgetting. Thus, if the frontal lobe becomes injured, even if the temporal lobes are

---

1   Lash, Marilyn. *The Essential Brain Injury Guide*. 5th ed. Vienna, VA: Academy of Certified Brain Injury Specialists, Brain Injury Association of America. 2016. Print.

spared, individuals may demonstrate significant memory loss due to an inability to correctly search for and find the memory.

Differential Diagnosis
Medical Disorders

- History of traumatic brain injury (TBI)
- Seizure disorders
- History of cerebrovascular accident (CVA)
- Chronic vitamin B deficiency
- Other cognitive dysfunctions: Attention, processing speed, executive function

Effects of Substances

- Chronic alcohol abuse leading to Korsakoff's syndrome
- Chronic abuse of cocaine, methamphetamine, marijuana, or heroin

Psychiatric Disorders

- Post-traumatic stress disorder (PTSD)
- Dissociative identity disorder (DID) and other dissociative disorders

Biomedical Approaches
Cholinergic Agents

- Physostigmine
- Cytidine-5-diphosphocholine
- Cholinesterase inhibitors (donepezil, rivastigmine, galantamine)

Catecholaminergic Agents

- Psychostimulants (methylphenidate, dextroamphetamine)
- Amantadine
- Bromocriptine
- Levodopa
- Selegiline

Other Agents

- Tricyclic antidepressants
- Other antidepressants (SSRIs, SNRIs, bupropion)

- Atomoxetine (SNRI)

- Dopamine receptor agonists: Pergolide, pramipexole, ropinirole

- Guanfacine

- Lamotrigine

- Memantine

- Improving attention, perception, and categorization skills

- External compensatory strategies— alarms, memory notebooks, digital devices

Chinese Medical Perspective: Impaired Memory (Jian Wang)

Impaired memory refers to either partial or total loss of memory about things which have happened either in the recent or distant past.

Relevant Western Diseases

Forgetfulness, amnesia

Chinese Medical Etiology

In Chinese medicine, memory impairment has a similar etiology to insomnia and profuse dreaming. There is either not enough nourishment of the Heart Shen or there is a harassing of the Heart Shen by some pathogen. Flaws quotes Zhu Dan-xi in saying, "Impaired memory is mostly due to essence spirit shortage and scantiness, [though] it may also have [i.e. be due to] phlegm."[2] Here it is implied that anxiety and overthinking may cause such essence spirit shortage and scantiness by damaging the Pericardium. A prenatal (pre-heaven) natural endowment or habitual bodily deficiency weakness due to overtaxation, enduring disease, immaturity or aging, overuse of certain medicines and drugs, or unrestrained sexual activity can all contribute to Kidney essence deficiency. Being deficient, Kidney essence then may fail to fill the "sea of marrow" and nourish the brain sufficiently.

Pattern Differentiation
Blood Stasis Internally Obstructing

Primary symptoms: Sudden onset of impaired memory that endures

Additional symptoms: Dry mouth with desire for fluids but no desire to swallow, chest oppression, abdominal fullness and pain exacerbated by pressure, black stools

---

2   Flaws, Bob and Lake, James. *Chinese Medical Psychiatry: a textbook and clinical manual: including indications for referral to Western medical services.* Boulder, CO: Blue Poppy. 2003. Print.

Tongue: Dark, purplish tongue, possibly static spots or macules, possibly tortuous and engorged sublingual veins

Pulse: Wiry (bowstring), choppy

Treatment principles: Quicken the Blood and transform stasis, open the portals and fortify the memory

Acupuncture treatment: HT-3, Si Shen Cong, SP-10, LI-4, SP-6

Herbal treatment:
Xue Fu Zhu Yu Tang Jia Jian (Drive Out Stasis in the Mansion of Blood Decoction Plus Modifications)
[Tao Ren 10g, Hong Hua 10g, Dang Gui 10g, Sheng Di Huang 12g, Chuan Xiong 6g, Chi Shao 10g, Zhi Ke 6–10g, Yu Jin 6g, Yuan Zhi 6–10g, Shi Chang Pu 6g]

Heart–Spleen Dual Deficiency

Primary symptoms: Impaired memory, sallow yellow complexion, lassitude of the spirit, heart palpitations, reduced sleep, profuse dreams

Additional symptoms: Shortness of breath, fatigue, poor appetite, loose stools, menstrual irregularities in females

Tongue: Pale, commonly enlarged tongue, white coat

Pulse: Fine, weak

Treatment principles: Fortify the Spleen and boost the Qi, supplement the Heart and nourish the Blood

Acupuncture treatment: GV-20, HT-7, BL-15, BL-20, ST-36

Herbal treatment: Gui Pi Tang Jia Jian (Restore the Spleen Decoction Plus Modifications)
[Bai Zhu 10g, Fu Shen 12g, Huang Qi 15g, Dang Shen 10g, Gan Cao 6g, Dang Gui 10g, Long Yan Rou 12g, Suan Zao Ren 15g, Yuan Zhi 10g, Yi Zhi Ren 15g, Mu Xiang 6–10g]

Modifications:
Heart Blood or Heart Yin deficiency predominant: Huang Qi; + Bai Zi Ren, Ye Jiao Yeng
Spleen Qi deficiency predominant: + Fu Ling, Huang Jing, Chen Pi; − Fu Shen

Kidney Essence Insufficiency

Primary symptoms: Impaired memory, absent-mindedness, lassitude of the spirit

Additional symptoms: Tendency to let the head fall forward, possible loose teeth, loss and/or early graying of the hair, low back and knee soreness and limpness, weak bones

Tongue: Pale tongue, white coat

Pulse: Vacuous or choppy

Treatment principles: Supplement the Kidneys and boost the essence

Acupuncture treatment: Si Shen Cong, BL-52, BL-23, SP-6, KI-3

Herbal treatment:

He Che Da Zao Wan Jia Jian (Placenta Great Fortifying Pills Plus Modifications) [Zi He Che 1g, Shu Di 12g, Niu Xi 12g, Du Zhong 10g, Gui Ban 20g, Gou Qi Zi 10g, Huang Jing 10g, Ren Shen 6–10g, Shan Yao 10g, Shan Zhu Yu 10g, Yuan Zhi 6–10g, Yi Zhi Ren 15g]

Heart and Kidney Not Communicating

Primary symptoms: Impaired memory, dizziness, tinnitus, heart palpitations, absent-mindedness

Additional symptoms: Low back and knee soreness and limpness, 5-palm heat, afternoon tidal heat, night sweats, vexation, insomnia

Tongue: Red tongue, scanty coat

Pulse: Fine, rapid

Treatment principles: Enrich the Kidneys, nourish the Heart, and promote the interaction between the Heart and Kidneys

Acupuncture treatment: Si Shen Cong, HT-6, BL-15, BL-23, KI-6, SP-6. Even technique

Herbal treatment:

Liu Wei Di Huang Wan Jia Wei (Six Ingredient Pill with Rehmannia Plus Modifications)
[Shu Di Huang 12g, Shan Yao 10g, Shan Zhu Yu 10g, Fu Ling 10g, Ze Xie 6–10g, Dan Pi 10g, Ren Shen 6–10g, Yuan Zhi 6–10g, Yi Zhi Ren 15g, Gui Ban 15g]

Modifications:

Heart Yang effulgence predominant: Use Zhen Zhong Dan Jia Jian (Pillow Elixer Plus Modifications)
[Gui Ban 15g, Mu Li 15g, Yan Zhi 10g, Shi Chang Pu 10g, Sheng Di 12g, Fu Shen 12g, Zhu Ye 10g]

Phlegm Qi Depression and Binding

Primary symptoms: Impaired memory, somnolence, dizziness or vertigo

Additional symptoms: Chest oppression, nausea, reduced food intake, profuse phlegm, sound of phlegm in the throat, spitting or hacking of phlegm, plum pit Qi

Tongue: Slimy white coat

Pulse: Wiry (bowstring), slippery

Treatment principles: Transform phlegm and quiet the spirit, rectify the Qi and resolve depression

Acupuncture treatment: HT-7, ST-40, ST-36, LI-4. Draining technique

Herbal treatment:
Wen Dan Tang Jia Jian (Warm the Gallbladder Decoction Plus Modifications) [Ban Xia 10g, Zhu Ru 10g, Zhi Shi 6–10g, Chen Pi 6–10g, Bai Zhu 10g, Fu Ling 10g, Dan Nan Xing 6g, Shi Chang Pu 6g, Gan Cao 3–6g]

Modifications:
Phlegm transforming into heat with dry mouth and throat, yellow phlegm, red complexion, red tongue: + Huang Lian, Huang Qin

Other Therapeutic Considerations
Orthomolecular Considerations

- Glutamic acid—200mg/day
- Vitamin B12—1mg/day
- Lecithin—2 tablespoons/day
- B-complex vitamin—50mg three times per day. A vitamin B deficiency will affect brain function

- Phosphatidylserine
- Vinpocetine (short-term memory)
- Resveratrol
- Pregnenolone

- Niacin—start with 100mg after each meal and increase up to 250mg until you feel a flushing of the skin. This stimulates blood circulation to the skin and head. Continue for trial period of three weeks. Niacin should only be used under a doctor's supervision as it can become toxic to the liver after several weeks

Phytotherapeutic Considerations

- Ginkgo biloba
- Ginseng root
- Gotu kola

Dietary Considerations

- Maintain a healthy diet. This includes using fresh, unprocessed foods. Eat daily servings of leafy green vegetables, whole grains, fresh fruits, and proteins with a minimum of animal fat. Keep intake of sugar foods and refined carbohydrates (such as white bread and white rice) to a minimum.

- Eliminate alcohol, smoking, and drug use.

Additional Considerations

- The effects of stress can be reduced through stress management and relaxation techniques such as visualization and meditation. Counseling is strongly encouraged.

- Get adequate rest and take naps as needed.

- Regular physical exercise—at least 30 minutes, three times a week. Consultation with a physician about a proper exercise program should be considered if one hasn't exercised for a while.

Research Studies

The therapeutic effects of acupuncture plus modified Bu Yang Huan Wu Tang were compared to a pharmaceutical medication in post-stroke cognitive dysfunction. The drug group received three tablets of piracetam, three times per day, for eight weeks. The Chinese medicine group received acupuncture at GB-20 and the extra point Gongxue located 1.5 cun below GB-20 six days a week and the herbal formula twice daily. The acupuncture plus herbs group achieved a 90 percent total treatment effective rate. The drug group achieved a 70 percent total effective rate. Bu Yang Huan Wu Tang was administered in the following modified version: Huang Qi, Dang Gui Wei, Chuan Xiong, Chi Shao, Tao Ren, Hong Hua, Di Long, E Zhu, Shi Chang Pu, Shui Zhi.[3]

---

3   Wang, Z.D., Xin, G.L., and Lin, F.Y. Clinical observation on nape acupuncture plus Bu Yang Huan Wu decoction for cognitive disorder after cerebral infarction. *Shanghai Journal of Acupuncture and Moxibustion*. 2013; 32(10). English summary obtained from www.healthcmi.com/Acupuncture-Continuing-Education-News/1698-acupuncture-alleviates-cognitive-dysfunction-after-stroke

Chapter 33

Executive Function

Executive function collectively refers to some of the most complex cognitive processes the human brain performs. Executive function operations are discussed in Chapter 10 on the frontal lobe and the prefrontal cortex. They include the following:

- Self-awareness
- Planning/organizing
- Goal setting
- Self-initiation
- Self-monitoring

- Self-evaluation
- Self-inhibition
- Change set
- Strategic behavior
- Working memory

In cases of a brain injury, problems can manifest in the following realms:

- Abstract thought
- Ability to analyze all aspects of a situation
- Lack of control over emotions
- Executing solutions
- Maintaining cognitive flexibility if one solution does not work

- Self-monitoring
- Impulsivity
- Disinhibition
- Hyperverbosity
- Considering all possible solutions to a problem

Executive function deficits may be present in all levels of injury severity and may impact all aspects of daily life. One's interpersonal, social, recreational, emotional, educational, and vocational life can all be significantly affected. Deficits in executive function are considered a critical determinant of functional outcome after a brain injury. Links have been established between the prefrontal cortex and virtually all other cortical and subcortical regions. Four distinct categories of function have been linked to specific regions of the prefrontal cortex, which are shown in Table 33.1.

TABLE 33.1 Categories of Frontal Executive Function

Dorsolateral prefrontal cortex	Executive cognitive functions	Spatial, temporal, and conceptual reasoning
Superior medial prefrontal cortex	Activation-regulating functions	Initiating and maintaining mental processes Monitoring response conflict
Ventromedial prefrontal cortex	Behavioral self-regulation functions	Emotional processing Mediation of stimulus–reward associations
Frontal polar regions	Metacognitive processes	Higher-order integrative aspects of personality, self-awareness, and social cognition Prospective memory: Complex multitasking

Dorsolateral Prefrontal Cortex

Focal injuries to this area will tend to result in difficulties in attention, working memory, planning, and reasoning. Phonemic and semantic fluency may decline. Diffuse axonal injury may cause executive cognitive functioning deficits whether or not there is direct frontal lobe injury. Higher-order functioning procedures may become apparent or increasingly so under situations of increased demand or task complexity.

Tests

Verbal fluency tasks (retrieval, monitoring, inhibition), Trail Making Test (part B) (divided attention), Wisconsin Card Sorting Test (concept formation/flexibility)

Superior Medial Prefrontal Cortex

This brain region provides an important activating function in initiating and sustaining mental processes at a high enough level to meet goal-directed tasks. Damage here can result in marked apathy or abulia (lack of will), and in severe cases of bilateral lesions can demonstrate an akinetic mutism. Deficits from injuries of a lesser degree have showed slowed reaction time on task tests or a slowed response/increased errors. The superior medial prefrontal cortex becomes engaged any time a cognitive task becomes more difficult and demands more performance monitoring. The anterior cingulate seems to be particularly relevant here in monitoring potential response conflicts such as in novel situations. The absence of such activation can contribute to an apathetic state.

Tests

Verbal fluency tasks, conflict trial of the Stroop color-naming test

Ventromedial Prefrontal Cortex

This region includes the orbitofrontal cortex and the adjacent ventral aspects of the medial prefrontal cortex. This makes up the limbic sector of the prefrontal cortex and tends to bear the brunt of a traumatic brain injury as it is vulnerable to both focal and diffuse effects. A lack of insight, impaired planning and decision making, social impropriety, a lack of empathy, and a dampened or poorly modulated emotional response tend to result from injury. A deficit in "social cognition" may also be apparent in which one lacks the ability to effectively interpret the behavior of others, make inferences about their feelings, beliefs, and intentions, conceptualize one's relationship to another, and guide one's behavior based on this information. Perception of facial expressions, voice, bodily gestures, social context, and the registering of negative emotions such as anger, sadness, disgust, and fear (yet not positive emotions) may be deficient. The ventromedial prefrontal cortex may play a role in such "self-conscious emotions" as embarrassment, shame, and pride. There may also be a striking dissociation between preserved intellectual ability on standard testing and a failure to apply this knowledge in less structured situations. An individual may be found to lack a "gut feeling" due to an inability to process emotionally related material.

Tests

Iowa Gambling Task (decision making), Frontal Systems Behavioral Scale

Frontal Pole

This lies in a position to fulfill a specialized, integrative role in relation to the other prefrontal cortex regions due to a unique cytostructure and reciprocal connections almost exclusively with higher-order association cortices. It receives processed, abstract information from other supramodal areas and seems to bridge prefrontal cortex functions with those of emotion, drive, and self-regulation. Future plans and goals, abstract reward concepts, and complex, real world multitasking (having a large overarching goal in mind while achieving smaller independent tasks) are thought to be processes in the frontal pole as well. It is also associated with the function of metacognition, explored in further detail below.

Treatment Options

- Cognitive rehabilitation—formal problem-solving training with applications in everyday situations and functional routines

- Speech–language pathologists

- Occupational therapists
- Neuropsychologists

Metacognition

This term refers to one's ability to reflect on, and be aware of, one's own cognitive functioning. This includes a perceived cognitive acuity that may not accurately represent what testing and observation by others reveals. In other words, an individual may think they cogitate better than they actually do. Intact metacognition would allow them to be aware of struggles they may experience with problem solving but still not be able to solve the problem. The term for diminished self-awareness and inability to recognize personal disability is anosognosia. Due to this being a higher-order cognitive function that reflects upon itself, metacognition has an integrative role for other aspects of executive functioning such as self-monitoring and information processing.

There are three levels of metacognitive impairment:

- Awareness of deficits caused by injury (memory deficits, delays in processing speed, etc.)
- Awareness of functional implications of these deficits
- Awareness to set realistic goals

Treatment Options

Cognitive rehabilitative approaches such as with an occupational therapist begin with external cueing, then move toward the patient internalizing the process.

Biomedical Approaches
Cholinergic Agents

- Physostigmine
- Cytidine-5-diphosphocholine
- Cholinesterase inhibitors (donepezil, rivastigmine, galantamine)

Catecholaminergic Agents

- Psychostimulants (methylphenidate, dextroamphetamine)
- Amantadine
- Selegiline
- Bromocriptine
- Levodopa

Other Agents

- Tricyclic antidepressants

- Other antidepressants (SSRIs, SNRIs, bupropion)

- Atomoxetine (SNRI)

- Memantine

- Dopamine receptor agonists: Pergolide, pramipexole, ropinirole

- Guanfacine

- Lamotrigine

Chinese Medical Perspective

Pattern differentiation can be based on coverage in the previous chapters on memory and attention impairment.

Chapter 34

Dementia

Dementia may be caused by structural damage to cerebral tissue or may result as a progressive decline in several dimensions of intellectual function that interfere substantially with the person's normal social or economic activities. A single brain trauma with diffuse injury to the tissue may incite dementia. Dementia can also develop as the result of multiple mild TBIs in which chronic traumatic encephalopathy (CTE) occurs. CTE is a rare, progressive, and degenerative condition of the central nervous system which typically follows repetitive brain trauma. This may be due to high-risk sports such as football or boxing. In this case, diffuse axonal injury causes a release of Tau proteins which are changed structurally by the metabolic breakdown of brain cells following trauma to create a chronic inflammatory state that causes a progressive degeneration of the central nervous system.

Etiology and Classification

Dementia may occur at any age, from any injury, in which enough impact is sustained to cause widespread damage to associative cortical areas.

Static Dementia

Stems from a single major injury (severe head injury)—nonprogressive.

Progressive Dementias

- *Alzheimer's disease*: Degenerative loss of cells, acetylcholine neurons affected, atrophy of the brain, senile plaques, neurofibrillary tangles, abnormally increased proteins in brain. Four major components: Heart disease of any kind, hypertension, diabetes, obesity. Some are now calling this a "type 3 diabetes" due to evidence of blood sugar correlates

- *Idiopathic, or simple, presenile dementia*: Alzheimer's-like changes, multiple infarcts, age of onset is abnormal

- *Multi-infarct dementia*: Small and large cerebral infarcts of varying age, step-wise intellectual dysfunction, neurological symptoms, depression

- *AIDS dementia*: Late-stage HIV with cognitive, emotional, motor deficits

- *Chronic progressive traumatic encephalopathy*: Progressive dementia from repeated head injury

Degrees of Severity

- *Mild cognitive impairment*: Memory problems better than expected for one's age

- *Medium-level Alzheimer's*: Hard to learn new things, difficulty performing tasks that involve multiple steps, impulsivity, paranoid thinking, forgets friends

- *Severe Alzheimer's*: Difficulty communicating, does not recognize family, sleeps a lot, loss of bowel/bladder control, loses weight

Symptoms

There are a number of warning signs that may point to the development of dementia (see Table 34.1) which can manifest as less severe symptoms of diagnostic criteria for dementia, which are shown in Table 34.2.

TABLE 34.1 Warning Signs of Dementia

Asking the same question repeatedly
Repeating the same story over and over again, word for word
Forgetting how to do an activity that used to be easy
Loss of ability to balance checkbook
Getting lost and misplacing things
Neglecting to bathe and wearing the same clothes over and over again
Reliance on someone else to answer questions and make decisions

TABLE 34.2 Signs and Symptoms

Slow disintegration of personality and intellect
Impaired insight and judgment
Loss of affect
Depression, paranoia, anxiety
Restricted interests, rigid outlook, difficulty with conceptual thinking
Difficulty acquiring new skills
Decreased initiative
Distractibility
Aphasia (speech disturbance), apraxia (motor), agnosia (recognition of perceptions)
Spatial disorientation
Memory impairment
Blunted affect
Deteriorated habits
Personality traits exaggerated
Insidious, progressive
Initially more of a problem for family

Diagnosis

- Memory impairment
- Aphasia, apraxia, agnosia, or disturbed executive function
- Continuing cognitive decline

Diagnostic Testing

- Complete Blood Count (CBC)
- Chem screen
- Thyroid function
- Serum B12
- Drug levels
- HIV
- CT scan
- EEG (wave slowing)—suggests that the hippocampus is working at a lower level

Differential Diagnosis

- Chronic alcohol use
- Vitamin B12 deficiency
- Drug side effects
- Primary psychiatric disorder
- Sometimes secondary to a treatable condition

Chinese Medical Perspective: Dementia

Dementia, or what has previously been referred to as "feeblemindedness" (a term that has now fallen out of favour), refers to a chronic or persistent disturbance of the intelligence characterized by mental sluggishness, lack of intelligence, foolishness, and/or clumsiness. When minor, it manifests as an abstraction of mind, diminished speech, mental torpor, or impaired memory. Severe cases may demonstrate absence of speech or muttering to oneself, deranged speech, crying or laughing for no reason, or no desire for food.

Relevant Western Diseases

> Alzheimer's disease, Pick's disease, cerebral atherosclerosis, transient ischemic attack, autism, hypertension, and Attention disorders

Chinese Medical Etiology

Dementia is an inability of the Shen to function correctly. In order for the Shen to be clear, there must be ample Qi within the Heart. Pathology may be due to malnourishment of the Heart by Blood, Yin, and/or Essence or some pathologic Qi cofounding the Shen, such as phlegm, dampness, or Blood stasis. Deficiencies which lead to malnourishment are Blood deficiency mixed with Qi depression, Liver Blood–Kidney Yin deficiency, and a deficiency and emptiness in the sea of marrow.

Aging is considered the main etiological factor for this disease. Overworking, mental exhaustion, and, in Chinese medicine, excessive sexual activity also are said to be factors that may cause this disease. In the elderly, the five Zang essences, especially Kidney essence, become depleted and fail to nourish the sea of marrow. Prenatal (pre-heaven) deficiency factors genetically passed from the parents are considered to be a weak constitution, poor nutritional status, alcohol and drug abuse, or an extreme fright during pregnancy which can injure the fetus and cause diminished intellectual ability. This deficiency may be noticeable even at a young age. Emotional disharmony, shock, or phlegm obstruct the Clear Yang cavity that causes Shen dysfunction. Birth trauma or physical injury are also considered factors which cause Qi and Blood stagnation to obstruct the clear cavity of the brain, causing Shen injury.

Pattern Differentiation
Qi Stagnation and Blood Stasis
Most cases have a history of traumatic injury or birth trauma.

> ***Primary symptoms***: Dementia, apathy, slowed reactions, sluggishness, fearfulness, flattened emotion and Shen numbness, depression and irritability, autism, diminished ability for socializing and learning

Additional symptoms: Insomnia, dream-disturbed sleep, dull and drooping eyes, may have headaches and dizziness, possible headache from short times of reading or watching screens for learning

Tongue: Purplish tongue, purple macules on tongue

Pulse: Deep, fine, wiry (bowstring), choppy

Treatment principles: Quicken the Blood, transform stasis, and boost the intelligence

Acupuncture treatment: SP-6, SP-8, SP-10, LI-4, LR-3, HT-7, BL-15, BL-17, GV-15, GV-17, GV-19, GV-20, GV-21, GV-24, Yintang

Herbal treatment:
Tong Qiao Huo Xue Tang Jia Jian (Open the Portals and Quicken the Blood Decoction Plus Modifications)
[Chi Shao 10g, Chuan Xiong 10–15g, Tao Ren 10g, Hong Hua 10g, Di Long 3g, Yu Jin 6g, Yuan Zhi 9g, Shi Chang Pu 6g, Ju Luo 10g, Da Zao 3pc]

Modifications:
Concomitant Qi and Blood deficiency + Dang Gui, Huang Qi

Phlegm Dampness Clouding the Mind

Primary symptoms: Mind abstraction, flat wooden affect, impoverished thinking and emotion, autism, lack of speech or speaking to oneself, disinclination to talk or to meet visitors, prefers staying alone, poor memory and thinking

Additional symptoms: Profuse phlegm, no appetite, heavy-headedness, chest and abdominal fullness and oppression, vomiting profuse phlegm, phlegm sounds in throat, pale complexion, shortness of breath, may not be able to take care of themselves in daily life, very sleepy and tired, may be overweight

Tongue: Swollen tongue with teeth marks, thick white coat

Pulse: Deep, weak, slippery

Treatment principles: Transform dampness and flush away phlegm, open the orifices and boost the intelligence

Acupuncture treatment: SP-3, SP-6, SP-9, ST-25, ST-36, ST-40, ST-41, HT-7, PC-7, CV-12, GV-22, Yintang

Herbal treatment: Zhi Mi Tang Jia Jian
[Ban Xia 10g, Chen Pi 10g, Bai Zhu 10g, Shen Qu 6g, Shi Chang Pu 10g, Fu Shen 12g, Yuan Zhi 6g, Ren Shen 3g, Dan Nan Xing 5g, Fu Zi 3g, Gan Cao 6g]

Qi Depression–Blood Deficiency

Primary symptoms: Dementia, emotional depression, possible insomnia with impetuosity and impatience

Additional symptoms: Frequent sighing, grief with a tendency to cry, chest and rib-side oppression distension, pale nails and lips

Tongue: Pale tongue

Pulse: Wiry (bowstring), fine

Treatment principles: Course the Liver and rectify the Qi, nourish the Blood and boost the intelligence

Acupuncture treatment: HT-7, LR-3, LR-8, LR-14, ST-36, Yintang

Herbal treatment:
Xiao Yao San He Gan Mai Da Zao Tang (Rambling Powder with Licorice, Wheat, and Jujube Decoction)
[Chai Hu 10g, Bai Shao 10g, Bai Zhu 10g, Dang Gui 10g, Fu Ling 10g, Bo He 3g, Sheng Jiang 3g, Da Zao 6pc, Fu Xiao Mai 15g, Gan Cao 10–15g]

Modifications:
Severe Liver depression + Yu Jin, He Huan Pi
Marked depressive heat − Sheng Jiang, Bo He; + Zhi Zi, Dan Pi
Insomnia + He Huan Hua, Suan Zao Ren

Liver Blood–Kidney Yin Deficiency

Primary symptoms: Dementia, lack of spirit in the eyes, motor ataxia, paraphasia

Additional symptoms: Dizziness, tinnitus, low back and knee soreness and limpness, numbness of the limbs with inhibited flexion and extension, possible 5-palm heat or night sweats, possible malar flushing and/or emaciation

Tongue: Red or pale tongue, red tip, scanty coat

Pulse: Fine, commonly wiry (bowstring), possibly rapid

Treatment principles: Supplement the Liver and nourish the Blood, enrich the Kidneys and boost the intelligence

Acupuncture treatment: GB-20, SP-6, KI-3, KI-4, BL-17, BL-18, BL-23, Si Shen Cong

Herbal treatment:
Da Bu Yuan Jian (Great Tonify the Primal Decoction)

[Shu Di 12g, Gou Qi Zi 10g, Shan Zhu Yu 10g, Du Zhong 10g, Ren Shen 3–6g, Shan Yao 10g, Yuan Zhi 10g, He Shou Wu 12g, Gan Cao 3g]

Sea of Marrow and Pre-Heaven Essence Deficiency

Problems may begin in childhood.

Primary symptoms: Dementia, poor memory, developmental slowing, the five developmental slowings (standing, walking, hair, teeth, language) and the five soft tissue weaknesses (head, neck, hands, feet, and mouth) in infants and children, late closure of the fontanelle in infants

Additional symptoms: Fragile bones, low back and lower limb soreness and weakness, inability to stand for a long period of time, unsteady walking, inability to hold up the head, a high level of Shen processing is slowed down, may age more rapidly than normal

Tongue: Pale tongue, scanty coat

Pulse: Fine, weak

Treatment principles: Supplement the Kidneys and foster the essence, fill the marrow and boost the intelligence

Acupuncture treatment: ST-36, KI-3, KI-4, KI-6, SP-6, BL-20, BL-23, BL-54, CV-6, GV-4, GV-20

Herbal treatment:

He Che Da Zao Wan Jia Jian (Placenta Great Construction Pills with Modifications) [Zi He Che 3g, Shu Di 12g, Gui Ban 12g, Niu Xi 10g, Du Zhong 10g, Mai Dong 12g, Tian Dong 12g, Gou Qi Zi 10g, Huang Jing 10g, Yuan Zhi 9g, Shi Chang Pu 9g, Lu Jiao Jiao 3g]

Other Therapeutic Considerations

Beneficial Activities to Boost Intelligence

- Learn a new language
- Puzzles, crosswords, brain games
- Play a musical instrument
- Listmaking
- New activities and new social environments

Orthomolecular Considerations

- Acetyl-L-carnitine—500mg TID
- Vitamin B3 (niacin)[1]
- Vitamin E—2000 IU/day

---

1   Marz, Russell. *Medical Nutrition from Marz: a textbook in clinical nutrition.* Portland, OR: Omni-Press. 1999. Print.

Phytotherapeutic Considerations

- Ginkgo biloba—80mg TID

- Curcumin-decreased inflammation—enough that it may inhibit neurofibrillary tangles

- Green tea

- Balm[2]

- Sage[3]

- Rosemary[4]

- Adaptogens: Ashwaghanda, ginseng, rhodiola[5]

Dietary Considerations

- Fruit/vegetable juice intake four to five times a week was shown to lower dementia risk fourfold

Research Studies

Di Huang Yin Zi not only significantly decreased the number of TUNEL-positive cells but also reduced the LDH release of the hippocampus of model rats. The Morris water maze test showed that the ability of the learning and memory of rats was dramatically impaired after ischemic brain injury. However, Di Huang Yin Zi ameliorated the impairment of the learning and memory of ischemic rats. Furthermore, western blotting and immunohistochemical data showed that the expression of extracellular-regulated protein and synaptophysin, which correlates with synaptic formation and function, decreased after ischemic insult.[6]

2   Perry, N., Court, G., Bidget, N., Court, J., and Perry, E. European herbs with cholinergic activities: potential in dementia therapy. *International Journal of Geriatric Psychiatry.* 1996; 11: 1063–1069. doi:10.1002/(SICI)1099-1166(199612)11:12<1063::AID-GPS532>3.0.CO;2-1

3   Perry, N., Court, G., Bidget, N., Court, J., and Perry, E. European herbs with cholinergic activities: potential in dementia therapy. *International Journal of Geriatric Psychiatry.* 1996; 11: 1063–1069.

4   Perry, N., Court, G., Bidget, N., Court, J., and Perry, E. European herbs with cholinergic activities: potential in dementia therapy. *International Journal of Geriatric Psychiatry.* 1996; 11: 1063–1069.

5   Yang, F-M., Dong, L-L., Cao, J., *et al.* Effects of rhodiola herb on behavior and the expression of Bcl-2 and bax protein in the hippocampus of vascular dementia rats. *Chinese Journal of Information of Traditional Chinese Medicine.* 2008-06. Web. http://en.cnki.com.cn/Article_en/CJFDTOTAL-XXYY200806022.htm

6   Hu, R., Yin, C-L., Wu, N., *et al.* Traditional Chinese herb Dihuang Yinzi (DY) plays neuroprotective and anti-dementia role in rats of ischemic brain injury. *Journal of Ethnopharmacology.* 2009 Jan 30; 121(3): 444–450. doi: 10.1016/j.jep.2008.09.035. Epub 2008, Oct 19.

Chapter 35

Language and Communication Dysfunction

A study of brain-injured individuals seven years out from a severe injury showed that nearly 50 percent reported some level of difficulty in speaking. Reports of difficulty in word finding can often follow a spectrum of any injury severity level; however, objective findings of communication deficits tend to accompany moderate-to-severe cases. Vulnerability to these deficits are both focal and diffuse.

Impairments include deficits in word retrieval, verbal associative fluency, and comprehension of complex auditory input. Conversational components can also be affected with difficulties in the pragmatic use of language, such as initiating and maintaining a specific topic of conversation, attending to the needs of the listener, or the use of indirect communication such as humor or sarcasm.

Anomic aphasia tends to be the most common form in which identifying objects and proper names, frequent paraphasias, and circumlocution (talking in circles) are found with preserved comprehension and repetition. Wernicke's (receptive) aphasia has also been observed, in which the ability to understand language is present. Other forms of aphasias are more rare. See Chapter 9 for a more extensive exploration of aphasia. Other speech disorders such as mutism, stuttering, and echolalia (repetition of speech) have also been known to occur. Speech apraxia can be present whereby an individual cannot effectively translate what they want to say into motor signals to initiate speech. Dysarthria, in which muscle weakness impacts the ability to speak, is relatively common following a TBI and may continue to be present after other language deficits subside. Many deficits are considered to have a reasonably good prognosis within the first year postinjury, particularly in cases of mild brain injury.

Language and communication dysfunctions cannot be viewed in isolation due to their neural substrates involving distributed networks which link prefrontal, perisylvian, and parietal language areas as well as other regions mediating broader aspects of communication such as one's non-dominant hemisphere. They reflect the interplay of primary receptive/ expressive language functions, other non-linguistic cognitive processes such as attention and working memory, and higher-order executive functions of the prefrontal cortex. Injury of the left prefrontal cortex has been associated with simplified, repetitive, and impoverished discourse. Right hemisphere prefrontal injury, on the other hand, may show an amplification of detail, insertion of irrelevant elements, and a tendency toward socially inappropriate speech.

Differential Diagnosis

Medical Disorders

- Delirium
- Dementia
- Cerebrovascular accident (CVA)
- Tic disorders

- Traumatic brain injury
- Seizure disorders
- CNS tumors

Psychiatric Disorders

- Schizophrenia and other psychotic disorders
- Acute mania in bipolar disorders or schizo-affective disorder
- Pervasive development disorders

Chinese Medical Perspective: Deranged Speech (Yan Yu Cuo Luan)

In Chinese medicine, deranged speech refers to incoherent, illogical, nonsensical speech.

Chinese Medical Etiology

Speech is considered to be derived from the function of the Heart organ system. When Heart Qi and Blood are excessive and exuberant, and the Heart Shen is quiet, the speech is orderly and coherent. However, when the Heart Qi and Blood are insufficient to construct and nourish the Shen and its functions, then the Shen may become disquieted. The functions of the Heart may lose their duty, and the speech may become deranged. Hence, deranged speech is primarily associated with either lack of nourishment of the Heart Shen or harassment and blockage of the Heart aperture by phlegm, heat, or static blood.

TCM Pattern Differentiation
Heart–Spleen Dual Deficiency

Primary symptoms: Deranged speech, disinclination to speak

Additional symptoms: Insomnia, heart palpitations, fatigue, lassitude of the spirit, cold hands and feet, a tendency to loose stools, poor appetite, a sallow yellow or pale white facial complexion, pale lips and nails, lack of strength

Tongue: Pale, fat tongue with teeth marks on edges

Pulse: Fine, weak, possibly slow

Treatment principles: Supplement the Heart and nourish the Blood, fortify the Spleen and boost the Qi

Acupuncture treatment: CV-23, HT-5, SP-6, ST-36, TW-8, BL-15, BL-20, GV-15

Herbal treatment: Gui Pi Tang Jia Wei (Restore the Spleen Decoction Plus Modifications)
[Huang Qi 10–15g, Dang Shen 10g, Bai Zhu 10g, Fu Shen 12g, Gan Cao 6–12g, Dang Gui 6–10g, Long Yan Rou 10g, Yuan Zhi 6–10g, Mu Xiang 6g, Shi Chang Pu 6g, Sheng Jiang 3g, Da Zao 3–5pc]

Yin Deficiency–Blood Dryness

Primary symptoms: Deranged speech, emotional lability, alternating joy and crying without apparent reason

Additional symptoms: Insomnia, heart palpitations, fatigue, a dry throat, possibly night sweats, agitation

Tongue: Red tongue, scanty dryish coat

Pulse: Fine, possibly rapid, possibly bowstring

Treatment principles: Enrich Yin and nourish the Blood, clear heat and quiet the Shen

Acupuncture treatment: SP-6, KI-3, HT-7, HT-5, TW-8, CV-23, BL-15, BL-17, GV-15

Herbal treatment:
Gan Mai Da Zao Tang Jia Jian (Licorice, Wheat, and Jujube Decoction Plus Modifications)
[Gan Cao 10–15g, Huai Xiao Mai 15–30g, Bai He 30g, Suan Zao Ren 12g, Zhi Mu 10g, Bai Shao 10g, Da Zao 10pc]

Liver Depression Qi Stagnation

Primary symptoms: Deranged speech, irritability, emotional depression

Additional symptoms: Taciturnity, chest oppression, rib-side distension

Tongue: Normal or slightly darkish tongue, thin white coat

Pulse: Fine, wiry (bowstring)

Treatment principles: Course the Liver and resolve depression

Acupuncture treatment: LR-3, LI-4, LR-14, CV-23, HT-5, TW-8, GV-15

Herbal treatment:
Si Ni San Jia Wei (Frigid Extremities Powder Plus Modifications)
[Chai Hu 6g, Zhi Ke 10g, Bai Shao 10g, Gan Cao 6g, Fo Shou 10g, Xiang Yuan 10g, Mei Gui Hua 10g, He Huan Hua 12g, Shi Chang Pu 6–10g]

Modifications:
Insomnia + Yuan Zhi, Suan Zao Ren

Phlegm Dampness Obstructing the Orifices

Primary symptoms: Deranged speech, muttering to oneself, slow reactions, mental-emotional confusion or abstraction

Additional symptoms: Dizziness and vertigo, nausea and vomiting, chest and abdominal oppression and fullness, profuse phlegm

Tongue: Swollen, fat tongue, slimy white coat

Pulse: Slippery, wiry (bowstring)

Treatment principles: Transform phlegm and dry dampness, open the orifices and quiet the Shen

Acupuncture treatment: ST-40, CV-12, ST-36, SP-9, CV-23, HT-5

Herbal treatment:
Dao Tan Tang (Guide Out Phlegm Decoction)
[Ban Xia 10g, Tian Nan Xing 10g, Zhi Shi 6g, Bai Zhu 10g, Fu Ling 10g, Chen Pi 6g, Yuan Zhi 6–10g, Shi Chang Pu 6g, Gan Cao 3–6g, Sheng Jiang 3g]

Modifications:
With Spleen Qi deficiency + Dang Shen, Huang Qi
Simultaneous Heart deficiency with insomnia and palpitations + Suan Zao Ren, Wu Wei Zi, Bai Zi Ren, Dang Shen

Phlegm Fire Harassing Above

Primary symptoms: Deranged speech, muttering to oneself, slow reactions, mental-emotional confusion or abstraction

Additional symptoms: Dizziness and vertigo, nausea and vomiting, chest and abdominal oppression and fullness, profuse yellow phlegm, irritability or even irascibility

Tongue: Red tongue, slimy yellow coat

Pulse: Slippery, wiry (bowstring), rapid

Treatment principles: Transform phlegm and clear heat, open the orifices and quiet the Shen

Acupuncture treatment: ST-40, ST-41, LR-2, CV-17, CV-12, CV-23, HT-5, TW-8, GV-15

Herbal treatment:
Huang Lian Wen Dan Tang Jia Wei (Coptis Decoction to Warm the Gallbladder Plus Modifications)
[Huang Lian 3–6g, Huang Qin 10g, Shi Chang Pu 6g, Dan Nan Xing 3–6g, Ban Xia 10g, Chen Pi 6–10g, Fu Shen 12g, Zhi Shi 6g, Zhu Ru 6–10g, Gan Cao 3–6g, Da Zao 3–5pc]

Blood Stasis Obstructing Internally

Primary symptoms: Deranged speech, especially premenstrually or postpartum in females with either dysmenorrheal or abdominal pain and scanty lochia

Additional symptoms: Possible menstrual irregularity, dark dusky facial complexion, headache, spider nevi, hemangiomas, or varicosities

Tongue: Purple red or possible static spots or macules; engorged, tortuous sublingual veins

Pulse: Wiry (bowstring), choppy, or bound

Treatment principles: Quicken the Blood and transform stasis, open the orifices and quiet the Shen

Acupuncture treatment: SP-10, SP-6, LI-4, CV-23, HT-5, TW-8, GV-15

Herbal treatment:
Tao Hong Si Wu Tang Jia Wei (Four Substance Decoction with Safflower and Peach Pit Plus Modifications)
[Tao Ren 10g, Hong Hua 10g, Shu Di 12g, Dang Gui 10g, Chi Shao 10g, Chuan Xiong 10–15g, Yuan Zhi 6–10g, Shi Chang Pu 6g]

Modifications:
Simultaneous Qi deficiency + Huang Qi, Dang Shen

Clinical Notes

- Shanshangdien ("upper thunder point"), located on the lateral side of the neck level with the Adam's apple between the sternal and clavicular heads of the SCM slightly inferior to LI-18, and Xiashangdien ("lower thunder point"), found slightly superior to GB-30 in the buttock region at the posterior tip of an equilateral triangle drawn from the greater trochanter and the iliac crest as the anterior two points, are two points worthy of consideration. According to Dr. John Chen and Dr. Hua Long Zhang, these points are "two very potent points reserved for those patients who have partial to complete paralysis."[1]

- The combination of HT-4, HT-5, SP-5 may be considered for stuttering.

- Bleeding the points Jin Yin (EX-HN 12) and Yu Ye (EX-HN 13) located below the tongue is considered, and is usually accompanied by body points such as KI-6, HT-5, CV-12, and CV-23. To this end, Michael Greenwood states: "KI-6 and CV-23 are said to open the Yin Qiao and Ren Mai, both of which travel to the face. HT-5 opens the Luo channel of the Heart, which penetrates the Heart and goes to the root of the Tongue. CV-23 is needled 2 cun toward the root of the tongue, to bring Qi to the Tongue, while bleeding the sublingual veins is designed to mitigate Blood stagnation."[2]

Research Studies

- Acupuncture was found effective for the treatment of aphasia after a stroke as patients were found to regain the ability to communicate through speech and written language at a similar rate as drug therapy patients. A combination of acupuncture with drug therapy produced optimal positive patient outcomes. Acupuncture, as a standalone therapy, produced a 46 percent total effective rate and donepezfil (a cognition-enhancing drug) produced a 50 percent total effective rate. Significantly, the combination of acupuncture with donepezfil produced a 77 percent total effective rate. Points used: CV-23, GV-15, GV-20, GV-24, Extra Point Laoguan, HT-5, KI-1.[3]

---

1   Chen, J. and Zhang, H-L. Treatment of neurodegenerative disorder. Acupuncture.com. 1997. Web. www.acupuncture.com/Conditions/alzandparkinson.htm

2   Greenwood, M. How do you treat poststroke aphasia with acupuncture in your practice? *Medical Acupuncture.* 2014; 26(5): 298–301.

3   Greenwood, M. How do you treat poststroke aphasia with acupuncture in your practice? *Medical Acupuncture.* 2014; 26(5): 298–301.

- A 2003 study from the University of Hong Kong on the fMRI of acupuncture was carried out on 17 healthy males. The acupuncture points stimulated were TW-8 and GV-15, both of which were called "language-implicated acupoints." This may have been a reference to other research on the effect of these acupoints on the brain's language centers.[4]

4   Li, A-P., Xiao, W-M., Wang, Y-M., and Xiong, X-P. A follow up study on poststroke aphasia recovery using acupuncture and donepezfil. *Journal of New Medicine.* 2013; 44(12). Web. Retrieved at www.healthcmi.com/Acupuncture-Continuing-Education-News/1677-acupuncture-rivals-drug-therapy-for-aphasia-recovery-after-stroke

Chapter 36

Anxiousness

Anxiety is a mood disorder characterized by apprehension, uncertainty, and fear directly out of proportion to any known cause. It can often be elevated to attacks of intense panic associated with physiologic changes. For further details on treating fear and worry see Chapter 44 on emotional lability and the seven emotions. Additionally, symptoms such as fatigue, irritability, muscle tension, restlessness, decreased concentration, and changes in sleep patterns often accompany these feelings. Other terms that may be used to describe this include "anxiety neurosis," "anxiety disorder," or "anxiety reaction." "Panic disorder" or a panic attack would also fall into the more extreme end of this category.

When the fear comes on intensely and suddenly, it is referred to as a panic attack. Other common symptoms accompanying a panic attack include heart palpitations, shortness of breath, trembling, a feeling of choking or suffocation, chest pain, abdominal symptoms, dizziness, loss of sense of reality, fear of losing control or dying, chills, hot flashes, or a feeling of numbness/tingling. Panic disorder describes repeated panic attacks followed by concern over future attacks or changes in behavior related to the panic attack.

Because individuals who have sustained a brain injury may experience impaired information processing speeds, difficulty with problem solving, or decreased ability to concentrate effectively, they may have a feeling of being overwhelmed when faced with decision-making situations or situations in which many things are occurring simultaneously. For this reason, parties, community outings, heavy traffic, or similar environments can induce a significant level of anxiety. Additionally, an individual may have anxiety or fear over falling and sustaining a further injury as a result of chronic pain. Memory impairments can induce anxiety in situations where individuals may forget where they are, what they may have been doing, or even which people are around them such as caregivers or even family members.

The Department of Veteran Affairs system found that approximately 25 percent of all veterans following active duty in Iraq and Afghanistan received a mental health diagnosis and 11 percent were found to have a form of mood disorder. One study found panic disorders occurring in a TBI population at a rate of 9.2 percent over 7.5 years. In genotype testing, there was evidence to support the presence of apolipoprotein E epsilon

4 (APOE*E4) as a predisposing factor to the development of psychiatric disorders after a severe TBI. The interactions between genetic polymorphisms and environmental influences such as early psychosocial adversity (e.g. history of abuse), life stress, and limited support structures may increase risk of development of mood disorders. Glutamate, with its role in excitotoxic injury and maladaptive stress responses, also plays a role in mood regulation via the hippocampus and prefrontal cortex. Significantly, lower hippocampal volumes have been found in individuals who have sustained a brain injury and developed mood disorders compared to those with similar injuries but no alterations in mood.

Anxiety can result from the conditions surrounding an injury, specific brain regions affected, damage to the neurotransmitter system, or any/all of the above. Anxiety coupled with depression tends to be demonstrated in the right hemisphere, in contrast to depression only, which tends to be shown in the left hemisphere.

Etiology

Anxiety can be physiological and/or psychological. There may be a genetic tendency present. The physiologic factors involved stem from arousal of the autonomic nervous system in the manner of a "fight or flight" response to fearful inner impulses and emotions. This stress response results in the characteristic body sensations often seen in a person in a panic attack.

Psychologic factors are individual to one's experience, but usually some sort of emotional stress precedes anxiety. The emotional stress may be easily identifiable (such as the loss of a job or relationship), or may be subconscious and harder to uncover, such as when hidden inner emotional drives of neediness, sexuality, and aggression are kept from the patient's conscious mind by psychological defenses. When these troubles are brought up by a social or environmental event that extremely stimulates the individual, the feelings of anxiety can represent their fear of losing control of these repressed conflicts and, in turn, their actions.

Another reason for anxiety is a known or subconsciously hidden trauma that certain situations or events can trigger, reverting the patient to the traumatic event and setting up the resulting fight or flight response.

Signs and Symptoms

- Severity of worry exceeds what the situation warrants
- Restlessness
- Fatigue
- Difficulty concentrating
- Irritability
- Muscle tension
- Insomnia

Diagnosis

At least three of the above signs.

Differential Diagnosis
Medical Disorders

- Hyperthyroidism or hypothyroidism
- Other endocrinological disorders (hyperparathyroidism, adrenal tumor, etc.)
- Cardiac arrhythmias
- Seizure disorders
- Hypoglycemia

Effects of Substances

- Alcohol abuse or illicit substance intoxication or withdrawal
- Medication side effects

Psychiatric Disorders

- Panic disorder with or without agoraphobia
- Generalized anxiety disorder (GAD)
- Post-traumatic stress disorder (PTSD)
- Obsessive–compulsive disorder (OCD)
- Social phobia and specific phobias
- Schizophrenia and other psychotic disorders

Biomedical Approaches

- Benzodiazepines
- SSRIs
- Psychotherapy
- Peer support or family therapy
- Biofeedback

Chinese Medical Perspective: Anxiety and Thinking (Shan You Si)

A class of psychiatric disorders characterized by persisting or recurrent fear that may or may not be associated with a specific object or situation. Anxiety is often accompanied by physiologic changes and behavior similar to those caused by fear. Anxiety disorders are the most common class of psychiatric disorders.

Relevant TCM Diseases

Fright and Fear (Jing Kong), Fright Palpitations (Jing Ji), Fearful Throbbing (Zheng Chong)

Chinese Medical Etiology

In Chinese medicine this disease is believed to be caused primarily by habitual deficiency of the righteous Qi and recurrent stimulation of the emotions. These internally damage the three organ systems of the Heart, Liver, and Spleen. This results in irregularity of the function of the viscera and bowels, disturbance in the flow of Qi and Blood, and thus substantial depletion and detriment. Unfulfilled desires or damage due to anger may result in Liver Qi stagnation and overthinking, and too much worry and anxiety may directly damage the Heart and Spleen.

Pattern Differentiation
Heart Qi Vacuity and Blood Stasis

Primary symptoms: Sudden onset of tension, fear, and dread, tension stretching from GV-14 to the head, a feeling of doom and approaching death causing incessant moaning, restless sitting, crying and sighing

Additional symptoms: Rapid distressed breathing, heart jumping rapidly, chest oppression, suffocating feeling in the chest, palpitations, shortness of breath, listlessness of the essence spirit, insomnia, profuse dreams

Tongue: Dark pale tongue, white coat

Pulse: Fine, weak, possibly bound or regularly intermittent

Treatment principles: Boost the Qi and nourish the Heart, quicken the Blood, free the flow of the vessels

Acupuncture treatment: LR-3, SP-10, LI-4, HT-7, PC-6, ST-36, BL-15, BL-17

Herbal treatment:
Tian Wang Bu Xin Dan (Emperor of Heaven's Special Pill to Tonify the Heart) [Sheng Di Huang 30g, Wu Wei Zi 10g, Dang Gui 15g, Tian Men Dong 15g, Mai Men Dong 15g, Bai Zi Ren 15g, Suan Zao Ren 15g, Ren Shen 10g, Xuan Shen 10g, Fu Ling 10g, Dan Shen 10g, Jie Geng 10g]

Modifications:
Suffocating oppressive feeling in the chest, possibly piercing pain: + Yu Jin, Gui Zhi, Qian Cao
Tension, disquietude, Heart Qi floating upward: + Long Gu, Zhen Zhu Mu, Mu Li
Emotional lability, tension, agitation, easy anger, headache, and dizziness due to Liver depression leading to fire: + Chai Hu, Zhi Zi, Huang Qin or add Dan Zhi Xiao Yao Wan
Liver depression with Spleen Qi and Blood deficiency without stasis: Use Xiao Yao Wan Jia Wei

Dan Zhi Xiao Yao Wan
[Mu Dan Pi, Zhi Zi, Chai Hu, Dang Gui, Bai Shao, Bai Zhu, Fu Ling, Gan Cao]

Liver Depression–Phlegm Fire

Primary symptoms: Emotional depression, anxiety, worry, sorrow, tension, vexation and agitation, easy anger

Additional symptoms: Tendency to sighing, insomnia, profuse dreams, chest and diaphragmatic fullness and oppression, bilateral rib-side distension and pain, profuse thick phlegm

Tongue: Red tongue, slimy yellow coat

Pulse: Wiry (bowstring), slippery, rapid

Treatment principles: Course the Liver and resolve depression, transform phlegm, clear heat

Acupuncture treatment: LR-2, PC-5, LI-4, ST-40, CV-17, CV-12

Herbal treatment:
Chai Hu Shu Gan San He Xiao Xian Xiong Tang (Bupleurum Course the Liver Powder Plus Minor Decoction [for Pathogens] Stuck in the Chest)
[Chai Hu 10g, Chen Pi 10g, Bai Shao 15g, Zhi Ke 10g, Gan Cao 6g, Chuan Xiong 6g, Xiang Fu 6g, Huang Lian 6g, Ban Xia 10g, Gua Lou 30g]

Modifications:
Heart vexation and disquietude, constipation, short reddish urine + Da Huang, Zhi Zi, Huang Qin
Headache, dizziness, red complexion, red eyes, irritability + Long Dan Cao, Ze Xie, Ju Hua, Jiang Can
Severe phlegm turbidity + Chuan Bei Mu, Ban Xia, Bai Zhu
Splitting headache with red complexion, stiff neck + Nui Xi, Shi Jue Ming, Xia Ku Cao

Heart Qi Stagnation and Blood Stasis

Primary symptoms: Episodes of anxiety and worry that endure for a long time, tension, wanness and sallowness, fearful throbbing, impaired memory, fear and dread, shaking, trembling

Additional symptoms: Torpid stagnant affect, chest area oppression, abdominal burping and belching or hiccup, dark stagnant complexion, dark greenish circles around the eyes

Tongue: Dark red tongue or static spots or macules

Pulse: Deep, wiry (bowstring); or fine, choppy

Treatment principles: Quicken the Blood, move stagnation, settle the Heart, quiet the Shen

Acupuncture treatment: LR-3, LI-4, SP-10, HT-7, PC-6, CV-17, BL-15, Yintang

Herbal treatment:
Xue Fu Zhu Yu Tang Jia Jian (Drive Out Stasis in the Mansion of Blood Decoction Plus Modifications)
[Dan Shen 15g, Dang Gui 15g, Chuan Xiong 10g, Chi Shao 10g, Tao Ren 12g, Hong Hua 10g, Chai Hu 15g, Zhi Ke 12g, Xiang Fu 15g, Yu Jin 15g, Long Chi 15g, Yuan Zhi 10g, Hu Po 6g, Gan Cao 6g]

Modifications:
Heart vexation and chaos, chaotic Qi and heat within the chest, tension, anxiety and worry, insomnia, profuse dreams: Use Zhu Sha An Shen Wan
[Zhu Sha, Huang Lian, Dang Gui, Sheng Di Huang, Gan Cao]

Heart–Spleen Dual Deficiency

Primary symptoms: Fear and dread, worry and anxiety, fright palpitations, insomnia, profuse dreams, impaired memory

Additional symptoms: Fatigue, lassitude of the spirit, lack of strength in the four limbs, scanty eating, loose stools, cold hands and feet, pale, somber, or sallow complexion, pale lips and nails

Tongue: Pale

Pulse: Fine, weak

Treatment principles: Fortify the Spleen, supplement the Heart, nourish Blood, quiet the Shen

Acupuncture treatment: ST-36, HT-7, PC-6, SP-6, BL-15, BL-17, BL-20

Herbal treatment:
Gui Pi Tang (Restore the Spleen Decoction)
[Bai Zhu 10g, Fu Shen 12g, Huang Qi 15g, Dang Shen 10g, Gan Cao 6g, Dang Gui 10g, Long Yan Rou 12g, Suan Zao Ren 15g, Yuan Zhi 10g, Mu Xiang 6–10g]

Modifications:
Nourish the Heart, nourish the spirit more + Bai Zi Ren
Settle, still, and quiet the spirit more + Long Gu, Mu Li

Yin Deficiency–Fire Effulgence

Primary symptoms: Fear and dread, susceptibility to fright, vexation and agitation

Additional symptoms: Dizziness, tinnitus, insomnia, palpitations, tidal heat, possible night sweats, malar flush, 5-palm heat, insomnia, dry mouth and throat, low back and knee soreness and weakness, nocturia that is scanty and yellow

Tongue: Red tongue, scanty coat

Pulse: Fine, rapid; or surging, rapid, rootless

Treatment principles: Clear the Heart and nourish Yin, settle fright, settle the Shen

Acupuncture treatment: KI-3, KI-7, SP-6, HT-6, PC-5, GV-20, Yintang

Herbal treatment:
Huang Lian E Jiao Tang (Coptis and Ass Hide Gelatin Decoction)
[Huang Lian 6–8g, Huang Qin 6g, E Jiao 9g, Bai Shao 6g]

Modifications:
Dry throat + Xuan Shen Mai Men Dong
Heart vexation + Zhi Zi, Zhu Ye
Pronounced fright susceptibility + Zhen Zhu Mu, Mu Li
Scanty, dark urine + Deng Xin Cao, Tong Cao

Clinical Notes

- Intradermal needles or ear seeds may be helpful at ear Shenmen or PC-6 to allow for stimulation of these points between appointments. Patients may also find this personally empowering as they can press or massage these points in the event that anxious feelings arise to aid in subduing symptoms.

- L-Theanine, an active ingredient in green tea, and available as a supplement, can be quite useful for patients as well, as it can be taken either in a low dose daily for general anxiety or symptomatically as needed. In the occurrence of panic attacks higher doses can be taken to abate symptoms. The relative safety, positive benefits on the brain (see Chapter 48), and low occurrence of side effects makes this an appealing option.

Other Therapeutic Considerations
Somatic Considerations

- Meditation
- Qigong/Tai Qi Chuan
- Yoga
- Exercise

Orthomolecular Considerations

- L-Theranine
- Phosphorus
- Lithium
- B vitamin complex (50mg BID)
- Calcium (1000mg/day, taken at bedtime)
- Magnesium (500mg/day)
- A daily multivitamin and mineral supplement

Phytotherapeutic Considerations

- Kava Kava (250mg TID for daytime anxiety)
- Valerian (150mg TID for daytime anxiety; for severe: 1 drop valerian oil to bath water)
- Ashwaganda (1 capsule or half a teaspoon of tincture BID)
- Bugleweed
- California poppy
- Catnip
- Chamomile
- Fennel
- Feverfew
- Ginkgo biloba
- Ginseng
- Hops
- Lemon balm
- Oats
- Passion flower
- Peppermint
- St. John's wort
- Skullcap
- Verben

Dietary Considerations

Maintain an overall healthy diet. Use fresh foods as close to the natural state as possible, avoiding prepackaged and processed foods. Eat daily servings of leafy green vegetables, whole grains (such as brown rice and millet), fresh fruit, and proteins with a minimum of animal fat. Drink at least eight cups of fluids daily.

Therapeutic foods:

- Increase foods that calm the Shen (Spirit), tonify the Heart, harmonize the Stomach and Spleen, clear Heat, and invigorate the Liver Qi
- Longan, oyster, rice, rosemary, wheat, wheat germ, mushroom
- Oatmeal
- Foods high in B-complex vitamins, oysters, celery, sesame seeds, tahini, calming foods, oatstraw juice and oats, collards, kelp, cherry, cucumber, corn, grapes, chicory, apples, kale, honey, mulberry, carrot

Avoid:

- Stimulants, especially those containing caffeine: coffee, chocolate, cola, black tea

- Foods with malic acids—most apples (apples without malic acid: Astrachan, Belleflower, Jonathan, Delicious); coffee, tea, fried foods, sugar and sweet foods

- Meat, alcohol, hot sauces, spicy foods, fatty foods, rich foods, salty foods, food additives, tobacco

Chapter 37

Depressive Disorders

Depression is considered a unipolar disorder characterized by mood disturbance, psychomotor dysfunction, and vegetative symptoms. It is classified as the uniform expression of the major affective disorders. Primary when it is the first mental disorder to appear in the patient, it is considered secondary when it appears with another psychiatric or medical condition. It may also be associated with aggressive behavior.

Reported prevalence of depressive disorders following a brain injury range from 6 percent up to 77 percent depending on the study and the data pool. Long-term studies indicate 44 percent of individuals with TBI were at a much higher risk of depression within 7.5 years of an injury. Severe injuries have shown lower rates of depression than more mild injuries. This seems to point to levels of self-awareness of symptoms playing a direct role in reports. Major depressive disorder is significantly associated with a comorbid anxiety disorder, with one study showing a 76.7 percent positive comorbidity. The compounding effect of depression with anxiety present tends to drastically prolong the duration of the depression, with one study showing that non-anxious depressive episodes had a median duration of 1.5 months, whereas an anxious depression had a median duration of 7.5 months. Apathy is also a common comorbidity.

Major depression has been shown to occur in lesions of the left dorsolateral frontal lobe, and/or left basal ganglia. Right hemisphere and parieto-occipital injuries demonstrated symptoms to a lesser degree. Diffuse axonal damage holds the possibility of progressing over weeks or months to impact vulnerable regions such as the neocortex, hippocampus, amygdala, thalamus, and striatum. Drevets argues that major depression could result from the deactivation of more lateral and dorsal frontal brain regions while an increase in activation of the ventral limbic and paralimbic structures, including the amygdala, occurs.[1]

---

1   Drevets, W., Price, J., and Furey, M. Brain structural and functional abnormalities in mood disorders: implications for neurocircuitry models of depression. *Brain Structure and Function.* 2008; 213(1–2): 93–118. doi:10.1007/s00429-008-0189-x

Cognitive abnormalities found in individuals with TBI remain consistent with left lateral prefrontal dysfunction. In athletes who have experienced a concussion and presented with depression there was a consistent finding of lowered activation of the dorsolateral prefrontal cortex and striatum as well as local gray matter loss.

A brain injury can affect neuromodulating systems, which can in turn affect mood. Depletion of serotonergic neurotransmission has been associated with affective disturbances, disinhibition, and aggressive behavior, and may play a role in depressive disorders. Alterations in dopamine transmission are associated with apathetic symptomology as well as impacting executive and memory functions. Brain injury can significantly impact the forebrain cholinergic system as well. Deficits in this system have been associated with behavioral changes including lack of motivation, agitation, disinhibition, and anhedonia.

Other factors such as social difficulties, job dissatisfaction, a low economic status, less education, or lack of personal relationships can increase the prevalence or severity of depressive states.

Etiology

Genetics

- Impaired limbic–diencephalon function
- Subcortical extrapyramidal structures and prefrontal connections

- Acetylcholine
- Norepinephrine, dopamine
- Serotonin

Physiologic

- Chronic pain or illness
- Chronic stress
- Hypoglycemia
- Hormonal imbalances

- Nutritional deficiencies (vitamin B6, B12, iron, thiamin, vitamin C)
- Aspartic acid excess
- Asparagine excess

Drug and Alcohol Abuse, Drug Reactions

- Steroids
- Digitalis
- Oral contraceptives

- Blood pressure medications
- Appetite suppressants
- Aspirin

Environmental

- Heavy metal exposure
- Industrial solvent exposure
- Toxin exposure

Personality

- Introversion
- Anxiety

Signs and Symptoms

- Depressed, irritable, anxious feelings
- Furrowed brows, slumped posture
- Monosyllabic speech
- Guilt
- Difficulty concentrating
- Recurrent thoughts of death and suicide
- Loss of interest
- Social withdrawal
- Helplessness, hopelessness
- Indecisiveness
- Inability to experience emotions
- Sleep disorders

Diagnosis

- Depressed mood
- Apathy/loss of interest
- Weight/appetite change
- Sleep disturbances
- Psychomotor change
- Guilt/worthlessness
- Cognitive dysfunction
- Suicidal ideation
- Hair analysis for heavy metals
- Norepinephrine imbalance: Motivation, energy, interest, concentration affected
- Serotonin imbalance: Impulsivity, change in sexual activity, appetite changes

Differential Diagnosis

- Adjustment disorder with depressed mood
- Frontal lobe syndrome
- Apathy
- Emotional lability
- PTSD

Melancholia/Anhedonia

- Endogenous depression
- Psychomotor slowing or agitation
- Anorexia, weight loss
- Guilt
- Loss of pleasure
- Insomnia

- Decreased libido
- Psychotic subtype in ~15 percent
- Delusions of having committed unpardonable crimes
- Accusatory hallucinatory voices
- Feelings of insecurity and worthlessness—persecution

Biomedical Approaches

- SSRIs
- Heterocyclic antidepressants

- 5-HT antagonists
- Psychotherapy

Chinese Medical Perspective: Depression Patterns (Yu Zheng)

"Yu" refers to any obstruction resulting from stagnation, stasis, accumulation, and retention. The broad concept of Yu Zheng encompasses clinical manifestations caused by stagnation of Qi, Blood, phlegm, fire, dampness, and food arising from internal organ dysfunction or from invasion by exogenous pathogenic influences. Clinical manifestations include melancholy, moodiness, despondence, depression, anxiety, irritability, or bouts of crying.

The Chinese term Dian, translated as withdrawal, refers to a torpid, flat, depressed affect with a tendency to taciturnity, uncommunicativeness, and solitariness. It may also include incoherent speech, a lowering of mental faculties, and even syncope and coma.

Relevant Biomedical Conditions

Depression, hysteria, schizophrenia, psychoneurosis, bipolar mood disorder, psychogenic psychosis, personality disorder, somatoform disorders, some hormonal and adolescent disorders

Chinese Medical Etiology

The Chinese medical understanding of the pathogenesis of depression emphasizes the Liver. The 18th-century text *Za Bing Yuan Xi Zhu* (Wondrous Lantern Peering into the Origin and Development of Miscellaneous Diseases) states, "All depression can be classified as a Liver disease." The Qing dynasty text *Zheng Zhi Hui Bu* (Complete Collection of Patterns and Treatments) states, "In all the many cases of depression, their cause is Qi which is not regulated or coursing. Treatment must first normalize the flow of Qi." Therefore, patients with depression tend to exhibit signs and symptoms of Liver Qi stagnation regardless of what other disease mechanisms are also at work.

An individual's prenatal (pre-heaven) disposition can also be an etiological factor. This dynamic establishes the constitutional state of the Shen, making it prone to injury. The status of the Shen is established by the prenatal condition. This causes to the Shen to be prone to injury or disharmonies at birth. A post-natal situation can be found in an individual's emotional disharmony. Strong constant emotional movement or emotion stimulants can negatively affect an unprepared Shen.

Early-stage: Emotional stress such as frustration, anger, and depression may cause Liver Qi stagnation. Qi is the motive force of metabolism. In a condition of prolonged Qi stagnation, other pathologies of Blood stasis, accumulation of dampness or phlegm, or food stagnation may arise. Over time these pathogenic factors may result in the accumulation of heat, creating fire conditions, and even further stagnation.

Later stage: Relatively more deficient. Constrained Liver Qi inhibits the Spleen's function, resulting in insufficient generation of Qi and Blood and malnourishment of the Heart Spirit. Deficiency of Heart Blood and Yin will lead to Kidney Yin deficiency with empty fire.

Pattern Differentiation
Stagnation of Liver Qi

Primary symptoms: Depression, mood swings, restlessness, chest, epigastric, abdominal, and hypochondriac distension and pain

Additional symptoms: Sighing, illogical speech, pain and distension relieved by belching and/or passing gas, dull affect, suicidal thoughts or self-injury, reduced appetite, menstrual irregularities

Tongue: Thin white or thin greasy coating

Pulse: Wiry (bowstring), slippery

Treatment principles: Soothe Liver, regulate Qi, relieve depression

Acupuncture treatment: [GV-20, GV-24] + BL-18, LR-3, PC-6, HT-7, ST-36, SP-4, CV-12, CV-17

Herbal treatment: Chai Hu Shu Gan San (Bupleurum Liver-Coursing Powder) [Chai Hu 6g, Bai Shao Yao 9g, Xiang Fu Zi 6g, Chuan Xiong 6g, Chen Pi 6g, Zhi Ke 6g, Zhi Gan Cao 3g]

Modifications:
Extreme depression, transformed heat, bitter taste, extreme anger, red tongue, rapid pulse: + Huang Qin, Huang Lian
With Spleen deficiency: Use Xiao Yao San Jia Jian (Augmented Rambling Powder)

Qi Stagnation turning into Fire

Primary symptoms: Easily agitated and irritable, hypochondriac distension and pain, chest oppression

Additional symptoms: Headache, red eyes, tinnitus, acid regurgitation, dry mouth, bitter taste in mouth, constipation, stomach upset, delirium, incoherent speech, uncontrolled behavior, delusions and hallucinations, insomnia, more active and goes outside, prefers cold drinks, dark-colored urine

Tongue: Red tongue, thin yellow coating

Pulse: Wiry (bowstring), rapid

Treatment principles: Clear Liver, drain fire, calm Stomach, regulate Qi, relieve depression

Acupuncture treatment: [GV-20, GV-24] + GB-34, GB-43, LR-3, LR-2, TW-6, PC-7, CV-13. Bleed LR-1

Herbal treatment: Dan Zhi Xiao Yao San (Moutan and Gardenia Free Wanderer Powder) + Zuo Jin Wan (Left Metal Pills)
[Chai Hu 9g, Bai Shao 12g, Dang Gui 9g, Bai Zhu 9g, Fu Ling 9g, Mu Dan Pi 9g, Shan Zhi Zi 9g, Zhi Gan Cao 6g, Sheng Jiang 3g, Bo He 3g]

Modifications:
Significant Stomach heat: voracious appetite, acid regurgitation, epigastric pain + Wu Zhu Yu 3g, Huang Lian 18g
Shen unsettled + Long Chi, Mu Li, Da Huang

Obstruction of Static Qi and Phlegm

Primary symptoms: Emotional depression, flat affect, plum-pit sensation in the throat that cannot be expectorated or swallowed

Additional symptoms: Chest and hypochondriac distension, costal pain, loss of appetite, paranoia, lots of worries, nonsensical speech, muttering to oneself, tendency to sigh, no thought for food or drink, tendency toward profuse phlegm, fibrocystic breasts in females

Tongue: White tongue, greasy or slippery coating

Pulse: Wiry (bowstring), slippery

Treatment principles: Regulate Qi to relieve constraint, resolve phlegm, relieve depression

Acupuncture treatment: [GV-20, GV-24] + CV-12, CV-17, CV-22, GV-26, HT-7, ST-40, LR-3, LR-14, PC-6

Herbal treatment:
Ban Xia Hou Po Tang (Pinellia and Magnolia Bark Decoction)
[Fa Ban Xia 12g, Hou Po 9g, Fu Ling 12g, Sheng Jiang 9g, Zi Su Ye 6g]
Shi Si Wei Wen Dan Tang (Ten Ingredient Decoction to Warm the Gallbladder)
[Ci Shi 12g, Zhi Shi Ying 12g, Tian Ma 10g, Chen Pi 10g, Ban Xia 12g, Dan Nan Xing 10g, Yuan Zhi 10g, Bai Zhu 10g, Fu Ling 12g, Shi Chang Pu 15g, Zhi Shi 10g, Zhu Ru 10g, Gan Cao 5g, Deng Xin Cao 1.5–3g]

Modifications:
With Spleen deficiency with fatigue, lassitude: + Dang Shen, increase Zhi Gan Cao
Lack of heat disturbing Heart: − Deng Xin Cao

Phlegm Dampness Obstruction

Primary symptoms: Depressed feelings, difficulty thinking, inattentiveness, a dull, flat affect

Additional symptoms: Slow movements, fatigue, lack of strength, cowering, solitariness, possible visual and auditory hallucinations, torpid food intake, heart vexation, insomnia

Tongue: Swollen with teeth marks on edges, slippery white coat

Pulse: Slippery or deep, slightly slow

Treatment principles: Warm Yang and fortify the Spleen, transform phlegm and open the orifices

Acupuncture treatment: [GV-20, GV-24] + CV-17, CV-12, PC-6, HT-7, ST-36, ST-40, BL-20, BL-21

Herbal treatment: Xiang Sha Liu Jun Zi Tang (Six Gentlemen Decoction Plus Aucklandia and Amomum) + He Li Zhong Tang Jia Wei (Regulate the Middle Pill Plus Modifications)
[Dang Shen 12g, Bai Zhu 10g, Fu Ling 20g, Gan Cao 10g, Mu Xiang 6g, Sha Ren 6g, Sheng Jiang 10g, Gan Jiang 10g, Chen Pi 10g, Ban Xia 10g, Cang Zhu 10g, Yuan Zhi 6g, Shi Chang Pu 10g, Huo Xiang 10g, Pei Lan 10g]

Modifications:
Pronounced Spleen deficiency with fatigue, lack of strength: + Huang Qi, Sheng Ma

Spleen deficiency affecting Kidneys with low back pain, excessive, frequent (possibly turbid) urination, and/or excessive white vaginal discharge: + Shan Yao, Bia Bian Dou

Blood Stasis Obstructing Internally

Primary symptoms: Emotional lability, irritability, suppressed anger, piercing lancinating headache

Additional symptoms: Speaking to oneself, torpid spirit, paranoia, delusional thinking, auditory and visual hallucinations, no desire, poor motivation, menstrual pain with dark clots, dark stagnant facial complexion, possibly painful areas of body

Tongue: Dark red with static macules or spots, possibly engorged tortuous sublingual veins

Pulse: Wiry (bowstring), choppy

Treatment principles: Rectify the Qi and resolve depression, quicken the Blood and transform stasis

Acupuncture treatment: [GV-20, GV-24] + BL-17, SP-10, LR-3, LR-8, BL-18

Herbal treatment: Xue Fu Zu Yu Tang Jia Wei (Drive out Stasis in the Mansion of Blood Decoction Plus Modifications)
[Tao Ren 10g, Hong Hua 10g, Dang Gui 10g, Sheng Di 10g, Chuan Xiong 6g, Chi Shao 6g, Jie Geng 5g, Chuan Niu Xi 10g, Chai Hu 3g, Zhi Ke 6g, Gan Cao 6g, Shui Zhi 6g]

Modifications:
Scanty speech and movement, lusterless complexion, fatigue and exhaustion + Huang Qi, Dang Gui

Yin and Blood Deficiency (Restless Organ Disorder)

Primary symptoms: Depression, hysteria, abnormal and unregulated emotional responses, mood swings, suspiciousness, trance-like mental state

Additional symptoms: Restlessness, disorientation, deafness, aphonia, convulsions, chest oppression, loss of consciousness

Tongue: Pale tongue, thin white coating

Pulse: Wiry (bowstring), thready

Treatment principles: Nourish the Heart, quiet the Shen, relieve depression

Acupuncture treatment: [GV-20, GV-24] + HT-7, SP-6, ST-36, LI-4, CV-14, PC-6

Herbal treatment: Gan Mai Da Zao Tang (Licorice, Wheat, and Jujube Decoction)
[Gan Cao 9g, Fu Xiao Mai 30g, Da Zao 10pc]

Heart and Spleen Dual Deficiency (Qi and Blood)

Primary symptoms: Pensiveness, palpitations, poor memory, confusion, insomnia, epigastric fullness and discomfort

Additional symptoms: Loss of appetite, loose stool, pale complexion, fatigue, excessive thinking, worry and anxiety, easily embarrassed, dreams frequently of ghosts, delusions and hallucinations, nonsensical speech, easily frightened, a predilection to sorrow and a desire to cry, flattened emotion, prefers staying alone

Tongue: Pale

Pulse: Weak, thready

Treatment principles: Tonify Spleen, nourish Heart, relieve depression

Acupuncture treatment: [GV-20, GV-24] + HT-7, ST-36, SP-3, SP-6, SP-10, CV-12, BL-15, BL-20, BL-43

Herbal treatment: Gui Pi Tang (Spleen-Returning Decoction)
[Huang Qi 9g, Ren Shen 9g, Bai Zhu 9g, Fu Shen 9g, Long Yan Rou 9g, Suan Zao Ren 9g, Mu Xiang 6g, Dang Gui 6g, Yuan Zhi 3g, Zhi Gan Cao 6g, Shang Jiang 3g, Da Zao 5pc]

Spleen–Kidney Yang Deficiency

Primary symptoms: Advanced age, bodily weakness, difficulty thinking, poor memory

Additional symptoms: Prefers staying alone, sluggishness, tiredness, inattentiveness, cowering, scanty speech, monologue, laughing by oneself, no thought for food and drink, diarrhea, bodily deficiency and lack of strength, lusterless facial complexion, fear of cold, chilled extremities

Tongue: Pale tongue, thin white coat

Pulse: Deep, fine, weak

Treatment principles: Warm and supplement the Spleen and Kidneys assisted by transforming phlegm and opening the orifices

Acupuncture treatment: [GV-20, GV-24] + BL-20, BL-21, BL-23, GV-4, SP-3, SP-6, KI-3, KI-7, CV-6, Yintang

Herbal treatment: Bu Gu Zhi Wan Jia Jian (Psoralea Decoction Plus Modifications)
[Huang Qi 15g, Dang Shen 12g, Bu Gu Zhi 12g, Rou Cong Rong 12g, Ba Ji

Tian 12g, Gan Cao 6g, Fu Ling 12g, Yuan Zhi 10g, Dang Gui 10g, Chuan Xiong 10g, Bai Zi Ren 12g, Suan Zao Ren 12g, Wu Wei Zi 10g, Rou Gui 6g]

Modifications:
With Blood stasis + Dan Pi, Yu Jin

Heart and Kidney Disharmony

Primary symptoms: Easily angered and irritable, dizziness, tinnitus, palpitations, insomnia

Additional symptoms: Weak and sore low back and knees, menstrual irregularities, nocturnal emissions

Tongue: Red tongue, scanty coating

Pulse: Thready, rapid

Treatment principles: Nourish Yin, clear heat, sedate the Heart, calm the spirit, relieve depression

Acupuncture treatment: [GV-20, GV-24] + HT-7, HT-5, BL-15, BL-23, KI-3, SP-6, CV-17, PC-6

Herbal treatment: Tian Wang Bu Xin Dan (Celestial Emperor Heart-Supplementing Elixir)
[Sheng Di Huang 30g, Tian Men Dong 12g, Mai Men Dong 12g, Suan Zao Ren 12g, Dang Gui 9g, Dan Shen 9g, Xuan Shen 9g, Ren Shen 6g, Fu Ling 6g, Wu Wei Zi 6g, Yuan Zhi 6g, Jie Geng 6g, Bai Zi Ren 12g]

Clinical Notes

- Electrical acupuncture has been found in clinical studies to be effective for the treatment of depression: Connect leads to GV-20 and GV-24 **or** GV-20 and Yin Tang. Set at 2 Hz continuous frequency; if anxiety is present with depression, set at 2/100 Hz mixed frequency

- May also consider internal/external dragon treatments

Other Therapeutic Considerations
Somatic Therapy Considerations

- Exercise is of tremendous benefit in improving one's mental health. At least 30 minutes three times per week should be engaged in physical exercise that will get the heart working vigorously such as brisk walking, aerobics, and swimming

- Meditation

- Qigong, Tai Qi Chuan

- Light therapy

Orthomolecular Considerations

- B vitamins (particularly B12)
- Amino acids
- Tryptophan
- Tyrosine
- Phenylalanine
- L-Theanine
- DHEA
- SAMe
- 5-HTP
- Magnesium
- Lithium
- Selenium
- Omega-3

Herbal Considerations

- St. John's wort (300mg TID)
- Kava-Kava (400–600mg BID)
- Lemon balm leaves (1 to 2 cups of tea per day for 1 to 2 weeks)
- Valerian
- Ginkgo biloba
- Licorice
- Siberian ginseng
- Damiana
- Basil
- Black hellebore
- Borage
- Clove
- Ginger
- Oat straw purslane
- Rosemary
- Sage
- Thyme
- Yohimbine
- He Shou Wu (Fo Ti)
- Culver's root
- Cayenne pepper (a quarter teaspoon TID; encapsulation may improve compliance)

Dietary Considerations
Eating Principles

- Consider food sensitivities

- Consume enough high-quality protein. Replace red meat with fish and chicken as much as possible and include beans, nuts, and seeds

- Hypoglycemic diet

- Treat hypothyroidism if present: Low thyroid function is a very common cause of depression

- Chelate heavy metals if present

- Avoid toxic fumes including cigarette smoke. Inhaling toxic fumes results in an increased level of cortisol and may exacerbate a pre-existing hypoglycemia. Cortisol decreases the uptake of tryptophan in the brain, resulting in decreased levels of serotonin

- Elimination/rotation diet, rotation diet, rotation diet expanded

Therapeutic Foods

- Foods high in omega-3 fatty acids: nuts, seeds, vegetable oils (safflower, canola, walnut, sunflower, flax seed), evening primrose oil, black currant oil

- Foods rich in vitamin B6

- Foods high in tryptophan: nuts, eggs, meat, fish, dairy

- If supplementing with tryptophan: include cofactors (vitamins B3, B6, and C) and wholewheat toast, bananas, walnuts, and pineapples that are high in serotonin

Specific Foods

Stagnant Liver Qi or stagnancy in the Liver channel:

- Foods that invigorate the Qi, Liver foods, sour foods, dispersing foods, foods that open channels

- Citrus peel, figs, honey

- Liver-cleansing foods: beets, carrots, artichokes, lemons, parsnips, dandelion greens, watercress, burdock root

Avoid:

- Hypoglycemia

- Foods containing tyramine if the patient is on MAO inhibitors. Cheese, chicken, liver, sardines, red wine, yeast, beer, soured cream, eggplant, and green bean pods should all be avoided

- Aspartame, which increases CNS tyrosine and phenylalanine while decreasing tryptophan availability—this results in decreased levels of serotonin in the brain

- Food intolerances; consider food sensitivities

- Meat, alcohol, hot sauces, spicy foods, fried foods, fatty foods, rich foods, salty foods

- Coffee, caffeine

- Sugar; diet high in simple carbohydrates, especially if indications of hypoglycemia

Research Studies

- A multi-centered collaborative study was conducted in which 241 inpatients with depression were recruited. Patients were randomly divided into two treatment groups: electro-acupuncture (EA) + placebo and an amitriptyline group. The results showed that the therapeutic efficacy of EA was equal to that of amitriptyline for depressive disorders (P > 0.05). Electro-acupuncture had a better therapeutic effect for anxiety somatization and cognitive process disturbance of depressed patients than amitriptyline (P < 0.05). Moreover, the side effects of EA were much less than those of amitriptyline (P < 0.001).[2]

- A meta-analysis of post-stroke depression reviewed 15 studies of 1096 patients. Comparison between the acupuncture group and Western medicine group concluded that there was a statistical difference in curative rate and remarkably effective rate, but no difference in effective rate.[3]

- Researchers from Jinan University (Guangzhou, China) conclude that acupuncture is effective for the alleviation of depression. In the study, the acupuncture treatment group achieved a total efficacy rate of 88.9 percent and the drug control group achieved an efficacy rate of 84.8 percent. Patients in the control group received administration of the pharmaceutical medication fluoxetine (Prozac). The researchers conclude that acupuncture slightly outperforms fluoxetine for the treatment of depression. In addition, acupuncture treatment displays certain advantages compared with antidepressant drugs. Acupuncture achieved a higher cure rate and the drugs had a significant adverse reaction rate.[4]

- After being exposed to a chronic unpredicted stress procedure for two weeks, rats were subjected to electro-acupuncture (EA) treatment, which was performed on acupoints GV-20 and GB-34, once every other day for 15 consecutive days (including eight treatments), with each treatment lasting for 30 minutes. The behavioral tests (i.e. forced swimming test, elevated plus maze test, and open-field entries test) revealed that EA alleviated the depressive-like and anxiety-like

2   Luo, H., Meng, F., Jia, Y., and Zhao, X. Clinical research on the therapeutic effect of the electro-acupuncture treatment in patients with depression. *Psychiatry and Clinical Neurosciences.* 1998; 52: S338–S340. doi:10.1111/j.1440-1819.1998.tb03262.x

3   Zhang, G-C., Fu, W-B., Xu, N-G., *et al.* Meta analysis of the curative effect of acupuncture on post-stroke depression. *Journal of Traditional Chinese Medicine.* 2012; 32(1): 6–11. http://dx.doi.org/10.1016/S0254-6272(12)60024-7

4   Bo, W. and Yi, X. Clinical observations on acupuncture treatment for depression. *Journal of Jinan University (Natural Science and Medicine Edition).* 2013; 34(6).

behaviors of the stressed rats. Immunohistochemical results showed that proliferative cells (BrdU-positive) in the EA group were significantly larger in number compared with the model group. Further, the results showed that EA significantly promoted the proliferation of amplifying neural progenitors (ANPs) and simultaneously inhibited the apoptosis of quiescent neural progenitors (QNPs).[5]

5   Yang, L., Yue, N., Zhua, X., *et al.* Electroacupuncture promotes proliferation of amplifying neural progenitors and preserves quiescent neural progenitors from apoptosis to alleviate depressive-like and anxiety-like behaviours. *Evidence-Based Complementary and Alternative Medicine.* 2014; 2014: 13 pages. Article ID 872568. http://dx.doi.org/10.1155/2014/872568

Chapter 38

Mania

A manic episode is indicated when an individual has a markedly elevated, expansive, or irritable mood for at least one week along with at least three of the following symptoms:

- Extremely amplified self-esteem
- Decreased desire for sleep
- Grandiose ideation

- Distractibility
- High-risk behaviors

Individuals may experience:

- Hyperactivity
- Distractibility, flightiness of ideas
- Hypersexuality, disinhibited sexuality
- Tangentality
- Delusions, usually of grandeur
- Confabulation

- Indiscriminate financial activity or irresponsibility
- Decreased need for sleep
- Pressured speech
- Emotional lability
- Increased aggression

While laughing and joking one moment, individuals may quickly become irritated, angered, enraged, destructive, or conversely tearful and depressed with slight provocation. That is, manic-depressive symptoms can occur, with mania predominating. Hence, bipolar affective disturbances may be due to waxing and waning abnormalities involving the right and left frontal lobes.

Relation to Brain Injury

It has been hypothesized that mania may relate to temporal basal polar lesions and multifocal lesions. This seems to be a more significant factor than the severity of the injury or other factors such as family history or social factors. When the right orbital and/or right lateral convexity are damaged by injury, tumor, or seizures, behavior often becomes inappropriate, labile, and disinhibited. Symptomatically, increased aggression with a lessened degree of euphoria may point to mania as a result of a brain injury compared to that stemming from other causes.

Differential Diagnosis

- Substance-induced mood disorder
- Psychosis associated with epilepsy
- Personality change as a result of brain injury

Biomedical Treatment

Lithium carbonate

Anticonvulsants

- Carbamazepine (Tegretol)
- Valproate (Depakote)
- Lamotrigine (Lamictal)
- Topiramate (Topamax)
- Clonazepam (Klonopin)

Antipsychotics

- Olanzapine (Zyprexa)
- Quetiapine (Seroquel)
- Risperidone (Risperdal)
- Aripiprazole (Abilify)
- Verapamil (calcium channel blocker)
- Benzodiazepines (short course)
- Psychotherapy

Chinese Medical Perspective: Mania (Kuang)

Withdrawal and mania, Dian and Kuang, are a Yin–Yang pair of conditions which can either exist separately or alternate back and forth between the two. Mania refers to an agitated, excited affect accompanied by inappropriate anger and/or laughing, mental, physical, and emotional restlessness, etc.

Relevant Western Diseases

Manic disorder, a manic episode in bipolar mood disorder, schizophrenia, delirium, psychoneurosis, psychogenic psychosis, and personality disorder

Diagnosis

- History of preliminary emotional or Shen injury

- Acute onset can create Shen confusion like irritability, delirium, hyperactivity, uncontrolled behavior, busy mind, and improper emotional expression

- No history of febrile disease or summer heat attack

- X-ray and CT scan exams have negative results; peripheral blood and spinal cord fluid exams are normal

Chinese Medical Etiology

In the early stage, Kuang syndrome is almost always due to fire or heat from the Liver, Heart, or Stomach and the clinical symptoms are very pronounced. In the late stage, the Yin energy and Blood become exhausted and cause a deficient condition. Some sources say that Blood stasis may also cause mania—in this case, heat has damaged the Blood to the degree that it has become static.

Pattern Differentiation
Liver Depression Transforming Fire

Primary symptoms: Emotional tension, agitation, irritability, easy anger, bouts of explosive, possibly violent anger

Additional symptoms: Chest, breast, rib-side, and abdominal distension and pain, menstrual irregularity and PMS, bitter taste in mouth, possible constipation, headache

Tongue: Red tongue; red or swollen tongue edges; thin, yellow, possibly slightly dry coat

Pulse: Wiry (bowstring), rapid

Treatment principles: Course the Liver and resolve depression, downbear fire and quiet the spirit

Acupuncture treatment: LR-2, GB-43, PC-8, PC-7, GV-14, PC-5

Herbal treatment:
Long Dan Xie Gan Tang Jia Jian (Gentiana Decoction to Drain the Liver)
[Long Dan Cao 6–10g, Chai Hu 6g, Huang Qin 10g, Huang Lian 3–4.5g, Bai Shao 10g, Zhi Zi 10g, Dan Pi 10g, Sheng Di 12g, Dang Gui 10g, Ze Xie 10g, Che Qian Zi 10g, Gan Cao 3g]

Modifications:
Heart palpitations and insomnia + Long Gu, Mu Li

Phlegm Fire Harassing Above

Primary symptoms: Impetuosity, rashness and impatience, breaking things and injuring other people, cursing and foul speech

Additional symptoms: Angry look in the eyes, red facial complexion, red eyes, bound constipated stools

Tongue: Red tongue, slippery yellow coat

Pulse: Wiry (bowstring), large, slippery, rapid

Treatment principles: Settle the Heart and flush phlegm, clear the Liver and drain fire

Acupuncture treatment: GV-14, GV-26, PC-6, PC-8, ST-40, LR-3

Herbal treatment:

Da Huang Huang Lian Xie Xin Tang Jia Wei (Drain the Epigastrium Decoction with Rhubarb and Coptis Plus Modifications)
[Da Huang 15g, Huang Qin 15g, Huang Lian 10g, Zhi Mu 15g, Zhi Zi 12g, Yu Jin 12g, Ban Xia 12g, Dan Nan Xing 10g, Tian Zhu Huang 10g, Shi Chang Pu 10g]

Yangming Heat Binding

Primary symptoms: Mania, agitation, improper emotional expression, non-stop laughing, excess self-esteem, boasting or talking big, deranged speech, singing aloud, climbing to high places, very creative at making up songs or forming ideas, frequent changing of ideas, illusions or hallucinations

Additional symptoms: Red facial complexion, body feels very hot like fire burning, tendency to strip off one's clothes, running around, more activity, no eating for days, thirsty and drinking cold water, recalcitrant constipation with dry bound stools, scanty reddish urine

Tongue: Red or purple tongue, thick and dry yellow or gray coat

Pulse: Deep, rapid, forceful

Treatment principles: Clear and drain the Yangming, calm the Shen, and quiet agitation

Acupuncture treatment: LI-4, LI-11, ST-40, ST-44, TW-6, GV-14, HT-5, PC-7, PC-8. Bleed: LU-11, LI-1, ST-45

Herbal treatment:

Da Cheng Qi Tang Jia Wei (Major Order the Qi Decoction Plus Modifications)
[Da Huang 15g, Huang Qin 12g, Mang Xiao 10g, Huo Po 15g, Zhi Shi 12g, Zhi Zi 12g, Lian Qiao 12g, Bo He 6g, Gan Cao 6g]

Modifications:
Thirst with desire to drink + Shi Gao, Zhi Mu

Heart and Kidney Not Communicating

Primary symptoms: Enduring, long-standing mania which is not too severe, laughing but less power than before, Shen irritability

Additional symptoms: Hoarse voice, lack of strength for activity and talking but keeps going at the same pace, vexation and agitation, insomnia, excessive speech, susceptibility to fear, 5-palm heat, afternoon tidal heat, dry mouth, constipation, scanty and dark urination, possibly malar flushing, possibly night sweats

Tongue: Red tongue; scanty, possibly yellow coat ("may be like mirror")

Pulse: Fine, wiry (bowstring), rapid; or deep, thready, rapid

Treatment principles: Supplement the Kidneys and nourish the Liver, downbear fire and quiet the Shen

Acupuncture treatment: SP-6, KI-2, KI-3, KI-6, LR-3, HT-7, GV-24, An Mian, Tai Yang, Si Shen Cong

Modifications:
Night sweats + HT-6
Heart palpitations + PC-6

Herbal treatment:
Er Yin Jian Jia Jian (Two Yin Tonic Plus Modifications)
[Sheng Di 12–15g, Mai Dong 15g, Xuan Shen 15g, Suan Zao Ren 12g, Fu Shen 12g, Huang Lian 6–10g, Mu Tong 10g, Deng Xin Cao 10g, Zhu Ye 10g, Dang Shen 12g, Shi Chag Pu 6g]

Blood Stasis and Heat Mutually Binding

Primary symptoms: Emotional lability, agitation, speaking to oneself, delusional thinking, auditory and visual hallucinations

Additional symptoms: Dark stagnant facial complexion, piercing lancinating headache

Tongue: Dark red with static macules or spots, possibly engorged, tortuous sublingual veins, and/or dryish, yellow coat

Pulse: Wiry (bowstring), rapid, possibly skipping

Treatment principles: Quicken the Blood and transform stasis

Acupuncture treatment: SP-10, SP-6, LI-4, LI-11, ST-25, GV-14

Herbal treatment:

Qin Lian Si Wu Tang Jia Wei (Four Substance Decoction with Scutellaria and Coptis Plus Modifications)

[Tao Ren 12g, Hong Hua 10g, Dang Gui 10g, Sheng Di 10g, Chuan Xiong 6g, Ci Shao 6g, Jie Geng 5g, Chuan Niu Xi 10g, Huang Lian 3–6g, Huang Qin 10–12g, Chai Hu 3g, Zhi Ke 6g, Gan Cao 6g, Shui Zhi 6g]

Modifications:

With constipation + Da Huang, Mang Xiao

Excitation and restlessness with agitated stirring + Dan Pi, Sheng Di

Restless sleep and depression, oppression, and discomfort + He Huan Pi, Ye Jiao

Classical Treatments

Diankuang caused by the one hundred pathologic factors: 13 Ghost Points—Sun Simiao

Kuang—one jumps and runs: CV-13, HT-7

Attack of Kuang: HT-3, PC-5, LI-11, SI-3, GB-1, KI-7

Hyperexcitation: ST-45, ST-42

Sudden hyperexcitation, hallucinations, violent sweats: PC-5

Attacks of hyperexcitation: HT-3, BL-43, CV-14, LR-8, CV-13, HT-7

Overexcitation from emotional agitation: GB-35, BL-18

Prolonged hyperexcitation, climbs up, sings, takes off clothes, runs: ST-45, ST-42, ST-40

Hyperexcitation becomes apoplexy (stroke): GB-39

Auricular Points

Shenmen, Point Zero, Sympathetic, Heart, Liver, Apex

Clinical Notes

- Patients exhibiting manic symptoms may have difficulty lying still long enough to perform a full body treatment. They may be verbose and flighty in both mind and bodily movements. It is possible that they may even remove needles that have been inserted, wanting to move and finding the increased sensation irritating. Auricular points may be helpful in an attempt to calm them quickly and possibly allow for a fuller treatment. Yintang or bleeding ear apex may also be helpful in this regard. Ear seeds may be helpful between treatments if the patient can keep them in.

- Massage at KI-1 may also be considered to help ground the patient and promote an inward and downward movement of Qi.

Chapter 39

Bipolar Disorder

Bipolar affective disorder (BAD) is characterized by mood disturbance involving periods of abnormally elevated mood (mania) and abnormally lowered mood (depression), psychomotor dysfunction, and vegetative symptoms. It has been found to be present in approximately 5 percent of the population and affects genders equally, though females tend to have depressive forms predominant while males tend to have manic forms more prevalent. In 85 percent of cases, depression dominates the personality cycle.

Bipolar disorder is associated with an enhanced sensitivity to dopamine, increased production of norepinephrine, serotonin, and dopamine, and an upregulation of glutamate. As discussed in the chapter on anxiety disorders, each of these neurotransmitter channels can be affected by a brain injury. Due to the heightened dopamine sensitivity, bipolar has additionally been linked to schizophrenic disorders.

Associations with increased white matter hyperintensities which tend to occur in demyelination, glial cell inflammation, brain ischemia-linked axonal loss, or aging brains have been noted. The prefrontal cortex and hippocampus have been demonstrated to have a 25–40 percent reduction in gray matter volume in individuals with BAD. Cerebellar atrophic changes may also occur which can stifle communication between limbic and cortex regions. There has also been an associated reduction of glucose and blood flow use. Decreased lymphocyte beta receptor functioning has also been found in depression and mania, but findings were inconclusive about whether this was a direct correlation or the result of a homeostatic regulation of peripheral beta receptors as a stress-induced increase.

Subtypes:

- Bipolar I—one or more manic episodes with a preceding hypomanic stage

- Bipolar II—one or more depressive episodes followed by one or more hypomanic episodes without full mania

- Cyclothymic disorder—chronic fluctuating mood disturbance with both depressive and hypomanic states

Etiology

- Brain injury
- Genetics
- Stressors
- Personality—extroverted, achievement oriented

Signs and Symptoms

- Twenty percent with unipolar develop bipolar within five years of onset of depression
- Sudden onset
- More psychomotor vegetation
- Depressive symptoms similar to unipolar depression
- Shorter cycles than unipolar depression—three to six months
- Hypersomnia
- A quick response to treatment for unipolar depression may be an indicator of unmanifested bipolar

Signs of Manic Psychosis

- Elation
- Irritability
- Hostility
- Rapid speech
- Extreme activity
- Lack of insight
- Believe they are at their best
- Paranoid delusions
- Racing thoughts
- Distractible
- Delusional grandiosity
- Auditory and visual hallucinations
- Need less sleep
- Inexhaustible, impulsive, excessive

Diagnostic Testing

- Ultrasound of the head
- CAT scan
- EEG
- Full blood count
- Thyroid and liver function tests
- Urine and creatine levels assessment

Biomedical Treatment

Lithium carbonate 300mg 2–5x/day, 0.3–0.8 mEq/L maintenance

Many side effects: tremor, muscle spasms, nausea, vomiting, diarrhea, thirst, polydipsia, polyuria, acne, psoriasis, hypothyroidism, nephrogenic diabetes, confusion, seizures, arrhythmia. Flaxseed oil helps decrease side effects (1–3 tbsp/day)

Anticonvulsants

- Carbamazepine (Tegretol)
- Valproate (Depakote)
- Lamotrigine (Lamictal)
- Topiramate (Topamax)

Antipsychotics

- Olanzapine (Zyprexa)
- Benzodiazepines (short course)
- Psychotherapy

Differential Diagnosis

Medical Disorders

- Endocrinologic diseases including thyroid and adrenal dysfunction
- Cancer
- Infectious diseases including HIV, hepatitis, and others
- Neurologic diseases including epilepsy and tumors

Effects of Substances

- Alcohol abuse or illicit substances
- Medication side effects

Psychiatric Disorders

- Major depressive episode
- Cyclothymic disorder
- Schizoaffective disorder
- Schizophrenia and other psychotic disorders
- Borderline personality disorder (and other personality disorders)

Possible Comorbidities

- Head trauma
- Substance abuse
- PTSD and obsessive compulsive disorder
- Eating disorders

Chinese Medical Approach: Mania and Withdrawal/Dian Kuang

Dian Kuang is a severe psychological condition characterized by extreme fluctuations between depressive psychosis and manic psychosis that are usually episodic and recurrent. Clinically, mania and withdrawal are not distinct disease entities; they are two aspects of one disorder and their clinical manifestations may be interchangeable.

Withdrawal/Dian is a form of depressive psychosis caused by Qi stagnation complicated by phlegm misting the Heart orifice; it is characterized by depression, apathy, incoherent speech, dementia, and subdued and non-violent behavior.

Mania/Kuang is caused by phlegm-fire harassing the Heart and is characterized by mental hyperactivity and manic behavior, manifesting with shouting, hostility, and violent behavior.

Relevant Biomedical Conditions

- Bipolar affective disorder (BAD)
- Schizophrenia
- Major depression
- Senile dementia
- Alzheimer's disease
- Brain tumor

Chinese Medical Etiology

Internal engenderment of (depressed) Qi, fire, phlegm, and stasis tend to be key elements. This disease tends to be located in the Heart, Liver, Spleen, and Kidneys. It can be divided into Yin and Yang, deficiency and excess. Most cases of this condition are considered due to a great fright, excessive stimulation by the seven emotions, and the five spirits (Wu Shen) transforming fire. This leads to fire exuberance and phlegm congestion, with Qi and Blood counterflow harassing and causing disruption of the Shen. This then results in mania. In terms of the depression pole of bipolar, worrying and thinking may become depressed, bound, and not able to extend themselves. An individual may have accumulated frustrated anger that has not been properly discharged. In either case, the Qi may become depressed and the Blood static, congealing and clouding the Shen.

Pattern Differentiation: Manic State
Liver Depression–Blood Heat Pattern

Primary symptoms: High spirits, tension, agitation, easy anger, difficulty thinking, rushing about, intrusiveness

Additional symptoms: Bilateral rib-side distension and pain, insomnia, profuse dreams, bitter taste, dry mouth

Tongue: Crimson tongue, scanty coat

Pulse: Wiry (bowstring), rapid

Treatment principles: Course the Liver and drain heat, resolve depression, quiet the Shen

Acupuncture treatment: LR-2, LI-4, LI-11, SP-10, HT-7, GB-20, GV-20

Herbal treatment:
Chai Hu Qing Gan Yin (Bupleurum Decoction to Clear the Liver)
[Chai Hu 10g, Zhi Zi 10g, Mu Dan Pi 15g, Su Geng 10g, Bai Shao 10g, Gou Teng 15g. Added later]

Liver Depression–Phlegm Fire Pattern

Primary symptoms: Emotional tension and agitation, excited, impetuous behavior

Additional symptoms: Bitter taste, raving, bilateral rib-side distension and pain, insomnia, profuse dreams, dizziness, headache, spitting yellow phlegm

Tongue: Red tongue, slimy yellow coat

Pulse: Wiry (bowstring), slippery, rapid

Treatment principles: Course the Liver and resolve depression, transform phlegm, drain fire

Acupuncture treatment: LR-2, ST-40, CV-12, CV-17, HT-7, PC-8, GB-20, GV-20. Strong stimulation

Herbal treatment:
Qing Qi Hua Tan Tang He Gun Tan Wan (Clear the Qi and Transform Phlegm Pill + Phlegm Expelling Pill)
Qing Qi Hua Tan Tang: [Chen Pi 10g, Xing Ren 10g, Zhi Shi 10g, Huang Qin 15g, Gua Lou 15g, Fu Ling 15g, Dan Nan Xing 15g, Ban Xia 12g]
Gun Tan Wan: [Meng Shi 9g, Da Huang 9g, Huang Qin 9g, Chen Xiang 1.5g]

Modifications:
Rash and impetuous and uncontrolled manic behavior: + Tie Luo, Ci Shi, Dai Zhe Shi
Constipation with yellowish red urine: + Da Huang, Mang Xiao
Headache and dizziness: + Ju Hua, Gou Teng, Bai Ji Li

Qi Stagnation and Blood Stasis

Primary symptoms: Emotional lability, changes in disease nature

Additional symptoms: Sometimes agitated and impulsive, manic speech, predilection to unstable anger, constant crying, laughing, singing, and swearing no matter who is present, dream-like confusion, aggression such as throwing of objects, chest-region fullness and oppression, piercing lancinating headache, red bloodshot eyes

Tongue: Dark purplish tongue, possible static macules or engorged sublingual veins

Pulse: Wiry (bowstring), choppy, possibly deep

Treatment principles: Quicken the Blood and transform stasis, rectify the Qi, resolve depression

Acupuncture treatment: LR-3, LI-4, SP-10, BL-15, BL-17, BL-18, GB-20, GV-20. Draining technique

Herbal treatment:
Dian Kuang Meng Xing Tang (From the Bad Dream of Psychosis Awakening Decoction)
[Tao Ren 24g, Chai Hu 10g, Chi Shao 20g, Mu Tong 10g, Da Fu Pi 10g, Che Pi 10g, Sang Bai Pi 10g, Xiang Fu 6g, Ban Xia 6g, Qing Pi 6g, Zi Su Zi 12g, Gan Cao 15g]

Modifications:
Excitation and restlessness: + Mu Dan Pi, Sheng Di Huang, Di Long
Insomnia and disquieted sleep: + Ku Shen, Ye Jiao Teng
Raving speech, hasty breathing, red complexion, bad breath, constipation: + Da Huang, Huang Lian
Rash, impetuous behavior and inability to control oneself: + Meng Shi, Chen Xiang
Severe psycho-emotional excitation: + Tie Luo, Meng Shi, Zhi Mu
Significant phlegm: + Wen Dan Tang (Gallbladder Warming Decoction)

Excessive Fire Injuring Yin

Primary symptoms: Prolonged manic psychosis, emotional instability, irritability, anxiety

Additional symptoms: Insomnia, fatigue, sometimes stillness, sometimes agitation, illogical speech, excessive speaking, easily frightened, panic attacks, palpitations, scanty and dark urine, 5-palm heat

Tongue: Red tongue, scanty or no coating

Pulse: Rapid, thready, wiry (bowstring)

Treatment principles: Nourish Yin, clear fire, quiet the Shen, stabilize emotions

Acupuncture treatment: [GV-24, GB-13, PC-4, PC-5] + KI-1, KI-3, LV-3, SP-6, HT-7, PC-6, GB-20, GV-20

Herbal treatment:

Er Yin Jian (Two Yin Brew)

[Sheng Di Huang 30g, Mai Men Dong 15g, Xuan Shen 15g, Huang Lian 10g, Mu Tong 10g, Zhu Ye 10g, Fu Shen 15g, Deng Xin Cao 5g, Suan Zao Ren 15g, Gan Cao 6g]

Modifications:

Excitation and restlessness: + Qian Jin Ding Zhi Wan

Heart vexation, chest oppression, sometimes aggravation, sometimes depression: + Chai Hu, Bai Shao, Xuan Fu Hua

Heart vexation, insomnia, excessive fear, long-standing susceptibility to fright without ceasing: + Dan Shen, Hu Po

Phlegm-Fire Disturbing the Heart

Primary symptoms: Acute onset with symptoms of manic and aggressive/destructive behavior, red eyes and face, insomnia, complete loss of appetite

Additional symptoms: Agitated, irritable, distending headache prior to episode, increased thirst with preference for cold drinks, dry mouth and throat, constipation

Tongue: Red tongue, yellow greasy coating

Pulse: Rapid, wiry (bowstring), slippery

Treatment principles: Purge fire, resolve phlegm, settle the Heart, drain Liver, stop mania

Acupuncture treatment: [GV-24, GB-13, PC-4, PC-5] + GV-14, GV-16, GV-26, LI-4, PC-6, PC-8, ST-40, LR-3

Herbal treatment:

Meng Shi Gun Tan Wan (Chlorite-Mica Phlegm-Shifting Pill) + Sheng Tie Luo Yin (Iron Flakes Beverage)

[Meng Shi, Da Huang, Huang Qin, Chen Xiang, Mang Xiao] +

[Tian Men Dong 9g, Mai Men Dong 9g, Zhe Bei Mu 9g, Dan Nan Xing 3g, Ju Hong 3g, Yuan Zhi 3g, Shi Chang Pu 3g, Lian Qiao 3g, Fu Ling 3g, Fu Shen 3g, Xuan Shen 4.5g, Dan Shen 4.5g, Gou Teng 4.5g]

Pattern Differentiation: Depressive State

Liver Qi Depression and Binding

Primary symptoms: Low spirits, many worries, susceptibility to anxiety, sorrow, hopelessness

Additional symptoms: Decreased movement, slowed reactions, rib-side distension and pain, abdominal distension, scanty eating, loose stools which are not crisp

Tongue: Pale

Pulse: Wiry (bowstring), slightly slow

Treatment principles: Course the Liver and resolve depression, rectify the Qi, harmonize the center

Acupuncture treatment: [GV-24, GB-13, PC-4, PC-5] + LR-3, LI-4, ST-36, CV-12, CV-14, CV-17

Modifications:
If phlegm: + ST-40

Herbal treatment:
Chai Hu Shu Gan Tang (Bupleurum Decoction for Spreading Liver Qi)
[Chai Hu 10g, Xiang Fu 10g, Zhi Ke 10g, Chen Pi 7g, Chuan Xiong 5g, Bai Shao 10g, Gan Cao 6g]

Modifications:
Qi depression is severe: + Yu Jin, Qing Pi
Five depressions complicating food, dampness, phlegm, blood, fire: + Yue Ju Wan
Sorrow, desire to commit suicide, muddled confused intelligence: + Su He Xiang Wan
Spleen and Blood deficiency more pronounced: Use Xiao Yao San
Spleen deficiency and/or Stomach disharmony are pronounced with depressive Lung heat and Stomach phlegm damp: Use Xiao Chai Hu Tang

Liver Blood Stasis and Stagnation

Primary symptoms: Emotional depression, suicidal thoughts/behavior, vexation and agitation, difficulty thinking, slowness making connections in the mind

Additional symptoms: Slow movement, a dark, dusky facial complexion, bilateral rib-side pain, blocked menstruation

Tongue: Dark-purplish tongue, possible static spots

Pulse: Wiry (bowstring), choppy

Treatment principles: Quicken the Blood and transform stasis, rectify the Qi, resolve depression

Acupuncture treatment: LR-3, LI-4, SP-10, SP-6, HT-7, PC-6, CV-17, CV-6. Mostly draining technique

Herbal treatment:
Xue Fu Zhu Yu Tang (Drive Out Stasis in the Mansion of Blood Decoction)
[Tao Ren 12g, Hong Hua 10g, Dang Gui 10g, Sheng Di Huang 10g, Chuan Xiong 6g, Chi Shao 6g, Jie Geng 5g, Chuan Niu Xi 10g, Chai Hu 3g, Zhi Ke 6g, Gan Cao 3g]

Modifications:
Heavy Qi depression with suicidal thoughts and behavior + Tao Hua, Yu Jin, Shi Chang Pu
Severe Blood stasis + Jiang Xiang, Chuan Shan Jia, Su Mu

Heart–Spleen Deficiency

Primary symptoms: Chronic depression, trance-like mental state, lack of interest, lack of contact with reality, self-blame, self-reproach

Additional symptoms: Decreased activity, excessive thinking/worry, timidity and fearfulness, incoherent speech, insomnia, impaired memory, fatigue, exhaustion, pale white or sallow yellow complexion, scanty eating, palpitations, loose stools

Tongue: Pale enlarged tongue, tooth marks, white coat

Pulse: Fine, weak

Treatment principles: Fortify the Spleen and nourish the Heart, boost Qi, supplement Blood

Acupuncture treatment: [GV-24, GB-13, PC-4, PC-5] + HT-7, SP-3, SP-6, ST-36, BL-15, BL-17, BL-20, CV-6

Herbal treatment:
Gui Pi Tang (Restore the Spleen Decoction)
[Ren Shen 9g, Huang Qi 9g, Bai Zhu 9g, Fu Ling/Shen 9g, Dang Shen 10g, Suan Zao Ren 9g, Long Yao Rou 9g, Ye Jiao Teng 6g, Mu Xiang 6g, Zhi Gan Cao 6g, Dang Gui 6g, Zhi Yuan Zhi 3g, Sheng Jiang 3g/5 slices, Da Zao 5pc]

Modifications:
Severe depression with poor sleep: + Yu Jin, Zhi Ke, He Huan Hua
Scanty eating with disinclination to speak: + Sha Ren, Chen Pi

Yang Xin Tang (Heart-Nourishing Decoction)
[Huang Qi 9g, Ren Shen 9g, Fu Ling 9g, Fu Shen 9g, Dang Gui 9g, Chuan

Xiong 6g, Zhi Ban Xia 6g, Bai Zi Ren 9g, Yuan Zhi 6g, Suan Zao Ren 15g, Wu Wei Zi 6g, Rou Gui 3g, Zhi Gan Cao 6g]

Spleen–Kidney Yang Deficiency Pattern

Primary symptoms: Essence spirit listlessness, low spirits, desire to stay lying down, scanty movement, diminished willpower, sorrow, ennui

Additional symptoms: Decreased sexual desire, impotence, seminal emission, clear/watery vaginal discharge and/or early menstruation, somber white complexion, cold limbs

Tongue: Pale puffy tongue, white coat, teeth marks

Pulse: Deep, fine

Treatment principles: Fortify the Spleen, boost Qi, warm Yang, supplement Kidneys

Acupuncture treatment: ST-36, CV-4, CV-6, BL-23, GV-4, BL-20, GV-20, moxa

Herbal treatment:
Wen Yang Xing Fen Tang (Warm the Yang and Excite Decoction)
[Dang Shen 15g, Shu Di Huang 15g, Xian Ling Pi 5g, Rou Cong Rong 15g, Gui Ban 15g, Fu Zi 10g, Huang Qi 10g, Gan Cao 10g, Rou Gui 6g, Gan Jiang 6g]

Modifications:
Devitalized spirit (scanty movement, short of breath, disinclination to speak, scanty eating): + Bai Zhu, Sheng Ma, Chen Pi, Mai Ya
Depression not resolved and decreased willpower: + Chai Hu, Yuan Zhi, Yu Jin, Zhi Ke
Slow and difficult thinking, slow, relaxed behavior, terminal urinary dribbling: + Tu Su Zi, Yi Zhi Ren, Wu Yao, Shi Chang Pu

Auricular points: Shenmen, Sympathetic, Point Zero, Heart, Liver

Clinical Notes

See Clinical Notes in Chapters 37 and 38 based on whether the patient is presenting with manic or depressive symptoms.

Other Therapeutic Considerations
Somatic Considerations

- Qigong
- Tai Qi Chuan

Orthomolecular Considerations

- EPA/DHA greatly stabilizes mood, stopping rapid mood cycling

- Lecithin (phosphatidylcholine) (15–30g) to prevent mania

- Vitamin C

- Vitamin E

- B vitamins

- L-Tryptophan is helpful in some studies, others not. High doses used—causes nausea

- 5-HTP has helped (50%) but can cause increase in serotonin-inducing mania—must be watched

- Multi-vitamin

Phytotherapeutic Considerations

- St. John's wort

- Skullcap

- Valerian

Dietary Considerations

Therapeutic foods:

- Increase foods that calm the Shen, tonify the Heart, and harmonize the Stomach and Spleen

- Increase foods rich in vitamin B-complex and vitamin C

- Longan, oyster, rice, rosemary, wheat, wheat germ, mushroom

- Stagnant Liver Qi or stagnancy in the Liver channel: Foods that invigorate the Qi, Liver foods, sour foods

- Dispersing foods, foods that open channels: Citrus peel, figs, honey

- Liver-cleansing foods: Beets, carrots, artichokes, lemons, parsnips, dandelion greens, watercress, burdock root

- Vitamin C foods

Avoid:

- Meat, alcohol, hot sauces, spicy foods, fried foods, fatty foods, rich foods, salty foods, coffee, caffeine, sweet foods and sugar

Chapter 40

Obsessive–Compulsive Disorder (OCD)

OCD is an anxiety disorder that is characterized by recurrent, ritualistic, unwanted, intrusive ideas, images, or impulses that seem weird, silly, nasty, or horrible (obsessions) with urges to do something that will lessen the discomfort of those obsessions (compulsions). In the general population, it affects approximately 1.6 percent of individuals within any six-month period. While not a widespread diagnosis following a brain injury, one study indicated an increased risk of 0.6 percent, with another showing rates as high as 15 percent. The subject warrants being covered as it can be a significant hindrance to one's navigation of life's demands and reintegration into society.

The most prominent symptoms following a brain injury seem to be behavioral repetition and obsessional symptoms. The increase in these activities may not lead to a formal diagnosis of obsessive–compulsive disorder.

The neurobiological basis of OCD stresses aberrant functioning of cortico–striatal–thalamic–cortical (CSTC) circuits. These circuits are distinct neural "loops," which originate from frontal cortical areas, pass through the basal ganglia (including the striatum) through either "direct" or "indirect" pathways, with a final projection through feedback projections to the thalamus. The "direct" and "indirect" basal ganglia pathways have, through glutamatergic and GABAergic neurotransmission, opposing actions on the thalamus that result in a disinhibition of thalamic activity. This increases both thalamic and frontal cortical activity and is theorized to be a contributing factor to OCD. Each is associated with either emotional, cognitive, or motor inputs. In individuals with OCD these circuits have been found to be hyperactive at rest and at times when symptoms are provoked. Treatment shows a normalization of this activity. Of particular note in OCD are circuits arising from the orbitofrontal cortex (OFC), the dorsolateral prefrontal cortex (DLPFC), and the anterior cingulate cortex (ACC). The OFC circuit acts in context-related processing and response inhibition. The DLPFC circuit is involved in working memory. The ACC circuit is responsible for emotional and reward processing. Over-activity of the orbitofrontal cortex, and its circuitry (the striatum) in particular, is believed to have a substantial role in the neurobiology of OCD.[1]

Signs and Symptoms

- Depression
- Repetitive, purposeful, intentional behaviors to balance obsessions: Washing, avoidance
- Psychotic disorders have loss of contact with reality

- Awareness that obsessions are not real and that compulsions are excessive (neurosis)
- Harm, risk, danger: Contamination, aggression, doubt

Differential Diagnosis
Medical Disorders

- CNS infection or injury
- Neurologic disorders, including Tourette's disorder, Parkinson's disease, and Huntington's disease

Other Tic Disorders

- History of cerebrovascular accident (CVA)

Psychiatric Disorders

- Obsessive–compulsive personality disorder
- Schizophrenia and other psychotic disorders

- Specific phobias
- Social phobias

Biomedical Approaches

- SSRIs
- Tryptophan
- Behavior therapy—structured cognitive–behavioral therapy

---

1   Vahabzadeh, A. and McDougle, C.J. Obsessive–Compulsive Disorder. In *Pathobiology of Human Disease*. Edited by Linda M. McManus and Richard N. Mitchell. San Diego, CA: Academic Press. 2014.

Chinese Medical Perspective

Relevant TCM Diseases

Vexation and agitation (Fan Zao), depression condition (Yu Zheng), impaired memory (Jian Wang), abject demeanor (Bie Die)

Chinese Medical Etiology

The Heart and Gallbladder's relationship to courage and, conversely, timidity can play a role in the development of symptoms akin to OCD. Also, the Gallbladder's relationship to decision making is a factor. If the Heart is overtaxed for an extended period of time, phlegm turbidity will accumulate and attack the Gallbladder. This will lead to Heart deficiency and Gallbladder timidity. The Heart is considered the sovereign organ which rules as emperor over the body-mind; when the Heart becomes deficient, one can no longer effectively control oneself. If the Gallbladder becomes weak, timidity develops and the ability to make decisions is lessened.

The second mechanism of this condition directly involves the Liver. If the emotions are repressed and depressed, disease will reach and affect the Liver. With Liver depression, the Qi eventually becomes stagnant. If this endures and is not resolved, then Qi stagnation will lead to Blood stasis involving the Gallbladder. This will inhibit and create aberrant decision making.

Pattern Differentiation

Heart–Gallbladder Qi Deficiency

Primary symptoms: Compulsive thoughts and actions, tension, worry and anxiety, inability to control oneself, easily frightened by touching things, fear and dread

Additional symptoms: Restlessness, susceptibility to excessive suspicion or paranoia, deficiency vexation, insomnia, dizziness or vertigo, possible profuse phlegm and/or plum pit Qi

Tongue: Pale tongue, white coat

Pulse: Fine or wiry (bowstring), fine

Treatment principles: Nourish the Heart and quiet the Shen, dry dampness, transform phlegm

Acupuncture treatment: HT-7, PC-6, ST-4, ST-36, CV-17, CV-12, GB-44

Herbal treatment:
Wen Dan Tang Jia Wei (Warm the Gallbladder Decoction Plus Modifications) [Ban Xia 15g, Zhu Ru 15g, Zhi Shi 10g, Chen Pi 10g, Sheg Jiang 10g, Gan

Cao 6g, Fu Shen 30g, Mai Men Dong 15g, Yuan Zhi 10g, Long Chi 21g, Shi Chang Pu 15g, Hu Po 6g]

Modifications:
Emotional tension and agitation, Heart vexation, easy anger + Chai Hu, Zhi Zi, Long Dan Cao
Stomach venter distension and oppression with torpid intake and scanty eating + Sha Ren, Mu Xiang, Ji Nei Jin
Insomnia and profuse dreams + Suan Zao Ren, He Huan Pi, Ye Jiao Teng
Compulsive reactive behavior and inability to control oneself + Ci Shi, Mu Li, Tian Men Dong

Qi and Blood Stasis and Stagnation

Primary symptoms: Compulsive behavior, inability to control one's thoughts, emotional lability, tension and agitation, stirring and fear

Additional symptoms: Dusky complexion, bilateral rib-side distension and pain or generalized body pain, piercing headache, insomnia, profuse dreams

Tongue: Pale tongue, white coat

Pulse: Fine or wiry (bowstring)

Treatment principles: Course the Liver and rectify the Qi, quicken the Blood, transform stasis

Acupuncture treatment: LR-3, LI-4, SP-10, HT-7, PC-6, BL-15, BL-17, GV-20, Yintang

Herbal treatment:
Xue Fu Zhu Yu Tang (Clear Stasis in the Mansion of Blood Decoction)
[Tao Ren 12g, Hong Hua 10g, Dang Gui 10g, Sheng Di Huang 10g, Chuan Xiong 6g, Chi Shao 10g, Niu Xi 10g, Jie Geng 6g, Chai Hu 3g, Zhi Ke 6g, Gan Cao 3g]

Modifications:
Compulsive reactive behavior, e.g compulsive handwashing + Gua Lou Gen, Gui Zhi, Bai Shao, Jiang Can
Obsessional thoughts and uncontrollable worries/anxieties + Shi Chang Pu, Tian Zhu Huang, Shi Xiang

Chapter 41

Schizophrenia

Schizophrenia is a severe disorder of thought characterized by distorted perceptions of reality, impaired reasoning, disorganized speech and behavior, and a lost capacity for the spontaneous experience of emotions. Delusional beliefs and auditory or visual hallucinations may also be present. Motivation is typically lacking with grossly impaired occupational and social functioning. Schizophrenics typically have a higher-than-chance occurrence of neurologic soft signs including diminished dexterity and increased blink reflex. Apraxia or inability to carry out tasks also tends to occur at a higher rate and is attributed to dysfunction of the right parietal lobe. Episodes are typically precluded by prodromes such as functional deterioration and atypical mood and behavior, delusions, and hallucinations.

The diagnosis of schizophrenia requires a course greater than six months. Shorter periods may be categorized as an associated psychotic disorder such as post-traumatic psychosis, schizophreniform disorder, brief psychotic disorder, delusional disorder, or schizoaffective disorder. One study proposed that the prevalence of schizophrenia following TBI increased by 2–5 times over the span of 10–20 years postinjury. Brain regions implicated in schizophrenia and post-traumatic psychosis such as the prefrontal cortex, temporal lobes, and hippocampus are ones which are particularly vulnerable to a TBI. Rates of psychosis following a brain injury vary from 0.7 percent to 9.8 percent. The degree of injury severity has been shown to have a significant impact on prevalence. A 10–15-year followup study of severe TBI found that 20 percent of individuals had developed psychosis. It is suggested that pediatric brain injury in particular may predispose to post-traumatic psychosis. Genetic predisposition and history of pre-morbid psychopathological disturbance play large roles in the likelihood of occurrence. Other neurological disorders such as prior injury to the brain, seizures, learning disabilities, birth complications, and ADD/ADHD also seem to be predisposing factors.

Neuro-psychological test data and functional brain-imaging studies reveal dysfunction in the temporal (40% of cases) and frontal lobes. These are the principal brain regions in language and executive functioning, including abstract reasoning. Injury to the left hemisphere appears to elicit a higher risk. Clinical similarities between schizophrenia and

TBI indicate orbitofrontal and dorsolateral prefrontal cortex and hippocampal pathology. Left temporal lobe involvement has been associated with delusions of passivity in which the individual feels as though they are being controlled or as if outside forces are acting upon them. It has also been speculated that the various symptoms of schizophrenia could result from disturbances in connectivity and disruption of cross talk among different regions of the brain. White matter deficits have been implicated with both positive and negative symptoms. A brain injury can impair an individual's ability to filter incoming sensory information, which is also a major characteristic of schizophrenia.

Etiology

- Genetic
- Prenatal and perinatal complications
- Viral CNS infections
- Maternal exposure to famine, influenza in second trimester of pregnancy
- Environmental stressors may trigger episodes

Signs and Symptoms
"Positive" Symptoms

- Excessive or distorted normal functions
- Delusions, hallucinations
- Bizarre behavior, thought disorder
- Movement disorders and agitated movements

"Negative" Symptoms

- Decrease or loss of normal functions
- Blunted affect
- Poverty of speech
- Anhedonia
- Asociality
- Negative symptoms are generally less common, if not entirely absent

Symptom clusters vary with schizophrenic subtypes. A summary of these subtypes is provided in Table 41.1.

TABLE 41.1 Symptom Patterns in Western Psychiatry

Paranoid subtype	Delusions or hallucinations, no disorganized or catatonic behavior
Disorganized subtype	Disorganized speech or behavior, inappropriate affect, no catatonic behavior
Catatonic subtype	Motoric immobility (including posturing) or excessive motor activity, extreme negativism, repeats words or actions of others
Undifferentiated subtype	Meets criteria of schizophrenia in general but no specific distinguishing symptoms
Residual subtype	Symptoms are present but in an undifferentiated form

Diagnosis

- Clinical
- Two or more signs for one month
- Social impairment for six months

Differential Diagnosis

See Table 41.2 for other psychotic disorders related to schizophrenia.

Medical Disorders

- CNS lesions including brain tumors
- Hyperthyroidism
- Systemic lupus erythematosus (SLE)
- Multiple sclerosis (MS)
- Delirium
- Dementia

Effects of Substances

- Alcohol or illicit substance intoxication or chronic use
- Side effects of certain medications including steroids, L-DOPA, others

TABLE 41.2 Psychotic Disorders Related to Schizophrenia

Schizophreniform disorder	Same symptom pattern as schizophrenia, symptoms last more than one month but less than six months
Brief psychotic disorder	Same symptom pattern as schizophrenia, symptoms last more than one day but less than one month
Delusional disorder	Non-bizarre delusions, symptoms last at least one month, never diagnosed schizophrenic
Schizoaffective disorder	Same symptom pattern as schizophrenia, in context of manic or depressive symptoms during the period of active psychosis
Substance-induced psychotic disorder	There is evidence that psychotic symptoms are due to the effects of a substance and the patient is not psychotic when not using that substance

Prognosis

Symptoms of schizophrenia may appear intermittently or continuously. Seventy percent of individuals will have subsequent episodes after the first episode, with symptoms worsening over the first five years, after which they reach a plateau. There is a 10 percent associated risk of suicide and an estimated decreased lifespan by ten years. There is also a moderate risk of violent behavior. Of affected individuals, approximately one-third improve while one-third become permanently incapacitated.

Biomedical Approaches
Antipsychotic Drugs

- Amisulpride (Solian)
- Olanzapine (Zyprexa)
- Resperidone (Resperdal)
- Clozapine (Clozaril)
- Quetiapine (Seroquel)
- Psychotherapy
- Support

Chinese Medical Perspective
Relevant TCM Diseases

> Withdrawal and mania (Dian Kuang), manic condition (Kuang Zheng), dementia (Chi Dai)

Chinese Medical Etiology

Causes of schizophrenia are considered closely related to the damage by the seven emotions and five minds (Wu Shen). Emotional stagnations may produce Qi depression, phlegm congelation, fire, Blood stasis, and other pathological changes which can cloud the Heart orifices and harass or cause chaos to the Shen, resulting in loss of psychological normalcy. The causes and mechanisms of schizophrenia may also be closely related to prenatal (pre-heaven) endowment and constitutional strength. If the righteous Qi exists internally and Yin is level (or calm) while Yang is activated, then psychological stimuli may cause psycho-emotional discomfort but will not cause disease. If one's constitution is habitually deficient, or if Yin or Yang are inclined in one direction or another, it may lead to the Shen easily being harassed.

Another important component in cases of schizophrenia is an increase in sensory input and one's ability to filter or process the incoming information. If the Earth phase is unable to take this input, process it, and transform it into digestible amounts, it will become overwhelming. This will create heat and fluid stagnation which develops into phlegm able to mist upward to cloud the mind.

Pattern Differentiation: Acute Episodes
Yang Disease Type

Primary symptoms: Excited, agitated stirring, visual hallucinations, delusions, difficulty thinking and disturbed, chaotic thoughts, odd, usually eccentric behavior

Additional symptoms: Form exuberant, body replete, red complexion and eyes, dry stools

Tongue: Red tongue, yellow coat

Pulse: Wiry (bowstring), rapid, forceful

Treatment principles: Drain fire, flush phlegm, quicken the Blood and dispel stasis, heavily settle and quiet the spirit

Acupuncture treatment: Alternate use of below with strong stimulation, draining technique.
CV-12, HT-7, SP-6
BL-15, BL-18, BL-20, ST-40

Herbal treatment:
Choose from the following as applicable.
Liver–Galbladder excess fire, psychomotor excitation prominent: Use Long Dan Xie Gan Tang
[Long Dan Cao 10–15g, Huang Qin 10g, Shan Zhi Zi 10g, Ze Xie 10g, Mu Tong 6g, Dang Gui 10g, Che Qian Zi 10g, Sheng Di Huang 10g, Chai Hu 6g, Gan Cao 6g]
Phlegm obstructing Heart orifices, turbid Qi clouding Heart: Use Di Dan Tang
[Fa Ban Xia 9g, Zhi Tian Nan Xing 6g, Chen Pi 9g, Zhi Shi 9g, Fu Ling 12g, Ren Shen 6g, Shi Chang Pu 9g, Zhu Ru 9g, Sheng Jiang 6g, Gan Cao 3g]

Blood stasis symptoms, excited, agitated stirring, delusions prominent: Use Dian Kuang Meng Xing Tang

[Tao Ren 24g, Chai Hu 10g, Chi Shao 20g, Mu Tong 10g, Da Fu Pi 10g, Che Pi 10g, Sang Bai Pi 10g, Xiang Fu 6g, Ban Xia 6g, Qing Pi 6g, Zi Su Zi 12g, Gan Cao 15g]

Phlegm fire harassing above, withdrawal and mania, agitation and mania prominent: Use Sheng Tie Luo Yin

[Tian Men Dong 9g, Mai Men Dong 9g, Zhe Bei Mu 9g, Dan Nan Xing 3g, Ju Hong 3g, Yuan Zhi 3g, Shi Chang Pu 3g, Lian Qiao 3g, Fu Ling 3g, Fu Shen 3g, Xuan Shen 4.5g, Dan Shen 4.5g, Gou Teng 4.5g]

Yin Disease Type

Primary symptoms: Flat affect, abnormally slow reactions, lack of will, difficulty thinking

Additional symptoms: Fatigued, body weak, Qi timidity, lassitude of the spirit, somber white complexion

Tongue: Pale

Pulse: Deep, fine

Treatment principles: Nourish the Blood and supplement the Heart, warm Yang and excite

Acupuncture treatment: Alternate use of the below treatments with an even technique.
GV-26, LU-11, SP-1, PC-7, ST-40
GV-16, GV-14, GV-12
CV-15, CV-13, CV-12, ST-40
GV-26, GV-16, PC-8, PC-7

Herbal treatment:
Choose from the following as applicable.
Qi and Blood deficiency, essence spirit listless: Use Yang Xin Tang
[Huang Qi 9g, Ren Shen 9g, Fu Ling 9g, Fu Shen 9g, Dang Gui 9g, Chuan Xiong 6g, Zhi Ban Xia 6g, Bai Zi Ren 9g, Yuan Zhi 6g, Suan Zao Ren 15g, Wu Wei Zi 6g, Rou Gui 3g, Zhi Gan Cao 6g]
Yang deficiency, chronic, simple, catatonic: Use Di Huang Yin Zi or Wen Yang Xing Fen Tang
[Dang Shen 15g, Shu Di Huang 15g, Xian Ling Pi 5g, Rou Cong Rong 15g, Gui Ban 15g, Fu Zi 10g, Huang Qi 10g, Gan Cao 10g, Rou Gui 6g, Gan Jiang 6g]

Pattern Differentiation: Remittent Stage

Liver Qi Depression

Primary symptoms: Emotional depression, dull affect, taciturnity, illogical speech, tendency to uncommon anger, suicidal thoughts, no desire to live, self-injury

Additional symptoms: Chest and rib-side fullness/oppression, tendency to sigh, no thought of food or drink, menstrual irregularity

Tongue: Dark tongue, thin white coat

Pulse: Wiry (bowstring)

Treatment principles: Drain and course the Liver and resolve depression

Acupuncture treatment: LR-3, PC-6, HT-7, LI-4, ST-36, CV-17

Herbal treatment:
Chai Hu Shu Gan San Jia Wei (Bupleurum Powder to Spread the Liver Plus Modifications)
[Chai Hu 12g, Xiang Fu 10g, Bai Shao 10g, Zhi Ke 10g, Chuan Xiong 6g, Yuan Zhi 10g, Su Geng 10g, Chen Xiang 6g, Gan Cao 3g]

Modifications:
Enduring or extreme depression transforming heat: + Huang Qin, Huang Lian
With Spleen-deficient loss of fortification: Use Xiao Yao San with additions and subtractions
Liver–Spleen disharmony with depressive heat: Use Dan Zhi Xiao Yao San or Xiao Chai Hu Tang

Phlegm Qi Depression and Binding

Primary symptoms: Emotional depression, a flat affect, paranoia, lots of worries, illogical speech, murmuring to oneself, laughing and crying without constancy

Additional symptoms: Tendency to sigh, chest and rib-side distension and fullness, no thought of food or drink, possible plum pit Qi, tendency toward profuse phlegm

Tongue: Slimy coat

Pulse: Wiry (bowstring), slippery

Treatment principles: Rectify the Qi and resolve depression, transform phlegm and open the orifices

Acupuncture treatment: GV-26, HT-7, PC-6, CV-12, ST-36, LR-2, ST-40

Herbal treatment:

> Shun Qi Dao Tan Tang He Kong Xian Dan Jia Jian (Rectify Qi and Eliminate Phlegm Decoction Plus Modifications)
> [Chen Pi 10g, Ban Xia 10g, Dan Nan Xing 10g, Fu Ling 15g, Xiang Fu 10g, Shi Chang Pu 15g, Mu Xiang 7g, Kuan Xian Dan 2–3 pills]

Modifications:

Chest and diaphragmatic fullness and oppression, profuse phlegm, drool in mouth: Use San Sheng San

Clouded Shen, dull affect, confused, chaotic speech: First use Su He Xiang Wan, then use Si Qi Tang + Dan Nan Xing, Yu Jin, Shi Chang Pu, Yuan Zhi

Qi depression transforming heat, insomnia, easy fright: Use Wen Dan Tang + Huang Lian combined with Bai Jin Wan

With spirit clouding and chaotic mind: Use Zhi Bao Dan

Phlegm Dampness Obstruction

Roughly corresponds to the simple type of schizophrenia.

Primary symptoms: Difficulty thinking, inattentiveness, a dull flat affect, slow movements, lack of strength, cowering, solitariness

Additional symptoms: Possible visual and auditory hallucinations, fatigue, torpid food intake, heart vexation, insomnia, laziness and passivity, lack of motivation, impaired social skills

Tongue: Swollen tongue with teeth marks, slimy white coat

Pulse: Slippery or deep, relaxed

Treatment principles: Warm Yang and fortify the Spleen, transform phlegm and open the orifices

Acupuncture treatment: GV-26, HT-7, PC-6, CV-12, SP-9, ST-36, ST-40, LR-2

Herbal treatment:

Xiang Sha Liu Jun Zi Tang He Li Zhong Tang Jia Wei (Six Gentlemen Decoction with Aucklandia and Amomum Plus Regulate the Middle Pill Plus Modifications)
[Dang Shen 12g, Bai Zhu 10g, Fu Ling 20g, Gan Cao 10g, Mu Xiang 6g, Sha Ren 6g, Sheng Jiang 10g, Gan Jiang 10g, Chen Pi 10g, Ban Xia 10g, Cang Zhu 10g, Yuan Zhi 6g, Shi Chang Pu 10g, Huo Xiang 10g, Pei Lan 10g]

Modifications:

Pronounced Spleen deficiency + Huang Qi, Sheng Ma

Kidney deficiency signs + Shan Yao, Bia Bian Dou

Phlegm Fire Harassing Upward

Roughly corresponds to the hebephrenic or disorganized type of schizophrenia.

Primary symptoms: Emotional tension and agitation, vivid hallucinations, childish or inappropriate behavior, excitable and compulsive behavior, breaking things and injuring other people, foul speech, disorganized thinking

Additional symptoms: Angry look in the eyes, red complexion, red eyes, bound constipated stools

Tongue: Red or crimson tongue, slimy yellow coat

Pulse: Wiry (bowstring), large, slippery, rapid

Treatment principles: Settle the Heart and flush phlegm, clear the Liver and drain fire

Acupuncture treatment: GV-14, GV-26, HT-5, PC-6, PC-8, ST-40, ST-43, ST-45, LR-2, LR-3

Herbal treatment:
Sheng Tie Luo Yin Jia Jian (Iron Filings Decoction Plus Modifications)
[Tie Luo 30–60g, Dan Nan Xing 10g, Bei Mu 12g, Ju Hong 12g, Shi Chang Pu 12g, Yuan Zhi 12g, Fu Shen 12g, Xuan Shen 12g, Tian Men Dong 12g, Mai Men Dong 12g, Lian Qiao 12g, Zhu Sha 1g]

Modifications:
Severe phlegm fire: + Meng Shi Shi Tan Wan
To clear Heart, open orifices: Can use An Gong Niu Huang Wan
Mainly Liver–Gallbladder fire: Use Dang Gui Long Hui Wan
Mainly Yangming heat: Use Da Cheng Qi Tang + Zao Jiao
Spirit mind clear but vexation, insomnia due to phlegm fire: Use Wen Dan Tang + Zhu Sha An Shen Wan

Heart–Spleen Dual Deficiency

Primary symptoms: Excessive thinking, worry and anxiety, dreaming of ghosts, confusion, heart palpitations, easily frightened, predilection to sorrow and a desire to cry, poor memory, difficulty thinking, sluggishness, illogical speech

Additional symptoms: Somber white complexion, fatigue, reduced food intake

Tongue: Pale

Pulse: Fine, forceless

Treatment principles: Fortify the Spleen and nourish the Heart, boost the Qi and quiet the spirit

Acupuncture treatment: BL-15, BL-20, PC-6, HT-7, ST-36

Herbal treatment:
Gui Pi Tang (Restore the Spleen Decoction)
[Dang Shen 12g, Bai Zhu 12g, Fu Shen 30g, Huang Qi 30g, Gan Cao 6g, Dang Gui 12g, Long Yan Rou 30g, Suan Zao Ren 30g, Yuan Zhi 6g, Mu Xiang 10g, Sheng Jiang 6g, Da Zao 6pc]

Modifications:
Excessive thinking, worry, anxiety, predilection to sorrow, fright, fear, restlessness, disturbed Heart spirit: Use Yang Xin Tang

Yang Deficiency Depletion

Roughly corresponds to chronic-type schizophrenia.

Primary symptoms: Advanced age, bodily weakness, or enduring disease that does not heal, resulting in Spleen disease reaching and damaging the Kidneys with difficulty thinking, sluggishness, inattention, cowering, scanty speech, and withdrawal

Additional symptoms: No thought for food or drink, bodily deficiency and lack of strength, lusterless complexion, fear of cold, chilled extremities

Tongue: Pale tongue, thin white coat

Pulse: Deep, fine, weak

Treatment principles: Warm and supplement the Spleen and Kidneys assisted by transforming phlegm and opening the orifices

Acupuncture treatment: BL-23, SP-4, GV-4, BL-20, BL-21, CV-4, CV-12, GV-20. Moxa

Herbal treatment:
Wen Yang Xi Fen Tang Jia Jian (Warm Yang and Excite Decoction Plus Modifications)
[Dang Shen 20g, Shu Di 15g, Fu Zi 10g, Rou Gui 10g, Rou Cong Rong 15g, Yin Yang Huo 15g, Gan Jiang 6g, Gui Ban 15g, Chen Pi 10g, Ba Xia 10g, Gan Cao 6g, Fu Ling 15g]

Modifications:
Severe phlegm blocking Heart orifices + Shi Chang Pu, Yuan Zhi
With Blood stasis + Dan Pi, Yu Jin
Pronounced Qi deficiency + Huang Qi, Shan Yao

Yin Deficiency with Deficiency Fire

Roughly corresponds to the catatonic type of schizophrenia.

Primary symptoms: Enduring manic disease gradually worsening, delusions and hallucinations, suspiciousness and hostility, fatigue, excessive speech, susceptibility to fright, emotional anxiety and tension, social withdrawal with feeling of loneliness, prolonged stupor

Additional symptoms: Occasional vexation, emaciated form, red complexion, 5-palm heat, dry mouth without desire to drink

Tongue: Red tongue, scanty or no coat

Pulse: Fine, rapid, possibly slippery

Treatment principles: Enrich Yin, downbear fire, quiet the Shen, and stabilize the mind

Acupuncture treatment: HT-7, PC-7, LR-3 → KI-1, SP-6, GV-24 → GV-23

Herbal treatment:
Er Yin Jian (Two Yin Pill)
[Sheng Di 30g, Mai Men Dong 12g, Xua Shen 12g, Fu Ling 12g, Suan Zao Ren 20g, Huang Lian 10g, Mu Tong 8g, Zhu Ye 12g, Deng Xin Cao 3g, Gan Cao 3g]

Modifications:
Dry stools + Huo Ma Ren, Yu Li Ren, Tao Ren
Dry mouth, torpid intake, no thought for food or drink + San Xian
Devitalized essence spirit with sluggish stirring + Tai Zi Ren, Huang Qi, Sheng Ma

Blood Stasis

Roughly corresponds to paranoid-type schizophrenia.

Primary symptoms: Emotional lability, sometimes agitated, sometimes still, speaking to oneself, torpid spirit, paranoia, delusional thinking, auditory and visual hallucinations, conflicting emotions

Additional symptoms: Dark stagnant complexion, loose association, piercing lancinating headache

Tongue: Dark red tongue, static macules or spots, possible engorged and tortuous sublingual veins

Pulse: Wiry (bowstring), choppy

Treatment principles: Rectify the Qi and resolve depression, quicken the Blood and transform stasis

Acupuncture treatment: HT-7, PC-6, SP-10, LI-4, BL-15, BL-17, BL-18, Ding Shen

Herbal treatment:

Xue Fu Zhu Yu Tang Jia Wei (Drive Out Stasis in the Mansion of Blood Decoction Plus Modifications)

[Tao Ren 12g, Hong Hua 10g, Dang Gui 10g, Sheng Di 10g, Chuan Xiong 6g, Chi Shao 6g, Jie Geng 5g, Chuan Niu Xi 10g, Chai Hu 3g, Zhi Ke 6g, Gan Cao 6g, Shui Zhi 6g]

Modifications:

Bitter taste in mouth, dry throat, short reddish urination, feeling of brewing heat internally + Mu Tong, Huang Qin

Excitation, restlessness, lack of calm + Dan Pi, Sheng Di

Restless sleep, depression, oppression, discomfort + He Huan Pi, Ye Jiao Teng

Scanty speech, scanty movement, lusterless complexion, fatigue + Huang Qi, Dang Gui

General Acupuncture Treatment

Primary acupuncture points

ST-40, SP-6, PC-5 → TW-6, CV-5, CV-13, GV-20 → Si Shen Cong, KI-1, BL-15, BL-18, BL-20, Ding Shen, HT-7, GB-20

Additional acupuncture points

GV-26, PC-6, Yen Tang, BL-44, GV-24, Hu Bian, GB-34, KI-4, PC-7, SI-16, LR-5, ST-36, CV-12, Bi Zhong, GV-26, CV-11, HT-5

Supplementary Points According to Symptom

Manic fits: + LR-1, GV-18, CV-15, PC-8, LU-11, LR-3, GV-26, LR-5, PC-6, LI-11, LR-8, HT-6, CV-24, SP-1, GV-23 → GV-20, LI-4 → SI-3, KI-3 → KI-1

Depression: + BL-15, BL-18, BL-20, BL-23, CV-14, PC-7, PC-8, KI-1, CV-17, LR-3, LR-2, Yin Tang, PC-6 → TW-5, LI-4 → PC-8

Auditory hallucinations: + SI-19, GB-2, TW-3, TW-17, SP-4

Visual hallucinations: + TW-17, BL-1, Yu Yao

Anxiety: + PC-6, LR-3, PC-8, CV-14

Obsessions: + GV-20, Tai Yang, Yin Tang

Forgetfulness: + GV-11, PC-6

Agitation, irritability, and excitability: + LR-3

Fear and fright: + BL-19, PC-4, CV-14

Poor appetite: + ST-36

Headache with dizziness (side effect of antipsychotics) + GV-20, Tai Yang, Yin Tang, LI-4, Ashi head points

Dizziness with tinnitus and limp, aching lumbus and knees (side effect of antipsychotics): + BL-23, KI-3

Amenorrhea and lactation (side effect of antipsychotics): + CV-4, BL-20, BL-23, ST-36, LI-4, LR-3, CV-3

Auricular Points

Primary: Kidney, Occiput, Heart, Stomach, Ear Shen Men, Central Rim, Subcortex, Sympathetic, Endocrine, Heart of Posterior Surface

Secondary: Brainstem, Adrenal Gland, External Ear, Internal Ear, Lesser Occipital Nerve, Neurasthenia Region

Research Studies

- Eight out of eleven participants completed a course of acupuncture treatment and all eleven reported positive benefits as a result of acupuncture, including improvements in the symptoms of schizophrenia, side effects of medication, energy, motivation, sleep, addictions, and other associated physical problems. However, participants' reports to the researcher and the acupuncturists varied at times and were often inconsistent between treatments, with participants revealing more information to the team towards the end of the study. In conclusion, the study indicated that patients diagnosed with schizophrenia would benefit from acupuncture treatment alongside conventional treatment.[1]

- A meta-analysis of 13 RCTs, all originating from China, met the inclusion criteria. One RCT reported significant effects of electro-acupuncture (EA) plus drug therapy for improving auditory hallucunations and positive symptoms compared with sham EA plus drug therapy. Four RCTs showed significant effects of acupuncture in response rate compared with antipsychotic drugs. Seven RCTs showed significant effects of acupuncture plus antipsychotic drug therapy for response rate compared with antipsychotic drug therapy. Two RCTs tested laser acupuncture against sham laser acupuncture. One RCT found beneficial effects of laser acupuncture on hallucination and the other RCT showed significant effects of laser acupuncture on response rate.[2]

1   Ronan, P., Robinson, N., Harbinson, D., and Macinnes, D. A case study exploration of the value of acupuncture as an adjunct treatment for patients diagnosed with schizophrenia: results and future study design. *Zhong Xi Yi Jie He Xue Bao*. 2011 May; 9(5): 503–514. Canterbury Christ Church University, Canterbury, Kent, UK.

2   Lee, M.S., Shin, B-C., Ronan, P., and Ernst, E. Acupuncture for schizophrenia: a systematic review and meta-analysis. *International Journal of Clinical Practice*. 2009; 63: 1622–1633. doi:10.1111/j.1742-1241.2009.02167.x

Chapter 42

Hallucinations

Hallucinations can result from injury to a particular cortical region or may occur secondary to tumors or seizures involving the occipital, parietal, frontal, or temporal lobe. They can also arise secondary to toxic exposure, high fevers, infections, exhaustion, starvation or extreme thirst, partial or complete hearing loss including otosclerosis, or with partial or complete blindness.

The degree of interpretative activity depends on the region involved and the type of processing performed there. Hallucinations thus become increasingly more complex as the disturbance expands from primary to association brain regions and as involvement moves from the occipital to anterior temporal regions (one of the major interpretative regions of the neocortex). In the primary regions simple hallucinary interpretations occur. Involvement of the association and multi-associational areas on the other hand causes one to hallucinate secondary to "feature detector" activation, and the individual will thus experience more complex, more realistic hallucinations.

Auditory Hallucinations

Auditory hallucinations have been associated with activity in Heschyl's gyrus, also known as the temporal gyrus, which acts as the primary auditory receiving area and association cortices. Tumors involving this area also give rise to similar, albeit transient hallucinations, including tinnitus. Individuals may complain that sounds seem louder and/or softer than normal, closer and/or more distant, strange, or even unpleasant. There is often a repetitive quality that causes the experience to be even more unpleasant. In some instances, the hallucination may become meaningful—such as the sound of footsteps, clapping hands, or music, most of which seem to have an actual external source. Brain injury/electrical stimulation may elicit sounds such as:

- Buzzing
- Clicking
- Ticking

- Humming
- Whispering
- Ringing

Most of these seem localized as though coming from the opposite side of the room.

Musical Hallucinations

Individuals with tumors and seizure disorders, particularly those involving the superior temporal gyrus, especially on the right side, have been reported to have also experienced musical hallucinations. Frequently, the same melody is heard over and over. In some instances, patients have reported the sound of singing voices, and individual instruments may be heard. Conversely, it has been frequently reported that lesions of the right temporal lobe may significantly impair one's ability to name or recognize melodies and musical pieces. It also seems to disrupt the ability to sense musical timing, the perception of timbre, loudness, and meter.

Verbal Hallucinations

With either right or left temporal destruction or stimulation (though left hemispheric function seems predominant), individuals may experience specific verbal hallucinations that may include:

- Single words
- Sentences
- Commands
- Advice

- "Distorted sentences"
- Distant conversations that can't quite be made out or incomprehensible words

Verbal hallucinations may also precede the onset of an aphasic disorder, such as the result of a developing tumor or other pathological process. Patients may complain of hearing "distorted sentences," "incomprehensible words," etc.

Although the majority of auditory neurons respond to auditory stimuli, about 25 percent also respond to visual stimuli, particularly those in motion. Visual responses have in fact been triggered from stimulation in the superior temporal lobe. These neurons are also involved in short-term memory, with injury to this area resulting in deficits. Electrical stimulation of these regions has induced both visual and complex auditory responses. Conversely, injury to the left and right superior temporal lobe can result in an inability to correctly perceive or hear complex sounds ("pure word deafness"). If limited to the right ear, agnosia for environmental and musical sounds may occur.

Simple Visual Hallucinations

The functional integrity of the temporal lobes, the inferior regions in particular, plays an important role in memorization and recollection of various auditory, visual, olfactory, and emotional experiences. When injured or disconnected from sources of input, one's ability to store information and draw visual–verbal mnemonic imagery from memory can be severely affected. When the middle temporal lobes and/or the limbic structures within (i.e. the amygdala and hippocampus) are artificially or abnormally activated, however, visual–

auditory imagery and a variety of emotional reactions can occur involuntarily. These can include complex hallucinations, dream-like states, confusional episodes, or an abnormal attribution of emotional significance to otherwise neutral thoughts and external experiences.

Occipital Lobe—Striate Cortex (Brodmann's Area 17)

Electrical stimulation, tumors, seizures, or trauma involving the striate cortex of the occipital lobe may produce simple visual hallucinations which are usually restricted to one half of the visual field. This is usually contralateral to the injury. These hallucinations may occur as:

- Sparks, stars, balls of fire

- Tongues of flames

- Colors and flashes of lights

Also:

- Objects may seem to become exceedingly large (macropsia) or small (micropsia)

- They may be blurred in terms of outline

- They may be stretched out in a single dimension

- Colors may become modified or even erased

- Sometimes, simple geometric forms may be reported

Complex Visual Hallucinations

Lesions and electrical stimulation involving the visual association areas (Brodmann's areas 18 and 19) can produce complex visual hallucinations that tend to be quite vivid and fully formed, so much so that they seem real. This is because there is a stream of visual information which becomes increasingly more complex as information is transmitted from the primary to secondary to association to multimodal areas in the temporal lobes where neurons fire in response to complex objects, including faces.

The anterior–inferior temporal regions, therefore, give rise to the most complex forms of imagery because cells in this area are specialized for the perception and recognition of specific forms. Moreover, structures such as the amygdala and hippocampus become activated, evoking memories and emotions as well. So much so that the experience may also become personally meaningful and include real individuals and real events that are produced from memory. Hippocampal stimulation was predominantly associated with either fully formed and/or memory-like hallucinations including feelings of familiarity, and secondarily with dream-like hallucinations.

Stimulation limited solely to the neocortex generally does not produce complex hallucinations unless the amygdala becomes activated. It appears that limbic activation, especially the amygdala, is necessary in order to bring a conscious perception of the activity in the temporal lobes. Interaction between the amygdala, hippocampus, and the neocortex is necessary for the individual to experience the hallucination, as it seems only when the neural activity envelops the neocortex of the temporal lobe that the individual becomes conscious of them.

Examples of complex hallucinations that have been reported include:

- Images of men, animals, various objects, and geometric figures

- Liliputian-type (miniature) individuals, with things appearing smaller (micropsias) or larger (macropsias) than they actually are

- Objects that seem to become telescoped/far away, or, when approached, objects that seem to loom and become exceedingly large

Complex hallucinations, although usually associated with tumors or abnormal activation of the visual association area, have also been reported with parietal–occipital, occipital–temporal, or inferior–temporal damage, or with lesions of the occipital pole and convexity. While simple hallucinations can regularly follow damage to either hemisphere, complex hallucinations are usually associated with right-sided cerebral lesions.

Hallucinations and the Interpretation of Neural Noise

When auditory hallucinations occur secondary to peripheral hearing loss, individuals often report hearing particular songs or melodies from their childhood. These may even be melodies they have forgotten over time. Similarly, individuals suffering from cortical blindness or those recovering from Wernicke's aphasia will frequently experience hallucinations. This seems to be a result of the interpretation of neural noise wherein the loss of input stimulates various brain regions to extract or assign meaningful significance to random neural events or whatever input is being received. This same hallucinatory experience can be found when an individual is placed in sensory-reduced environments or even when movement is restricted.

Conversely, hallucinations can also result from increased levels of neural noise. If a cortical area is abnormally activated, that area may begin interpreting its own neural activity. Neurons which interpret facial, word, and object recognition may become simultaneously activated—as well as all associated memories. In so doing, the brain attempts to interpret this as an experience.

Chinese Medical Perspective
Chinese Medical Etiology

Hallucinations may be associated with disturbances of the Hun and, by extension, the Liver and Gallbladder organs. The Hun acts as a Yang entity, coming and going, yet is rooted by a sufficient Liver Yin. Heart fire with phlegm can also generate hallucinations as the Shen becomes unsettled and the phlegm mists upward to cloud or distort the mind.

General Acupuncture Points

GV-20 → GB-18, HT-4, LR-8, LR-5

Auditory hallucinations: TW-19, TW-17

Visual hallucinations: SI-6, GB-37

Olfactory hallucinations: LI-20, ST-44

Gustatory hallucinations: Hai Quan, CV-7

Tactile hallucinations: PC-6, ST-40[1]

Research Studies

Sixty patients were selected for randomized real electro-acupuncture treatment or sham electro-acupuncture treatment. Patients in the real electro-acupuncture group experienced greater improvement in the Psychotic Symptom Rating Scales Auditory Hallucination Subscale total score, Physical Characteristics factor score, and the Positive and Negative Syndrome Scale positive symptom score than the sham electro-acupuncture group at both week four and week six. The clinical response rates in the real electro-acupuncture group and sham electro-acupuncture group were 43.3 percent and 13.3 percent respectively. It was concluded that electro-acupuncture might provide improvement in auditory hallucinations and positive symptoms for patients with schizophrenia who are partially responsive or non-responsive to risperidone monotherapy.[2]

1   Rossi, Elisa. *Shen: Psycho-Emotional Aspects of Chinese Medicine.* Edinburgh, London: Elsevier Churchill Livingstone. 2007. Print.

2   Cheng, J., Wang, G., Xiao, L., *et al.* Electro-acupuncture versus sham electro-acupuncture for auditory hallucinations in patients with schizophrenia: a randomized controlled trial. *Clinical Rehabilitation.* 2009; 23(7): 579–588. doi: 10.1177/0269215508096172

Chapter 43

Post-Traumatic Stress Disorder (PTSD)

The after-effect of a stressful situation can cause a chronic complex of emotional and physical symptoms in which one re-experiences an overwhelming traumatic event. This causes intense fear, helplessness, horror, and avoidance of stimuli associated with the trauma.[1] PTSD awareness has seen an upsurge in recent decades and correlations with brain injuries within military populations, and community or mass traumas.

The national prevalence in the United States is an estimated 7–9 percent of the population being affected. This percentage increases in populations with a higher risk of repeated exposure to traumatic events such as paramedics, firefighters, etc., ranging from 17 to 22 percent. If the individual has sustained a head injury, either due to an automobile accident or some other cause, sample rates ranged from 13 to 33 percent of those developing some degree of PTSD. Military personnel are estimated to range in rates from 10 to 30 percent, with combat exposure further increasing the risk and being a primary determinant compared to deployment without combat exposure.[2] Due to the increased numbers of blast injuries, head injuries and PTSD are becoming increasingly comorbid occurrences. A summary of factors which play a role in the development of PTSD is provided in Table 43.1. A 2008 study found that 43.9 percent of personnel who reported a TBI with loss of consciousness met the criteria for PTSD.

PTSD acts as a continuation and magnification of anxiety-related symptoms which fit into three primary symptom clusters—re-experiencing, avoidance symptoms, and hyperarousal.

---

1   Evidence-based Synthesis Program (ESP) Center, Durham Veterans Affairs Healthcare System. *Efficacy of Complementary and Alternative Medicine Therapies for Posttraumatic Stress Disorder.* August 2011. Web. www.hsrd. research.va.gov/publications/esp/cam-ptsd-REPORT.pdf. Retrieved 2017, Oct 17.

2   Committee on the Assessment of Ongoing Effects in the Treatment of Posttraumatic Stress Disorder; Institute of Medicine. *Treatment for Posttraumatic Stress Disorder in Military and Veteran Populations: Initial Assessment.* Washington DC: National Academies Press. 2012. Web. http://cdn.govexec.com/media/gbc/docs/pdfs_edit/071712bb1. pdf. Retrieved 2017, Oct 17.

In order to meet diagnostic criteria, these symptoms must be present for at least one month and impair the individual's ability to function in a social, occupational, or other important life arena. Diagnostic criteria are provided in Table 43.2.

TABLE 43.1 Factors in the Development of PTSD

Pre-traumatic factors	Ongoing life stress or demographics
	Lack of social support
	Young age at time of trauma
	Pre-existing psychiatric disorder
	Low socio-economic status, education level, intelligence, gender
	Prior trauma exposure (reported abuse in childhood, report of other previous traumatization, report of other adverse childhood factors)
	Family history of psychiatric disorders
Peritraumatic or trauma-related factors	Severe trauma
	Type of trauma (interpersonal traumas such as torture, rape, or assault convey a high risk of PTSD)
	High perceived threat to life
	Community (mass) trauma
	Peritraumatic dissociation
Post-traumatic factors	Ongoing life stress
	Lack of positive social support
	Negative social support (e.g. negative reactions from others)
	Bereavement
	Major loss of resources
	Other factors, including children at home and distressed spouse

TABLE 43.2 Diagnostic Criteria for PTSD

Activity	**Related Symptoms**
Exposure to or witnessing of a threatening event	Intense fear
	Feeling of helplessness
	Horror
	Symptoms of re-experiencing
Recurrent or intrusive memories	Nightmares
	Sense of reliving the trauma
	Psychological or physiological distress when reminded of the trauma
Avoidance	Inability to recall parts of the trauma
	Withdrawal
	Emotional numbing

Increased autonomic arousal	Sleep disturbance
	Irritability
	Hypervigilance
	Difficulty concentrating
	Exaggerated startle response

Many symptoms that present in cases of PTSD are similar to or are also found in brain injuries such as cognitive impairments (poor attention and memory), behavioral components (impulsivity, disinhibition), and emotional changes (emotional lability, depression). Secondary effects such as social isolation, difficulty in interpersonal relations, and impairments in functioning in home and work environments may also become problematic. This overlap in symptoms can make differential diagnosis difficult. Table 43.3 compares these symptom clusters. It is possible that the similarities in symptomology relate to similarities in brain regions and functions affected by both conditions, as discussed below. In cases where both are present, it has been proposed that a brain injury compromises the individual's ability to cope with the stress of PTSD through disinhibition of executive function, while PTSD compromises the ability to navigate some of the cognitive difficulties that can follow a brain injury. As a result, this interplay can be difficult for an individual to manage. Silver states the best explanation of the dynamic between the two disorders is "that the unique interface between the central nervous system and concurrent psychological distress leads to signs and symptoms that are characteristic of both post-concussion and PTSD. In addition, this relationship is dynamic, and the relative contributions of etiological factors contributing to the symptoms change over time."[3]

TABLE 43.3 Comparison of Symptoms between PTSD and Brain Injury

PTSD	Found in Both PTSD and Brain Injury	Brain Injury
Flashbacks	Fatigue	Headache
Avoidance	Irritability	Nausea/vomiting
Hypervigilance	Insomnia	Photophobia or noise sensitivity
Nightmares	Depression	Vision problems
Re-experiencing	Cognitive deficits	

Brain regions often affected by PTSD tend to overlap with those most commonly affected by a brain injury as well. Among these are the medial prefrontal cortex, anterior cingulate cortex, temporal region, hippocampus, and the amygdala. It has been proposed that PTSD is characterized by an exaggerated amygdaloid response coupled with impairments in regulation of the medial prefrontal cortex (hypoactivation in the dorsal and rostral anterior cingulate

---

3   Silver, Jonathan, Yudofsky, Stuart, and McAllister, Thomas. *Textbook of Traumatic Brain Injury*. Washington, DC: American Psychiatric Pub. 2011. Print.

and ventromedial prefrontal cortex), which fails to inhibit the heightened fear reactions of the amygdala. It has been further hypothesized that impairment of executive function due to injury of the frontal lobe increases the perseverance of the re-experiencing effect. Hippocampal atrophy has also been correlated to PTSD, as demonstrated by volumetric studies and magnetic resonance spectroscopy. This seems to be a phenomenon that occurs primarily in the right hemisphere in Vietnam combat veterans, with an 18 percent decrease. Interestingly, this hippocampal atrophy was demonstrated to be a left hemisphere occurrence in women who experienced childhood sexual abuse. This atrophy does not occur within the first six months postinjury, but rather a while after the event, and does not seem to occur in children.

Neurochemical changes associated with PTSD involve many neurotransmitter pathways. The role of serotonergic pathways in this process has a significant body of evidence. The regions most sensitive to serotonin include the limbic system and frontal–subcortical circuits. SSRIs have often been used for PTSD symptoms, as benefits have been demonstrated. These SSRIs also modulate the release of norepinephrine which directly impacts startle response, the prefrontal cortex inhibition of the amygdala, and release with recollection of the traumatic event, all of which create a feedback loop of consolidation of the memory. Additionally, GABA has been demonstrated to be downregulated, and the excitotoxic neurotransmitter glutamate, increased. Acetylcholine regulation may also be impacted and has a significant effect on cognitive symptoms due to its supporting role in the reticular formation involved in arousal and attention, the entorhinal–hippocampal formation involved in declarative memory, and the frontal–subcortical circuits involved in executive functioning.

Endocrine changes associated with PTSD show that individuals tend to have low cortisol levels with high levels of corticotropin-releasing factor (CRF). This is interesting, as a classic stress response involves elevated levels of CRF, ACTH, and cortisol. This was originally attributed to the idea of adrenal fatigue following the acute injury, but emergency room studies have shown low-to-normal levels of cortisol as well. It has been shown that those with PTSD have an increased number of glucocorticoid receptors and that these receptors demonstrated increased sensitivity. These changes allow for greater inhibition of cortisol via negative feedback at the pituitary gland, with less ACTH released and the subsequent attenuation of cortisol. Primary effects on the central nervous system of blast injuries were indicated by elevated levels of eicosanoids and stress hormones. There is also emerging evidence that the state of one's gut health may play a role in the development of PTSD, with an unhealthy microbiome increasing risk.[4]

It has been proposed that postinjury amnesia, particularly in severe brain injuries, may act as a "protective mechanism" against the development of PTSD, as most cases with severe TBI do not meet the criteria for PTSD. It is mild cases of brain injury that seem to demonstrate the highest rates of PTSD development. As discussed in Chapter 12, anti-hypertensive pharmaceuticals have also been shown to reduce PTSD risk.

---

4   Hemmings, S.M.J., Malan-Müller, S., van den Heuvel, L.L. *et al.* The microbiome in posttraumatic stress disorder and trauma-exposed controls. *Psychosomatic Medicine.* 2017; 79 (8): 936. doi:10.1097/PSY.0000000000000512

Etiology

Although a traumatic event is the trigger for the anxiety disorder known as PTSD, not all people experiencing traumatic events acquire the continued acute emotional responses to it.

Another factor in the development of PTSD, outside of the traumatic event, is the person's own innate ability to cope with the stress. While some soldiers become "battle-fatigued" following combat, others emerge from battle exhilarated by the encounter. It is hard to determine who exactly is at highest risk for development of PTSD in situations of severe stress (like soldiers before going to battle, or survivors of a massive natural disaster). Many physically and mentally "strong" people will be affected by the overwhelming stress, while some appearing physically or mentally "weak" can rise to the occasion and remain relatively unaffected in the long term. This is likely due to the numerous factors beyond fortitude of the mind that have been discussed in this chapter, many of which are neurobiologically set. For this reason, all who encounter stressors should be made aware of any personality, emotional, or physical changes that might signify the beginnings of PTSD.

Signs and Symptoms

- Depression
- Re-experience of some traumatic event:
  - Nightmares
  - Flashbacks
- Persistent avoidance of stimuli
- Increased arousal
- Anger or irritability

Types of Stressors That Can Induce PTSD

- Threat to one's life or physical integrity
- Serious threat or harm to one's children, spouse, other close relatives, or friends
- Destruction of one's home or community
- Seeing another person who is mutilated, dying, or dead
- Being the victim of physical violence (including child abuse)

Biomedical Approaches

- Antidepressants (SSRIs):
  - Fluoxetine
  - Sertraline
  - Paroxetine

- Mood stabilizers—lamotrigine

- Atypical antipsychotics—lanzapine

- Beta-blockers—propranolol

- Psychotherapy:

  ° Cognitive–behavioral (individual and group, trauma focused, or traditional)

  ° Exposure therapy

  ° Stress management

Chinese Medical Perspective

Dr. Joe Chang states that the most commonly involved patterns are those of excess, especially in the Heart and Liver.[5] Most common signs tend to be anger, frequent panic attacks, anxiety, left arm numbness, heaviness in the chest, and dream-disturbed sleep as the autonomic nervous system seems affected.

Underlying deficiency patterns, generally of the Spleen or Kidney, often emerge after balancing the excesses. The adrenals may also be drained, with signs of fatigue, loss of interest in everyday activity, memory loss, poor digestion/appetite, or low back pain. Dr. Chang strongly recommends an integrative approach to treating PTSD with a focus on both the patient and environment/social relationships surrounding them.

Acupuncture Mechanisms in PTSD

- Redirects blood flow from the limbic system to the prefrontal cortex

- Balances the sympathetic and parasympathetic responses

- Inhibits the amygdala to alleviate hypervigilance

- Reduces epinephrine production to down-regulate the sympathetic response

- Initiates endorphin secretion to reduce pain[6]

Pattern Differentiation
Liver Qi Stagnation

> ***Primary symptoms***: Hyperarousal aggravated by suppressed emotions (anxiety, overthinking, anger, sorrow), depression, irritability, labile mood

5   Chang, J.C., Wang, W., and Jiang, Y. *The Treatment of PTSD with Chinese Medicine: an integrative approach* = Zhong xi yi jie he zhi liao chuang shang hou ying ji zhang ai. Beijing: People's Medical Publishing House. 2010.

6   Resko, E. and Sigrist, E. *Treating PTSD with Chinese Medicine: a manual for practitioners*. Oregon College of Oriental Medicine. Web. http://library.ocom.edu/images/student_research/macom/ErinReskoErikaSigrist.pdf

Additional symptoms: Distending pain in chest/hypochondria, hiccups/sighing, poor appetite, insomnia, globus hystericus, possible abdominal masses. Women: irregular menses, dysmenorrhea, distending breast pain

Tongue: Red tongue, thin white coat

Pulse: Wiry (bowstring) or slippery

Treatment principles: Soothe Liver, regulate Qi

Acupuncture treatment: GB-34, LR-3, TW-6, PC-6, LR-13, LR-14

Herbal treatment:
Chai Hu Shu Gan San (Bupleurum Powder to Spread the Liver)
[Chai Hu 6g, Bai Shao 9g, Xiang Fu 6g, Chuan Xiong 6g, Chen Pi 6g, Zhi Ke 6g, Zhi Gan Cao 3g]

Liver Qi Stagnation Leading to Fire

Primary symptoms: Hyperarousal, irritability, severe headaches, nightmares

Additional symptoms: Dizziness, red eyes/complexion, tinnitus, bitter taste, dry throat, thirst (cold), burning, pain in hypochondria, insomnia, dry stools, dark urine

Tongue: Red tongue, yellow coat

Pulse: Wiry (bowstring), rapid

Treatment principles: Clear Liver fire, move Liver Qi, calm Shen

Acupuncture treatment: GB-34, LR-2, TW-6, PC-6, LR-13, LR-14

Herbal treatment:
Jia Wei Xiao Yao San (Augmented Rambling Powder)
[Chai Hu 9g, Dang Gui 9g, Bai Shao 9g, Bai Zhu 9g, Fu Ling 9g, Zhi Gan Cao 4.5g, Mu Dan Pi 9g, Zhi Zi 9g]

Heart Fire

Primary symptoms: Hypervigilance, irritability, vexation, insomnia (trouble falling asleep)

Additional symptoms: 5-center heat, dizziness, tinnitus, lower back pain, seminal emission, red complexion, mouth/tongue ulcers, dry mouth, delirious speech, mania, dry stools, painful (dark yellow) urination

Tongue: Red tongue, dry coat

Pulse: Thready, rapid

Treatment principles: Clear heat, calm Shen

Acupuncture treatment: HT-7, HT-8, HT-9, CV-15, SP-6, KI-6, LI-11, GV-19, GV-24

Herbal treatment:
Dao Chi San Jia Jian (Guide Out the Red Powder Plus Modifications)
[Huang Lian 3–6g, Huang Qin 10g, Mu Tong 6–10g, Sheng Di 12g, Dan Zhu Ye 10g, Zhi Zi 10g, Deng Xin Cao 3g, Gan Cao Shao 10g, Lian Xin 2g]

Phlegm Fire Rising to Heart and Gallbladder

Primary symptoms: Hyperarousal, insomnia, intrusive images/disturbing dreams of the traumatic event, easily frightened, frequent nightmares, excessive and random speech

Additional symptoms: Dizziness, stuffiness and fullness in abdomen, bitter taste, nausea, vomiting, excessive exercising, aggression, poor appetite, sticky/greasy sensation in mouth, sputum

Tongue: Red tongue, yellow, greasy coat

Pulse: Wiry (bowstring) or rapid, slippery

Treatment principles: Clear heat, resolve phlegm, calm Shen

Acupuncture treatment: PC-5, HT-7, HT-8, PC-7, CV-15, ST-40, SP-6, BL-20, GV-20, GV-24, GB-13 (may also consider the use of Sun Si Miao's 13 Ghost points)

Herbal treatment:
Wen Dan Tang (Warm the Gallbladder Decoction)
[Fa Ban Xia 6g, Zhu Ru 6g, Zhi Shi 6g, Chen Pi 6g, Gan Cao 6g, Fu Ling 9g, Sheng Jiang 2pc, Da Zao 3pc]

Heart and Spleen Deficiency

Primary symptoms: Hypervigilance, insomnia, emotional disturbance, mental fatigue, palpitation, timidity

Additional symptoms: Poor memory, poor appetite, pale lips/complexion, dizziness

Tongue: Pale tongue, thin white coat

Pulse: Thready, weak

Treatment principles: Nourish Heart Blood, tonify Spleen Qi

Acupuncture treatment: HT-7, PC-6, CV-4, CV-12, CV-14, CV-15, BL-17, BL-20, ST-36, SP-3, SP-6

Herbal treatment:
Gui Pi Tang (Restore the Spleen Decoction)
[Ren Shen 9g, Huang Qi 9g, Bai Zhu 9g, Fu Ling/Shen 9g, Dang Shen 10g, Suan Zao Ren 9g, Long Yao Rou 9g, Ye Jiao Teng 6g, Mu Xiang 6g, Zhi Gan Cao 6g, Dang Gui 6g, Zhi Yuan Zhi 3g, Sheng Jiang 3g/5 slices, Da Zao 5pc]

Heart and Gallbladder Deficiency

Primary symptoms: Timidity, trouble falling asleep, frequent nightmares, fear of experiencing traumatic event

Additional symptoms: Palpitations, difficulty making decisions, dizziness, blurred vision, shortness of breath, fatigue

Tongue: Pale tongue, white coat

Pulse: Thready, wiry (bowstring)

Treatment principles: Tranquilize the mind, calm the Shen

Acupuncture treatment: HT-7, SP-6, GB-40, PC-6, An Mian, BL-15, BL-18, BL-19, BL-47, CV-6, CV-17

Herbal treatment:
An Shen Ding Zhi Wan Jia Jian (Spirit-Quieting Mind-Stabilizing Pill Plus Modifications)
[Fu Ling 9g, Fu Shen 9g, Yuan Zhi 6g, Ren Shen 9g, Long Gu 30g, Shi Chang Pu 6g, Suan Zao Ren 12g, Hu Po 1g]
Gan Mai Da Zao Tang (Licorice, Wheat, and Sour Jujube Decoction)
[Gan Cao 9g, Fu Xiao Mai 30g, Da Zao 10pc]

Auricular Protocols

NADA: Shenmen, Sympathetic, Liver, Kidney, Lung
Battlefield acupuncture: Shenmen, Point Zero, Omega 2, Thalamus, Cingulate Gyrus
Auricular trauma protocol: Shenmen, Point Zero, Hypothalamus, Hippocampus, Amygdala, Master Cerebral

Auricular Point Indications

- Sympathetic: Balances autonomic nervous system

- Shenmen: Psychospiritual vitality, balance to Heart channel, hypersensitivity to needles

- Kidney: Warms freeze response, finds safety in self, restores vitality/reserves

- Liver: Softens anger/hypervigilance, freeze/fight response

- Hypothalamus: Stimulates parasympathetic nervous system, triggers HPA axis, important for attention/vigilance/arousal

- Amygdala: Modulates expression of anger/fear/aggression/irritability

- Hippocampus: Memory encoding/emotional experiences. Important for memory/concentration. Eases mind's grip on traumatic memory, brings relief to hyperarousal/intrusive images

- Master cerebral: Psychoemotional/psychosomatic disorders, emotions around pain and chronic pain. Zones for limbic system (memory, emotions, compulsive behavior) and prefrontal cortex (concentration, decision making, initiating action)

- Point zero—moves mind/body/emotions toward homeostasis

Other Therapeutic Considerations
Somatic Therapy Considerations

- Aerobic exercise: Regular exercise helps minimize stress

- Qigong

- Tai Qi Chuan

- Trauma release exercises (TRE)

- Eye movement desensitization and reprocessing (EMDR)

- Body-based psychotherapies (Bioenergetics, Reichian therapy, Hakomi, Core Energetics, etc.)

Phytotherapeutic Considerations

- Panax ginseng
- Valerian
- Sumbul
- Skullcap

- Hops
- Wild oats
- Passion flower

Dietary Considerations

Therapeutic foods:

- Increase foods that calm the Shen, tonify the Heart, and harmonize the Stomach and Spleen

Avoid:

- Meat, alcohol, hot sauces, spicy foods, fried foods, fatty foods, rich foods, salty foods, coffee, caffeine, sweet foods and sugar

Research Studies

- A systematic review synthesized evidence from seven studies which met criteria with 709 total participants included. Studies compared acupuncture with treatment as usual (TAU), sham acupuncture, a passive waitlist control, cognitive–behavioral therapy, and paroxetine. Statistically significant effects in favor of acupuncture (as adjunctive or monotherapy) were found versus any comparator for PTSD symptoms at postintervention. Safety data suggested that acupuncture is not associated with any serious adverse events. No systematic differences by type of acupuncture were found in those comparing such data. Potential benefits of acupuncture for PTSD and depression symptoms were identified compared with control groups in the months following treatment.[7]

- Fifty-five service members meeting research diagnostic criteria for PTSD were randomized to usual PTSD care (UPC) plus eight 60-minute sessions of acupuncture conducted twice weekly or to UPC alone. Outcomes were assessed at baseline and 4, 8, and 12 weeks post-randomization. It was found that Mean improvement in PTSD severity was significantly greater among those receiving acupuncture than in those receiving UPC. Acupuncture was also associated with significantly greater improvements in depression, pain, and physical and mental health functioning. The study concluded acupuncture as being effective for reducing PTSD symptoms.[8]

- One hundred and thirty-eight patients with earthquake-caused PTSD who enrolled were randomly assigned to an electro-acupuncture group and an oral paroxetine group. The electro-acupuncture group was treated by scalp electro-acupuncture on Baihui (GV-20), Sishencong (EX-HN-1), Shenting (GV-24), and Fengchi (GB-20). The efficacy and safety of the electro-acupuncture on treatment of 69 PTSD

7   Grant, S., Colaiaco, B., Motala, A., *et al. Needle Acupuncture for Posttraumatic Stress Disorder (PTSD): a systematic review.* Santa Monica, CA: RAND Corporation, 2017. Web. www.rand.org/pubs/research_reports/RR1433.html

8   Engel, C-C., Cordova, E-H., Benedek, D-M., *et al.* Randomized effectiveness trial of a brief course of acupuncture for posttraumatic stress disorder. *Medical Care.* 2014 Dec; 52(12 Suppl 5): S57–64. doi:10.1097/MLR.0000000000000237

patients were evaluated using the Clinician-Administered PTSD Scale (CAPS), Hamilton Depression Scale (HAMD), Hamilton Anxiety Scale (HAMA), and Treatment Emergent Symptom Scale (TESS). Efficacy in the electro-acupuncture group was found significantly better than that in the paroxetine group.[9]

- A systematic review of randomized controlled trials showed the following: "One high-quality RCT reported that acupuncture was superior to wait list control and therapeutic effects of acupuncture and cognitive-behavioral therapy (CBT) were similar based on the effect sizes. One RCT showed no statistical difference between acupuncture and selective serotonin reuptake inhibitors (SSRIs). One RCT reported a favorable effect of acupoint stimulation plus CBT against CBT alone. A meta-analysis of acupuncture plus moxibustion versus SSRI favored acupuncture plus moxibustion in three outcomes," suggesting "that the evidence of effectiveness of acupuncture for PTSD is encouraging."[10]

- The *Journal of Mental and Nervous Diseases* published a study evaluating the possible efficacy and acceptability of acupuncture for PTSD. People diagnosed with PTSD were randomized to either an empirically developed acupuncture treatment (ACU), a group cognitive–behavioral therapy (CBT), or a wait-list control (WLC). The primary outcome measure was self-reported PTSD symptoms at baseline, end treatment, and three-month follow-up. Compared with the wait-list group, acupuncture provided large treatment effects for PTSD similar in magnitude to the cognitive–behavioral group. Symptom reductions at end treatment were maintained at three-month follow-up for both interventions.[11]

9   Wang, Y., Hu, Y-P., Wang, W-C., Pang, R-Z., and Zhang, A-R. Clinical studies on treatment of earthquake-caused posttraumatic stress disorder using electroacupuncture. *Evidence-Based Complementary and Alternative Medicine.* 2012; 2012: 7 pages. Article ID 431279. doi:10.1155/2012/431279

10   Young-Dae Kim, In Heo, Byung-Cheul Shin, *et al.* Acupuncture for posttraumatic stress disorder: a systematic review of randomized controlled trials and prospective clinical trials. *Evidence-based Complementary and Alternative Medicine: eCAM.* 2013; 2013: 615857.

11   Hollifield, M., Nityamo, S-L., Warner, T., and Hammerschlag, R. Acupuncture for posttraumatic stress disorder: a randomized controlled pilot trial. *Journal of Nervous and Mental Disease.* 2007 Jun; 195(6): 504–513. doi:10.1097/NMD.0b013e31803044f8

Chapter 44

Behavioral Changes and Emotional Lability

Behavioral changes can often be a problematic sequela of a brain injury, impacting one's social interactions with family, friends, support systems, employers, and others. This may be to the degree of losing these relationships altogether. This results in a sense of loneliness or isolation. At times, they may further result in consequences such as substance abuse, incarceration, homelessness, psychiatric hospitalization, and victimization.

These changes may be temporary or last a lifetime. Many individuals coming out of a coma display a period of increased irritability, confusion, physical restlessness, disorientation, and confabulation. Some individuals will develop a quick temper following their injury in which they may often yell, curse, hit, kick, and throw things. These can be triggered by feelings of frustration, being misunderstood, isolation, or difficulty in concentration. These have been conceptualized as pre-morbid traits exacerbated in the face of now overwhelming stimuli. Some will develop an involuntary expression of the opposite emotion of that which they are actually feeling, such as laughing when they are in fact sad. This can cause a lot of difficulty in their interactions with others and frustration for both parties. A pseudobulbar effect, also known as emotional incontinence, can develop in which emotions spontaneously arise without any particular event or trigger to which it is associated.

Following the occurrence of a brain injury, the individual may experience a type of "maturation arrest" in which subsequent development becomes stalled at the maturation level they were at prior to the time of injury. Developmental models of psychoneurological development may help a practitioner to understand some behaviors that appear immature or undeveloped for one's age or as if they remain "locked in" to a particular stage of development.[1] This will be further discussed in Chapter 46.

---

1   Chapman, S.B. Neurocognitive stall: a paradox in long term recovery from pediatric brain injury. *Brain Injury Professional*. 2006; 3(4): 10–13.

Common Neurobehavioral Complications of Brain Injury

- Aggression
- Agitation/irritability
- Apathy
- Denial of deficits
- Childish behavior
- Poor self-awareness
- Loss of sense of self
- Disinhibition
- Eating disturbances
- Flat affect/restricted emotions

- Inability to recognize emotions
- Impulsivity
- Lability/emotional instability
- Poor initiation
- Poor judgment and reasoning
- Dysphoria
- Delusions
- Euphoria
- Aberrant motor behavior
- Psychosis (rare)

Lezak[2] described five primary attributes to personality alterations that can occur after a TBI:

- Impaired social perceptiveness
- Impaired self-control and regulation
- Stimulus-bound behavior
- Emotional change
- Inability to learn from personal experience

Neurophysiological bases for such changes are dependent upon the site of injury and the extent of damage done. Diffuse axonal injuries may result in an "unplugging" of the neural networks from one another and a decrease in interaction with the remainder of the CNS during functional activities. The ventromedial prefrontal cortex mediates between emotional and moral cognition. Moral judgment is associated with activation of the right temporal cortex, lenticular nucleus, and the cerebellum; whereas judgments not containing emotional significance show activation of the frontopolar cortex and medial frontal gyrus. Reactions and psychological defenses in response to noxious stimuli stem from an interaction between the limbic-mediated drives, paralimbic cortical inhibition, and contextual relations tied to past events/experiences. Some individuals will find that they are much more driven toward sensation-seeking behaviors. That is, they become "adrenaline junkies"—seeking out activities that provide a "rush." This is neurophysiologically linked to frontal activity. Orbitofrontal injuries often demonstrate behavioral changes such as impulsivity, euphoria, and manic symptoms, as well as the pseudobulbar effect mentioned earlier. Specific traits

---

2   Lezak, M.D. Living with the characterologically altered brain injured patient. *Journal of Clinical Psychiatry*. 1998; 39: 592–598.

have been researched and documented to correlate with particular brain regions that are outlined in Table 44.1.

Neurochemically, it has been postulated that dopamine receptor activity may relate to vigilance, expectation, and reward. The serotonergic circuits have been implicated in hostility as this pertain to those with a type A personality. There has also been a shown correlation between high-circulating levels of catecholamines and their metabolites with positive post-TBI outcome levels. Many neurotransmitters are involved in aggressive behavior, including norepinephrine, dopamine, acetylcholine, and GABA. Norepinephrine enhances aggressive behavior, as can elevated levels of dopamine and acetylcholine. Lowered levels of ser0tonergic activity and GABA, as an inhibitory neurotransmitter, have been associated with increased aggression or, rather, a disinhibition of aggressive impulses.

TABLE 44.1 Brain Regions Associated with Personality Traits

Trait	Association
Aggression	Reduced cingulate cortex volume and activity
Conditioned memory storage	Cerebellum
Decision values	Central orbitofrontal activation
Dispassionate analysis	Increased anterior cingulate activity
Emotional bias in moral decisions	Ventromedial and orbitofrontal prefrontal cortices activation
Emotional memory storage	Amygdala
Empathy/self-reflection	Insula activation
Extroversion	Reduced dorsolateral prefrontal cortex, anterior cingulate, and thalamus activity
Goal values	Medial orbitofrontal activation
Insightful/"eureka" moments	Increased superior temporal gyrus activity
Mistrust/disbelief	Reduced insula activity
Novelty seeking	Increased hippocampus and striatum activity
Optimism	Increased amygdala and anterior cingulate activity
Personal awareness of mental state	Medial prefrontal cortex
Personal space boundaries	Motor, somatosensory, cingulate, and parietal cortices
Prediction errors	Ventral striatum (caudate–putamen) activation
Punctuality/subjective time sense	Substantia nigra, basal ganglia, and prefrontal circuits
Reflective/comparing	Lateral prefrontal cortex activation
Self-monitoring/guiding behavior	Cingulate cortex
Social avoidance/fear/anxiety	Increased amygdala activity
Social comfort/safety	Increased striatal activity
Trust/belief	Increased ventromedial prefrontal cortex activity
Perceived unfairnes	Increased insula activity

The extent to which these behavioral changes or difficulties manifest is dependent on a number of factors, including severity of the injury, personality characteristics prior to the injury, learning style, intelligence, and influences of one's current environment. These environmental factors may include level of stimulation, familiarity to the individual with whom they are interacting, availability of support, and demands upon the individual, among others. Possible methods of controlling these environmental factors are listed in Table 44.2.

TABLE 44.2 Possible Methods of Controlling Environmental Factors

Reducing noise and other extraneous stimuli
Limit visitor numbers and time
Eliminating TV and technology
Incorporate familiar objects
Repeat routines for familiarity
Provide a sense of safety (veiled beds, blankets, soft lap belts, padded hand mitts, etc.)

Behavior Assessment

A number of variables are assessed in measuring behavior, including frequency, rate, duration, latency, and the percentage of time that behaviors are properly conducted when asked. These are shown in Table 44.3.

TABLE 44.3 Variables in Measuring Behavior

Name	Measure	Considerations
Frequency	Count how many times a behavior occurs	Best for behaviors with a distinct start and end (striking, attending a group, asks for assistance, etc.)
Rate	Point per unit of time	Can help bring perspective to frequency (10x/hour vs. 10x/week)
Duration	How long behavior lasts from start to end	e.g. yelling, hand-washing
Latency	Time between stimulus and response	e.g. time between a verbal cue and initiation of action
Percent correct	Number of correct responses out of total possible number of responses	e.g. number of times one correctly completes a task vs. how many total attempts

Indirect

- Interviews
- Checklists

Possible downsides: Individuals may intentionally or unintentionally misreport or exaggerate due to awareness deficits or impaired memory.

Direct: Direct Observation of the Individual

- Functional analysis/assessment
- Minnesota Multiphasic Personality Inventory (MMPI)
- Millon Clinical Multiaxial Inventory
- Personality Assessment Inventory
- Millon Behavioral Health Inventory
- Millon Behavioral Medicine Diagnostic
- Four-term contingency

Differential Diagnosis

- Preinjury drug and substance abuse
- Coexisting anxiety and depressive disorders
- Drug effects and side effects:
    - Alcohol, cocaine, amphetamines
    - Stimulating antidepressants
    - Antipsychotics
    - Anticholinergic medications
- Epilepsy (ictal, postictal, and interictal)
- Alzheimer's disease
- Delirium (hypoxia, electrolyte imbalance, anesthesia and surgery, uremia, etc.)
- Infectious disease (encephalits, meningitis, pneumonia, UTI)
- Metabolic disorders (hyperthyroidism, hypothyroidism, hypoglycemia, vitamin deficiency)

Biomedical Approaches

- Counseling/verbal therapies (see Table 44.4 for types of procedure-learning teachings)

- Use of a notebook/compensatory device

- Reinforcement protocols and behavioral treatments

Aggression

- Antipsychotics: Olanzapine, haloperidol

- Sedatives/hypnotics: Benzodiazepines—may rarely cause increased hostility, aggression, or rage

- Anti-anxiety: Buspirone, clonazepam

- Anti-convulsants: Carbamazepine, oxcarbazepine

- Anti-manic: Lithium

- Antidepressants: Trazadone, sertraline, fluoxetine

- Stimulants: Amantadine, methylphenidate

- Anti-hypertensives: propranolol, nadolol, pindolol

TABLE 44.4 Possible Teaching Methods for Procedures Learning

Task analysis	List of very specific steps involved in completing a task. Breaks larger tasks into smaller components
Shaping	Reinforcing actions that loosely resemble target behavior and easier to display by the individual
Prompting and cueing	Individual is supported to display a correct response with visual, audible, or tactile prompts
Fading	Individual learns to produce the same response under gradually changing conditions with less support over time
Generalization	The individual begins to respond similarly to different stimuli or situations they have not been trained in
Discrimination	Individual responds differently to similar stimuli based on situation

De-escalation Techniques When Working with Behavioral Disorders

These techniques may be helpful in situations that become very emotional, tense, or even hostile while working or interacting with an individual:

- Active listening: Good eye contact, paraphrasing, restating, clarification

- Orientation: To person, place, time, and purpose of activity

- Redirection: Decreasing the stress of the task at hand; moving to a known or preferred skill

- Setting limits: Remaining calm; outlining all expectations and clearly defining consequences, both positive and negative outcomes, stating positive outcomes first

- Withdrawing attention: Ignoring off-task behavior; helping the individual realize the relationship between attention and calm interactive behavior

- Contracting: Clearly defining the parameters of expectation

Chinese Medical Perspective: Irritability (Yi Nu)

Irritability or Yi Nu translates literally as "easy anger" and refers to an emotional disposition to easily becoming angry or irritated. This frequently is not under the person's volitional control. If this anger is even more pronounced, it then is referred to as "great anger" or irascibility. The disease mechanisms are the same in both cases and merely a matter of degree. Additionally, the individual may present with one or more of the following: frequent emotional changes, improper emotional expression, a long-existing emotional stimulant and stressor, or an acute emotional outburst.

Chinese Medical Etiology

Anger is the emotion associated with the Liver organ system and the wood phase in the five-element system. Disease mechanisms which produce easy anger or irritability are thus associated with this organ system. In each case there is the presence of Liver depression. This is an accumulation of pent-up Qi/unfulfilled desires within the individual. When this culminates to a certain degree, any additional stimuli may cause this pent-up Qi to rush outward by over-coursing and over-discharging. This further damages the Liver and inhibits its Qi mechanism.

Pattern Differentiation
Liver Depression Qi Stagnation

Primary symptoms: Irritability, depression, taciturnity

Additional symptoms: Chest and rib-side distension and pain, belching, low appetite, talkative, insomnia, worried and sensitive, suspicious of small things, body aches and stiffness, frequent sighing, dymenorrhea or irregular menstruation

Tongue: Dark or normal color, thin white coat

Pulse: Wiry (bowstring), tense

Treatment principles: Course the Liver and rectify the Qi

Acupuncture treatment: LR-1, LR-3, LR-6, LR-14, PC-6, LI-4, HT-7, TW-6, Yintang

Modifications:
Liver depression and Qi stagnation severe: + LR-14, BL-18
Irascibility is severe: + GV-24
Severe chest oppression: + CV-17

Herbal treatment:
Chai Hu Shu Gan San Jia Jian (Bupleurum Powder to Soothe the Liver Plus Modifications)
[Chai Hu 10g, Zhi Ke 10g, Bai Shao 10g, Dang Gui 10g, Chuan Xiong 6–10g, Xiang Fu 10g, Chuan Lian Zi 3–6g, He Huan Pi 12g]

Modifications:
Liver depression/Spleen deficiency: Use Xiao Chai Hu Tang (Minor Bupleurum Decoction) or Xiao Yao San (Rambling Powder)

Liver–Gallbladder Fire Flaring

Primary symptoms: Irritability, vexation and agitation, red face and eyes

Additional symptoms: Rib-side pain, bitter taste in mouth, dry mouth, possible headache or vertigo

Tongue: Red body, yellow tongue

Pulse: Wiry (bowstring), rapid

Treatment principles: Clear the Liver and drain Gallbladder fire

Acupuncture treatment: LR-2, GB-41, ST-44, PC-5

Herbal treatment:
Xie Qing Wan Jia Jian (Drain the Green Pill Plus Modifications)
[Long Dan Cao 6g, Zhi Zi 10g, Huang Qin 10g, Da Huang 3–6g, Dang Gui 10g, Chuan Xiong 6–10g, Qiang Huo 10g, Fang Feng 10g, Gan Cao 3g, Bo He 3–6g, He Huan Pi 10g]

Modifications:
Severe vexation and agitation: + Huang Lian
Severe rib-side pain: + Chai Hu, Chuan Lian Zi, Yan Hu Suo
Severe headache and vertigo: + Xia Ku Cao
Severe red eyes: + Ju Hua

Liver Blood–Kidney Yin Deficiency

Primary symptoms: Irritability, dizziness, depressed, feels like anger is held inside

Additional symptoms: Low back and knee soreness and limpness, dry skin and throat, dry rough eyes, 5-palm heat, possible night sweats, malar flush, afternoon tidal heat, insomnia, profuse dreams

Tongue: Red or pale tongue, red tip, scanty coat

Pulse: Fine, rapid; or floating, rapid

Treatment principles: Supplement the Kidneys and enrich Yin, nourish the Blood and soothe the Liver

Acupuncture treatment: LR-3, LR-8, SP-6, KI-2, KI-3, KI-6, KI-7, KI-9, KI-27, Yintang

Herbal treatment:
Qi Ju Di Huang Wan Jia Wei (Lycium Fruit, Chrysanthemum, and Rehmannia Pill Plus Modifications)
[Shu Di 12g, Shan Yao 10g, Shan Zhu Yu 10g, Ze Xie 6g, Dan Pi 10g, Gou Qi Zi 10–12g, Ju Hua 10g, Huang Bai 10g, Long Gu 12g]

Frequent Joy (Shan Xi)

The concept of frequent joy relates to frequent, inappropriate, or nervous laughter or laughing without reason. It is a type of excited, manic affective state or propensity. Also pertinent to assessing this state is the presence of frequent emotional changes, improper emotional expression, the presence of a long-term emotional stimulant and stressor, or an acute emotional outburst.

Differential Diagnosis

Medical Disorders

Neurologic disorders, including multiple sclerosis (MS), encephalomyelitis, and others

Psychiatric Disorders

Bipolar disorder, schizophrenia or psychotic disorders, certain personality disorders

Chinese Medical Etiology

Joy is the affect or emotion associated with the Heart organ system and the fire phase. If any type of pathologic heat harasses the Heart spirit, it may manifest as frequent joy. The main specific types of pathogenic heat or fire causing this condition are Heart fire effulgence, non-interaction between the Heart and Kidneys, phlegm fire harassing the Heart, and Liver depression effulgent fire.

Pattern Differentiation
Heart Fire Effulgence

Primary symptoms: Frequent laughing without reason, wild or incoherent speech, feeling of happiness and excitement, joyful to everything

Additional symptoms: Overdressing, insomnia, frequent dreams with happy, colorful scenes, vexation and agitation, thirst with a desire for chilled drinks, sores in the mouth and on the tip of the tongue, hot, painful, urgent, and/or reddish urine, red facial complexion

Tongue: Red tongue with red dots or ulceration

Pulse: Rapid

Treatment principles: Clear the Heart and drain fire

Acupuncture treatment: HT-7, HT-8, HT-9, PC-8, SP-2, SP-6, ST-25, ST-40, ST-44, GB-8, GV-20

Herbal treatment:
Xie Xin Dao Chi San Jia Jian (Drain the Epigastrium and Guide Out the Red Decoction)
[Huang Lian 3–6g, Huang Qin 10g, Mu Tong 6–10g, Sheng Di 12g, Dan Zhu Ye 10g, Zhi Zi 10g, Deng Xin Cao 3g, Gan Cao Shao 10g, Lian Xin 2g]

Heart and Kidney Not Communicating

Primary symptoms: Frequent laughing without reason in a chronic situation, low energy, monologue, happiness, emaciation, dreams at night, frequent sexual dreams, prone to startling

Additional symptoms: Low back and knee soreness and limpness, insomnia, profuse dreams, vexatious 5-palm heat, afternoon tidal heat, night sweats, seminal emission, tinnitus, scanty yellow urine

Tongue: Red body, scanty coat

Pulse: Fine, rapid, floating, or surging

Treatment principles: Supplement the Kidneys and enrich Yin, clear the Heart and downbear fire

Acupuncture treatment: BL-15, BL-17, KI-3, KI-6, KI-7, HT-6, HT-7, PC-4, PC-6, SP-6, CV-14

Herbal treatment:
Huang Lian E Jiao Tang Jia Wei (Coptis and Ass Hide Gelatin Decoction Plus Modifications)
[Huang Lian 6g, Huang Qin 10g, E Jiao 10g, Bai Shao 10g, Ji Zi Huang 1pc, Shi Chang Pu 10g, Yuan Zhi 6–10g, Shu Di Huang 12–15g]

Modifications:
Insomnia with profuse dreams + Mu Li, Long Gu
Severe vexation and agitation + Lian Xin, Bai Zi Ren, Suan Zao Ren
Seminal emission + Huang Bai, Zhi Mu
Night sweats + Gui Ban, Shan Zhu Yu

Phlegm Fire Harassing Above

Primary symptoms: Frequent laughing without reason, drooling when laughing, profuse phlegm

Additional symptoms: Vexation and agitation, bitter taste in mouth, heart palpitations, impaired memory, and susceptibility to fright during sleep

Tongue: Slippery, yellow coat

Pulse: Slippery, rapid

Treatment principles: Flush phlegm and downbear fire, clear the Heart and quiet the spirit

Acupuncture treatment: ST-40, ST-44, GV-14, HT-7, GV-20

Herbal treatment:
Huang Lian Wen Dan Tang Jia Jian (Warm the Gallbladder Decoction with Coptis Plus Modifications)
[Ban Xia 10g, Che Pi 10g, Gan Cao 6g, Zhi Shi 10g, Zhu Ru 10g, Fu Ling 12g, Sheng Jiang 3g, Huang Qin 10g, Huang Lian 3–6g, Shi Chang Pu 6g]

Liver Depression–Effulgent Fire

Primary symptoms: Frequent laughing without reason, changeable moods, irritability, impatience, frequent nightmares

Additional symptoms: Disturbed sleep, chest and rib-side fullness and distension, red eyes

Tongue: Red

Pulse: Wiry (bowstring), rapid

Treatment principles: Course the Liver and rectify the Qi, clear heat and discharge fire

Acupuncture treatment: HT-7, PC-5, LR-2, GB-41, ST-44

Herbal treatment:
Xie Gan An Shen Tang (Drain the Liver and Calm the Spirit Decoction)
[Long Dan Cao 6–10g, Zhi Zi 10g, Chai Hu 6–10g, Huang Qin 10g, Huang Lian 3–6g, Sheng Di 12g, Dang Gui 10g, Gan Cao 3g]

Heart Qi Deficiency and Blood Stagnation

Primary symptoms: Laughing in chronic and frequent situations, monologue, spacing out

Additional symptoms: Weakness, lassitude, low or no motivation, palpitations, easily startled, head and body aches, low or no concentration, shortness of breath

Tongue: Purplish tongue, thin coat, purplish dots

Pulse: Wiry (bowstring), choppy

Treatment principles: Nourish the Heart Qi, move Blood, and dispel stasis

Acupuncture treatment: HT-5, HT-7, CV-14, CV-17, SP-4, SP-6, SP-10, GV-20, GV-24

Herbal treatment:
[Ren Shen 12g, Bai Zhu 12g, Fu Shen 9g, Dang Shen 12g, Gan Cao 5g, Shu Di Huang 15g, Dang Gui 9g, Bai Shao 9g, Chuan Xiong 9g, Bai Zi Ren 9g, Zhi Gan Cao 3g]

Anxiety and Thinking (Shan You Si)

This refers to a tendency to worry or of excessive thinking. Worry and anxiety, preoccupation, and obsessional thinking are the key symptoms of this disorder. Other factors in diagnosis include frequent emotional changes, improper emotional expression, the presence of a long-term emotional stimulant and/or stressor, or an acute emotional outburst.

Differential Diagnosis
Medical Disorders

- History of traumatic brain injury
- Infection or injury of CNS
- Tourette's disorder

- Neurologic disorders including Parkinson's disease and Huntington's disease

- History of cerebrovascular accident (CVA)

Psychiatric Disorders

- Obsessive–compulsive disorder (OCD)

- Obsessive–compulsive personality disorder

- Schizophrenia, catatonic subtype, other psychotic disorders

- Major depressive episode

- Specific or social phobias

Chinese Medical Etiology

Thinking is the emotional state associated with the Spleen organ system and the earth phase. Therefore, overthinking is said to damage the Spleen and "bind" the Qi. This binding inhibits the Spleen's Qi mechanism of transforming and transporting, and hinders the rising of the clear and refined Qi.

Pattern Differentiation
Spleen and Stomach Qi Deficiency

Primary symptoms: Overthinking all the time, no appetite, bloated abdomen after eating a small amount of food

Additional symptoms: Low energy and tired quickly, feeling sleepy but difficulty falling asleep, waking up frequently at night, loose stool, diarrhea, dizziness, vertigo, very heavy/weak feeling in extremities

Tongue: Pale tongue, very thin coat

Pulse: Deep, weak

Acupuncture treatment: SP-3, SP-6, ST-25, ST-40, ST-42, CV-6, CV-11, GB-8, GV-20

Herbal treatment:
[Huang Qi 12g, Ren Shen 9g, Bai Zhu 9g, Cang Zhu 9g, Chai Hu 9g, Fu Shen 12g, Yuan Zhi 9g, Da Zao 3pc, Gan Cao 5g]

Liver–Spleen Disharmony

Primary symptoms: Persistent anxiety and preoccupation, prone to obsession, moodiness, vexation, irritability, and being suspicious

Additional symptoms: Chest oppression, breast/rib-side distention, poor appetite, loose stools, possible painful diarrhea, insomnia, menstrual irregularities and PMS

Tongue: Pale, fat, may also be somewhat dark or dull in color

Pulse: Wiry (bowstring)

Treatment principles: Course the Liver and rectify the Qi, fortify the Spleen and boost the Qi

Acupuncture treatment: LR-3, LR-13, LR-14, SP-4, SP-13, ST-25, ST-36, ST-40, CV-12

Herbal treatment:
Si Ni San Jia Wei (Frigid Extremities Decoction Plus Modifications)
[Chai Hu 10g, Bai Shao 10g, Bo He 6g, Mei Gua Hua 6g, Xiang Fu 6–10g, Bai Zhu 10g, Dang Shen 10g, Gan Cao 6g]

Heart–Spleen Dual Deficiency

Primary symptoms: Persistent anxiety and preoccupation, obsessional thinking, poor memory, no concentration

Additional symptoms: Shortness of breath, disinclination to talk, lassitude of the spirit, heart palpitations, insomnia, waking up frequently, anxiety dreams at night, sensitive to sounds, lights, and emotional stimulants, torpid intake, loose stools, sallow yellow or pale white facial complexion, pale lips and nails

Tongue: Pale, fat tongue; thin coat

Pulse: Fine, weak, deep

Treatment principles: Fortify the Spleen and boost Qi, nourish the Heart and relieve anxiety

Acupuncture treatment: BL-15, BL-20, SP-3, SP-4, SP-6, HT-3, CV-6, CV-11, CV-14, CV-17, GV-20

Herbal treatment:
Gui Pi Tang Jia Jian (Restore the Spleen Decoction Plus Modifications)
[Bai Zhu 10g, Fu Shen 10g, Huang Qi 10–15g, Suan Zao Ren 12g, Yuan Zhi 6–10g, Mu Xiang 6–10g, Dang Gui 10g, Dang Shen 10g, Yu Jin 10g]

Modifications:
Insomnia + He Huan Pi, Bai Zi Ren
Severe Heart Blood deficiency + Bai Shao, E Jiao, Bai Zi Ren
Epigastric distension and nausea due to phlegm-damp + Ban Xia, Chen Pi, Zhi Ke

Lung–Spleen Qi Deficiency

Primary symptoms: Anxiety and preoccupation, moodiness, sorrow, a desire to cry, lassitude of the spirit

Additional symptoms: Fatigue, chest oppression, shortness of breath, faint voice, sweating on slight exertion, possible persistent weak cough provoked by talking or exertion, cold hands and feet, loose stools, torpid intake

Tongue: Pale, fat tongue; thin coat

Pulse: Fine, weak

Treatment principles: Fortify the Spleen and boost the Qi, supplement the Lungs and relieve anxiety

Acupuncture treatment: BL-13, BL-43, CV-4, CV-6, ST-36

Herbal treatment:
Bu Fei Tang (Restore the Lung Decoction)
[Dang Shen 10g, Huang Qi 10–15g, Shu Di 12g, Wu Wei Zi 10g, Zi Wan 10g, Bai Zhu 10g, Chen Pi 3g, Gan Cao 3–6g]

Modifications:
Loose stools or diarrhea with poor appetite + Fu Ling
Food stagnation with loss of appetite, abdominal distension, loss of taste + Mai Ya, Shen Qu, Shan Zha
Spontaneous perspiration + Fu Xiao Mai, Ma Huang Gen

Frequent Sorrow (Shan Bei)

This refers to uncontrollable low spirits and a tendency toward grieving, melancholy, and crying or a desire to cry. It may be marked by frequent emotional changes, improper emotional expression, a long-term emotional stimulant and/or stressor, or an acute emotional outburst.

Chinese Medical Etiology

Sorrow is the affect or emotion associated with the Lung organ system and the metal phase. Tears are considered the fluid of the Liver. As such, Chinese medicine attributes the causes of sorrow, grief, melancholy, and crying to these two organs. If, due to any reason, the Lungs become deficient, they may lose control over their functions, including the production and control of sorrow.

Internally generated heat flaring upward may also disturb the Lungs and cause sorrow and crying. This is most commonly depressive heat, and can be complicated by Lung Qi and/or Heart Blood deficiency due to a concomitant Spleen Qi deficiency.

Pattern Differentiation
Heart–Lung Deficiency

Primary symptoms: Grief with a tendency to crying, heart palpitations, shortness of breath, fatigue

Additional symptoms: Possibly an enduring, weak cough commonly provoked by exertion or talking, runny nose with clear, watery snivel, a tendency to catch a cold, faint voice, sweating on slight exertion

Tongue: Pale tongue, thin coat

Pulse: Fine, weak

Treatment principles: Supplement the Heart and Lung Qi

Acupuncture treatment: PC-7, PC-5, BL-13, BL-15, BL-20, BL-42. Alternate using BL-15 and BL-20 each treatment

Herbal treatment:
Bu Fei Tang Jia Jian (Restore the Lung Formula Plus Modifications)
[Ren Shen 6–12g, Huang Qi 10–15g, Shu Di 12g, Wu Wei Zi 10g, Bai Zi Ren 12g, Suan Zao Ren 12g, Fu Shen 12g, Gan Cao 6–10g]

Modifications:
Profuse sweating + Fu Xiao Mai, Bai Zhu
Borborygmus, torpid intake, and loose stools + Bai Zhu, Chen Pi

Liver Fire Invading the Lungs

Primary symptoms: Frequent sorrow and susceptibility to crying alternating with irritability, generally acute onset, suspicious of everything, taciturnity

Additional symptoms: Eructation, chest and rib-side pain and distension, frequent sighing, shortness of breath, coughing, depression, head and body aches, no appetite, insomnia, PMS, bitter taste in mouth

Tongue: Dark or reddish tongue, white, yellow, or dryish coat

Pulse: Wiry (bowstring), rapid

Treatment principles: Course the Liver and resolve depression, clear the Lungs and drain fire

Acupuncture treatment: LR-2, LR-3, LR-14, BL-18, BL-13, LU-1, LU-5, LU-7, BL-42, BL-47, CV-17, GV-20

Herbal treatment:
Si Ni San Jia Jian (Frigid Extremities Powder Plus Modifications)

[Chai Hu 10g, Zhi Ke 10g, Bai Shao 10g, Qing Pi 6g, Zhi Zi 6–10g, Huang Qin 10g, Bo He 6g, Jie Geng 10g, Xing Ren 6–10g, He Huan Pi 10g, Yu Jin 6g, Gan Cao 10g]

Modifications:
Concomitant Spleen deficiency: May use Xiao Chai Hu Tang Jia Wei (Minor Bupleurum Decoction Plus Modifications)
[Chai Hu 10g, Dang Shen 10g, Huang Qin 10g, Yuan Zhi 6–10g, Wu Wei Zi 6–10g, Gan Cao 6g, Ban Xia 10g, Da Zao 3–5pc, Sheng Jiang 3g]

Heart Deficiency–Lung Heat

Primary symptoms: Grief and crying for no reason, melancholy, mental abstraction, heart vexation

Additional symptoms: Insomnia, flushed red facial complexion, heat and sweating in palms and feet

Tongue: Red tongue, scanty coat

Pulse: Wiry (bowstring), fine, rapid

Treatment principles: Nourish Yin and downbear fire, supplement the Heart and quiet the spirit

Acupuncture treatment: KI-3, HT-6, PC-6, SP-6, BL-15, BL-23, BL-43

Herbal treatment:
Gan Mai Da Zao Tang Jia Wei (Licorice, Wheat, and Jujube Decoction Plus Modifications)
[Gan Cao 10–15g, Xiao Mai 20–45g, Da Zao 6pc, Tian Dong 12g, Mai Dong 12g, Bai Shao 10g, Bai He 10g, Fu Shen 12g, Huang Qin 10g, He Huan Hua 10–15g, Suan Zao Ren 12g]

Lung and Spleen Qi Deficiency

Primary symptoms: Feeling of sad mood constantly, depression, crying often and tearing is more often, vulnerable emotion

Additional symptoms: Chest tightness and oppression, low voice and cough, low appetite, losing weight, low energy, staying alone

Tongue: Pale tongue, thin coat

Pulse: Thin, weak

Acupuncture treatment: LU-1, LU-3, LU-5, LU-9, SP-3, SP-6, CV-6, CV-17, GV-20

Herbal treatment:

Bu Zhong Yi Qi Wan Gan Mai Da Zao Tang (Tonify the Middle and Augment the Qi Decoction with Licorice, Wheat, and Jujube Decoction)

[Huang Qi 20g, Bai Zhu 12g, Ren Shen 12g, Dang Gui 9g, Chen Pi 9g, Sheng Ma 6g, Chai Hu 9g, Zhi Gan Cao 5g, Da Zao 9g, Fu Xiao Mai 9g, Gan Cao 9g]

Susceptibility to Fear and Fright (Shan Kong, Shan Jing)

Susceptibility to fear (Shan Kong) refers to an emotional state of anticipation of the feeling of danger or discomfort that is often not founded or is unreasonable. It is the fear of something which is not currently present but which causes fear about the future, as in paranoia. Susceptibility to fright (Shan Jing) is an emotional state of becoming easily startled or frightened by minor occurrences or even nothing at all.

Western Psychiatric Conditions Associated with Fear and Fright

Susceptibility to fear:

- Generalized anxiety

- Agoraphobia

- Psychosis with anxiety

- Adjustment disorder with anxiety

- Specific social phobias

Susceptibility to fright:

- Panic attacks, triggered

- Panic disorder, triggered

- Post-traumatic stress disorder (PTSD)

- Phobias with panic symptoms

Differential Diagnosis
Medical Disorders

- Neurologic disorders

- Endocrine disorders

- Toxic exposure

- Other medical disorders

Effects of Substances

- Alcohol and illicit substance intoxication or withdrawal
- Side effects or discontinuation effects on medication

Psychiatric Disorders

- Panic disorder with or without agoraphobia
- Social phobia
- Specific phobias
- Post-traumatic stress disorder (PTSD)
- Generalized anxiety disorder (GAD)
- Schizophrenia and other psychotic disorders
- Personality disorders

Chinese Medical Etiology

Fear and fright are the affects associated with the Kidney organ system and the water phase. Therefore, Kidney deficiency can manifest as a susceptibility to fear. Prenatal (pre-heaven) Essence insufficiency, immaturity or aging, enduring disease, overtaxation, unrestrained sexual activity, and overuse of certain medicines and drugs can consume the Jing and cause insufficiency, resulting in fear. With susceptibility to fright there is an exaggerated startle reflex. This startling is considered a type of unsettled movement of Qi or wind.

Pattern Differentiation
Kidney Essence Insufficiency

Primary symptoms: Susceptibility to fear, heart palpitations

Additional symptoms: Low back and knee soreness and limpness, lassitude of the spirit, dizziness, tinnitus, feeling like head is empty, heart vexation, reduced sleep, seminal emission, night sweats, may have long disease history

Tongue: Red tongue, scanty coat

Pulse: Fine, weak

Treatment principles: Supplement the Kidneys, fill the essence, and fortify the mind

Acupuncture treatment: BL-15, BL-23, BL-52, KI-3, KI-7, KI-9, KI-27, CV-4, CV-6, CV-7, CV-21, LU-9, SP-6, GV-20

Herbal treatment:
Liu Wei Di Huang Wan Jia Wei (Six Ingredient Pill with Rehmannia Pill Plus

Modifications)

[Shu Di 15g, Shan Zhu Yu 12g, Shan Yao 12g, Fu Ling 10g, Ze Xie 6g, Dan Pi 10g, Yuan Zhi 10g, Gui Qi Zi 10g, Mai Dong 10g, Wu Wei Zi 10g]

Modifications:

Severe night sweats, insomnia, profuse dreams + Suan Zao Ren, Bai Zi Ren

Kidney Yang deficiency with impotence, seminal emission, and chilled limbs + Lu Jiao, Rou Gui

Qi and Blood Deficiency

Primary symptoms: Intermittent susceptibility to fear

Additional symptoms: Heart palpitations, shortness of breath, pale white facial complexion, pale lips and nails, fatigue, lack of strength, aversion to wind, spontaneous perspiration

Tongue: Pale tongue, thin coat

Pulse: Fine, weak

Treatment principles: Supplement the Qi, nourish the Blood, and quiet the spirit

Acupuncture treatment: HT-7, SP-6, SP-10, ST-36, KI-3, KI-7, BL-15, BL-17, CV-4, CV-6, CV-17, GV-20

Herbal treatment:

Ba Zhen Tang Jia Wei (Eight Gentlemen Decoction Plus Modifications)

[Dang Shen 10g, Bai Zhu 10g, Fu Ling 10g, Shu Di 12g, Bai Shao 10g, Dang Gui 10g, Chuan Xiong 6–10g, Shi Chang Pu 6g, Yuan Zhi 6g, Gan Cao 5g, Long Yan Rou 6g, Gou Qi Zi 5g]

Modifications:

Insomnia: + Suan Zao Ren, Fu Shen

Spontaneous sweating: + Huang Qi, Fu Xiao Mai

Heart–Gallbladder Qi Deficiency

Primary symptoms: Timidity, paranoia, susceptibility to fear and fright, indecisiveness when decision making is needed, inability to control oneself, prone to being startled

Additional symptoms: Dislike of meeting people or dating, sensitive to some sounds and light, headache, rib-side discomfort, heart palpitations, possible heart vexation and/or insomnia, profuse dreams, possible profuse phlegm and/or plum pit Qi, low appetite, menstrual disorders

Tongue: Pale tongue, thin coat

Pulse: Slightly bowstring, weak, possibly slippery or soft

Treatment principles: Supplement the Qi, nourish the Heart, and quiet the Gallbladder

Acupuncture treatment: GV-24, GB-8, GB-13, GB-35, GB-40, LR-3, LR-8, LR-13, LR-14, CV-4

Herbal treatment:
Shi Wei Wen Dan Tang (Ten Ingredient Formula to Warm the Gallbladder) [Dang Shen 10g, Fu Ling 10g, Zhi Gan Cao 3–10g, Chen Pi 6g, Ban Xia 10g, Yuan Zhi 10g, Suan Zao Ren 12g, Zhi Shi 6g, Shu Di 12g, Wu Wei Zi 10g]

Liver Depression Blood Deficiency

Primary symptoms: Susceptibility to fright, irritability, vexation and agitation

Additional symptoms: Breast, chest, abdominal, and rib-side distension and fullness especially during premenstrual period, dizziness, headache, moodiness, pale white facial complexion and pale nails, scanty, delayed, or blocked menstruation

Tongue: Pale tongue, thin coat

Pulse: Fine, wiry (bowstring)

Treatment principles: Course the Liver and rectify the Qi, nourish the Blood and quiet the spirit

Acupuncture treatment: PC-7, PC-6, LR-3, LR-14, ST-36

Herbal treatment:
Xiao Yao San (Rambling Powder)
[Chai Hu 10g, Dang Gui 10g, Bao Shao 10g, Bai Zhu 10g, Fu Ling 10g, Gan Cao 6g, Bo He 3–6g, Sheng Jiang 3g, Da Zao 3pc, Long Gu 12g, Mu Li 12g]

Modifications:
Severe Blood deficiency: + Shu Di
Liver depression transforming into fire with dryness, red eyes, and severe susceptibility to fright: − Bo He, Sheng Jiang; + Zhi Zi, Dan Pi
Severe breast or rib-side distenstion and pain: + Chuan Lian Zi, Yan Hu Suo

Liver Blood–Kidney Yin Deficiency

Primary symptoms: Susceptibility to fright, vexation, reduced sleep

Additional symptoms: Pale white facial complexion, dizziness, lower back pain, afternoon tidal heat, night sweats, 5-palm heat

Tongue: Red or pale tongue, red tip

Pulse: Fine, wiry (bowstring), possibly rapid

Treatment principles: Nourish the Blood and enrich Yin, quiet the spirit and relieve fright

Acupuncture treatment: HT-6, BL-15, BL-17, BL-18, SP-6, KI-3

Herbal treatment:
Gui Shao Di Huang Tang Jia Jian (Rehmannia Decoction with Tanguei and Peony Plus Modifications)
[Dang Gui 10g, Bao Shao 10g, Shu Di 12g, Shan Yao 10g, Fu Shen 10g, Sha Zhu Yu 10g, Ze Xie 6g, Dan Pi 6–10g, Suan Zao Ren 12g, Bai Zi Ren 12g]

Modifications:
Marked deficiency heat + Zhi Mu, Huang Bai

Phlegm Fire Harassing Upward

Primary symptoms: Susceptibility to fright, heart palpitations

Additional symptoms: Vertigo and dizziness, vexation, insomnia, headache, dryness and bitterness in the mouth, profuse commonly yellow phlegm

Tongue: Red tongue, slippery yellow coat

Pulse: Slippery, rapid

Treatment principles: Clear heat and transform phlegm, quiet the Heart and calm the spirit

Acupuncture treatment: PC-7, GB-41, CV-12, ST-40

Herbal treatment:
Huang Lian Wen Tang (Coptis Decoction to Warm the Gallbladder)
[Ban Xia 10g, Zhu Ru 10g, Zhi Shi 6g, Chen Pi 6–10g, Fu Ling 10g, Huang Lian 3–6g, Gan Cao 3g]

Modifications:
Concomitant Liver depression + Chai Hu, Chuan Lian Zi
Vomiting + Pi Pa Ye, increase Zhu Ru
Severe fright + Mu Li, Long Gu

Heart Fire

Primary symptoms: Susceptibility to fright, heart vexation

Additional symptoms: Flushed red facial complexion, red eyes, sores in the mouth and on tip of the tongue, preference for chilled drinks, disturbed sleep, difficult burning dark-colored urination

Tongue: Red tongue, thin yellow coat

Pulse: Rapid

Treatment principles: Clear the heat, discharge fire, and relieve fright

Acupuncture treatment: PC-8, SI-7, HT-7, KI-4

Herbal treatment:
Xie Xin Dao Chi San Jia Jian (Drain the Epigastrium and Guide Out the Red Decoction Plus Modifications)
[Mu Tong 5g, Sheng Di 12g, Huang Lian 6g, Zhu Ye 10g, Deng Xin Cao 3g, Lian Xin 3g, Long Chi 12g, Zhen Zhu Mu 12g, Gan Cao 6g]

Vexation and Agitation (Bu An Jing, You)

In Chinese medicine, vexation refers to an annoyance attributed to an oppressive heat in the chest. Agitation refers to a restlessness of the limbs. Vexation is a subjective symptom, while agitation is an objectively observable sign. The two, despite their differences, are generally considered one disease state as they often coexist and share etiologies.

Differential Diagnosis
Medical Disorders

- Parkinson's disease
- History of cerebrovascular accident
- Brain tumors
- Hyperthyroidism

Effects of Substances

- Alcohol or illicit substance intoxication or withdrawal
- Akathisia as a side effect of antipsychotic medications
- Side effects or discontinuation effects on medication

Psychiatric Disorders

- Generalized anxiety disorder
- Conversion disorder
- Depression and other mood disorders
- Bipolar disorder, manic phase
- Schizophrenia, psychotic disorders
- Post-traumatic stress disorder (PTSD)

- Social phobia and specific phobias
- Personality disorders

Pattern Differentiation
Exterior Cold–Depressed Heat

Primary symptoms: Vexation and agitation, generalized body pain, fever

Additional symptoms: Aversion to cold, no sweating, headache, slight thirst

Tongue: Thin, yellowish white coat

Pulse: Floating, tight, rapid

Treatment principles: Resolve the exterior and scatter cold, clear heat and eliminate vexation

Acupuncture treatment: HT-8, SI-7, BL-12, LI-4, LI-11

Herbal treatment:
Da Qing Long Tang Jia Jian (Major Blue-Green Dragon Decoction)
[Ma Huang 10g, Gui Zhi 6g, Gan Cao 6g, Xing Ren 10g, Shi Gao 25g, Sheng Jiang 3g, Da Zao 3pc, Dan Dou Chi 10g]

Yangming Excess Heat

Primary symptoms: Vexation and agitation, high fever, sweating, coarse breathing, thirst, constipation with dry bound stools

Additional symptoms: Abdominal fullness; pain in the abdomen exacerbated by pressure; in severe cases, delirium

Tongue: Dry yellow/dry black coat

Pulse: Surging, large/deep, excess

Treatment principles: Clear heat, engender fluids, and greatly precipitate heat binding

Acupuncture treatment: LI-4, ST-44, TW-6, ST-37, BL-21, KI-2. Draining technique

Herbal treatment:
Bai Hu Tang Jia Wei (White Tiger Decoction Plus Modifications)
[Shi Gao 25g, Zhi Mu 10g, Gan Cao 6g, Geng Mi 10g, Dan Dou Chi 10g, Zhi Zi 10g]

Gallbladder Depressed Fire

Primary symptoms: Vexation and agitation, alternating cold and heat

Additional symptoms: Chest and rib-side fullness and oppression, bitter taste in mouth, inhibited urination

Tongue: Normal or red tongue, half yellow, half white coat

Pulse: Wiry (bowstring), rapid

Treatment principles: Harmonize the Shaoyang, clear heat, and eliminate vexation

Acupuncture treatment: LR-14, GV-14, PC-5, GB-41

Herbal treatment:
Xiao Chai Hu Tang Jia Jian (Minor Bupleurum Decoction Plus Modifications) [Chai Hu 12g, Huang Qin 10g, Dang Shen 10g, Ban Xia 10g, Zhi Gan Cao 6g, Qing Hao 10g, Zhi Zi 10g, Long Gu 12g, Mu Li 12g, Sheng Jiang 5g]

Heat Entering the Nutritive and Blood Levels

Primary symptoms: Vexation and agitation, insomnia, fever which is worse at night, mania in severe cases

Additional symptoms: Macules or eruptions on the skin, blood ejection (hemetemesis, epistaxis, hematuria, hemafecia, etc.)

Tongue: Crimson

Pulse: Fine, rapid

Treatment principles: Clear heat, cool the Blood, and eliminate vexation

Acupuncture treatment: HT-8, PC-8, BL-40 (bleed), LI-11, KI-1

Herbal treatment:
Qing Ying Tang Jia Jian (Clear the Nutritive Level Decoction Plus Modifications) [Shui Niu Jiao 25g, Sheng Di 12g, Xuan Shen 10–15g, Zhu Ye 10g, Mai Dong 12g, Dan Pi 10g, Dan Shen 10g, Huang Lian 6g, Jin Yin Hua 10–12g, Lian Qiao 10–12g]

Modifications:
Severe skin eruptions or blood ejection: − Jin Yin Hua, Lian Qiao; + Zhi Zi, Chi Shao; increase Sheng Di to 20g

Diaphragm Heat

Primary symptoms: Deficiency vexation

Additional symptoms: Insomnia, burning sensation in the region of the heart, chest and diaphragm glomus and oppression with a desire to vomit

Tongue: Thin yellow coat

Pulse: Rapid

Treatment principles: Clear the diaphragm and eliminate vexation

Acupuncture treatment: LI-5, ST-44, BL-17, HT-8, PC-3

Herbal treatment:
Zhi Zi Dou Chi Tang Jia Wei (Gardenia and Prepared Soybean Decoction Plus Modifications)
[Zhi Zi 10g, Dan Dou Chi 10g, Bo He 6g, Gan Cao 3g]

Modifications:
Severe internal heat: + Shi Gao

Phlegm Fire Harassing Above

Primary symptoms: Vexatious heat in the heart and agitation, sound of phlegm in the throat, spitting sticky thick phlegm

Additional symptoms: Dyspnea, heavy-headedness, vertigo, chest oppression, abdominal distension, nausea, vomiting

Tongue: Slippery yellow coat

Pulse: Slippery, rapid

Treatment principles: Clear heat, transform phlegm, and eliminate vexation

Acupuncture treatment: PC-8, ST-44, LI-11, GV-14, ST-40

Herbal treatment:
Huang Lian Wen Dan Tang Jia Jian (Warm the Gallbladder Decoction with Coptis Plus Modifications)
[Ban Xia 10g, Zhu Ru 10g, Zhi Shi 6g, Chen Pi 10g, Gan Cao 3g, Fu Ling 10g, Sheng Jiang 3g, Da Zao 3pc, Huang Lian 6g, Huang Qin 10g]

Liver Depression Creating Heat

Primary symptoms: Irritability

Additional symptoms: Bitter taste in mouth, rib-side distension and pain, breast distension and pain, menstrual irregularity in females

Tongue: Red tongue, yellow coat

Pulse: Wiry (bowstring), rapid

Treatment principles: Course the Liver and rectify the Qi, clear heat and resolve depression

Acupuncture treatment: LR-2, LR-3, LI-4, LI-11, ST-36

Herbal treatment:
Dan Zhi Xiao Yao San (Augmented Rambling Powder)
[Chai Hu 10g, Bai Shao 10g, Dang Gui 10g, Bai Zhu 10g, Fu Ling 10g, Dan Pi 10g, Zhi Zi 10g, Gan Cao 6g]

Heart Fire Flaring

Primary symptoms: Vexation and agitation, heart palpitations

Additional symptoms: Insomnia, urgent, choppy, painful urination, sores in the mouth and tip of tongue

Tongue: Red or red-tipped tongue

Pulse: Wiry (bowstring), rapid

Treatment principles: Clear the Heart and downbear fire, disinhibit urination and quiet the spirit

Acupuncture treatment: PC-8, HT-8, CV-4, ST-39, SI-2

Herbal treatment:
Dao Chi San Jia Wei (Guide Out the Red Powder Plus Modifications)
[Sheng Di 12g, Mu Tong 10g, Deng Xin Cao 10g, Huang Lian 6g, Zhu Ye 6g, Gan Cao 6g, Hu Po 1g]

Modifications:
Hematuria: + Huan Lian Cao, Xiao Ji
Simultaneous Yin deficiency: + Shi Hu, Zhi Mu

Yin Deficiency with Deficiency Heat

Primary symptoms: Deficiency vexation and agitation, insomnia, heart palpitations, profuse dreams

Additional symptoms: Low back/knee soreness/limpness, 5-palm heat, afternoon tidal heat, malar flushing, dry throat/mouth

Tongue: Red tongue, scanty coat

Pulse: Fine rapid, floating rapid, or surging rapid

Treatment principles: Nourish Yin, downbear fire, and eliminate vexation

Acupuncture treatment: HT-6, KI-7, KI-2, KI-3, ST-41

Herbal treatment:
Predominant effulgent fire: Use Huang Lian E Jiao Tang (Coptis and Ass Hide

Gelatin Decoction)

Predominant Yin deficiency: Use Zhi Bai Di Huang Wan (Anemarrhena, Phellodendron, and Rehmannia Decoction)

Heat and Stasis Mutually Binding

Primary symptoms: Vexation and agitation, chest, breast, or abdominal pain which is severe, fixed in location, worse at night, and associated with feelings of burning heat

Additional symptoms: Spider nevi, reddish purple lips and facial complexion, hemagiomas and varicosities, abnormal vaginal bleeding in females with clots mixed in with bright red blood

Tongue: Reddish purple tongue with static spots or macules, possible yellow coat

Pulse: Wiry (bowstring), rapid, possibly choppy

Treatment principles: Quicken the Blood and transform stasis, clear heat and eliminate vexation

Acupuncture treatment: SP-10, SP-6, BL-17, HT-7, PC-6

Herbal treatment:

Qin Lian Si Wu Tang Jia Wei (Four Substance Decoction with Scute and Coptis Plus Modifications)

[Huang Qin 10g, Huang Lian 3–4.5g, Tao Ren 10g, Hong Hua 10g, Dang Gui 10g, Sheng Di 12g, Chuan Xiong 6–10g, Chi Shao 10g, Chuan Niu Xi 10g, Dan Shen 10g, Chai Hu 6–10g, Zhi Ke 6g, Gan Cao 3g]

Yin Deficiency Heat Affecting Yang

Primary symptoms: Red facial complexion as if rouged, no aversion to cold, chilly breath, faint respiration, symptoms similar to mania, vexation and agitation, restlessness

Additional symptoms: Desire to sit in water or in a Yin, cool place, reversal chilling of the four limbs, long clear urination, loose stools with undigested food, oral thirst but no desire to drink or possible liking for hot drinks

Tongue: Dark pale tongue, moist glossy coat

Pulse: Deep, fine

Treatment principles: Break Yin and rescue Yang, stem counterflow and scatter cold

Acupuncture treatment: ST-36, CV-8, CV-4. Moxa

Herbal treatment:

Tong Mai Si Ni Tang (Unblock the Pulse Decoction for Frigid Extremities)
[Fu Zi 10g, Gan Jiang 4.5g, Gan Cao 6g]

Use of Luo Vessels in Emotional Lability

Use Yin Luo points to work on a person's level of "armoring" being affected:
Moods (Wei-Qi level)—LU-7 and LR-5
Suppression (Ying-Qi level)—PC-6 and SP-4
Repression (Yuan-Qi level)—KI-4 and TW-5
Plum blossom these points (those for the appropriate level) in an infinity pattern—start with side of body with the dominant symptoms. If unsure what level the person is at, do *all* levels (mood, suppression, and repression). In brain injury cases, any of these levels may be affected. If there is significant psychological trauma as well, then suppression and repression may be more of a concern.

Use Yang Luo points for a patient's emotional disposition, tonifying the Yuan-source point of the organ's Yin-paired meridian first:
Anger = GB-37 + LR-3
Anxiety = SI-7 + HT-7
Obsession = ST-40 + SP-3
Grief/depression = LI-6 + LU-9
Fear = BL-58 + KI-3

Chapter 45

Substance Abuse

Substance abuse, both pre- and postinjury, is a very significant factor that requires assessment and appropriate treatment if present. In the United States alcoholism is estimated to affect 15 percent of the general population, while drug addiction ranges from 9 to 20 percent. In medical populations substance abuse numbers increase to between 25 and 50 percent, while those with psychiatric disorders climb to an incredible 50–75 percent. Treatment populations are disproportionally male, made up of 75 percent male to 25 percent female. Average ages for treatment are 30–35 years in males and 25–30 years in females. Two-thirds of TBIs involve motor vehicle accidents. Fifty percent of fatal motor vehicle accidents in the US are associated with drugs or alcohol. Individuals with a brain injury may become addicted to medications such as opioids or turn to illicit drugs/alcohol as a means of self-medicating or attempting to deal with feelings of depression, anxiety, or social isolation.

According to Silver, if alcohol or drug addiction (or both) are implicated in a brain injury, it has likely been a problem that preceded or led up to an injury.[1] History of substance abuse has been associated with poorer neuropsychological outcomes, greater likelihood of repeat injuries, and higher risk of late deterioration.[2] Frequent complications that may arise include drug–drug interactions, drug overdose, increased sensitivity to medication effects, and increased seizure risk. Cognitive and emotional aspects may also be affected, including increased lack of behavioral control, hallucinations, delusions, anxiety, or depression. This is especially true in relation to drug seeking or withdrawal symptoms. Differentiation between symptomology may become difficult as lethargy, agitation, confusion, disorientation, and respiratory depression after intoxication or overdose are similar to symptoms that may follow a brain injury.

Alcohol and other depressant drugs can cause depression and suicidal and homicidal thinking during intoxication. Anxiety, hyperactivity, hallucinations, and/or delusions can

---

1   Silver, Jonathan, Yudofsky, Stuart, and McAllister, Thomas. *Textbook of Traumatic Brain Injury.* Washington, DC: American Psychiatric Pub. 2011. Print.

2   Corrigan, J. Substance abuse as a mediating factor in outcome from traumatic brain injury. *Archives of Physical Medicine and Rehabilitation.* 1995 Apr; 76(4): 302–309.

arise during withdrawal. Stimulant drugs can cause anxiety, hallucinations, and delusions during intoxication while possibly eliciting depression and suicidal thinking during withdrawal. The compounded effects of a brain injury and substance abuse may be additive in nature. Hemodynamic depression, blood–brain barrier disruption, and changes in homeostasis are additional factors if intoxication is present at the time of injury. Those hospitalized as a result of brain injury and who are alcohol or drug users tend to have a longer period of hospitalization. Symptoms of agitation have also been shown to be longer lasting. Those who were intoxicated before sustaining an injury have been shown to have a lower global cognitive score at the time of hospital discharge than those not intoxicated. It is also possible that cognitive deficits such as inattention and poor concentration, short-term memory, and information processing speed may be further adversely affected.

Tobacco smoking tends to prevent the immune system from working properly and increases susceptibility to disease. In addition, a burning cigarette transmits a large amount of reactive molecules (called free radicals) that can bind and destroy cells within the body. Cigarette smoking has been implicated in causing or worsening depression, high blood pressure, osteoporosis, arthritis, and heart disease, acting as a stimulant to the heart and the nervous system. Withdrawal from nicotine includes symptoms such as restlessness, constipation, sweating, headaches, irritability, hunger, and inability to concentrate. Interestingly, a study on rat models showed that intermittent administration of nicotine attenuated cognitive deficits related to nicotinic cholinergic receptor dysfunction following a brain injury.[3] Chronic nicotine use, however, is associated with degeneration of one half of the fasciculus retroflexus which affects emotional control, sexual arousal, REM sleep, and seizure activity.[4] Smokers who have sustained a mild brain injury have been shown to have lessened improvement in processing speed, visuospatial learning and memory, visuospatial skills, and global neurocognition compared to non-smokers.[5]

Chronic exposure to alcohol or drugs has been shown to result in changes to limbic pathways. Homeostatic states seem to be affected whereby a new set point, known as alleostasis, may be responsible for intense cravings. Alcohol-induced atrophy of the limbic, cerebellar, and frontal structures has been shown through neuroimaging. Those with a combination of both brain injury and substance dependence showed greater degrees of atrophic changes than each condition on their own. GABA may be downregulated, while N-methyl-D-aspartate may be upregulated due to chronic alcohol exposure.

3   Verbois, S.L., Hopkins, D.M., Scheff, S.W., and Pauly, J.R. Chronic intermittent nicotine administration attenuates traumatic brain injury-induced cognitive dysfunction. *Neuroscience.* 2003 Jul 16; 19(4): 1199–1208. doi:10.1016/ S0306-4522(03)00206-9

4   University of California, Los Angeles. Nicotine causes selective degeneration in brain, UCLA neuroscientists report. *ScienceDaily.* 2000 Nov 13. www.sciencedaily.com/releases/2000/11/001110073314.htm

5   Duazzo, T., Abadjian, L., Kincaid, A. *et al.* The influence of chronic cigarette smoking on neurocognitive recovery after mild traumatic brain injury. *Journal of Neurotrauma.* 2013 Jun 1; 30(11): 1013–1022. doi:10.1089/ neu.2012.2676

Diagnosis

- Preoccupation with acquiring alcohol or drugs

- Compulsive use of drugs despite adverse consequences

- Pattern of relapse or inability to cut down despite adverse consequences

- Three of the following occurring at any time in the same 12-month period:

  ◦ Tolerance

  ◦ Withdrawal

  ◦ Substance taken in larger amounts or longer period than intended

  ◦ Persistent desire or unsuccessful attempts to cut down or control use

  ◦ Significant time spent in substance acquisition, use, or recovering from effects

  ◦ Reduction or halting of important social, occupational, or recreational activities

  ◦ Use is continued despite awareness of having a persistent physical or psychological problem likely caused or exacerbated by the substance

- Screening: Brief Michigan Alcohol Screening Test (Brief MAST), CAGE questionnaire

- Family history is best predictor for onset of alcoholism and drug addiction

Biomedical Approaches

- Benzodiazepines (alchohol, sedative withdrawal—those with a shorter half life such as lorazepam)

- Opioid agonists ("anti-craving"): Naltrexone, acamprosate (alcohol)

- Disulfiram (alcohol—causes distressing side effects when alcohol is consumed including nausea, vomiting, and headache)

- Diazepam (benzodiazepine withdrawal)

- Phenobarbital (sedative withdrawal)

- Clonidine (opiates)

- Methadone (opiates)

- Abstinence

- Confrontation of denial

- Support groups/12-step programs (e.g. Alchoholics Anonymous, Narcotics Anonymous)

- Group therapy

Note: Individuals with a brain injury seem to have reduced tolerance to a wide variety of medications, particularly sedatives, and doses are often reduced to allow for the increased sensitivity.

Chinese Medical Perspective
Chinese Medical Etiology

Drug dependence may be physiological—the state of adapting to a drug associated with the development of tolerance and clinically seen by a withdrawal or abstinence syndrome; or psychological—feelings of contentment while on the drug, therefore creating a strong desire to experience repeated drug administrations to achieve pleasure or avoid pain. The phenomenon, therefore, may be metabolically or psychologically based.

Acupuncture Treatment for Substance Abuse
Auricular Points

- NADA protocol: Sympathetic, Shenmen, Liver, Kidney, Lung/Heart

- Smoking: Sweetbreath—midway between LU-7 and LI-5

13 Ghost Points

The 13 ghost points may be used in cases of addiction in accordance to the teachings of Jeffrey Yuen, as the use of substances over time overtakes the clarity of the Shen and gradually depletes the body's Yin resources.[6]

1st Trinity

Involves an initial build-up of phlegm and the beginnings of psychological dysfunction and disorientation with the world; used mainly for heat and wind conditions and may involve a sore throat.

> *GV-26* (Ghost Palace): Said to affect one's genetic predispositions and sense of humanity. Used for inappropriate, spontaneous laughter or crying, fatigue, and/or epilepsy

> *LU-11* (Ghost Faith): Said to attend to worldly affairs and undertakings. Used for epilepsy, sore throat, clearing heat in the channel

---

6   Isabella III, N. and Ma, T. 13 ghost points. Web. www.point-to-point-acupuncture.com/files/13_GHOST_POINTS.pdf. Retrieved 2017, Oct 17.

SP-1 (Eye of the Ghost): Associated with the Earth phase and one's body. Used for feelings of disorientation within the world, epilepsy, and resuscitation

2nd Trinity

Involves life attitudes that become less flexible—becoming set in one's ways, not having a decisive direction. Wind can become an issue with uncontrollable movements or paralysis.

PC-7 (Ghost Heart): Earth point on fire meridian: an intense craving for material possessions, dampness and phlegm harassing the Heart, alternating and frequent laughing/crying, irritability

BL-62 (Ghost Path): Opening point for Yang Qiao Mai to address how one walks into the world and one's constitution. Begins to believe the same thing and walk the same path as the "ghost." Used for epilepsy, paralysis, headache

GV-16 (Ghost Pillow): Addresses one's flexibility and ability to adapt to change. The "ghost" is able to access the brain. Used for "ghost ridged tongue," lockjaw, loss of voice, headache

3rd Trinity

The level where many addicts get stuck at by using substances to try to instill fire.

ST-6 (Ghost Bed): The ability to look at suffering and not ignore it. Located at the jaw—lockjaw, mouth deviation, trigeminal neuralgia. Addresses the ability to "chew" the world. The person has become fully possessed by the "ghost"

CV-24 (Ghost Market): Deals with one's ability to appreciate one's own resources/Yin. The "ghost" has begun to absorb and consume Yin resources, causing wasting disease and emaciation. Dark urine and nosebleeds occur in the body's attempt to rid the body of the "ghost"

PC-8 (Ghost Cave): Deals with acknowledging one's true passion in life. Paranoia can develop due to not having a firm self-image or not embracing Yin resources. Self-destructiveness may occur. Fevers, sweating, and heat in the Blood level

4th Trinity

GV-23 (Ghost Hall): Involves the ability to embrace one's self. The "ghost" has taken over. Phlegm begins to significantly block the collaterals. Severe nasal congestion, poor vision, dizzy spells, Alzheimer's disease

CV-1 (Ghost Store): Also relates to the ability to embrace one's self. The Yin becomes fully consumed. Urinary/defecation blockage or incontinence, menstrual issues, prolapse

LI-11 (Ghost Leg): Pertains to the world as a reflection of the self, being responsible for one's own emotions, outlook, and role in society. There is no longer communication with the outside world. High fever, vomiting

Yintang

Used for chronic and acute childhood fright wind (epilepsy), fright spasm, insomnia, stress, and melancholia.

Other Treatment Considerations
Somatic Considerations

- Stress management and relaxation techniques such as visualization and meditation

- Counseling and support groups

- Regular exercise—at least 30 minutes three times per week, e.g. brisk walking, aerobics, swimming

- Saunas and steam baths

Orthomolecular Considerations

- A multivitamin can be taken daily

- Glutamine—500 to 1000mg four times per day between meals to reduce craving for nicotine and other drugs

- B-complex vitamins—25 to 50mg a day to help reduce stress and tiredness

- Vitamin C—1000mg four times a day for a week, then 1000mg twice a day

Phytotherapeutic Considerations
Alcohol:

- *Oats*: Help overcome habit

- *Cayenne*: Delirium tremens steadies patient, promotes sound sleep

- *Chamomile*: Sedative

- *White fringetree*: Gastrointestinal or hepatic disorders

- *Hops*: Delirium tremens, excitement—aids digestion

- *Goldenseal*: Helps to overcome cravings

- *Passion flower*: Insomnia; sedative

- *Skullcap*: Delirium tremens, nervine, insomnia, nightmares, restlessness

- *American ginseng*: Modulates effects of some drugs and protects against eurotoxicity

Drug withdrawal:

- *Oats*: Help overcome habit (alcohol, morphine, opium)

- *Panax ginseng*: Promotes detoxification, protects mood and

cognition, attenuates withdrawal symptoms

- *Chamomile*: Sedative

- *Skullcap*: Muscle twitchings

Smoking:

- *Lobelia*: Aids withdrawal symptoms (stimulates nicotinergic receptors), expectorant

- *Bitter-berry (Chokeberry)*: Sedative, quiets irritation of mucosa

- *Milk thistle*: Clears toxins

- *Valerian*: Reduces anxiety and irritability and aids relaxation

- *Sweetflag*: Nerve tonic, helps overcome habit

- *Fennel*: Helps expel mucous secretions

- *Catnip*: Nervous irritability

- *Passion flower*: Nervine, insomnia

- *Licorice root*: Irritations of mucosa

- *Skullcap*: Nervine

- *Kola-nut*: Depressive states, melancholia

- *Coltsfoot*: To substitute habit

Dietary Considerations
Alcohol Withdrawal

Eating principles: Once stabilized, a short alkaline fast is recommended but needs to be highly supervised. Good dietary habits are a must.

Therapeutic foods:

- Increase foods that cool the Blood, clear Heat, and soothe the Liver: beets and beet tops, bamboo shoots, spinach, banana, grapefruit, mulberry, persimmon, strawberry, white mushroom, apple, ginseng, white fungus

- Daikon radish, pear, mandarin orange, black soybeans, dandelion, burdock, chlorophyll, artichokes, garlic, onions

- Increase zinc-rich foods, magnesium-rich foods, foods with vitamins B1 and B6; in beginning detoxification, supply with enough fruit juices to get lift when needed and enough liquid

- Dandelion tea

Avoid:

- Cinnamon and other Heating foods, spicy foods, coffee (long term), sweets and sugary foods, high-fat diet, fried foods, candies, simple carbohydrates, fatty foods, rich foods, chocolate, nuts, smoking, stress, constipation, hot foods, chili, spicy foods

Smoking and Drug Detoxification

- All alcohol detoxification applies and fasting is recommended. For smoking detoxification, increase all foods rich in vitamin A

- An alkalinizing diet to reduce nicotine cravings is recommended

Additional Recommendations

- Create a deadline and decide on the date one begins to quit. This should be a time when there is minimal life stress and strain.

- Establish a new routine. Changing one's routine will help break up old habit patterns that are associated with substance use.

- Fill the time that used to be spent using a substance with other activities and associations. Examples may include hobbies, starting a diary, reading, sewing, gardening, remodeling, learning a new skill or craft, creative arts activities, listening to music, taking music lessons, joining clubs, taking classes, or other social activities.

- If any of the withdrawal symptoms are causing extreme discomfort or seem to be getting worse even though several days have passed since you started to quit, consider a medical examination.

- Nicotine: Quitting all at once has been shown to be a more successful strategy than just tapering down usage. Without cigarettes, the nicotine will clear out of the body in about 48 hours. This will help diminish cravings and give the body systems a chance to heal. Lobelia can be very helpful during this detoxification stage.

Chapter 46

Special Considerations in Pediatric and Adolescent Brain Injuries

According to the Centers for Disease Control and Prevention, traumatic brain injury is the leading cause of death and acquired disability of children and teens in the United States. The two largest at-risk groups are those 0–4 years and adolescents aged 15–19. In children aged 0–15, the estimated incidence of acquired brain injury is 738 per 100,000 children, with almost half a million emergency-room visits each year. Between 80 and 90 percent of these are considered mild, 7–8 percent are considered moderate, and 5–8 percent are considered severe, with the majority of lesions occurring in the dorsolateral frontal, orbitofrontal, and frontal lobe white matter.[1]

In those 0–4 years old, most cases are due to falls. These young children are, however, also more susceptible to abusive head trauma (AHT), previously known as "shaken baby syndrome" (SBS). Older children and teens are more likely to sustain a concussion as a result of sport injuries, falls, being struck by something, or motor vehicle accidents. Outcomes of recovery are dependent on many factors, including time of injury, the developmental state of the brain at the time of injury, and the extent of injury. Evidence shows that young children are just as, if not more, susceptible to the effects of a brain injury than older children. There is a higher incidence of diffuse injury and cerebral swelling (44%) compared to adults. This results in increased likelihood of cranial hypertension. Post-traumatic seizures are of particular relevance as well, as prevalence within the first week of injury is twice as likely

---

1   Lash, Marilyn. *The Essential Brain Injury Guide.* 5th ed. Vienna, VA: Academy of Certified Brain Injury Specialists, Brain Injury Association of America. 2016. Print.

(10% vs. 5%) to occur compared to adults.[2] The prognosis for acquiring new skills is worse the younger a child is at the time of injury.

New Psychiatric Disorders

There has been a recorded 54–63 percent incidence of new psychiatric disorders in children with severe TBI and a 10–21 percent incidence in children with mild or moderate TBI approximately two years after injury. Predictors of these developing include severity of the injury, preinjury psychiatric disorders, preinjury family function, family psychiatric history, socioeconomic status, preinjury intellectual function, and preinjury adaptive function. The most consistent of these was preinjury and postinjury family function, including family burden and family distress.[3] Tentative support for a bidirectional influence of both child behavior and family function after a TBI has been demonstrated. Common psychiatric disturbances that occur after a brain injury are found in Table 46.1.

TABLE 46.1 Psychiatric Disturbances Following Brain Injury

Disturbance	Associated Regions	Other Factors
Attention-deficit/ hyperactivity disorder	Right putamen, thalamus, orbital frontal gyrus	Preinjury family functioning Not associated with injury severity, family function, socioeconomic status, family stressors, family psychiatric history, gender, or lesion area
Personality change due to TBI	Superior frontal gyrus, frontal white matter	Affective instability, aggression, disinhibited behavior, apathy, paranoia Approximately 40 percent incidence in severe injury Associated with adaptive and intellectual functioning decrements
Post-traumatic stress disorder (reexperiencing)	Right limbic area (including cingulum) lower lesion fraction	Injury severity, socioeconomic disadvantage, and mood or anxiety disorder at time of injury
Post-traumatic stress disorder (hyperarousal)	Left temporal lesions and lower frequency of orbitofrontal lesions	Injury severity, socioeconomic disadvantage, and mood or anxiety disorder at time of injury
Obsessions	Mesial prefrontal and temporal lesions	Psychosocial adversity, higher prevalence in females

---

2   Silver, Jonathan M., Yudofsky, Stuart C. and McAllister, Thomas W. *Textbook of Traumatic Brain Injury.* Washington, DC: American Psychiatric Pub. 2011. Print.

3   Schoenbrodt, L. (ed.) *Children with Traumatic Brain Injury: a parent's guide.* Bethesda, MD: Woodbine House. 2001. Print.

Disturbance	Associated Regions	Other Factors
Obsessive–compulsive disorder	Frontal and temporal lobes	Psychosocial adversity, higher prevalence in females
Anxiety disorder	Superior frontal gyrus, frontal white matter	May include overanxious disorder, specific phobia, separation anxiety disorder, avoidant disorder Associated with preinjury anxiety symptoms and younger age at time of injury
Mania/hypomania	Frontal and temporal lobes	Increased injury severity, family history of major mood disorders

Neurocognitive Development and Arrest

Children's brains are still developing and continue to generally go through significant spikes of maturation through the age of 22. During these peaks, new neural connections increase dramatically within particular cortical regions and diffusely throughout the brain. The age, location of the child on the spectrum of development, and location of injury at the time it is sustained can delay or arrest further development or learning of new skills. This has been referred to as "neurocognitive stall" by Chapman.[4] Peak development ages have been shown to occur at approximately 0–1 years, 3–5 years, 7–10 years, 14–15 years, 17–19 years, and lastly at approximately 21–22 years of age.

The time between birth and approximately five years old is when the developing brain goes through the most dramatic formation of new neural pathways and connections. For this reason, young children who suffer a brain injury within this age range tend to have poorer overall outcomes. During this time, the most apparent development occurs in the lower brain functions of the brainstem and cerebellum as well as the limbic system associated with normal emotional development. Due to the progressive development of brain regions, preschoolers who sustain a frontal lobe injury will often appear unaffected shortly after the injury. As they age, however, and the frontal region becomes more prominent in the individual's conscious state and cognitive functioning, the injured area may not develop or function properly. This can result in long-term psychosocial and behavioral problems as well as serious learning, behavioral,and emotional problems as the child grows older and more independent cognitive behavior is expected of them. This can be misconstrued or misdiagnosed as a learning disability or a behavioral disorder rather than the effect of an injury to the brain.

Between the ages of three and five all regions of the brain undergo a rapid growth in neural connections in which visuospatial, visuo-auditory, and executive functions all show

---

4   Chapman, S.B. Neurocognitive stall: a paradox in long term recovery from pediatric brain injury. *Brain Injury Professional*. 2006; 3(4): 10–13.

synchronous development. Here the child refines formal operational skills in abilities to form images, use words, place things in a particular order, and problem solve. The sensory motor region of the brain peaks at about age six as the operational functioning of rationale, logic, and mathematical thinking becomes more available.

Around the ages of seven to ten the frontal executive functions begin to rapidly accelerate in development. This involves elaboration of visuo-spatial functions and visuo-auditory regions. By age ten the child is generally suited to perform formal operations such as calculations and the perception and placement of meaning to familiar objects.

At the ages of approximately 14–15 the visuo-auditory, visuo-spatial, and somatic systems tend to reach their maturational peak within a one-year interval of one another. The dialectic ability to review formal operations, find flaws within them, and create new ones becomes more readily available. At this time, social development and the establishment of a firm peer system outside of the family structure also tends to become more apparent as self-identity is explored and developed.

By ages 17–19 the young individual tends to begin questioning information they are given, will reconsider it based on experience, and form a new hypothesis where necessary while incorporating their own ideas. This tends to continue until the mid-twenties, a time when mylenation of the frontal cortex becomes complete.

In the context of the eight-circuit model of consciousness, as explored in my previous book *Circuits and Shen: Models of the Evolution of Consciousness and Chinese Medicine*, these age ranges roughly correlate to the bio-survival (0–2 years), emotional–territorial (2–5 years), neuro-semantic (7–10 years), and the socio-sexual circuits (12–19 years). An in-depth exploration of each of these stages is beyond the scope of this text. Table 46.2 is a simplified reference of the "lower" four earthly circuits. The "higher" four heavenly circuits can also come into play with certain mental–emotional concerns following a brain injury such as mania and schizophrenia. For a more thorough investigation of these concepts and treatment approaches refer to *Circuits and Shen*.

TABLE 46.2 First Four "Earthly" Circuits of Consciousness

Circuit	Approximate Age of Standard Development	Developmental Attributes	Chinese Organ System Associations
Bio-survival	0–2 years	Basic survival mechanisms, ability to thrive, eating, sleeping, digestion, nurturing bond, undifferentiated from everything else, particularly primary nurturing figure, fear Imprint: safety (approach) vs. danger (avoidance) Neural connections most active: brainstem, cerebellum	Water/Kidney

Circuit	Approximate Age of Standard Development	Developmental Attributes	Chinese Organ System Associations
Emotional–territorial	2–5 years	Establishment of boundaries between self and external world, learning to control and manipulate the world, basic reproductive drives, tantrums, anger, lack of empathy for others, narcissism Imprint: dominance vs. submissiveness Neural connections most active: limbic system	Wood/Liver
Neuro-semantic	7–10 years	Formal operations, problem solving, map making, linear rationale, mathematics, organization and list making, logic and "left-brained" thinking Imprint: intellectualism and rationality Neural connections most active: parietal, frontal lobes	Earth/Spleen
Socio-sexual	12–19 years	Social and peer support groups, separation from family unit and further ego establishment, sexuality, charisma, conformity, and upholding societal morals and norms Imprint: social and sexual intelligence and roles Neural connections most active: prefrontal lobes	Fire/ Pericardium/ Triple Warmer

Causes of Pediatric and Adolescent Brain Injury

Non-traumatic

- Brain tumors

- Anoxia/hypoxia

- Infections: Cerebral vascular accidents (stroke)—often secondary to another disease such as sickle cell disease or arteriovenous malformation (AVM)

- Toxic substance/environmental exposure

Abusive Head Trauma (AHT, Previously Known as "Shaken Baby Syndrome")

Often committed by a frustrated caregiver or parent in response to crying, temper tantrums, or issues with developmental milestones such as toilet training. If an infant is violently shaken, the head sustains multiple impacts involving chin to chest and the back of the head whipping back to impact the upper back, causing coup and contrecoup injuries.

- Most common in infants 0–5 years of age

- Accounts for an estimated 50–80 percent of head trauma-related deaths in those under two years old

- Study of 10,555 survivors showed 77 percent were under one year of age (60% male, 40% female)

- Higher risk in infants with excessive crying from birth to four months

- Seventy-one percent of individuals responsible were male caregivers (in those who admitted the abuse)—56 percent being biological fathers, 16 percent being a mother's boyfriend, 15 percent being the child's biological mother. Because of this familial tendency, it is important to assess risk of continued abuse and provide information, resources, and support connections

Diagnostics

Medical professionals look for:

- Subdural hemorrhage or hematoma

- Cerebral edema

- Retinal hemorrhage: Present in 85 percent of AHT/SBS

Prognosis

Poor—70–85 percent survive with long-term disabilities such as behavioral problems, learning disabilities, blindness, deafness, seizures, and cerebral palsy; 15–30 percent of cases are fatal.

Concussion and Mild Brain Injury

Hundreds of thousands of teen athletes each year are thought to sustain a concussion annually. While most of these are mild, with the individual making a complete recovery, approximately 10 percent of these athletes will experience persistent symptoms including problems with attention, memory, fatigue, sleep, headaches, dizziness, irritability, or personality changes. When these symptoms become chronic and persist for extended periods of time it is referred to as post-concussion syndrome (PCS). This can cause difficulties in their academic as well as athletic performance. School, family, and social life can all be impacted as a result.

If the individual continues their athletic activities too soon without allowing for a full recovery, they can experience "second impact syndrome," which can be fatal or cause severe disability as a result of cerebral swelling or subdural hematoma. Another risk of a secondary impact is chronic traumatic encephalopathy (CTE), a progressive degenerative disease which includes dementia, memory loss, aggression, confusion, and depression. While symptomatically CTE appears similar to Alzheimer's disease, the two seem to vary in the disease process. CTE has been demonstrated to stem from physiological changes in the brain tissue, including a unique build-up of abnormal Tau proteins.

Fortunately, in recent years, awareness of the impact of concussions on youth has resulted in increased education of educators, coaches, and parents. By 2015 all 50 states had enacted concussion laws governing youth sports, most of which contain guidelines on how to approach a suspected concussion and when to remove a player until evaluated by a medical professional, as rest and recovery are essential. This may include staying home from school for a period of time, while restricting time spent text messaging, playing video games, and utilizing a computer for extended periods of time.

Educational Need Considerations

Some children who sustain a brain injury will require special accommodations in their educational environment. Areas where impairment may impact education are listed in Table 46.3. At times these are basic interventions in the classroom. Others may need a formal plan put into place as part of their general education. This is referred to as a 504 Accommodation Plan in which there is a specially designed individual approach to their education via the legal plan of the Individual Education Plan (IEP) process. Public schools are federally mandated to provide a free, appropriate public education through special education supports and services, Thomas W. called Specialized Academic Instruction (SAI), to children with eligible disabilities.

The 504 Accommodation Plan is intended to eliminate discrimination against students with disabilities and may address possible options such as:

- Preferential seating
- Extended time on tests or assignments
- Tests given in a quiet or alternate setting
- Word banks being provided during tests
- Additional rest breaks
- Shortened assignments
- Visual aids

- Books on CD or text-to-speech
  software

Possible instructional strategies in the classroom are provided in Table 46.4.

TABLE 46.3 Areas of Possible Impairment Impacting Education

Motor impairments	Gross and fine motor, strength, coordination, speed Rigidity, tremors, spasticity, ataxia, apraxia
Physical effects	Disruption in growth, eating disorders, development of diabetes, thermal dysregulation
Feeding	Dysphagia
Sensory impairments	Vision, hearing, difficulty with worksheets, completion of only half of an assignment sheet due to visual neglect, disorientation, slow to produce written material
Communication impairments	Expressive and receptive movement, pragmatic, taking turns in conversation, inability to summarize/articulate thoughts, indefinite wording/talking around a subject, difficulty or inability to understand metaphors and figurative speech, difficulty in word retrieval
Cognitive impairments	Attention: Easily distracted, delayed response to questions, difficulty staying on topic, unable to complete task without prompting, blurts out answers inappropriately, fatigued by mid-afternoon
	Memory: Remembering assignments/materials, learning routines, homework tasks, unable to recall content of material, prospective, difficulty remembering two to three-step directions, repeated exposure necessary
	Executive functioning/higher learning: Difficulty with organization and completion of long-term assignments, unable to sequence necessary steps to obtain goal, unable to problem solve as issues arise, difficulty drawing conclusions from facts, difficulty evaluating and altering performance
Academic	Learning difficulties, inability to take notes while listening, difficulty copying information from board
Fatigue	Physical and cognitive
Medical issues	Seizures, headache, pain, orthopedic issues
Social–emotional or behavioral difficulties	Irritability/easily frustrated, disinhibition, socially inappropriate actions or words, emotional lability, difficulty fitting in with peers, easily misled by peer pressure, misperception of social cues or interactions, impulsivity to leave seat/classroom, lack of awareness or denial of impairments, appears unmotivated, withdrawal, depression, apathy, rigidity in thinking or behavior

| Family difficulties | Difficulty interacting, stress upon family, abuse, neglect, or needs not being met at home |
| Post-school concerns | Vocational issues, housing issues |

Fewer than 2 percent of children 0–19 years old with a brain injury are referred for special education programs, placing the onus on public schools to ensure the child's education. One study found that close to 60 percent of children with a TBI fail to receive any school-based services due to delayed effects of the injury and a failure to recognize a need for continued monitoring after an injury. This can make the schooling process quite difficult and frustrating for the individual. As of this publication the majority of states lack an organized approach to school re-entry following a pediatric brain injury—exceptions including Kansas, Pennsylvania, Oregon, and Texas.

TABLE 46.4 Possible Instructional and Compensatory Strategies

Attention and concentration	Clear learning objectives
	Short, concise instructions
	Shorten assignments; divide work into small sections
	Minimize distractions
	Non-verbal attention cues
	Additional breaks
	Reward on-task behavior
Memory and learning processing	Learning objectives for each lesson
	Link new information to relevant prior knowledge
	"My turn, our turn, your turn" teaching method (modeling, guided practice, independent practice)
	Hands-on learning opportunities
	Frequent repetition and summation of information
	Utilization and education in using graphic organizers
	Memory devices
	Extra set of books for home
	Direct instruction curriculum materials
Organization	Templates for assignments, projects, papers
	Visual schedule
	Assistance with homework planner, backpack check
	Assignments and notes provided on school website
	Utilize different-colored notebooks for each subject
	Break long-term projects into specific timelines for each part
Following directions	Oral and written instruction
	Highlight written instruction
	Task-analyze directions into simple steps

Auditory–perceptual	Limit amount of information presented
	Speak at a slower pace, with pauses
	Provide visuals to accompany verbal information
	Use a peer to repeat oral instructions
Visual–perceptual	Limit amount of information on page
	Use large print
	Present materials on a slant
	Longer viewing times
	Seating close to front of classroom
	Arrows or cue words for orientation
	Maps or teach student to navigate schedule
Motor–physical	Assistive technology and adapted devices to provide access
	Allow extra time for tasks and changing classes
	Adapted physical education

Related Services for Children and Adolescents

- Speech–language pathology
- Auditology services
- Interpreting services
- Psychological services
- Physical therapy
- Occupational therapy
- Recreation, including therapeutic recreation
- Early identification and assessment of disabilities in children
- Counseling services, rehabilitative counseling
- Orientation and mobility services (for visual impairment)
- Medical services for diagnostics or evaluation
- School health and nursing services
- Social work services in schools
- Parent counseling and training

Resources[5]

Web

BrainSTEPS (Strategies Teaching Educators, Parents and Students) Child and Adolescent Brain Injury School Re-entry Program
www.brainsteps.net

---

5   Lash, Marilyn. *The Essential Brain Injury Guide.* 5th ed. Vienna, VA: Academy of Certified Brain Injury Specialists, Brain Injury Association of America. 2016. Print.

Lash and Associates Publishing/Training, Inc.—educational books, DVDs, and tip cards
www.lapublishing.com

Project Optimal Traumatic Brain Injury Program—online self-study program providing advanced, specialized training for education specialists
www.innovative-learning.com/projectoptimal/?pg=traumatic-brain-injury

Print

Blosser, J.L., DePompei, R. *Pediatric Traumatic Brain Injury: Proactive Intervention.* 2nd ed. Clifton Park, NY: Delmar Learning; 2003

DePompei, R., Blosser, J., Savage, R., Lash, M. *Back to School after Mild Brain Injury or Concussion.* Youngsville, NC: Lash and Associates Publishing/Training, Inc.; 2011

Lash, M., Wolcott, G., Pearson, S. *Signs and Strategies for Educating Students with Brain Injuries.* Wake Forest, NC: Lash and Associates Publishing/Training, Inc.; 2005

Lebby, P.C., Asbell, S.J. *The Source for Traumatic Brain Injury: Children and Adolescents.* East Moline, IL: LinguiSystems; 2007

Max, J.E., Ibahim, F., Levin, H. Neuropsychological and psychiatric outcomes of traumatic brain injury in children. *Cognitive and Behavioral Abnormalities of Pediatric Diseases.* Edited by R. Nass, Y. Frank. New York: Oxford University Press; 2010

Savage, R., Wolcott, G. *Educational Dimensions of Acquired Brain Injury.* Austin, TX: Pro-Ed; 1994

Ylvisaker, M. *Traumatic Brain Injury Rehabilitation: Children and Adolescents.* 2nd ed. Boston, MA: Butterworth, Heinemann; 1998

Chapter 47

Special Considerations in Military Populations

The Department of Defense (DoD) did not begin surveying traumatic brain injury until 2006. Between this time and 2012 over 229,000 service members were diagnosed with TBI. Those returning from Operation Iraqi Freedom (OIF) were reported to have had an approximate 22 percent incidence. Most of these cases were mild with an expected full recovery, with an 8 percent incidence of persistent symptoms.[1] Certain Military Occupational Specialties (MOS) within the military increase one's risk of sustaining a TBI, including infantry, Explosive Ordinance Device (EOD) personnel, and special forces. Outside of field operations, injuries to the brain can occur in training accidents, such as in rappelling, shooting, parachuting, other specialty activities, or from operating within closed-in spaces such as tanks or submarines.

Fifty-five percent of combat injuries were found to be related to blast injuries, 27 percent were found to be from "multiple mechanisms," and 7 percent the result of vehicular injuries. Those who experienced penetrating injuries are at a higher risk for cerebral vasospasm and pseudoaneurysm than those who have sustained a blunt TBI. Forty-three percent of those with TBI had a psychiatric disorder noted in their records, with PTSD being the most common. For more details on PTSD, refer to Chapter 43.

The differences in the military healthcare system from the civilian system creates different approaches to diagnostic and treatment protocols which are helpful to be familiar with if working regularly with service member populations. The complexity of the DoD and VA healthcare systems, and the high prevalence of comorbidities such as PTSD, can make the recovery process particularly challenging. Creating a supportive environment of people who can understand the challenges upon service members as they struggle with conflicting feelings about their combat experience, military status, and their injuries is critical for their

---

1   Silver, Jonathan M., Yudofsky, Stuart C. and McAllister, Thomas W. *Textbook of Traumatic Brain Injury.* Washington, DC: American Psychiatric Pub. 2011. Print.

psychosocial healing. This can include a wide range of support from family members, healthcare providers, therapists, and peer counselors.

Blast Injuries

Blast injuries, or blast-induced neurotrauma (BINT), are a common mechanism of injury in recent wars and are often referred to as the signature wounds of Operation Iraqi Freedom (OIF) and Operation Enduring Freedom (OEF). These accounted for nearly 55 percent of combat injuries, including from IEDs, rocket-propelled grenades, mortars, mines, bombs, and grenades. In most cases this involves a combination of both blunt and blast injury co-occurring with a sudden vehicular deceleration or impact with another object. Concussive blasts can impact the body at a velocity beyond the speed of sound at up to 670m/s (2414 km/h). This is quickly followed by a very high-velocity wind capable of evisceration or disintegration. Individuals positioned between a blast and a building often suffer from injuries two to three times the degree of injury of a person in an open space, as explosions near or within hard solid surfaces become amplified by two to nine times due to shockwave reflection. The hierarchy categories of blast injuries are summarized in Table 47.1.

BINT is considered to represent a unique clinical entity caused by interwoven mechanisms of systemic, local, and cerebral responses to blast exposure. Brain trauma mechanisms include:

- Direct interaction with the head through direct passage of the blast wave through the skull and/or causing acceleration and/or rotation of the head

- Transfer of kinetic energy from the blast wave through large blood vessels in the abdomen and chest to the central nervous system

Blast exposure has been reported to cause brain edema and considerable metabolic disturbances in the brain, including significantly decreased glucose, magnesium, and ATP concentrations; increased lactate concentration and lactate/pyruvate ratio; and an impaired sodium and potassium function. This points to an overall pattern of energy failure or an imbalance between the body's energy demands and available energy, as well as an impairment in neuronal cell membrane permeability. Swelling of neurons, an astroglial response, and myelin debris in the hippocampus have also been found in animal studies, while immunohistochemical analyses have shown significant damage to the neuronal cytoskeleton of the temporal cortex, cingulate gyrus, the piriform cortex, dentate gyrus, and in the CA1 region of the hippocampus over seven days after blast exposure. Oxidative stress, changes in antioxidant–enzyme defense systems, and later cognitive deficits have also been seen.

Evidence is accumulating that a primary blast injury affects organs which have fluid interfaces such as the lungs and liver, allowing for the transfer of the kinetic energy and sudden pressure increases. This causes a vagal reflex which leads to apnea, rapid breathing, bradycardia, hypotension, and dilatation of the peripheral blood vessels that results in lowered blood pressure. These are frequently observed immediate symptoms after blast exposure and may increase risk of cerebral hypoxemia. The autonomic nervous system and neuroendocrine–immune systems also become activated as a result,[2] along with diffuse axonal injury in the brain and spinal cord. Prevention proves difficult, however, as body armor, while protecting from shrapnel and penetrating injuries (secondary and tertiary blast injuries) and undoubtedly increasing survival rates, actually establishes an improved contact surface for shock-front–body interaction and energy transfer. It also serves as a reflecting surface that concentrates the power of an explosion as the blast wave resonates internally.[3]

TABLE 47.1 Hierarchy of Blast-Related Injuries

Primary blast injury	Direct impact to the body of blast force
Secondary blast injury	Injury due to energized debris (projected or falling) or shrapnel
Tertiary blast injury	The displaced body impacts the ground, wall, or other object
Quarternary blast injury	Inhalation of gases or other toxic substances

Diagnostics/Assessment

- In 2006 the Defense and Veterans Brain Injury Center (DVBIC) developed an operational definition of traumatic brain injury in military operations. It is described as "an injury to the brain resulting from an external force and/or acceleration/deceleration mechanism from an event such as a blast, fall, direct impact, or motor vehicle accident which causes an alteration of mental status typically resulting in the temporally related onset of symptoms such as: headache, nausea, vomiting, dizziness/balance problems, fatigue, trouble sleeping, sleep disturbances, drowsiness, sensitivity to light/noise, blurred vision, difficulty remembering, and/or difficulty concentrating"[4]

- Military Acute Concussion Evaluation (MACE)

- Standardized Assessment of Concussion (SAC): Assesses four cognitive domains—orientation, immediate memory, concentration, memory recall

- Brief Traumatic Brain Injury Screen (BTBIS)

2   Silver, Jonathan, Yudofsky, Stuart, and McAllister, Thomas. *Textbook of Traumatic Brain Injury*. Washington, DC: American Psychiatric Pub. 2011. Print.

3   Cernak, I. and Noble-Haeusslein, L. Traumatic brain injury: an overview of pathobiology with emphasis on military populations. *Journal of Cerebral Blood Flow and Metabolism*. 2010; 30(6): 1262. Web. https://doi.org/10.1038/jcbfm.2009.203

4   Menon, D.K., Schwab, K., Wright, D.W., and Maas, A.I. Position statement: definition of traumatic brain injury. *Archives of Physical Medicine and Rehabilitation*. 2010; 91(11): 1637–1640.

- Combat stress screening:
  - ◦ Neuropsychological Assessment (20-minute assessment required for any service member preparing for deployment)
  - ◦ Neurobehavioral Symptom Inventory (NSI): Able to assess most common TBI symptoms
  - ◦ State-Trait Anxiety Inventory (STAI): Mood and sleep scale
  - ◦ Automated Neuropsychological Assessment Metrics (ANAM): Mood and sleep scale
  - ◦ ANAM Simple Reaction Time and Continuous Performance subtests: Objective assessment of cognitive performance
  - ◦ Repeatable Battery for the Assessment of Neuropsychological Status
- Stateside screening occurs through the Post-Deployment Health Assessment (PDHA) and Post-Deployment Health Reassessment (PDHRA)

Standard Treatment Methods

According to Clinical Practice Guidelines (CPG) in deployment settings, these are:

- Symptom management: Pharmacological intervention, glasses, etc.
- Education: Educational materials, flyers, national website
- Implementation of duty restrictions
- MEDEVAC to hospital or continental United States as necessary[5]

Standard levels of medical care within the military are summarized in Table 47.2.[6]

TABLE 47.2 Levels of Medical Care

Level I	Other service members in field, Battalion Aid Stations (BAS): Observation, rest, non-critical symptom management
Level II	Mobile, basic medical care, basic diagnostics, holding limited to 72 hours
Level III	Combat Support Hospital: Highest in-field care. Full surgical and intensive care capabilities, CT scans and diagnostics

5   The Management of Concussion–Mild Traumatic Brain Injury Working Group. *VA/DoD Clinical Practice Guideline for the Management of Concussion–Mild Traumatic Brain Injury.* 2016. https://www.healthquality.va.gov/guidelines/Rehab/mtbi/mTBICPGFullCPG50821816.pdf

6   Lash, Marilyn. *The Essential Brain Injury Guide.* 5th ed. Vienna, VA: Academy of Certified Brain Injury Specialists, Brain Injury Association of America. 2016. Print.

| Level IV | Non-battlefield facilities such as Landstuhl Regional Medical Center in Germany, MRI, neurology evaluation |
| Level V | Stateside facilities comparable to Level I trauma centers |

Stateside treatment is through primary care according to VA-DoD concussion management guidelines. Those with severe or penetrating injuries are managed according to civilian TBI guidelines.[7]

- A VA Polytrauma System of Care (PSC) team develops individual follow-up plans for each veteran after discharge

- Case workers, clinical psychologists, neuropsychologists, social workers, etc.

- Civilian partnership programs for model community reintegration may be sought and can be helpful

- Community Integrated Rehabilitation (CIR): e.g. DVBIC (Defense and Veterans Brain Injury Center), residential community programs, comprehensive holistic day treatments, home-based programs

Medical Evaluation and Discharge

When a service member has experienced a TBI which renders them unable to perform required duties, they may be retired from the military under a medical discharge. This process involves evaluation by both the Medical Evaluation Board (MEB) and the Physical Evaluation Board (PEB). The MEB first determines whether the service member's long-term medical condition allows them to continue to meet medical retention standards as well as having military physicians clearly document medical conditions and limitations that may exist as a result. These findings are considered informal and are then referred to the PEB who will formally determine if one is fit to continue service and eligibility for disability compensation. The PEB will recommend one of the following:

- Return to duty (with or without assignment limitations)

- Placement on the temporary disabled/retired list (TDRL)

- Separation from active duty

- Medical retirement

---

7   Silver, Jonathan, Yudofsky, Stuart, and McAllister, Thomas. *Textbook of Traumatic Brain Injury*. Washington, DC: American Psychiatric Pub. 2011. Print.

If medical retirement is determined, the PEB rates the disability on a 0–100 percent scale in increments of 10 percent according to the VA Schedule for Rating Disabilities.[8]

Emotional Impact of Unit Separation and Peer Support

Removal from one's unit or cohort can often increase anxiety and the likelihood of PTSD. Medical evacuation removes the service member from their primary support system as well as bringing on feelings of guilt about abandoning their brothers and sisters in arms. For this reason, many service members will not report or present for medical attention and opt to "tough it out." This increases the overall likelihood of medical errors, subsequent injury, and possible psychological distress should a post-concussion syndrome develop.

Concerns upon Returning Home

As with any brain injury case, one's family life can be greatly impacted following an injury. A service member may or may not be able to participate in discussions and decisions in their medical treatment and recovery expectations. Family members may have to suddenly adjust to the service member experiencing symptoms that can range from mild memory impairment to being minimally responsive and bed bound. This can often be a complex process of adapting, coping, and grieving. The service member may have difficulty successfully engaging in treatment due to a tendency to forget appointments, forget to take medications, the inability to drive to a doctor's office, or general confusion.

Emotional changes may also have an impact on others upon return. Mood lability and irritability can lead to lowered tolerance of frustrations dealing with their condition, with possible emotional outbursts toward family members and healthcare providers. Aggressiveness and disinhibition can elicit fear, confusion, or discomfort in both family and providers unfamiliar with TBI. In those for whom PTSD is a compounding factor, hypervigilance, increased anxiety, difficulty accommodating to civilian social structures (or relative lack of structure in comparison to the military), and re-experiencing of traumatic events ("flashbacks") may be difficulties. Due to the potential of one's experiences being of a very violent nature, frequently where one's life is in immediate danger, reactions and re-experiencings may also be amplified and potentially violent in themselves.

Common Comorbidities

Comorbidities and polytraumas can be particularly frequent in military populations, which can at times delay the detection of a brain injury. A multifocal approach to treatment will often be most effective. Common comorbidities include:

---

8   McCrea, M., Pliskin, N., Barth, J., *et al.* Official position of the military TBI task force on the role of neuropsychology and rehabilitation psychology in the evaluation, management, and research of military veterans with traumatic brain injury. *The Clinical Neuropsychologist.* 2008; 22(1): 10–26. http://dx.doi.org/10.1080/13854040701760981

- Chronic pain, especially in polytraumas

- Depression

- Anxiety

- Substance abuse

- PTSD—a study showed up to 44 percent of service members with concussion met criteria[9]

Resources[10]

Veterans Crisis line: 1-800-273-8255. Press 1

Defense and Veterans Brain Injury Center
www.dvbic.org

Defense Center for Excellence for Psychological Health and TBI
www.dcoe.health.mil

US Air Force Center of Excellence for Medical Multimedia: TBI
www.traumaticbraininjuryatoz.org

Mental Wellness Program including TBI Issues for Post-deployment
www.dvbic.org/service-members---veterans/care-coordination.aspx

Brainline.org
www.brainline.org

National Intrepid Center of Excellence
www.wrnmmc.capmed.mil/NICoE/SitePages/index.aspx

Military TBI Care Coordination Program
www.dvbic.org/service-members---veterans/care-coordination.aspx

Overview of VA TBI Rehabilitation Programs
www.polytrauma.va.gov/understanding-tbi

Returning Veterans Project (Oregon/Washington)
www.returningveterans.org/resources

---

9 Brady, K.T., Tuerk, P., Back, S.E., Saladin, M.E., Waldrop, A.E., and Myrick, H. Combat posttraumatic stress disorder, substance use disorders, and traumatic brain injury. *Journal of Addiction Medicine.* 2009; 3(4): 179–188. doi:10.1097/ADM.0b013e3181aa244f

10 Silver, Jonathan M., Yudofsky, Stuart C., and McAllister, Thomas W. *Textbook of Traumatic Brain Injury.* Washington, DC: American Psychiatric Pub. 2011. Print.

Chapter 48

Other Considerations of Brain Injury Care: Diet and Exercise

Neurochemical disruptions that result from the impact of an injury, and the subsequent movement of the brain within the skull, can alter cerebral metabolism. Ionic equilibrium across membranes may become disrupted with an increase in extracellular potassium and glutamate, with a resulting intracellular increase in calcium. Cellular glucose uptake increases, called hyperglycolysis, occurring within eight days in order to meet necessary cellular energy to reestablish homeostasis. This is followed by a long period of glucose metabolic depression. The magnitude and duration of this depression increases with severity and age of injury. Increases in reactive oxygen species (ROS) and correlated DNA damage further contributes to problems in glucose processing and subsequent cortical functioning.[1]

Select diets and exercise can modulate levels of molecules important for synaptic plasticity, such as brain-derived neurotrophic factor (BDNF). This affects normal function and recovery events following brain insults. BDNF is a neurotrophin known as a regulator of survival, growth, and differentiation in neurons during development. It is now known that BDNF functions to translate activity into synaptic and cognitive plasticity as well as being able to modulate the efficacy of neurotransmitter release, stimulate synthesis of vesicle-associated proteins, and regulate transcriptional factors. The hippocampus is capable of inducing a rapid potentiation of glutamate-mediated synaptic transmission and long-lasting potentiation of dentate gyrus connections. Functional blocking of BDNF has been demonstrated in impaired learning and memory in rats. BDNF, but not nerve growth factor

---

1   Prins, M. and Matsumoto, J. The collective therapeutic potential of cerebral ketone metabolism in traumatic brain injury. *The Journal of Lipid Research*. 2014 Dec; 55: 2450–2457.

(NGF) or neurotrophin-3 (NT-3), seems to play a role in consolidating long-term memories as well.[2, 3]

Fasting has been studied in rat models of cortical injury. Results showed that fasting for 24 hours, but not 48 hours, after a moderate, but not severe, injury showed neuroprotection with significant tissue sparing, maintenance of cognitive functioning, and improvement of mitochondrial function. Biomarkers for oxidative stress and calcium loading were shown to be decreased as well and is believed to be the result of ketosis rather than hypoglycemia. Ketone administration after a moderate injury also showed tissue sparing.[4] TBI patients who were fasted or maintained on a ketogenic-like diet to minimize hyperglycemia have also demonstrated significantly lower plasma glucose and lactate concentrations, elevated β-hydroxybutyrate levels, and better urinary nitrogen balance compared to a normal diet.

It has thus been argued that whether ketosis is achieved by starvation or administration of a ketogenic diet, the common underlying conditions of low plasma glucose in the presence of ketones have consistently shown neuroprotective effects after a brain injury and that maintenance of "normoglycemia" may not be the optimal approach postinjury.[5] A combination of ketone administration and hypertonic saline has also been shown to potentially provide an added control of intracranial pressure with improved cerebral metabolism.[6] Little exploration into specific dosing, timing, and route/duration of administration has been done, however, so caution should be taken in administering this method as side effects include dehydration, hypoglycemia, and less commonly nutrient deficiency, decreased bone density, immune dysfunction, cardiomyopathy, and elevated mean blood cholesterol with a prolonged ketogenic diet.[7]

General Brain Food Considerations

Leafy greens: Kale, romaine lettuce, Swiss chard

Spinach

Beets

2   Griesbach, G., Hovda, D., and Gomez-Pinilla, F. Exercise-induced improvement in cognitive performance after traumatic brain injury in rats is dependent on BDNF activation. *Brain Research.* 2009; 1288: 105–115. doi:https://doi.org/10.1016/j.brainres.2009.06.045

3   Lee, J., Duan, W., Long, J.M., *et al.* Dietary restriction increases the number of newly generated neural cells, and induces BDNF expression, in the dentate gyrus of rats. *Journal of Molecular Neuroscience.* 2000; 15: 99–108. https://doi.org/10.1385/JMN:15:2:99

4   Davis, L.M., Pauly, J.R., Readnower, R.D., Rho, J.M., and Sullivan, P.G. Fasting is neuroprotective following traumatic brain injury. *Journal of Neuroscience Research.* 2008; 86: 1812–1822. doi:10.1002/jnr.21628

5   Prins, M. Diet, ketones, and neurotrauma. *Epilepsia.* 2008; 49: 111–113. doi:10.1111/j.1528-1167.2008.01852.x

6   Davis, L.M., Pauly, J.R., Readnower, R.D., Rho, J.M., and Sullivan, P.G. Fasting is neuroprotective following traumatic brain injury. *Journal of Neuroscience Research.* 2008; 86: 1812–1822. doi:10.1002/jnr.21628

7   White, H. and Venkatesh, B. Clinical review: ketones and brain injury. *Critical Care.* 2011; 15: 219. https://doi.org/10.1186/cc10020

Sweet potato	Bone broth
Cauliflower, broccoli	Egg yolks
Avocados	Extra virgin olive oil
Coconut oil	Nuts, especially walnuts
Dark chocolate	Beans
Blueberries	

Dietary and Supplementary Considerations
Omega-3 Fatty Acids

Fish-derived omega-3 fatty acids have been shown to counteract deterioration in cognition and synaptic plasticity after traumatic brain injury. Docosahexaenoic acid (DHA) has been found to be a key component of neuronal membranes at sites of signal transduction at the synapse. Evidence suggests that DHA serves to improve neuronal function by supporting synaptic membrane fluidity and function, regulating gene expression and cell signaling. Omega-3 fatty acids also appear to reduce oxidative stress damage that results from trauma, indicating their possibility in facilitating the recovery process. Recently, DHA dietary supplementation in conjunction with exercise has been shown to have beneficial effects on synaptic plasticity and cognition in rodents under normal conditions.[8]

Vitamin E

Vitamin E, found in certain oils, nuts, and spinach, functions as an antioxidant in reducing free radicals in the brain that would otherwise impede the optimal function of neurons. Vitamin E has shown positive effects on memory performance in older people. An animal study demonstrated a correlation between the amount of vitamin E ingested and improved neurologic performance, survival, and brain mitochondrial function.[9]

Dietary Polyphenols

Polyphenols can be broadly divided into two categories: flavonoids and non-flavonoids. Although numerous studies have reported flavonoid-mediated neuroprotection, there is little information about the interaction of flavonoids or their metabolites with the blood–brain barrier. The flavonoid epigallocatechin gallate has been reported to enter the brain after gastric administration. The citrus flavonoids naringin and hesperetin readily cross the

---

8   Wu, A., Ying, Z., and Gomez-Pinilla, F. Docosahexanoic acid dietary supplementation enhances the effects of exercise on synaptic plasticity and cognition. *Neuroscience*. 2008; 155(3): 751–759.

9   Navarro, A., Gómez, C., María-Jesús Sánchez-Pino, M-J., *et al*. Vitamin E at high doses improves survival, neurological performance, and brain mitochondrial function in aging male mice. *American Journal of Physiology—Regulatory, Integrative and Comparative Physiology*. 2005 Nov; 289(5). doi:10.1152/ajpregu.00834.2004

blood–brain barrier, whereas the less lipophilic glucuronide or glycoside conjugates do not do so as easily.[10]

Berries

Berries are a rich source of phenolic compounds as well as anthocyanins, proanthocyanidins, and other flavonoids. A significant positive correlation between serum anthocyanin content and postprandial antioxidant status has been observed.[11] In mice supplemented with blueberry extract, the concentrations of hippocampal extracellular signal-regulating kinase (ERK) and striatal and hippocampal protein kinase C receptor (PKCR) were higher than in mice supplemented with a control diet. Both protein kinase C and ERK have been shown to be involved in early and late stages of memory formation.[12] These results indicate that blueberry extract supplementation might prevent cognitive and motor deficits through various neuronal signaling pathways.

Curcumin

There is substantial evidence indicating that curcumin has antioxidant, anti-inflammatory, and antiamyloid activities. For instance, curcumin could inhibit lipid peroxidation, activate glutathione transferase, or induce heme oxygenase-1. When fed to older mice with advanced amyloid accumulation, curcumin reduced amyloid beta levels and plaques. In this study, low (160ppm) and high (500ppm) doses of curcumin significantly lowered oxidized proteins and interleukin, I-beta, whereas low doses reduced plaque burden.[13] Follow-up studies demonstrated that curcumin could cross the blood–brain barrier, targeting senile plaques and disrupting existing plaques.[14]

Green Tea

Green tea is rich in flavonoids, with the main compounds being epigallocatechin-gallate (-)-epigallocatechin, (-)-epicatechin, and (-)-epicatechin-3-gallate. Catechin intake has been associated with a wide variety of beneficial health effects. The prevention of cerebrovascular

10   Slemmer, J.E., Shacka, J.J., Sweeney, M.I., and Weber, J.T. Antioxidants and free radical scavengers for the treatment of stroke, traumatic brain injury and aging. *Current Medicinal Chemistry*. 2008 Feb; 15(4): 404–414. https://doi.org/10.2174/092986708783497337

11   Mazza, G., Kay, C.D., Cottrell, T., and Holub, B.J. Absorption of anthocyanins from blueberries and serum antioxidant status in human subjects. *Journal of Agricultural and Food Chemistry*. 2002; 50(26): 7731–7737.

12   Micheau, J. and Riedel, G. Protein kinases: which one is the memory molecule? *Cellular and Molecular Life Sciences*. 1999; 55(3): 534–548.

13   Lin, G.P., Chu, T., Yang, F., *et al*. The curry spice curcumin reduces oxidative damage and amyloid pathology in an Alzheimer transgenic mouse. *Journal of Neuroscience*. 2001; 21(21): 8370–8377.

14   Garcia-Alloza, M., Borelli, L.A., Rozkalne, A., *et al*. Curcumin labels amyloid pathology in vivo, disrupts existing plaques, and partially restores distorted neuritis in an Alzheimer mouse model. *Journal of Neurochemistry*. 2007; 102(4): 1095–1104.

diseases or stroke has been demonstrated, and although there is no significant outcome relative to tea consumption to Alzheimer's disease case control, there are several studies showing that green tea extract may protect neurons from A-beta-induced damages.[15, 16, 17] A minimizing effect of the accumulation of eicosanoids and oxidative damage has been shown in reperfusion-induced brain injury along with a reduction in neuronal cell death.[18]

Resveratrol

Resveratrol found in grapes, red wine, and berries has been the focus of a number of studies demonstrating its antioxidant, anti-inflammatory, antimutagenic, and anticarcinogenic effects.[19, 20, 21] Recently it has been found that resveratrol can mimic dietary restriction and trigger sirtuin proteins.[22] The sirtuin enzymes are a phylogenetic family of enzymes that break down nicotinamide adenine dinucleotide (NAD)-dependent protein deacetylation. In yeast, sir2 is essential for lifespan extension by caloric restriction and a variety of other stresses, including increased temperature, amino acid restriction, and osmotic shock.

Citicoline

An acetylcholine precursor which readily crosses the blood–brain barrier, citicoline has been shown in animal studies to prevent TBI-induced neuronal loss in the hippocampus, decrease cortical contusion volume, and improve neurologic recovery. It additionally enhances cerebral mitochondrial lipid metabolism and phospholipid synthesis. Protection of the cerebral cortex and hippocampus occurs by decreasing edema and blood–brain barrier breakdown. In humans, studies have shown increased cerebral blood flow, decreased infarct

15   Bastianetto, S., Yao, Z.X., Papadopolous, Z.X., *et al.* Neuroprotective effects of green and black teas and their catechin gallate esters against beta-amyloid-induced toxicity. *European Journal of Neuroscience.* 2006; 23(1): 55–64.

16   Choi, Y.T., Jung, C.H., Lee, S.R., *et al.* The green tea polyphenol (-)-epigallocatechin gallate attenuates beta-amyloid-induced neurotoxicity-cultured hippocampal neurons. *Life Sciences.* 2001; 70(5): 603–614.

17   Levites, Y., Amit, T., Youdim, M.B., and Mandel, S. Neuroprotection and neurorescue against abeta: toxicity and PKC-dependent release of nonamloidogenic soluble precursor protein by green tea polyphenol (-)-epigallocatechin-3-gallate. *Federation of American Societies for Experimental Biology Journal.* 2003; 17(8): 952–954.

18   Hong, J-T., Ryu, S-R., Hye Jin Kim, H.J., *et al.* Neuroprotective effect of green tea extract in experimental ischemia-reperfusion brain injury. *Brain Research Bulletin.* 2000; 53(6): 743–749. https://doi.org/10.1016/S0361-9230(00)00348-8

19   De la Lastra, C.A. and Villegas, I. Resveratrol as an anti-inflammatory and anti-aging agent: mechanisms and clinical implications. *Molecular Nutrition and Food Research.* 2005; 49(5): 405–430.

20   Jang, M., Cai, L., Udeani, G.O., *et al.* Cancer chemopreventative activity of resveratrol, a natural product derived from grapes. *Science.* 1997; 275(5297): 218–220.

21   Soleas, G.J., Diamandis, E.P., and Goldbert, D.M. Resveratrol: a molecule whose time has come? And gone? *Clinical Biochemistry.* 1997; 30(2): 91–113.

22   Baur, J.A. and Sinclair, D.A. Therapeutic potential of resveratrol: the in vivo evidence. *Nature Reviews Drug Discovery.* 2006; 5(6): 493–506.

volume, accelerated recovery of consciousness, and improved recovery of cognitive, memory, verbal, and motor deficits.[23]

Huperzine A

An extract of Chinese club moss, this is a potent selective reversible acetylcholinesterase inhibitor. Being rapidly absorbed and easily crossing the blood–brain barrier, it has demonstrated positive outcomes in vascular dementia and age-related cognitive decline.[24]

Pine Needle

Pre-treatment with pine needle extract has shown increases in the proliferating cells and immature neurons against hippocampal neurogenesis suppressed by scopolamine. This study also showed gene and protein facilitation of BDNF and modulation of cholinergic activity via the CREB-BDNF pathway.[25] Another study demonstrated pine needle polyphenols significantly increased total antioxidative capacity, glutathione peroxidase, and super oxide dismutase activity, while nitric oxide and nitric oxide synthase activity were decreased, showing a significant relieving effect on learning, memory, and spontaneous activities.[26]

Acetyl-L-Carnitine

This protects against neurotoxicity and is synergistic with lipoic acid in enhancing the cholinergic system and facilitating uptake of acetylcoenzyme A into mitochondria during fatty acid oxidation. Improved energy, neural stamina, and cognitive function have been reported.[27]

SAMe

A naturally occurring condensation of methionine and ATP, SAMe maintains cellular membrane integrity in repairing damaged proteins and maintaining fluidity of the lipid

23   Silver, Jonathan M., Yudofsky, Stuart C., and McAllister, Thomas W. *Textbook of Traumatic Brain Injury*. Washington, DC: American Psychiatric Pub. 2011. Print.

24   Silver, Jonathan M., Yudofsky, Stuart C., and McAllister, Thomas W. *Textbook of Traumatic Brain Injury*. Washington, DC: American Psychiatric Pub. 2011. Print.

25   Lee, J-S., Kim, H-G., Lee, H-W., *et al*. Hippocampal memory enhancing activity of pine needle extract against scopolamine-induced amnesia in a mouse model. *Scientific Reports*. 2015; 5: 9651. doi:10.1038/srep09651

26   Wang, C., He, L., Yan, M., *et al*. Effects of polyprenols from pine needles of Pinus massoniana on ameliorating cognitive impairment in a d-galactose-induced mouse model. *AGE*. 2014; 36: 9676. https://doi.org/10.1007/s11357-014-9676-6

27   Silver, Jonathan M., Yudofsky, Stuart C., and McAllister, Thomas W. *Textbook of Traumatic Brain Injury*. Washington, DC: American Psychiatric Pub. 2011. Print.

bilayer in nerve cell membranes. It also generates glutathione, the body's major antioxidant, and enhances the function of the dopamine system.[28]

Creatine

Animal studies have shown enhanced cellular energy in brain injuries with creatine. Amelioration of headaches, fatigue, and dizziness in children and adults who have sustained a TBI has also been noted.[29]

Nutrition for Neurotransmitters[30]

Below is a list of nutrients that support neurotransmitter production. Neurotransmitters are the communication signals of the nervous system, and by increasing and maintaining the healthy production of neurotransmitters the brain can function properly and more effectively.

GABA Enhancement/Glutamate Lowering
Magnesium

> Blocks excessive stimulation from glutamate. It will decrease excito-toxicity when there is too much glutamate in the brain (often seen in those with MS, chronic pain, anxiety, seizures, and/or mood disorders). It has also been shown to be neuroprotective in animal models of brain injury
>
> *Dietary sources*: pumpkin seeds, sesame seeds, spinach, Swiss chard, black beans, pinto beans, milk of magnesia, epsom salt baths

Organic Sulfur

> Necessary component to generate GABA
>
> *Dietary sources*: garlic, leeks, onion, chives, cabbage, kale, collards, broccoli, cauliflower, radishes, kohlrabi

Taurine

> Taurine has been shown to help prevent epileptic seizures and be useful in the prevention of cardiac arrhythmias, atherosclerosis, and congestive heart failure.

---

28   Silver, Jonathan M., Yudofsky, Stuart C., and McAllister, Thomas W. *Textbook of Traumatic Brain Injury.* Washington, DC: American Psychiatric Pub. 2011. Print.

29   Wahls, Terry L. *Minding My Mitochondria: how I overcame secondary progressive multiple sclerosis (MS) and got out of my wheelchair.* Iowa City, Iowa: TZ Press. 2010. Print.

30   Zurmohle, U., Herms, J., Schlingensiepen, R., *et al.* Changes in the expression of synapsin I and II messenger RNA during postnatal rat brain development. *Experimental Brain Research.* 1996; 108(3): 441–449.

It has been suggested that 1–2g/day in divided doses may help GABA production in a strategy to protect the brain or assist in the treatment of mood disorders

Dietary sources: Fish and shellfish

Glutathione

Very important to the generation of GABA. It is manufactured inside the cell, from its precursor amino acids: glycine, glutamate, and cysteine

Dietary sources: Must be manufactured from its precursors, particularly cysteine. Garlic, onions, and cruciferous vegetables such as broccoli, kale, collards, cabbage, cauliflower, and watercress can help increase production

N-Acetyl Cysteine (NAC)

Considered the most cost-effective strategy to increase intracelluar glutathione and is a key component in the generation of GABA

Dietary sources: Poultry, yogurt, egg yolks, red peppers, garlic, onions, broccoli, brussels sprouts, other cruciferous vegetables, oats, wheat germ, asparagus, avocado

Milk Thistle

A powerful antioxidant that supports the brain, liver, and kidneys in animal studies by preventing the depletion of glutathione. Silymarin is the active compound in milk thistle and is considered helpful in the detoxification process of the liver as well as protecting the liver from toxins

Dietary sources: Milk thistle seeds

Turmeric

A powerful antioxidant, anti-inflammatory, and antiamyloid substance. Turmeric is believed to inhibit lipid peoxidation, activate glutathione S-transferase, or induce heme oxygenase. Studies have demonstrated that turmeric could cross the blood–brain barrier, targeting senile plaques and disrupting existing plaques

Dietary sources: Curry, used as a spice

Selenium

Selenium is a co-factor for the enzyme glutathione peroxidase, which helps generate glutathione in the mitochondria and has been shown to be neuroprotective

Dietary sources: Fish, mushrooms, tofu, free-range chicken, turkey, venison

Norepinephrine Lowering Substances
Theanine

Shown to be neuroprotective as well as improving cognition and concentration and reducing anxiety and depression

Dietary sources: Green tea—particularly matcha tea

Serotonin Enhancement
Aerobic Exercise

Physical activity boosts the brain's serotonin levels. Thirty minutes of activity will elevate one's serotonin.

Vitamin D

Many adolescents, adults, and elderly individuals are vitamin D deficient. In addition to being important in brain development, vitamin D provides important support to immune function, lowers the risk of autoimmune disorders, lowers the risk of cancer, and is important in maintaining normal mood.

Vitamins and Supplements for Mitochondrial Health

The following is a list of vitamins that support mitochondrial function and brain function. Mitochondria are within every cell of the body and act as the energy producers within the cell and help optimize neural function.

Thiamine (Vitamin B1)

Thiamine supports mitochondrial function within the brain by aiding the production of ATP. Thiamine is also an important co-factor, along with vitamin B12, in helping the brain cells make myelin to insulate the nerve. As it is excreted by the kidneys, and generally not stored in the body, it is important to have a steady supply in one's diet

Dietary sources: Tuna, sunflower seeds, black beans, peas, pinto beans, lentils, lima beans, sesame seeds

Riboflavin (Vitamin B2)

Riboflavin is part of the FADH complex of enzymes used by mitochondria to convert the energy stored in food to the energy stored in ATP to be used by the body. It is also a critical nutrient for the elimination of toxins

Dietary sources: Almonds, fish, broccoli, asparagus. Most foods derived from plants or animals contain at least small quantities of riboflavin

Niacinamide (Vitamin B3)

Niacinamide is an important nutrient for brain health. It is a key nutrient for mitochondria. An ample supply of niacinamide makes the generation of ATP more efficient and reduces the level of free radicals

Dietary sources: Wheat germ, mushrooms, organ meats, tuna, salmon

Pyridoxine (Vitamin B6)

Vitamin B6 is involved in many aspects of neurological activity. It is very important in forming many neurotransmitters, including serotonin and GABA

Dietary sources: Garlic, tuna, cauliflower, mustard greens, bananas, celery, cabbage, crimini mushrooms, asparagus, broccoli, kale, collard greens, brussels sprouts, cod, chard

Cobalamin (Vitamin B12)

The body requires cobalamin in order to make hemoglobin and is also necessary, along with vitamin B6, for brain cells to effectively make myelin, the protective sheath around nerve cells

Dietary sources: Animal products, including fish, meat, poultry, eggs, milk, and milk products

Vitamin E

Vitamin E functions as an antioxidant, reducing free radicals in the brain that would otherwise impede the optimal function of neurons. Vitamin E has shown positive effects on memory performance in older people. An animal study demonstrated a correlation between the amount of vitamin E ingested and improved neurologic performance, survival, and brain mitochondrial function

Dietary sources: Oils, nuts, spinach

Folic Acid

Folate is essential for normal brain function. It helps prevent hyperhomocysteinemia, which is associated with increased risk of cardiovascular disease, Parkinson's, Alzheimer's, and other dementias

Dietary sources: Green leafy vegetables, asparagus, citrus fruit juices, legumes, fortified cereals

Co-enzyme Q

Co-enzyme Q is an important ingredient in the mitochondrial process to generate ATP and it is a potent intracellular antioxidant

Dietary sources: Wheat germ, dark green leafy vegetables like kale and spinach, organ meats

Alpha-Lipoic Acid

Several studies suggest that the use of alpha-lipoic acid may help reduce pain, burning, itching, tingling, and numbness in people who have nerve damage caused by diabetes

Dietary sources: Spinach, broccoli, beef, yeast (especially brewer's yeast), kidney and heart organ meats

L-Carnitine

Structurally related to the B vitamins, L-carnitine assists mitochondria in using fatty acids as an energy source. It also helps improve muscle strength in neuromuscular-disorder-affected individuals and has been associated with decreased oxidative stress and decreased aging in animal studies. L-Carnitine and alpha-lipoic acid have been shown to be a potent combination, providing protection to mitochondria and reducing aging in animals

Dietary sources: Dairy products, red meat (raw or very rare is best for absorption)

Creatine Monohydrate

Creatine functions to increase the availability of ATP. It acts by donating a phosphate ion during ATP production to increase the availability of ATP. Several studies have shown that taking additional creatine has been neuroprotective to a variety of insults and has helped maintain and improve muscle strength in people with Parkinson's and the frail elderly

Dietary sources: Fish, red meat, wild game

General Dietary Recommendations According to Organ System in Chinese Medicine

Lung/Large Intestine

Beneficial: Adzuki beans, anise, basil, caraway seeds, cardamom, carrots, cauliflower, cayenne pepper, celery, Chinese cabbage, cinnamon, clove, cooked apples, cooked pears, dill, garlic, ginger, ginseng, grapes, green onions, honey, horseradish, leeks, licorice, lotus root mustard greens, oatmeal, olives, onions, orange peel, paprika, parsley, pepper (black), sweet rice, tangerines, walnut

Avoid: Alcohol, beef, cigarettes, coffee, dairy products, fried foods, greasy food, oily food, raw pears, pork, raw or iced food/drink, sugar

If thick yellow phlegm and damp-heat, avoid: baked goods, citrus fruit and fruit juice, fermented food, nuts and nut butters, spicy and pungent food, vinegar, yeast bread

Spleen/Stomach

Beneficial: Adzuki beans, apples (sweet), apricots, bean curd, butter, congees, cooked vegetables, dates, figs, garlic, ginseng, grapefruit peel, grapes, honey, kombucha, mandarin oranges, mustard green, oats, pineapple, pumpkin, raspberries, spices, squash, warm water/tea

Avoid: Candy, celery, dairy products, fruit juice, ice cream, ice water and cold liquids, pork, radishes, soda, spicy foods, sugar, tofu

If damp-heat, avoid: baked goods, citrus fruit and fruit juice, fermented food, nuts and nut butters, spicy and pungent food, vinegar, yeast bread

Heart/Small Intestine

Beneficial: All fruit, asparagus, basil, black beans, brussels sprouts, buckwheat, celery, cherries, chives, cinnamon, crab apples, dandelion, dark leafy greens, dill, endive, figs, grapes, kidney beans, lettuce, mung beans, olive oil, oysters, paprika, parsley, persimmons, quinces, raspberries, red lentils, salmon, soup, squash, vegetables

Avoid: Bacon, butter, candy, canned vegetables, carrot soup, fried foods, high-fat snack, hot dogs, ice cream, lard mayonnaise, potato chips, red meat, salt, saturated fats, sugar, whole milk

Kidney/Bladder

Beneficial: Adzuki beans, barley, beef kidney, beef, blackberries, blueberries, boysenberries, buckwheat, chestnuts, chives, cinnamon bark, clove, concord grapes, cranberries, cucumbers, dulce, egg yolk, fennel, green beans, kale, kelp, kidney beans, lamb, lentils, lotus root, miso, mung beans, peanuts, peas, pinto beans, pumpkin seeds, radish leaf, raspberries, salt (in moderation), sesame seeds, soybeans, tangerines, tofu, water, watermelon

Avoid: Alcohol, artificial sweeteners, bacon, buttermilk, canned soup, canned vegetables, cigarettes, coffee, corned beef, dairy products, frozen dinners, ham, hot dogs, "hot" foods, oatmeal, pickles, potato chips, pungent foods, recreational drugs, salt (in excess), sausage, stimulants

Liver/Gallbladder

Beneficial: Applesauce, artichokes, avocados, basil, beef, beets, blackberries, black-eyed peas, broccoli, burdock, cabbage, celery, chicken livers, chives, coconut milk, cucumbers, dandelion, goji berries, green lentils, hawthorn fruit, kefir, kelp, leeks, lychees, mung beans, nori, peppermint, plums, pomegranates, quinces, rosemary, sesame seeds, sorrel, summer squash, triticale, zucchini

Avoid: Alcohol, bacon, barbecued foods, banned soup, banned vegetables, coffee, fatty foods, frozen dinners, greasy foods, nuts, potato chips, pretzels, red meat (excess), salty foods, sausage, sour foods, sugar and sweets

If damp-heat, avoid: baked goods, citrus fruit and fruit juice, fermented food, nuts and nut butters, spicy and pungent food, vinegar, yeast bread

General Dietary Recommendations According to Pattern Differentiation in Chinese Medicine

Lung Organ System

Lung Qi Deficiency

Common symptoms: Fatigue, weak voice with no desire to talk, yawning, weak respiration, weak cough or no cough, difficult breathing, head hair that comes out easily, dry skin, hypersensitivity leading to anxiousness and antisocial behavior, thumb fatigue, exhausted appearance, bright white face

Foods to Supplement

> *Grains*: Job's tears
>
> *Vegetables*: Yam
>
> *Fruit*: Grape
>
> *Dairy*: Cheese
>
> *Poultry*: Crane

Organ: Beef lung

Spice: Peach blossoms

Foods to Avoid

Fruit: Peach, lemon, banana

Lung Yin Deficiency

Common symptoms: Low or hoarse voice, low grade tidal fever, feeling of fire rising in the body at night, red cheeks, 5-palm heat, flushing, spontaneous sweats, night sweats, dry and painful throat, dry cough with little to no phlegm, bloody sputum, appetite loss, emaciated appearance, watery stools

Foods to Supplement

Vegetables: Asparagus, watercress

Fruit: Apple, date, sweet orange

Dairy: Cheese

Poultry: Inner membrane of chicken eggshell

Animal: Turtle shell

Sweeteners: Honey

Herbs: Hemp

Foods to Avoid

Fruit: Peach

Stomach Organ System
Deficient Cold Stomach

Common symptoms: Lethargy, perpetual fatigue, pale and withered face, sweats easily, daytime sweating, lack of sensitivity along Heart meridian, hurried breathing, difficult breathing with exertion, pain around lower front or back of chest, palpitations with mental or physical exertion, arrhythmia

Foods to Supplement

Seeds and nuts: Chestnut

Vegetables: Sweet potato

Seafood: Eel, trout, grass carp

Dairy: Fresh sheep's milk

Beverage: Brandy (in moderation)

Spices: Garlic, raw ginger, cinnamon, fennel seeds, cardamom seeds, red pepper

Foods to Avoid

Grain: Millet, buckwheat

Vegetables: Water chestnut, radish, watercress, lettuce, bok choy

Fruit: Watermelon, lemon

Seafood: Crab

Sweetener: Sugarcane

Spleen Organ System
Spleen Qi Deficiency

Common symptoms: Lethargy, sleepiness, lack of energy, excess thinking or brooding, mental unrest and fatigue, tendency to remain alone and not talk to others, craving for sweets, weak limbs, emaciation, muscular atrophy, weak joints, poor appetite, uncomfortable feeling after eating, vomiting, belching, indigestion, slight abdominal pain better with touch, loose stools

Foods to Supplement

Grains: Rice, sweet rice, barley, Job's tears, millet, oats, broomcorn

Seeds and nuts: Sesame, chestnut, lotus

Legumes: Peas, soybean, stringbean

Vegetables: Onions, carrots, pumpkin, squash, yam/sweet potato, leeks, turnip, rutabaga, parsnip, kuzu root, lotus root, arrowroot, mustard greens, millet sprouts, coconut meat

Fruit: Apple, cherry, salted peach, raisin, red and black date, fig

Fruit peels: Sweet orange, red outer layer of tangerine peel

Seafood: Sardine, anchovies, mackerel, sturgeon, whitefish, butterfish, carp, eel, octopus, cuttlefish, shark fin

Poultry: Chicken, turkey, goose, pheasant, pigeon, crane

Animal: Rabbit, lamb, beef, ham

Organ: Chicken gizzard, beef, lamb, and pork stomach

Sweetener: Amasake

Spice: Mustard seed

Foods to Avoid

Grain: Buckwheat

Seeds and nuts: Black sesame, plum kernel

Legumes: Broadbean, mungbean powder

Vegetables: Bamboo shoots

Fruit: Plum, banana, grapefruit, loquat, tea melon

Dairy: Milk, cheese

Poultry: Duck

Animal: Green turtle and shell

Oil: Sesame

Condiment: Vinegar, ice

Spleen Yang Deficiency

Common symptoms: Edema, ascites, scleroderma, frostbite, mental depression, weak limbs, weak body, poor circulation in the legs and feet, cold limbs, heaviness of the legs, swelling of the extremities, difficulty moving the big toes, coldness in the back and hip area, spine pain, a tendency to round the back and slouch, stiff shoulders, excess salivation, no appetite, inability to digest food and drink, fullness and distension after meals, continuous abdominal pain that feels better with heat, pressure, and food, watery stools with undigested food, clear cold dysentery, difficult urination, leukorrhea

Note: Also use Spleen Qi deficiency dietary guidelines

Foods to Supplement

Legumes: Black soybeans

Vegetables: Scallions, garlic leaf, chive, seaweed, mustard leaf

Seafood: Herring, sardine, carp

Poultry: Chicken

Animal: Mutton

Organ: Chicken gizzard, beef, lamb, and pork stomach

Sweetener: Sorghum

Spice: Mustard seed, fresh and dried ginger, cinnamon, red and black pepper

Foods to Avoid

> *Grain*: Sweet rice, unroasted millet
>
> *Vegetables*: Salads, watercress, water chestnut, radish, bitter endive, purslane, mungbean sprouts, kelp, agar, seagrass
>
> *Fruit*: Watermelon, muskmelon, persimmon, trifoliate oranges, juices, citrus
>
> *Poultry*: Duck egg
>
> *Condiment*: Excess salt or liquid with meals

Spleen Blood Deficiency

Common symptoms: Pale face, restlessness, dissatisfaction, memory loss, palpitations, heart pain, inability to obtain nourishment

Note: Also use Spleen Qi deficiency dietary guidelines

Foods to Supplement

> *Vegetables*: Cooked lotus root, coconut meat, spinach
>
> *Fruit*: Red date, grape, longan
>
> *Seafood*: Mussels, fresh oyster, cuttlefish, sea cucumber
>
> *Poultry*: Chicken egg
>
> *Animal*: Pork leg
>
> *Organ*: Beef, pork, and lamb liver
>
> *Sweetener*: Amasake
>
> *Spice*: Nutmeg

Foods to Avoid

> *Vegetables*: Water chestnut

Spleen Dampness

Common symptoms: Aching, weak, and heavy body, hesitancy to move, inability to lie down peacefully, skin eruptions that contain fluid, weakness of the extremities, pale gums, dry and sticky mouth, inability to taste food, sweet taste in the mouth, tendency to drink while eating, weak respiration, oppression in the chest, scanty urination

Note: Also use Spleen Qi and Yang deficiency dietary guidelines

Foods to Supplement

Grains: Barley, Job's tears, corn, rye

Seeds and nuts: Chestnut

Legumes: Adzuki bean, kidney bean, broadbean

Vegetables: Scallion, garlic, button mushroom, kohlrabi, radish, turnip, pumpkin, mustard greens, lamb's quarters

Fruit peels: Red outer layer of tangerine peel

Seafood: Anchovy, shrimp, perch, mackerel

Poultry: Chicken

Animal: Rabbit, lamb, beef, ham

Organ: Chicken gizzard

Foods to Avoid

Legumes: Soybeans, tofu

Seeds and nuts: Black sesame, pine

Fruit: Olives

Seafood: Clams, mussels, octopus, sardines, carp, shark

Dairy: Milk products

Poultry: Eggs, duck, goose

Animal: Pork, excess red meat

Oil: Honey, excess sugar

Condiment: Excess salt

Heart Organ System
Heart Qi Deficiency

Common symptoms: Lethargy, perpetual fatigue, pale and withered face, sweats easily, daytime sweating, lack of sensitivity along Heart meridian, hurried breathing, difficult breathing with exertion, pain around lower front or back of chest, palpitations with mental or physical exertion, arrhythmia

Foods to Supplement

Grains: Corn

Organ: Lamb heart

Sweetener: Honey

Beverage: Coffee (in moderation)

Spice: Red pepper, mace

Foods to Avoid

Poultry: Chicken egg whites

Heart Yang Deficiency
Common symptoms: Tendency for fatigue, dislike of cold, gray ashen face, timidity, lack of willpower, cold limbs, cold/pain in left shoulder and arm, left shoulder and arm weakness, poor appetite, upper abdominal weakness

Foods to Supplement

Meat: Lamb

Organ: Lamb heart

Beverage: Coffee, brandy (in moderation)

Spice: Red pepper

Foods to Avoid

Vegetables: Water chestnut, radish

Poultry: Chicken egg whites

Heart Blood Deficiency
Common symptoms: Tendency for fatigue, dislike of cold, gray ashen face, timidity, lack of willpower, cold limbs, cold/pain in left shoulder and arm, left shoulder and arm weakness, poor appetite, upper abdominal weakness

Foods to Supplement

Fruit: Red and black dates

Meat: Beef

Organ: Lamb heart

Beverage: Coffee (in moderation)

Foods to Avoid

> *Vegetables*: Water chestnut

Heart Yin Deficiency

Common symptoms: Agitation, restlessness, anxiety, nervous tension, forgetfulness, stammering, insomnia, excess dreaming, disturbed sleep, sensitive skin, night sweats, warmth and sweat in the palms and soles of the feet, pulling sensation in the tongue, dry throat, hoarse voice, tends to constantly clear throat, shoulder pain, palpitations, spermatorrhea

Foods to Supplement

> *Grain*: Wheat
>
> *Seeds and nuts*: Lotus seed
>
> *Fruit*: Lotus fruit
>
> *Organ meat*: Chicken liver

Heart Fire

Common symptoms: Restless sleep, insomnia, irritability, incessant laughing, delirious speech, agitation, impulsiveness, red face, burning eyes, thirst, burning tongue, bloody cough or vomit, shortness of breath, hot and melancholic chest, agitation/heat in the Heart, dark yellow or bloody urination

Foods to Supplement

> *Seeds and nuts*: Chestnut
>
> *Vegetables*: Eggplant
>
> *Fruit*: Peach, pear peel
>
> *Beverage*: Liquor
>
> *Herbs*: Safflower, peach blossoms, cherry root, lotus blossom, ginseng, hops, rosemary, thyme

Foods to Avoid

> *Seeds and nuts*: Walnut
>
> *Seafood*: Sardine
>
> *Herbs*: Garlic, dill seed, fennel seed, mustard seed, red chili, black pepper, chive seed, star anise

Phlegm Obstructing the Heart

Common symptoms:

- Cold Phlegm: Sudden blackouts, inward, restrained and foolish manner, tendency to stare at walls and mutter to oneself, inability to speak, drooling

- Phlegm with Heat: Hyperactivity, agitation, aggression, tendency to move, crying or laughing without reason, loquaciousness, abnormal speech, violent behavior—lashing out toward others or immediate environment

Foods to Supplement

Vegetables: Asparagus, lettuce, mustard greens

Seafood: Shrimp

Organ meat: Chicken gallbladder

Herbs: Mustard seed, plantain, spinach seed, cinnamon (cold)

Foods to Avoid

Seeds and nuts: Almond

Fruit: Persimmon

Dairy: Fresh milk

Sweetener: Honey, brown sugar

Kidney Organ System

Kidney Yin Deficiency

Common symptoms: Night sweats, hot flashes, insomnia, forgetfulness, frequent and urgent urination, fatigue from overwork, tinnitus, blurry vision, dry mouth and throat, redness of cheeks and ears, 5-palm heat, dry stool, hemorrhoids, premature ejaculation, wet dreams, uterine bleeding or amenorrhea, weakness, stiffness or soreness of the lower back, paralysis, sciatica, anxiety, restlessness, impatience, constant complaining, thin and shriveled constitution, prone to inflammation, idiopathic low grade fevers, vertigo, abnormal hair loss, inflammation of the breast

Foods to Supplement

Grains: Whole wheat

Seeds and nuts: Chestnut, walnut, black sesame seed

Legumes: Black beans

Vegetables: String bean, potato, sea vegetables

Fruit: Strawberry, raspberry

Seafood: Mussels, oysters, dried scallops, prawns, perch

Poultry: Pigeon eggs

Animal: Turtle shell, beef marrow

Organ: Beef, pork, and lamb kidneys, chicken and lamb liver

Spice: Chive seeds

Foods to Avoid

Legumes: Black-eyed peas

Fruit: Tangerine peel

Beverages: Liquor, coffee

Spice: Chives, garlic, mustard seed, dill seed, anise, cardamom seed, fresh and dried ginger, red chili, black pepper

Herbs: Peppermint

Kidney Yang Deficiency

Common symptoms: General debilitation. Fondness of laying down and sleeping, fear of cold, bright white or dark complexion, resting perspiration, vitiligo, difficulty walking with a tendency to stumble, suspended growth, coldness of limbs, weakness of knees and feet, sciatica, coldness and soreness of lower back, aching bones, arthritis, dizziness, deafness, hearing loss, tinnitus, pale lips, dry mouth with thirst, loose teeth, urge to urinate immediately after drinking fluids, copious clear urination, dribbling urination, night urination, impotence, premature ejaculation, orchitis, idiopathic swelling, ascites

Foods to Supplement

Grains: Oats

Seeds and nuts: Chestnut, walnut

Legumes: Black-eyed peas, fenugreek seeds

Vegetables: Carrot, sea vegetables

Fruit: Crab apple, grape, raspberry

Seafood: Carp

Animal: Pork or ox tail, mutton

Herbs: Parsley, garlic, dry ginger, star anise, red chili

Foods to Avoid

General: Ice

Legumes: Tofu

Vegetables: Water chestnut, radish

Fruit: Watermelon

Beverages: Coffee

Kidney Dampness

Common symptoms: Many indications of Kidney Yang deficiency plus particularly puffy skin lacking elasticity, heaviness of the body, idiopathic swelling, edema, ascites, orchitis

Foods to Supplement

Grains: Corn

Seeds and nuts: Chestnut, walnut

Legumes: Peas, soybean, kidney beans

Vegetables: Chinese cabbage, squash

Fruit: Melon, grapes, dates

Fruit peel: Watermelon peel

Seafood: Sardine, anchovy, whitefish

Organ: Pork kidney and intestine

Foods to Benefit Abdominal Water

Grain: Barley

Seeds and nuts: Black sesame, plum kernel

Legumes: Adzuki bean, mung bean, black soybean

Vegetables: Cucumber, watercress, seaweed

Fruit: Plum

Seafood: Clam, frog, carp

Poultry: Duck

Herbs: Plantain, shepherd's purse

Foods to Benefit Swelling of Skin and Joints

Legumes: Adzuki bean, kidney bean

Vegetables: Scallion, eggplant

Seafood: Frog, shark

Poultry: Duck

Spice: Ginger, mustard seed, savory

Gallbladder Organ System
Gallbladder Excess Heat

Common symptoms: Fatigue from overwork, restlessness, restless sleep, insomnia, stupor, chills and fever, neck spasm, shoulder pain, stiff muscles and limbs, inability to turn the body, temple headaches, migraines, deafness, sore or itchy throat, bitter taste in mouth, vomiting bitter-tasting material, burning pain and distension in the flanks and chest, excessive responsibility, pushing and overconcentration to the point of unproductive work, impatience, tendency to become easily upset and angered

Foods to Supplement

Grains: Wheat germ

Legumes: Broadbean

Vegetables: Celery, cucumber, turnip, lamb's quarters

Seafood: Gold carp

Animal: Cow's gallbladder

Herbs: White pepper

Foods to Avoid

Animal: Pork

Liver Organ System
Liver Blood Deficiency

Common symptoms: Pale lusterless face, lack of energy, easily fatigued, desire to lie down and close the eyes, tendency to stumble, lack of exercise, exaggerated need for food and rest, no appetite, inability to gain weight, tendency to be easily poisoned, dizziness, fainting spells, lack of determination, tendency to be overcome with fear, inability to face the world, depression, stiff muscles, spasms, numbness, weak joints, hazy vision, spots in the vision, lack of sexual energy or interest, impotency, prostate problems, irregular or insufficient menses

Foods to Supplement

Seeds and nuts: Black sesame

Vegetables: Chive, mushroom

Fruit: Strawberry, raspberry, mulberry, grape, fresh longan

Seafood: Mussels, perch

Animal: Pork leg

Herbs: Angelica Sinensis (Dang Gui), lycium, chive seeds

Foods to Avoid

Vegetables: Water chestnut

Herbs: Peppermint

Liver Yin Deficiency

Common symptoms: Insomnia, giddiness, general itching, depression, nervous tension, oversensitivity to details, easily upset, irritability, short-temperedness, headaches, eye problems, blurred vision, dry eyes with spots, light sensitivity, double vision, near-sightedness, night blindness, partial blindness, palpitations, menopausal problems, tendency to inflammation, idiopathic low-grade fever, afternoon tidal fever, red cheeks, 5-palm heat

Foods to Supplement

Vegetables: Agar

Seafood: Whitebait

Foods to Avoid

Beverages: Coffee, alcohol

Liver Qi Stagnation

Common symptoms: Irritability, oversensitivity, plum-like sensation in the throat, tightness in the neck, breast, neck, or flank, painful menses, irregular menses, swollen breasts especially during menses, difficult breathing, coughing or vomiting with blood, depression, frustration, overly stressed, repressed emotions manifesting inappropriately, quick to anger—displaying emotions without control (e.g. screaming)

Foods to Supplement

Seeds and nuts: Black sesame

Vegetables: Celery, scallion, leek, garlic, kohlrabi, beets, cabbage, coconut milk, kelp, nori

Fruit: Plum, mulberry, trifoliate orange, peach, longan, lycium

Fruit peels: Green sweet orange peel

Beverages: Amasake

Seafood: Mussels

Organ: Beef and chicken liver

Herbs: Dillseed, basil, bayleaf, ginger, black pepper, marjoram, rosemary, safflower, saffron

Foods to Avoid

Fruit: Sour orange

Beverages: Alcohol, coffee, caffeinated drinks

Liver Qi Stagnation Invading the Spleen

Common symptoms: Liver Qi stagnation symptoms with additional nausea, vomiting, sour belching, nervous stomach, abdominal pain and distension, gas and gas pain, diarrhea or constipation, hemorrhoids, hernia

Foods to Supplement

Grains: Brown rice, barley

Legumes: Soybean, broadbean

Seeds and nuts: Chestnut, peanut

Vegetables: Lettuce

Fruit: Lemon, red and black dates, trifoliate orange

Flowers: Chrysanthemum, plum blossom

Seafood: Whitefish, gold carp

Poultry: Goose

Animal: Ham

Organ: Chicken gizzard, lamb and pork stomach

Herbs: Fennel seed, cherry leaf, corncob, squash vine, string bean root

Foods to Avoid

Vegetables: Mushroom, potato

Liver Fire

Common symptoms: High fever without cause, restless and agitated sleep, insomnia, accumulated fatigue due to never-ending drive, excessive alcohol and sugar consumption, irritability, frequent and violent fits of anger, splitting headache, migraines, convulsions, heat sensation in the head with flushed face, various bleeding symptoms, hallucinations, deafness, sudden tinnitus, swollen and painful red eyes, excessive tearing, eyelid tremors, Conjunctivitis, dryness of mouth/throat, bitter taste in mouth, cough with or without blood, constipation, hemorrhoids, dark, scanty, sometimes bloody urination, urethral discharge, prostate problems, scrotal diseases, excessive erections, inflammation of the sexual organs, sacral pain

Foods to Supplement

Legumes: Soy milk

Vegetables: Celery, asparagus, lettuce, watercress, Chinese cabbage, agar

Fruit: Plum, grapefruit, pomegranate, olive

Poultry: Duck egg

Organ: Cow's gallbladder

Foods to Avoid

Vegetables: Coconut milk

Beverages: Alcohol, coffee

Spices: All hot, fiery spices

Herbs: Peppermint

Liver Wind

Common symptoms: Liver fire symptoms plus pulsating headaches, extreme dizziness, unconsciousness, stroke, hemiplegia, trembling, spasms, tetany, convulsions, extreme stiffness of neck and limbs, back pain, rigidity, numbness or spasms of the limbs, abnormal walking, side pain, deviation of the eyes, lips, or tongue, facial paralysis, tinnitus, difficulty moving eyes, difficulty speaking

Foods to Supplement

Legumes: Peas

Seeds and nuts: Pine nuts

Vegetables: Lettuce

Fruit: Mulberry

Poultry: Chicken egg yolk

Animal: Pork leg

Foods to Avoid

Grains: Sweet rice

Seafood: Crab, trout

Poultry: Chicken

Spices: Star anise

Exercise and Neural Repair

Much like a healthy diet, physical activity is thought to benefit neuronal function by increasing brain-derived neurotrophic factor (BDNF) levels and reducing oxidative stress. More specifically, exercise has been found to play an important role in the regulation of neurite development,[31] maintenance of the synaptic structure,[32] axonal elongation,[33] and neurogenesis[34] in the adult brain. Studies have indicated that physical activity displays long-lasting changes in the morphology and function of the nervous system, suggesting that a lifestyle that implements regular exercise can lead to a brain that is more resistant to insults. Postinjury application of exercise seems promising in facilitating recovery, though more studies are necessary to determine when, and to what extent, it should be integrated into a client's lifestyle. Exercise applied after experimental traumatic brain injury has been shown to have beneficial effects, but the effects seem to depend on the postinjury resting period and the severity of the injury. Recent work has demonstrated that different types of exercise

---

31   Zurmohle, U., Herms, J., Schlingensiepen, R., *et al.* Changes in the expression of synapsin I and II messenger RNA during postnatal rat brain development. *Experimental Brain Research*. 1996; 108(3): 441–449.

32   Vaynman, S., Ying, Z., and Gomez-Pinilla, F. Exercises induces BDNF and synapsin I to specific hippocampal subfields. *Journal of Neuroscience Research*. 2004; 76(3): 356–362.

33   Molteni, R., Wu, A., Vaynman, S., *et al.* Exercise reverses the harmful effects of consumption of a high-fat diet on synaptic and behavioral plasticity associated to the action of brain-derived neurotrophic factor. *Neuroscience*. 2004; 123(2): 429–440.

34   Van Praag, H., Kempermann, G., and Gage, F.H. Running increases cell proliferation and neurogenesis in the adult mouse dentate gyrus. *Nature Neuroscience*. 1999; 2(3): 266–270.

seem to have greater stimulation of specific brain regions.[35] While preliminary, these findings are outlined in Table 48.1.

TABLE 48.1

Exercise type	Brain Region	Functions
Aerobic Exercise	Hippocampus	Memory
Sports Drills	Prefrontal cortex/basal ganglia	Attention, multitasking, inhibition
Yoga	Frontal lobe, insula	Integration of thoughts and emotion
Weight lifting	Prefrontal cortex	Complex thinking, reasoning, multitasking, problem-solving
High intensity intervals	Hypothalamus	Appetite regulation

Essential Oils

Essential oil qualities can vary greatly in character, ranging from antibacterial, antiviral, and anti-inflammatory natures to an immunostimulant with hormonal, glandular, emotional, circulatory, and calming effects, and a memory and alertness enhancer, that have been documented.[36, 37] The stimulation properties of these oils are said to lie in their structure, which closely resembles actual hormones.[38] The mechanism of their action is said to involve integration of essential oils into a biological signal of the receptor cells in the nose when inhaled. The signal is then transmitted to limbic and hypothalamic regions of the brain via the olfactory bulb. These signals cause the brain to release neurotransmitters like serotonin, norepinephrine, etc. to link the nervous system and other body systems to elicit a healing response.[39] The olfactory bulb has demonstrated persistent neurogenesis in adults.[40] This, coupled with the connections to the limbic system and hippocampus, may point to

35   Beal, T. *Five Different Physical Exercises That Affect the Brain in Very Different Ways.* Preventativedisease.com. 2016, Jun 14. Web. http://preventdisease.com/news/16/061416_Five-Different-Physical-Exercises-Affect-Brain-Different-Ways.shtml. Retrieved 2017, Oct 17.

36   Svoboda, K.P. and Deans, S.J. Biological activities of essential oils from selected aromatic plants. *Acta Horticulture.* 1995; 390: 203–209.

37   Svoboda, K., Hampson, J., and Hunter, E.A. Production and bioactivity of essential oils in secretory tissues of higher plants. *Proceedings of World Aromatherapy II Conference of National Association for Holistic Aromatherapy (NAHA).* 1998 Sep 25–28; 105–127.

38   Colgate, S.M. and Molyneux, R.J. *Bioactive Natural Products Detection, Isolation and Structural Determination.* Florida: CRC Press. 1933. Print.

39   Ali, B., Al-Wabel, N.A., Shams, S., *et al.* Essential oils used in aromatherapy: a systemic review. *Asian Pacific Journal of Tropical Biomedicine.* 2015 Aug; 5(8): 601–611. https://doi.org/10.1016/j.apjtb.2015.05.007

40   Altman, J. Autoradiographic and histological studies of postnatal neurogenesis. IV. Cell proliferation and migration in the anterior forebrain, with special reference to persisting neurogenesis in the olfactory bulb. *Journal of Complementary Neurology.* 1969; 137: 433–457. doi:10.1002/cne.901370404

particular scents and stimulation of the bulb, potentially altering the cognitive operations of memories or traumas. The matter of essential oils is a common question given the rise in their popularity in recent years. While I do not frequently use them clinically, below are a few oils which may be further explored in relation to brain injury.

Bergamot

A study demonstrated bergamot essential oil to reduce neuronal damage caused in vitro by excitotoxic stimuli and that this neuroprotection was associated with the prevention of injury-induced engagement of critical death pathways. In addition to preventing reactive oxygen species accumulation and activation of calpain, bergamot oil seemed to counteract the deactivation of Akt kinase and the consequent activation of glycogen synthase kinase-3β (GSK-3β). This was hypothesized to be the result of oil monoterpene hydrocarbons.[41]

Basil

Basil is a top-note oil which is listed as a nervine, CNS stimulant, and adrenal restorative. It is said to increase the guardian Qi, tonify the Kidney Yang, and rectify the brain. From these functions, it is indicated for concussion, fatigue, exhaustion, nervous depression, anxiety, memory loss, and shock.[42]

Frankincense/Boswellia

Frankincense is a base-note oil that, among other things, is said to act as a nervous restorative, antidepressant, antioxidant, and immunostimulant. In herbal form frankincense is known as Ru Xiang and is used in Chinese medicine frequently for its anti-inflammatory, analgesic, and wound-healing properties indicated for traumas of many types. As an oil, some of its indications include irritability, restlessness, sensory overstimulation, nightmares, mental confusion or weakness, neurasthenia, and menstrual irregularities. It is said to invigorate the Blood and calm the Shen by harmonizing the Yi and Hun.[43]

Vetiver

Vetiver is a base-note oil well regarded as having a relaxant or grounding effect in overstimulation conditions. It is listed as being indicated for anxiety, fear, hypersensitivity, overexcitement, delusion, and paranoia. It is also said to reduce basal ganglia and cingulate system hyperfunctioning and resolve temporal lobe dysregulation. Obsessions and compulsions are also listed as being conditions that may benefit. It is said to be a neuroendocrine restorative, assisting in hormonal or central nervous system deficiencies including fatigue,

---

41   Corasaniti, M.T., Maiuolo, J., Maida, S., *et al.* Cell signaling pathways in the mechanisms of neuroprotection afforded by bergamot essential oil against NMDA-induced cell death in vitro. *British Journal of Pharmacology.* 2007; 151(4): 518–529. doi: 10.1038/sj.bjp.0707237

42   Holmes, Peter. *AROMATICA: a clinical guide to essential oil therapeutics.* London: Jessica Kingsley Publishers. 2017. Print.

43   Holmes, Peter. *AROMATICA: a clinical guide to essential oil therapeutics.* London: Jessica Kingsley Publishers. 2017. Print.

chronic neurasthenia, insomnia, and hysteria. Additionally, it is indicated for a wide range of menstrual concerns. Chinese medical functions are said to include invigorating Blood, tonifying the Blood and essence, augmenting the Qi by tonifying the Spleen, nourishing Kidney Yin, and regulating Heart Qi to harmonize the Shen. A study of its chemical constituents concluded that vetiver oil may suppress inflammatory responses including nitric oxide production and cell apoptosis by regulating the expression of the inflammation-related enzymes heme oxygenase-1, inducible nitric oxide synthase, and cyclooxygenase-2 (inducible cyclooxygenase) and the inflammatory cytokines tumor necrosis factor-α, interleukin-1β, and interferon-β.[44]

Lavender

A top/middle note, lavender oil has been studied extensively, and there is growing evidence that it is of benefit in several neurological disorders. Several animal and human studies suggest anxiolytic, mood stabilizer, sedative, analgesic, and anticonvulsive and neuroprotective properties. Rat studies have shown that lavender oil diminishes glutamate-induced neurotoxicity, thus having a neuroprotective effect on cerebral ischemic injury[45, 46] as well as decreasing neurological deficit scores, infarct size, and the levels of mitochondria-generated reactive oxygen species and attenuated neuronal damage.[47] Chinese medical literature lists its actions as regulating in dysregulation conditions, a relaxant in overstimulation conditions, and mildly euphoric in acute shock conditions, speculating that it may reduce limbic system and basal ganglia hyperfunctioning while resolving temporal lobe dysfunction. In this sense, it is indicated for hypomania, PTSD, panic attacks, insomnia, irritability, depression, anxiety, feeling mentally overwhelmed, shock, and trauma.

Orange

Orange essential oil, a top note, has been found to have CNS depressant-like effects in mice. A study examined the effects on fear, memory, and immune-cell activation in a mouse model of PTSD using Pavlovian Fear Conditioning. Mice showed no difference in freezing up when fear stimuli were introduced, but when tested for extinction retention 48 hours later the treatment group experienced a significant decrease in freezing behavior versus control. This suggests that orange oil may affect extinction of fear memories.[48]

44   Chou, S-T., Lai, C-P., Lin, C-C., and Shih, Y. Study of the chemical composition, antioxidant activity and anti-inflammatory activity of essential oil from Vetiveria zizanioides. *Food Chemistry*. 2012; 134(1): 262–268. https://doi.org/10.1016/j.foodchem.2012.02.131

45   Koulivand, P.H., Khaleghi Ghadiri, M., and Gorji, A. Lavender and the nervous system. *Evidence-based Complementary and Alternative Medicine: eCAM*. 2013; 2013: 681304. doi:10.1155/2013/681304

46   Büyükokuroğlu, M.E., Gepdiremen, A., Hacimüftüoğlu, A., and Oktay, M.J. The effects of aqueous extract of Lavandula angustifolia flowers in glutamate-induced neurotoxicity of cerebellar granular cell culture of rat pups. *Ethnopharmacology*. 2003 Jan; 84(1): 91–94.

47   Wang, D., Yuan, X., Liu, T., Liu, L., Hu, Y., Wang, Z., and Zheng, Q. Neuroprotective activity of lavender oil on transient focal cerebral ischemia in mice. *Molecules*. 2012 Aug 15; 17(8): 9803–9817.

48   Moshfegh, C., Swiercz, P., Hopkins, L., and Marvar, P. Effects of essential oil on fear memory and the immune response: a potential alternative therapy for post-traumatic stress disorder (PSTD). *The FASEB Journal*. 2016 Apr; 30(1): Supplement 1238.5.

Point Indications Relating to the Brain According to George Soulié de Morant

Lung Meridian

LU-1 Zhong Fu (Central Workshop): Tonifies temporal–parietal lobe, medulla, automaton–parrot, inferior spinal cord

LU-2 Yun Men (Door of the Clouds): Tonifies three nervous centers, three psychologies

LU-3 Tian Fu (Heavenly Workshop): Tonifies temporal–parietal lobes, parrot [Hun]

LU-4 Xia Bai (Close to the Whiteness): Tonifies temporal–parietal lobes, automaton–parrot [Hun]

LU-5 Chi Ze (Elbow Crease): Disperses cerebellum, primate [Po]

LU-6 Kong Zui (Deepest Hollow): Tonifies temporal–parietal lobes

LU-7 Lie Que (Broken Sequence): Tonifies posterior part of frontal lobes, cerebellum, medulla oblongata, spinal cord, psychology

LU-8 Jing Qu (Passage for the Meridian): Tonifies cerebellum, mid spinal cord

LU-9 Tai Yuan (Supreme Abyss): Tonifies mid-brain, spinal cord

LU-10 Yu Ji (Area of the Fish): Tonifies cerebellum, upper spinal cord

LU-11 Shao Shang (Lesser Merchant): Tonifies cerebellum, spinal cord

Large Intestine Meridian

LI-1 Shang Yang (Yang of the Merchants): Tonifies inferior occipital lobes, temporal–parietal lobes, pituitary and thyroid glands

LI-2 Er Jian (Second Interval): Disperses inferior occipital, inferior frontal lobes

LI-3 San Jian (Third Interval)

LI-4 He Gu (Bottom of the Valley): Tonifies three nervous centers, three sense organs, opposite pituitary

LI-5 Yang Xi (Little Valley of Yang): Tonifies frontal lobes, spinal cord

LI-6 Pian Li (Lateral Succession): Tonifies brain, cerebellum, medulla oblongata, spinal cord

LI-7 Wen Liu (Warm Dwelling): Tonifies temporal–parietal lobes

LI-8 Xia Lian (Inferior Angle): Tonifies opposite brain

LI-9 Shang Lian (Superior Angle): Tonifies opposite and central inferior lateral side of the brain, opposite spinal cord

LI-10 San Li (Arm Third Mile): Tonifies posterior frontal lobes

LI-11 Qu Chi (Swamp of the Curve): Tonifies all nervous centers, the three endocrines, and three levels of the psyche

LI-12 Zhou Liao (Hollow of the Elbow): Tonifies posterior frontal lobes

LI-13 Wu Li (Fifth Mile)

LI-14 Bi Nao (Deltoid and Arm):

LI-15 Jian Yu (Deltoid of the Shoulder): Tonifies the posterior frontal, temporal–parietal lobes

LI-16 Ju Hu (Big Bone): Tonifies inferior frontal lobes

LI-17 Tian Ding (Celestial Cauldron)

LI-18 Fu Tu (Suddenness Tamed)

LI-19 He Liao (Hollow of Cereals)

LI-20 Ying Xiang (Encountering Perfumes)

Stomach Meridian

ST-1 Cheng Qi (Receiver of Tears): Tonifies inferior occipital lobe, eyes

ST-2 Si Bai (Four Whitenesses): Tonifies inferior occipital lobe

ST-3 Ju Liao (Great Hollow): Tonifies eye

ST-4 Di Cang (Silo, Granary of Earth): Tonifies medulla oblongata, spinal cord

ST-5 Da Ying (Great Meeting): Tonifies cerebellum

ST-6 Jia Che (Maxillary): Tonifies anterior temporal lobes, eyes

ST-7 Xia Guan (Lower Barrier): Tonifies anterior temporal lobe

ST-8 Tou Wei (Chain of the Head): Tonifies occipital lobes, eyes

ST-9 Ren Ying (Human Meetings or External Sensations): Tonifies posterior part of inferior frontal lobe, anterior temporal lobe

ST-10 Shui Tu (Sudden Water): Tonifies posterior part of frontal lobes

ST-11 Qi She (Home of Energy): Tonifies cerebellum, pons

ST-12 Que Pen (Basin of the Point)

ST-13 Qi Hu (Sidegate of Energy): Tonifies temporal–parietal lobes

ST-14 Ku Fang (House of Treasure): Tonifies anterior frontal lobes, superior occipital lobes, medulla oblongata, spinal cord

ST-15 Wu Yi (Draft-screen of the Bedroom): Tonifies cerebellum, inferior spinal cord

ST-16 Ying Chunag (Window of the Chest): Tonifies medulla

ST-17 Ru Zhong (Middle of the Breast)

ST-18 Ru Gen (Base of the Breast)

ST-19 Bu Rong (Not at Ease)

ST-20 Cheng Man (Receive Fullness): Tonifies cerebellum

ST-21 Liang Men (Door with Beam): Tonifies hypothalamus (anterior), parasympathetic

ST-22 Guan Men (Door of the Barrier): Tonifies medulla oblongata, spinal cord

ST-23 Tai Yi (Great Curvature): Tonifies posterior part of the mid-brain (sympathetic)

ST-24 Hua Rou [Men] (Sliding Flesh Gate): Tonifies anterior opposite frontal lobes

ST-25 Tian Shu (Celestial Axis): Tonifies temporal–parietal lobes, automaton–parrot [Hun], superior occipital lobes, primate [Po]

ST-26 Wai Ling (Exterior Hill)

ST-27 Da Ju (Large Eminence): Tonifies superior occipital lobes, primate [Po], posterior frontal lobes

ST-28 Shui Dao (Way of Water): Tonifies opposite eye, posterior frontal lobes

ST-29 Gui Lai (Recurrence, Periodicity): Tonifies superior occipital lobes, primate [Po], eyes

ST-30 Qi Chong (Assaults of Energy): Tonifies temporal–parietal lobes, superior occipital lobes, automaton–parrot [Hun], primate [Po]

ST-31 Bi Guan (Barrier to Articulation): Tonifies spinal cord

ST-32 Fu Tu (Lying Hare): Tonifies superior part of the posterior frontal lobes and middle part same side, medulla oblongata, spinal cord

ST-33 Yin Shi (Market in Shadow): Tonifies cerebellum, opposite side of superior part of the posterior and frontal lobes, middle part same side, medulla oblongata, opposite spinal cord

ST-34 Liang Qiu (Hill of the Roof-Beams)

ST-35 Du Bi (Calf's Nose)

ST-36 Zu San Li (Leg Three Miles): Tonifies nerves, governor vessel

ST-37 Shang Lian (Upper Edge): Tonifies opposite superior occipital lobes, primate [Po], spinal cord same side

ST-38 Tiao Kou (Mouth in Pieces): Tonifies superior posterior frontal lobes

ST-39 Xia Lian (Lower Angle): Tonifies temporal–parietal lobes, automaton–parrot [Hun]

ST-40 Feng Long (Abundance and Prosperity): Tonifies opposite mid-brain, opposite frontal lobes; evolved man

ST-41 Jie Xi (Enlarging Valley): Tonifies posterior central lobes, sympathetic system, superior occipital lobes, primate

ST-42 Chong Yang (Yang Assault): Tonifies temporal–parietal lobes, eyes, medulla, spinal cord

ST-43 Xiang Gu (Hollowed Valley): Tonifies opposite mid-brain, opposite inferior eye

ST-44 Nei Ting (Interior Pavilion): Tonifies temporal–parietal lobes, medulla oblongata, spinal cord, automaton–parrot

ST-45 Li Dui (Cruel Payment): Disperses temporal–parietal lobes, automaton–parrot [Hun], superior occipital lobes, primate [Po]

Spleen Meridian

SP-1 Yin Bai (Hidden Whiteness): Tonifies anterior frontal lobes

SP-2 Da Du (Great Capital): Tonifies anterior frontal lobes, inferior occipital lobes

SP-3 Tai Bai (Supreme Whiteness): Tonifies anterior frontal lobe, evolved man [Shen]

SP-4 Gong Sun (Son of the Prince): Tonifies frontal lobe, lower spinal cord

SP-5 Shang Qui (Mound of the Merchant): Disperses evolved man [Shen], frontal lobes

SP-6 San Yin Jiao (Reunion of 3 Yin): Tonifies frontal lobes, cerebellum, pons, spinal cord

SP-7 Lou Gu (Valley of the Outflow): Tonifies cerebellum

SP-8 Di Ji (Celestial Elasticity)

SP-9 Yin Ling Quan (Source of the Internal Plateau): Tonifies cerebellum, pons

SP-10 Xue Hai (Sea of Blood)

SP-11 Ji Men (Portal of the Winnowing Machine): Tonifies posterior frontal lobes, lower spinal cord

SP-12 Chong Men (Door of Assaults)

SP-13 Fu She (House of Workshops): Tonifies occipital lobe

SP-14 Fu Jie (Knot of the Abdomen)

SP-15 Da Heng (Great Transverse): Tonifies anterior frontal lobes, evolved man [Shen]

SP-16 Fu Ai (Mourning of the Abdomen)

SP-17 Shi Dou (Cave of Nourishment)

SP-18 Tian Xi (Celestial Flow)

SP-19 Xiong Xiang (Region of the Chest)

SP-20 Zhou Rong (Circulating Blood)

SP-21 Da Bao (Large Envelope): Tonifies posterior frontal lobes, cerebellum, medulla oblongata, sense organs

Heart Meridian

HT-1 Ji Quan (Source of the Axis): Tonifies opposite frontal lobes

HT-2 Qing Ling (The Immateriality of Sky): Tonifies opposite frontal lobes

HT-3 Shao Hai (Smaller Sea): Tonifies three nervous centers, three endocrines, three levels of the psyche, eyes

HT-4 Ling Dao (Way of Immateriality): Tonifies three nervous centers, three levels of the psyche, three endocrines, three sense organs

HT-5 Tong Li (Village of Passage): Tonifies anterior frontal lobes, evolved man [Shen]

HT-6 Yin Xi (Valley of Yin): Tonifies cerebellum, pons, medulla oblongata, spinal cord, opposite eye

HT-7 Shen Men (Door of the Evolved): Tonifies opposite brain, spinal cord

HT-8 Shao Fu (Lesser Workshop): Tonifies cerebellum, pons

HT-9 Shao Chong (Lesser Attack): Tonifies frontal lobes, governor meridian, opposite eye

Small Intestine Meridian

SI-1 Shao Ze (Smaller Marsh)

SI-2 Qian Gu (Anterior Valley): Tonifies posterior frontal lobes

SI-3 Hou Xi (Posterior Vale): Tonifies dorsal spinal cord same side, opposite brain, GV-22, inferior posterior frontal lobes, cerebellum, spinal cord, lateral eye

SI-4 Wan Gu (Wrist Bone): Tonifies spinal cord, governor vessel; disperses occipital lobes, mid-brain

SI-5 Yang Gu (Yang External Valley): Tonifies opposite brain

SI-6 Yang Lao (Help for the Aged): Tonifies opposite eye, opposite inferior occipital lobe

SI-7 Zhi Zheng (Correct Limb): Tonifies opposite mid-brain, opposite mid-height of spinal cord

SI-8 Xiao Hai (Small Sea): Tonifies medulla oblongata, spinal cord, opposite lateral eye

SI-9 Jian Zhen (True Shoulder): Tonifies posterior frontal lobes

SI-10 Nao Shu (Ascent of the Deltoid)

SI-11 Tian Zong (Heavenly Ancestors)

SI-12 Cheng Feng (To Ride the Wind)

SI-13 Qu Yuan (Curve of the Wall)

SI-14 Jian Wai (Outside the Shoulder): Tonifies temporal–parietal lobes

SI-15 Jian Zhong (Middle of the Shoulder): Tonifies temporal–parietal lobes, occipital lobes

SI-16 Tian Chuang (Celestial Window): Tonifies inferior frontal lobes, temporal–parietal lobes, lateral eye

SI-17 Tian Rong (Celestial Face): Tonifies occipital lobes, opposite lateral eye

SI-18 Quan Liao (Cheek Bone Hole): Tonifies inferior frontal and temporal–parietal lobes, inferior occipital lobes, lateral eye

SI-19 Ting Gong (Hollow of the Cheek): Tonifies medulla and spinal cord

Bladder Meridian

BL-1 Jing Ming (Clarity of the Pupils): Tonifies inferior occipital lobe

BL-2 Zan Zhu (Tight Bamboo): Tonifies opposite inferior occipital lobes

BL-3 Mei Chong (Attack on the Eyebrows)

BL-4 Qu Cha (Minister of the Curve): Tonifies inferior spinal cord, temporal–parietal lobes

BL-5 Wu Chu (Five Places): Tonifies superior posterior frontal lobes

BL-6 Cheng Guang (Receives Light): Tonifies inferior occipital lobe

BL-7 Tong Tian (Communicates with the Sky): Tonifies opposite inferior occipital lobe

BL-8 Luo Que (Track of the Veins): Tonifies temporal–parietal, posterior frontal lobes

BL-9 Yu Zhen (Pillow of Jade): Tonifies inferior occipital lobes

BL-10 Tian Zhu (Celestial Column): Tonifies the parasympathetic system, anterior mid-brain

BL-11 Da Zhu (Great Shuttle): Tonifies medulla oblongata, spinal cord, thoracic spine, governor vessel

BL-12 Feng Men (Door of Wind): Tonifies mid-brain (parasympathetic), eye same side

BL-13 Fei Shu (Assent of the Lungs)

BL-14 Jueyin Shu (Assent of the Least Yin)

BL-15 Xin Shu (Assent of the Heart)

BL-16 Du Shu (General Assent Point)

BL-17 Ge Shu (Assent of the Diaphragm): Tonifies temporal–parietal lobes

BL-18 Gan Shu (Assent of the Liver): Tonifies temporal–parietal lobes

BL-19 Dan Shu (Assent of the Gallbladder): Tonifies temporal–parietal lobes

BL-20 Pi Shu (Assent of the Spleen)

BL-21 Wei Shu (Assent of the Stomach)

BL-22 San Jiao Shu (Assent of the Triple Warmer)

BL-23 Shen Shu (Assent of the Kidney): Tonifies superior occipital lobe, primate [Po]

BL-24 Qi Hai Shu (Assent of the Sea of Qi)

BL-25 Da Chang Shu (Assent of the Large Intestine)

BL-26 Guan Yuan Shu (Assent of the Origin of the Barrier)

BL-27 Xiao Chang Shu (Assent of the Small Intestine)

BL-28 Pang Guang Shu (Assent of the Bladder)

BL-29 Zhong Lu Shu (Assent of the Central Vertebrae)

BL-30 Bai Huan Shu (Assent of the Sphincter): Tonifies cerebellum

BL-31 Shang Liao (Superior Hole)

BL-32 Ci Liao (Second Hole)

BL-33 Zhong Liao (Central Hole)

BL-34 Xia Liao (Lower Hole)

BL-35 Hui Yang (Reunion of the Yang)

BL-36 Cheng Fu (Receives Support)

BL-37 Yin Men (Door of Propensity)

BL-38 Fu Xi (Superficial Vale)

BL-39 Wei Yang (Exterior of the Delegate)

BL-40 Wei Zhong (Middle of the Delegate): Tonifies governor vessel, evolved man [Shen], superior occipital lobes, primate [Po]

BL-41 Fu Fen (Adjoining Division)

BL-42 Po Hu (Portal of the Primate): Tonifies primate [Po]

BL-43 Gao Huang Shu (Vital Centers): Tonifies three nervous centers, three endocrine glands

BL-44 Shen Tang (Room of the Evolved): Tonifies temporal–parietal and frontal lobes

BL-45 Yi Xi (Cries of Pain): Tonifies mid-brain (?)

BL-46 Ge Guan (Barrier of the Diaphragm)

BL-47 Hun Men (Door of the Automaton–Parrot): Tonifies automaton–parrot [Hun]

BL-48 Yang Gang (Firmness of Yang)

BL-49 Yi She (Home of the Imagination)

BL-50 Wei Cang (Storehouse of the Stomach): Tonifies cerebellum

BL-51 Huang Men (Door of the Vital Centers): Tonifies medulla oblongata, spinal cord

BL-52 Zhi Shi (Home of the Decision-Will): Tonifies medulla oblongata, spinal cord

BL-53 Bao Huang (Vital of the Uterus)

BL-54 Zhi Bian (Beside the Row): Tonifies central brain, medulla oblongata

BL-55 He Yang (Reunites the Yang): Tonifies mid-brain

BL-56 Cheng Jin (Receives the Muscles): Tonifies cerebellum

BL-57 Cheng Shan (Receives the Mountain): Tonifies cerebellum

BL-58 Fei Yang (Gliding Flight): Tonifies posterior frontal lobes

BL-59 Fu Yang (Additional Yang): Tonifies opposite superior occipital lobes

BL-60 Kun Lun (Mount Kunlun): Tonifies parathyroid glands; disperses all nervous centers (especially mid-brain): endocrines (except parathyroids), levels of the psyche

BL-61 Pu Can (Help of the Servant): Tonifies mid-brain (thalamus)

BL-62 Shen Mai (Perforating Vessel): Tonifies brain

BL-63 Jin Men (Gate of Gold): Tonifies anterior frontal lobe; disperses mid-brain

BL-64 Jing Gu (Bone of the Capital): Tonifies posterior inferior frontal lobes

BL-65 Shu Gu (Linking Bones): Disperses cerebellum, spinal cord

BL-66 Tong Gu (Communicating Valley): Tonifies medulla oblongata, frontal lobes, upper spinal cord

BL-67 Zhi Yin (Extreme Yin): Tonifies posterior frontal lobes, posterior hypothalamus (sympathetic)

Kidney Meridian

KI-1 Yong Quan (Bubbling Source): Tonifies medulla oblongata, spinal cord, superior occipital lobes, primate [Po]

KI-2 Ran Gu (Valley of Approbation): Disperses medulla oblongata, spinal cord

KI-3 Tai Xi (Supreme Vale): Enhanced connectivity between the superior temporal gyrus and postcentral gyrus

KI-4 Da Zhang (Big Bell): Tonifies superior occipital lobe, primate [Po], spinal cord

KI-5 Shui Quan (Water Source): Tonifies superior occipital lobes, cerebellum

KI-6 Zhao Hai (Mirroring Ocean): Tonifies cerebellum, pons, lower spinal cord

KI-7 Fu Liu (Flows Again): Tonifies superior occipital lobes, primate [Po], medulla oblongata, spinal cord

KI-8 Jiao Xin (Mutual Confidence): Tonifies posterior frontal lobes, spinal cord

KI-9 Zhu Bin (Built Riverbank): Tonifies superior occipital lobes, primate [Po], lower GV vessel

KI-10 Yin Gu (Valley of Yin): Tonifies cerebellum, pons, spinal cord, lateral eye same side

KI-11 Heng Gu (Transverse Bone): Tonifies superior occipital lobes, lower spinal cord, primate

KI-12 Da He (Great Respectability): Tonifies superior occipital lobes, primate [Po], opposite lateral side of eye

KI-13 Qi Xue (Point of Energy): Tonifies brain, cerebellum, spinal cord, lateral side of eye

KI-14 Si Man (Four Plentitudes): Tonifies mid-brain opposite, spinal cord, eye same side

KI-15 Zhong Zhu (Central Flow): Tonifies anterior frontal lobes, inferior lateral side of the eye

KI-16 Huang Shu (Assent of the Vital Centers): Tonifies posterior frontal lobes, spinal cord, opposite eye

KI-17 Shang Qiu (Turning of the Merchants): Tonifies cerebellum, pons, eye same side

KI-18 Shi Guan (Stone Barrier): Tonifies temporal–parietal lobes, spinal cord, eye same side

KI-19 Yin Du (Yin Capital): Tonifies cerebellum, pons, spinal cord, eye same side

KI-20 Tong Gu (Communicating Valley): Tonifies cerebellum, pons, spinal cord, eye same side

KI-21 You Men (Obscure Door): Tonifies temporal–parietal lobe, medulla oblongata, spinal cord

KI-22 Bu Lang (Veranda of the Steps): Tonifies cerebellum, lower part of the eye

KI-23 Shen Feng (Mark of the Evolved Man): Tonifies anterior mid-brain (vagus, anterior hypothalamus)

KI-24 Ling Xu (Emptiness of the Immaterial): Tonifies anterior frontal lobes

KI-25 Shen Cang (Treasure of the Evolved Man): Tonifies anterior frontal lobe, medulla oblongata, spinal cord

KI-26 Yu Zhong (In Doubt): Tonifies cerebellum, lower spinal cord

KI-27 Shu Fu (Workshop of the Assent Points): Tonifies three nervous centers, three endocrines, three levels of the psyche

Pericardium Meridian

PC-1 Tian Chi (Celestial Pool): Tonifies cerebellum, pons, opposite eye

PC-2 Tian Quan (Celestial Source): Tonifies mid-brain, cerebellum, medulla oblongata, spinal cord, eye

PC-3 Qu Ze (Pool of the Curve)

PC-4 Xi Men (Door of the Vale): Tonifies temporal–parietal lobes, automaton–parrot [Hun]

PC-5 Jian Shi (Intercalary Messenger): Tonifies occipital lobes, primate [Po]

PC-6 Nei Guan (Internal Barrier): Tonifies cerebellum, spinal cord

PC-7 Da Ling (Great Plateau): Tonifies cerebellum

PC-8 Lao Gong (Palace of Fatigue): Tonifies sympathetic system, endocrine system, superior occipital lobes, inferior frontal lobes, spinal cord; disperses parasympathetic system

PC-9 Zhong Chong (Central Assault): Tonifies temporal–parietal lobes, automaton– parrot [Hun]

Triple Warmer Meridian

TW-1 Guan Chong (Assault on the Barrier): Tonifies temporal–parietal lobes, mid-height of spinal cord

TW-2 Ye Men (Door of the Humors): Tonifies opposite brain, lower spinal cord, temporal– parietal lobes

TW-3 Zhong Zhu (Central Islet): Tonifies brain, spinal cord

TW-4 Yang Chi (Pool of Yang)

TW-5 Wai Guan (Barrier of the Yang): Tonifies three levels of the psyche, three sense organs, mid-brain, spinal cord, sympathetic system

TW-6 Zhi Gou (Ditch like a Fork): Tonifies posterior frontal lobes, mid-brain, cerebellum, spinal cord

TW-7 Hui Zong (Reunion of the Ancestors): Tonifies temporal–parietal lobes, automaton– parrot [Hun], spinal cord, opposite thyroid gland

TW-8 San Yang Luo (Secondary Vessel of the 3 Yang): Tonifies posterior frontal and temporal lobes same hemisphere, temporal–parietal lobes

TW-9 Si Du (Four Trenches): Tonifies temporal–parietal lobes

TW-10 Tian Jing (Celestial Well): Disperses cerebellum, medulla oblongata, spinal cord, mid-brain (thalamus)

TW-11 Qing Leng Yuan (Abyss of Limpid Cold)

TW-12 Xiao Luo (River During the Thaw): Tonifies posterior frontal lobes, spinal cord

TW-13 Nao Hui (Reunion of the Deltoid)

TW-14 Jian Liao (Hollow of the Shoulder): Tonifies opposite lateral eye

TW-15 Tian Liao (Celestial Hollow): Tonifies cerebellum

TW-16 Tian You (Celestial Opening): Tonifies opposite lateral eye

TW-17 Yi Feng (Wind Screen)

TW-18 Qi Mai (Vessel of Stupidity): Tonifies anterior part of eye same side

TW-19 Lu Xi (Breath of the Cheeks): Tonifies posterior and inferior frontal lobes, medulla oblongata, opposite spinal cord, anterior eye same side

TW-20 Jiao Sun (Descendants of the Horns): Tonifies thyroid, eye, opposite occipital lobes

TW-21 Er Men (Door of the Ear): Tonifies anterior temporal–parietal lobes, eye

TW-22 He Liao (Silo, Hollow of Cereals): Tonifies eye

TW-23 Si Zhu Kong (Bamboo Thread): Tonifies lower opposite frontal lobes

Gallbladder Meridian

GB-1 Tong Zi Liao (Hole in the Pupil): Tonifies spinal cord same side, opposite occipital lobes, opposite retina

GB-2 Ting Hui (Reunion of Hearing): Tonifies superior occipital lobes

GB-3 Ke Zhu Ren (Host and Guest): Tonifies occipital lobes, lateral side of the opposite posterior eye

GB-4 Han Yan (Heavy Chin): Tonifies upper posterior frontal lobes same side, medulla oblongata, rectus externus of the same side eye

GB-5 Xuan Lu (Suspended Skull): Tonifies opposite side of medulla oblongata, both eyes

GB-6 Xuan Li (Suspended Hundredth): Tonifies eye (oblique muscles)

GB-7 Qu Bin (Twisted Bun): Tonifies occipital lobes, spinal cord, eye

GB-8 Shuai Gu (Valley of the Assembly): Tonifies spinal cord, opposite temporal–parietal lobes

GB-9 Tian Chong (Sky Assault): Tonifies opposite inferior occipital lobes

GB-10 Fu Bai (Superficial Whiteness): Tonifies inferior occipital lobes, eye same side

GB-11 Qiao Yin (Yin of the Opening): Tonifies lower opposite brain, eye same side

GB-12 Wan Gu (Final Bone [mastoid]): Tonifies opposite superior posterior frontal lobes, eye

GB-13 Ben Shen (Fundamental Evolved Man): Tonifies posterior frontal lobes opposite and inferior, opposite spinal cord

GB-14 Yang Bai (Extended Whiteness): Tonifies inferior opposite occipital lobes, eye: opposite rectus externus

GB-15 Lin Qi (Near to Tears): Tonifies posterior eye, inferior occipital lobes

GB-16 Mu Chuang (Window of the Eye): Tonifies eye (especially lateral)

GB-17 Zheng Ying (Correct Stage)

GB-18 Cheng Ling (Receives the Immaterial): Tonifies opposite inferior frontal lobes

GB-19 Nao Kong (Hollow of the Brain): Tonifies half brain opposite (meninges), medial part of the eye same side

GB-20 Feng Chi (Marsh of Winds): Tonifies sympathetic system, governor vessel, posterior mid-brain (posterior hypothalamus), pons, medulla oblongata, spinal cord, three endocrines, opposite eye

GB-21 Jian Jing (Well of the Shoulder): Tonifies opposite side of the brain, three psychological pulses, three endocrines

GB-22 Yuan Ye (Abyss of the Axilla): Tonifies lower posterior frontal lobes

GB-23 Zhe Jin (Brusque Muscles): Tonifies opposite side of the brain, spinal cord, eye same side

GB-24 Ri Yue (Sun and Moon): Tonifies cerebellum

GB-25 Jing Men (Door of the Capital): Tonifies medulla, spinal cord, eyes

GB-26 Dai Mai (Belt Vessel): Tonifies brain, medulla, spinal cord

GB-27 Wu Shu (The Five Pivots): Tonifies posterior frontal lobes

GB-28 Huan Tiao (To Jump into a Hoop): Tonifies posterior frontal lobes, spinal cord

GB-29 Ju Liao (Stays in the Hole): Tonifies mid-brain

GB-30 Wei Dao (Path of the Parallels): Tonifies mid-brain

GB-31 Feng Shi (Wind Market)

GB-32 Xia Du (Lower Torrent): Tonifies cerebellum, lower spinal cord

GB-33 Xi Yang Guan (External Barrier of the Knee): Tonifies temporal–parietal lobes

GB-34 Yang Ling Quan (Source of the External Plateau): Tonifies posterior frontal lobes, cerebellum, medulla oblongata, eyes; "reunion of the spinal cord"

GB-35 Yang Jiao (Crossing the Yang): Tonifies medulla oblongata; disperses anterior frontal lobes

GB-36 Wai Qiu (Curve Toward the Exterior): Tonifies posterior frontal lobes, mid-brain, opposite governor vessel

GB-37 Guang Ming (Brilliant Light): Tonifies medulla oblongata same side, eyes

GB-38 Yang Fu (Help for the Yang): Disperses superior occipital lobes, primate [Po], eye same side; tonifies evolved man [Shen]

GB-39 Xuan Zhong (Suspended Bell): Tonifies posterior frontal lobes, bone marrow

GB-40 Qiu Xu (Fair of the Hill): Tonifies superior occipital lobes, primate [Po], spinal cord; enhanced connectivity between the superior temporal gyrus and anterior insula

GB-41 Lin Qi (Ready to Cry): Tonifies inferior occipital lobes, spinal cord, thyroid

GB-42 Di Wu Hui (Fifth Reunion of the Earth): Tonifies temporal–parietal lobes, eye

GB-43 Xia Xi (Narrowed Valley): Tonifies superior occipital lobes, primate [Po]

GB-44 Qiao Yin (Yin of the Opening): Tonifies temporal–parietal lobes, opposite eye

Liver Meridian

LR-1 Da Dun (Great Abundance)

LR-2 Xing Jian (Acting Interval): Disperses cerebellum, medulla oblongata, lower spinal cord, opposite eye

LR-3 Tai Chong (Supreme Assault): Tonifies temporal–parietal lobes, automaton–parrot [Hun]

LR-4 Zhong Feng (Central Seal): Tonifies brain, medulla oblongata, spinal cord, three endocrines

LR-5 Li Gou (Wormwood Hollow): Tonifies cerebellum, pons, posterior frontal lobes. Opposite cerebellum: if insufficient, spasms: tonify; if excess, weakness: disperse

LR-6 Zhong Du (Central Capital): Tonifies posterior frontal lobes, temporal–parietal lobes, opposite eye

LR-7 Xi Guan (Barrier of the Knee): Tonifies posterior frontal upper lobes opposite, lower part same side

LR-8 Qu Quan (Source of the Curve): Tonifies cerebellum

LR-9 Yin Bao (Envelope of the Yin): Tonifies cerebellum, spinal cord

LR-10 Wu Li (Fifth Mile): Tonifies mid-brain, cerebellum, lower spinal cord

LR-11 Yin Lian (Yin Angle): Tonifies anterior frontal lobes

LR-12 Yang Shi (Arrows for Sheep)

LR-13 Zhang Men (Great Door): Tonifies opposite side brain, cerebellum, medulla oblongata, spinal cord opposite

LR-14 Qi Men (Door of the Epoch): Tonifies anterior and posterior frontal lobes

Conception Vessel Meridian

CV-1 Hui Yin (Reunion of the Yin): Tonifies governor vessel

CV-2 Qu Gu (Bone Curve, Pubis): Tonifies inferior left occipital lobe

CV-3 Zhong Ji (Central Pole): Tonifies three nervous centers, three levels of the psyche, three endocrines (except parathyroids)

CV-4 Guan Yuan (Origin of the Barrier): Tonifies anterior frontal lobe, opposite eye, evolved man [Shen]

CV-5 Shi Men (Stone Door): Tonifies opposite mid-brain (stiopallidum)

CV-6 Qi Hai (Ocean of Energy): Tonifies nervous centers, three endocrines, three levels of the psyche, three sense organs

CV-7 Yin Jiao (Crossing of the Yin)

CV-8 Shen Guan (Barrier for the Evolved Man): Tonifies opposite brain, three levels of the psyche, three endocrines, three sense organs

CV-9 Shui Fen (Division of the Waters): Tonifies medulla oblongata, dorsal spine

CV-10 Xia Wan (Lower Stomach)

CV-11 Jian Li (Established Village)

CV-12 Zhong Wan (Central Stomach): Tonifies occipital lobes, parasympathetic system

CV-13 Shang Wan (Upper Stomach): Tonifies temporal–parietal lobes

CV-14 Ju Guan (Great Barrier)

CV-15 Jiu Wei (Pigeon's Tail): Tonifies corpus callosum, opposite lateral eye; disperses anterior frontal lobes, temporal–parietal lobes, evolved man [Shen], parrot [Hun]

CV-16 Zhong Ting (Central Pavilion): Tonifies cerebellum, spinal cord

CV-17 Shan Zhong (Middle of the Chest): Tonifies cerebellum, medulla oblongata

CV-18 Yu Tang (Room of Jade): Tonifies pituitary gland

CV-19 Zi Gong (Purple Palace)

CV-20 Hua Gai (Flowered Cover): Tonifies mid-brain (anterior hypothalamus, vagus), thyroid gland

CV-21 Xuan Ji (Armillary Sphere): Tonifies cerebellum

CV-22 Tian Tu (Celestial Spring): Tonifies thyroid same side, cerebellum

CV-23 Lian Quan (Source of the Angle)

CV-24 Cheng Jiang (Recieves the Noodles): Tonifies posterior frontal lobes

Governor Vessel Meridian

GV-1 Chang Qiang (Prolonged Stiffness): Tonifies governor vessel, spinal cord, medulla oblongata, superior occipital lobe, primate [Po]

GV-2 Yao Shu (Assent Point of the Lumbar): Tonifies governor vessel

GV-3 Yao Yang Guan (Barrier of the Yang): Tonifies governor vessel, mid-brain opposite, all the nerves

GV-4 Ming Men (Gate of Destiny): Tonifies governor vessel, cerebellum, inferior occipital lobes, eye

GV-5 Xuan Shu (Axis of Suspension): Tonifies governor vessel, superior occipital lobes, primate [Po]

GV-6 Ji Zhong (Middle of the Vertebrae): Tonifies governor vessel, posterior frontal lobes, cerebellum, spinal cord

GV-7 Zhong Shu (Central Axis): Tonifies governor vessel

GV-8 Jin Suo (Contraction of the Muscles): Tonifies governor vessel, anterior frontal lobes

GV-9 Zhi Yang (Maximum Yang): Tonifies governor vessel, anterior frontal lobes, evolved man [Shen]

GV-10 Ling Tai (Terrace of the Immaterial): Tonifies governor vessel, medulla oblongata

GV-11 Shen Dao (Way of the Evolved Man): Tonifies governor vessel, anterior frontal lobes, evolved man [Shen], eyes

GV-12 Shen Zhu (Pillar of the Body): Tonifies governor vessel, brain, spinal cord

GV-13 Tao Dao (Way of Ovens): Tonifies governor vessel, medulla oblongata, spinal cord, eyes

GV-14 Da Zhui (Great Hammer) (C-7–pituitary): Tonifies pituitary (deficiency), its 13 hormones and all the endocrines, vagus, adrenals, thyroids, parathyroids, three nervous centers

GV-15 Ya Men (Door of Muteness): Tonifies governor vessel, spinal cord, temporal–parietal lobes

GV-16 Feng Fu (Wind Workshop): Tonifies governor vessel, adrenals, anterior and central brain (vagus)

GV-17 Nao Hu (Little Brain Barrier): Tonifies governor vessel, cerebellum, lateral eye same side

GV-18 Qiang Jian (Stiff Interval): Tonifies all energy of the governor vessel, medulla oblongata, superior occipital lobes, primate

GV-19 Hou Ding (Posterior Summit of the Head): Tonifies governor vessel, superior occipital lobes, primate, eye

GV-20 Bai Hui (One Hundred Meetings): Tonifies governor vessel, superior occipital lobes, primate [Po], anterior mid-brain, parasympathetic

GV-21 Chang Hui Qian Ding (Anterior Summit): Tonifies governor vessel, temporal–parietal lobes, automaton–parrot [Hun]

GV-22 Chang Hui (Meeting of the Brain): Tonifies the opposite brain, Yang energy of the whole body

GV-23 Shang Xing (Superior Star): Tonifies governor vessel, opposite cerebellum, eyeball same side

GV-24 Shen Ting (Palace of the Evolved Man): Tonifies opposite frontal lobes, evolved man [Shen], opposite eye

GV-25 Su Liao (Simple Hole): Tonifies governor vessel

GV-26 Ren Zhong (Man's Center): Tonifies governor vessel, anterior and posterior frontal lobes, pituitary gland with C-8

GV-27 Dui Dan (Prominent Extremity): Tonifies governor vessel, mid-brain

GV-28 Yin Jiao (Crossing of the Gums): Tonifies governor vessel, eyes

Indications by Region/Category

Frontal Lobes

General tonifying: LI-5, ST-40 (opposite), SP-4, SP-5, SP-6, HT-1 (opposite), HT-2 (opposite), HT-9, BL-44, BL-58, BL-66, LR-14, GV-24

General dispersing: GB-35, CV-15

Posterior region: LU-7, LI-10, LI-12, LI-15, ST-9, ST-10, ST-27, ST-28, ST-32 (opposite), ST-33 (opposite), ST-38, SP-11, SP-21, SI-2, SI-3, SI-9, BL-5, BL-8, BL-64, BL-67, KI-8, KI-16, TW-6, TW-8 (same side), TW-12, TW-19, GB-4 (same side), GB-12 (opposite), GB-13 (opposite), GB-22, GB-27, GB-28, GB-34, GB-36, GB-39, LR-5, LR-6, LR-7 (opposite), LR-11, CV-24, GV-6, GV-26

Superior region: ST-32 (opposite), ST-33 (opposite), ST-38, BL-5, GB-4 (same side), GB-12 (opposite), LR-7 (opposite)

Anterior region: ST-14, ST-24 (opposite), SP-1, SP-2, SP-3, SP-15, HT-5, BL-63, KI-15, KI-24, KI-25, GB-35 (disperses), CV-4, CV-15 (disperses), GV-8, GV-9, GV-11, GV-26 inferior region, LI-2, LI-16, ST-9, SI-3, SI-16, SI-18, BL-64, PC-8, TW-19, TW-23 (opposite), GB-13 (opposite), GB-18 (opposite), GB-22

Mid-Brain

General tonifying: LU-9, ST-23 (posterior/sympathetic), ST-40 (opposite), ST-41 (posterior central lobes), ST-43 (opposite), SI-4, SI-7 (opposite), BL-10 (anterior), BL-12 (parasymp.), BL-45, BL-54, BL-55, KI-14 (opposite), KI-23 (anterior/vagus), PC-2, TW-5, TW-6, GB-29, GB-30, GB-36, LR-10, CV-5 (stiopallidum), CV-20 (vagus), GV-3 (opposite), GV-16 (vagus), GV-20 (anterior), GV-27

General dispersing: BL-60, BL-63, TW-10

Hypothalamus: ST-21 (anterior), BL-67 (posterior/sympathetic), KI-23 (anterior), GB-20 (posterior), CV-20 (anterior)

Pituitary: LI-1, LI-4 (opposite), CV-18, GV-14 ("and its 13 hormones"), GV-26 (w/C-8)

Thalamus: BL-61, TW-10 (disperses)

Temporal–Parietal Lobes

Tonifying: LU-1, LU-3, LU-6, LI-1, LI-7, LI-15, ST-13, ST-25, ST-30, ST-39, ST-42, ST-44, SI-14, SI-15, SI-16, SI-18, BL-4, BL-8, BL-17, BL-18, BL-19, BL-44, KI-18, KI-21, PC-4, PC-9, TW-1, TW-2, TW-7, TW-8, TW-9, TW-21 (anterior), GB-8 (opposite), GB-33, GB-42, GB-44, LR-3, LR-6, CV-13, CV-15, GV-15, GV-21

Dispersing: ST-45

Temporal lobes only: ST-6 (anterior), ST-7 (anterior), ST-9 (anterior), KI-3 (enhanced connectivity between the superior temporal gyrus and postcentral gyrus), TW-8 (same hemisphere), GB-40 (enhanced connectivity between the superior temporal gyrus and anterior insula)

Occipital Lobe

General tonifying: ST-8, SP-13, SI-15, SI-17, PC-5, TW-20 (opposite), GB-1 (opposite), GB-3, GB-7, CV-12

Dispersing: LI-2 (inferior), SI-4, GB-38 (superior)

Superior region: ST-14, ST-25, ST-27, ST-29, ST-30, ST-37 (opposite), ST-41, ST-45, BL-23, BL-40, BL-59 (opposite), KI-1, KI-4, KI-5, KI-7, KI-9, KI-11, KI-12, PC-8, GB-2, GB-40, GB-43, GV-1, GV-5, GV-18, GV-19, GV-20

Inferior region: LI-1, ST-1, ST-2, SP-2, SI-6 (opposite), SI-18, BL-1, BL-2 (opposite), BL-6, BL-7 (opposite), BL-9, GB-9 (opposite), GB-10, GB-14 (opposite), GB-15, GB-41, CV-2 (left side), GV-4

Cerebellum

Tonifying: LU-7, LU-8, LU-10, LU-11, LI-6, ST-5, ST-11, ST-15, ST-20, ST-33, SP-6, SP-7, SP-9, SP-21, HT-6, HT-8, SI-3, BL-30, BL-50, BL-56, BL-57, KI-5, KI-6, KI-10, KI-13, KI-17, KI-19, KI-20, KI-22, KI-26, PC-1, PC-2, PC-6, PC-7, TW-6, TW-15, GB-24, GB-32, GB-34, LR-5 (opposite: if insufficient, spasms: tonify; if excess, weakness: disperse), LR-8, LR-9, LR-10, LR-13, CV-16, CV-17, CV-21, CV-22, GV-4, GV-6, GV-17, GV-23

Dispersing: LU-5, BL-65, TW-10, LR-2

Pons

Tonifying: ST-11, SP-6, SP-9, HT-6, HT-8, KI-6, KI-10, KI-17, KI-19, KI-20, PC-1, GB-20, LR-5

Medulla Oblongata

Tonifying: LU-1, LU-7, LI-6, ST-4, ST-14, ST-16, ST-22, ST-32, ST-33, ST-42, ST-44, SP-21, HT-6, SI-8, SI-19, BL-11, BL-51, BL-52, BL-54, BL-66, KI-1, KI-7, KI-21, KI-25, PC-2, TW-19, GB-4, GB-5 (opposite), GB-20, GB-25, GB-26, GB-34, GB-35, GB-37, LR-4, LR-13, CV-9, CV-17, GV-1, GV-10, GV-13, GV-18

Dispersing: KI-2, TW-10, LR-2

Autonomic Nervous System

Sympathetic tonifying: ST-41, PC-8, TW-5, GB-20

Parasympathetic tonifying: ST-21, BL-10, CV-12, GV-20

Parasympathetic dispersing: PC-8

Spinal Cord

Tonifying: LU-1 (inferior), LU-7, LU-8 (mid), LU-9, LU-10 (upper), LU-11, LI-5, LI-6, LI-9 (opposite), ST-4, ST-14, ST-15 (inferior), ST-22, ST-31, ST-32, ST-33 (opposite), ST-37 (same side), ST-42, ST-44, SP-4 (lower), SP-6, SP-11 (lower), HT-6, HT-7, SI-3 (dorsal same side), SI-4, SI-7 (opposite mid-height), SI-8, SI-19, BL-4 (inferior), BL-11 (especially thoracic), BL-51, BL-52, BL-65,

BL-66 (upper), KI-1, KI-2, KI-4, KI-6 (lower), KI-7, KI-8, KI-10, KI-11 (lower), KI-13, KI-14, KI-16, KI-18, KI-19, KI-20, KI-21, KI-25, KI-26 (lower), PC-2, PC-6, PC-8, TW-1 (mid-height), TW-2 (lower), TW-3, TW-5, TW-6, TW-7, TW-12, TW-19 (opposite), GB-1 (same side), GB-7, GB-8, GB-13 (opposite), GB-20, GB-23, GB-25, GB-26, GB-28, GB-32 (lower), GB-34 ("reunion point"), GB-40, GB-41, LR-4, LR-9, LR-10, LR-13 (opposite), CV-9 (dorsal), CV-16, GV-1, GV-6, GV-12, GV-13, GV-15

Dispersing: TW-10, LR-2 (lower)

Thyroid Gland

Tonifying: LI-1, TW-7 (opposite), TW-20, GB-41, CV-20, CV-22, GV-14

Governor Vessel

Tonifying: ST-36, HT-9, SI-4, BL-11, BL-40, KI-9 (lower), GB-20, GB-36 (opposite), CV-1, GV-1, GV-2, GV-3, GV-4, GV-5, GV-6, GV-7, GV-8, GV-9, GV-10, GV-11, GV-12, GV-13, GV-14, GV-15, GV-16, GV-17, GV-18 ("all GV energy"), GV-19, GV-20, GV-21, GV-23, GV-24, GV-25, GV-26, GV-27, GV-28

Eyes

Tonifying: ST-1, ST-3, ST-6, ST-8, ST-28 (opposite), ST-29, ST-42, ST-43 (opposite inferior), HT-3, HT-6 (opposite), HT-9 (opposite), SI-3 (lateral), SI-6 (opposite), SI-8 (opposite lateral), SI-16 (lateral), SI-17 (opposite lateral), SI-18 (lateral), BL-12 (same side), KI-10 (lateral same side), KI-12 (opposite lateral), KI-13 (lateral), KI-14 (same side), KI-15 (inferior lateral), KI-16 (opposite), KI-17 (same side), KI-18 (same side), KI-19 (same side), KI-20 (same side), KI-22 (lower part), PC-1 (opposite), PC-2, TW-14 (opposite lateral), TW-16 (opposite lateral), TW-18 (ant. same side), TW-19 (ant. same side), TW-20, TW-21, TW-22, GB-1 (opposite retina), GB-3 (opposite posterior lateral), GB-4 (same side rectus externus), GB-5, GB-6 (oblique muscles), GB-7, GB-10 (same side), GB-11 (same side), GB-12, GB-14 (opposite rectus externus), GB-15 (posterior), GB-16 (especially lateral), GB-19 (medial same side), GB-20 (opposite), GB-23 (same side), GB-25, GB-34, GB-37, GB-38 (same side), GB-42, GB-44 (opposite), LR-6 (opposite), CV-4 (opposite), CV-15 (opposite lateral), GV-4, GV-11, GV-13, GV-17 (same side lateral), GV-19, GV-23 (same side), GV-24 (opposite), GV-28

Dispersing: LR-2 (opposite)

Brain (General)

Tonifying: LI-6, LI-8 (opposite), LI-9 (opposite and central inferior lateral side), HT-7 (opposite), SI-3 (opposite), SI-5 (opposite), BL-62, KI-13, TW-2 (opposite), TW-3, GB-11 (lower opposite), GB-19 (opposite), GB-21 (opposite), GB-23 (opposite), GB-26, LR-4, LR-13 (opposite), CV-8 (opposite), GV-12, GV-22 (opposite)

Dispersing: N/A

Three Nervous Centers

Tonifying: LU-2, LI-4, LI-11, HT-3, HT-4, BL-43, KI-27, CV-3, CV-6, GV-14

Dispersing: N/A

Three Psychic Centers

Tonifying: LU-2, LU-7 ("psychology"), LI-11, HT-3, HT-4, KI-27, TW-5, GB-21, CV-3, CV-6, CV-8

Dispersing: BL-60

Three Sense Organs

Tonifying: LI-4, SP-21, HT-4, TW-5, CV-6, CV-8

Dispersing: N/A

Wu Shen (Five Spirits/Three Levels of the Psyche)

Shen (evolved man)

Tonifying: ST-40, SP-3, SP-15, HT-5, BL-40, GB-38, CV-4, CV-15, GV-9, GV-11, GV-24

Dispersing: SP-5

Hun (automaton–parrot)

Tonifying: LU-1, LU-4, ST-25, ST-30, ST-39, ST-44, ST-45, BL-47, PC-4, PC-9, TW-7, LR-3, CV-15, GV-21

Dispersing: N/A

Po (primate)

Tonifying: LU-5, ST-25, ST-27, ST-29, ST-30, ST-37, ST-41, ST-45, BL-23, BL-40, BL-42, KI-1, KI-4, KI-7, KI-9, KI-11, KI-12, PC-5, GB-40, GB-43, GV-1, GV-5, GV-18, GV-19, GV-20

Dispersing: GB-38

Other Notable Indications

Tonifies nerves: ST-36, GV-3

Tonifies GV-22: SI-3

Tonifies meninges: GB-19

Tonifies marrow: GB-39

Tonifies corpus callosum: CV-15

Tonifies all Yang energy: GV-22

Appendix B

Relevant Individual Herbs

Neuroprotective Properties of Select Chinese Herbs

A large concern in a brain injury is the damage done to the tissue itself and the diffusion of injury due to inflammation and endogenous cytotoxicity causing more injury over time. Specific research has been done on several traditional Chinese medicinals and their regulating effects on protection of the brain and neural tissue. The following is a summary of some of this research.

Yu Jin (Radix Curcumae, Curcumin), Jiang Huang (Rhizoma Curcumae Longae, Turmeric), Curry Powder

The bright yellow color in curry powder is from the ground root of turmeric (a relative of ginger). Its main active constituent, which is also bright yellow in color, is curcumin. Curcumin has been under investigation for numerous potential benefits, including antiviral, anticancer, and anti-inflammatory activity. Studies have indicated potential benefits for Alzheimer's disease and in Parkinson's disease by a direct effect of decreasing amyloid pathology.[1] Curcumin has been shown to effectively lower oxidative damage, cognitive deficits, synaptic marker loss, and amyloid deposition. Curcumin proved to be immunomodulatory, simultaneously inhibiting cytokine and microglial activation indices related to neurotoxicity.[2] Animal studies have demonstrated that in cases of global cerebral ischemia both intravenous and supplementation diet (2.0g/kg) significantly attenuated ischemia-induced neuronal death and glial activation as well as decreased lipid peroxidation, mitochondrial dysfunction, and apoptotic indices. This ultimately reduced oxidative stress and the signaling cascade leading to apoptotic cell death.[3] Biochemical changes correlated well with its ability to ameliorate changes in locomotor activity after trauma.

---

1   Ringman, J.M., Frautschy, S. A., Cole, G. M. *et al.* A potential role of the curry spice curcumin in Alzheimer's disease. *Current Alzheimer Research.* 2005; 2(2): 131–136.

2   Cole, G.M., Morihara, T., Lim, G. P., *et al.* NSAID and antioxidant prevention of Alzheimer's disease: lessons from in vitro and animal models. *Annals of the New York Academy of Sciences.* 2004; 1035: 68–84.

3   Wang, Q., Sun, A., Simonyi, A., *et al.* Neuroprotective mechanisms of curcumin against cerebral ischemia-induced neuronal apoptosis and behavioral deficits. *Journal of Neuroscience Research.* 2005; 82(1): 138–148.

Dan Shen (Salvia Miltiorrhiza)

The benefits of salvia for promoting circulation, particularly capillary microcirculation, and for alleviating fibrosis have been extensively described with research over several decades.[4] Continuing investigation suggests neuroprotective effects from the herb and its active components which include tanshinones and salvianic acid. These compounds are being studied especially in relation to Parkinson's disease and stroke. In a transient focal cerebral ischemia model, TsIIA (16mg/kg) readily penetrated the blood–brain barrier and, 24 hours after middle cerebral artery occlusion, brain infarct volume was reduced by 30 percent and 37 percent following treatment with TsIIA and TsIIB respectively. The reduction in brain infarct volume was accompanied by a significant decrease in the observed neurological deficit.[5] A study of salvianic acid A (SA) found it capable of protecting diverse kinds of cells from damage caused by a variety of toxic stimuli that is likely due to its antioxidative properties and anti-apoptotic activity. It concluded that "data indicated that SA might provide a useful therapeutic strategy for the treatment of progressive neurodegenerative disease such as Parkinson's disease."[6]

Huang Qin (Scutellaria Baicalensis)

The flavonoids of scutellaria have been studied extensively because they show a potent and broad therapeutic benefit with no signs of toxicity in moderately high clinical doses. Baicalin, baicalein, and wogonin have been isolated and evaluated for anti-inflammatory and neuroprotective actions. They have mainly been tested in models of brain damage associated with stroke. Wogonin is a potent neuroprotector which has shown inhibition of inflammatory activation of cultured brain microglia and thus microglial cytotoxicity by diminishing lipopolysaccharide-induced tumor necrosis factor-alpha (TNF-alpha), interleukin-1beta, and nitric oxide (NO) production. The neuroprotective effect of wogonin was further demonstrated using both transient global ischemia and kainate injection. In both animal models wogonin conferred neuroprotection by attenuating the death of hippocampal neurons, and the neuroprotective effect was associated with inhibition of the inflammatory activation of microglia.[7] Another study on focal ischemic brain injury in rats found that wogonin, intraperitoneally administered at a dosage of 20mg/kg at 30 minutes before and four hours after the surgery, reduced infarct areas in the cerebral cortex as well as the striatum. The total volume of infarction was significantly reduced. Behavioral deficits at 24 hours after the surgery were also significantly improved. It concluded that "the neuroprotective effects of wogonin provide strong pharmacological basis for the use of wogonin or Scutellaria baicalensis in the treatment of stroke."[8] Baicalin is a flavonoid derivative from Scutellaria baicalensis with various pharmacological effects. Recently, the neuroprotective effect of baicalin was reported, finding that it had a protective effect on ischemic-

4   Dharmananda, S. *Salvia and the History of Microcirculation Research in China*. www.itmonline.org/arts/salvia.htm. Institute for Traditional Medicine. 2001 Aug. Web.

5   Lam, B.Y., Lo, A. C., Sun, X., *et al*. Neuroprotective effects of tanshinones in transient focal cerebral ischemia in mice. *Phytomedicine*. 2003; 10(4): 286–291.

6   Wang, X.J. and Xu, J.X. Salvianic acid A protects human neuroblastoma SH-SY5Y cells against MPP+-induced cytotoxicity. *Neuroscience Research*. 2005; 51(2): 129–138.

7   Lee, H., Kim, Y. O., Kim, H., *et al*. Flavonoid wogonin from medicinal herb is neuroprotective by inhibiting inflammatory activation of microglia. *FASEB Journal*. 2003; 17(13): 1943–1944.

8   Cho, J. and Lee, H.K. Wogonin inhibits ischemic brain injury in a rat model of permanent middle cerebral artery occlusion. *Biological and Pharmaceutical Bulletin*. 2004; 27(10): 1561–1564.

like or excitotoxic injury in rat hippocampal slices, which may have been partly related to inhibition of PKC(alpha) translocation.[9] Scutellaria has also demonstrated amelioration of blood–brain barrier permeability in breaches due to injury.

Ren Shen (Panax Ginseng)

Ginseng is one of the most widely used of all traditional Chinese herbs. Laboratory investigations with isolated ginsenosides have demonstrated its pharmacological potential, and its neuroprotective effects are now being investigated.[10] One study found that after 18 days two primary ginsenosides increased neurite outgrowth in the absence of nerve growth factor (NGF), suggesting neurotrophic and selective neuroprotective actions that may contribute to the reported enhancement of cognitive function.[11] A Korean study specifically emphasized nitric oxide and cytokines, which have been implicated in chronic brain inflammation, and concluded that one of the ginsenosides, Rb1, "exerted a significant inhibitory effect on this proinflammatory repertoire" and that "neurodegenerative diseases such as Alzheimer's disease, which is caused primarily by cell death due to chronic inflammation and cell stress, might be controlled by proper doses of non-toxic, natural Rg1 and Rb1."[12, 13] Ren Shen acts on endocrine and immunological functions, metabolism, enhancement of general physical and mental health, decreased mortality rates in some diseases, and lower PGE levels and higher serum cAMP levels. In terms of influence on intelligence, ginsenosides promote reflexes, reactions, memory, and thinking processes. Through MAO inhibition it is beneficial in the synthesis of neural transmitters, thus enhancing overall brain function.

Shi Chang Pu (Acori Tatarinowii)

Acorus is indicated to open the mind, calm the Shen, aid in resuscitation, and clear fuzzy cognition. In studies, it has been demonstrated as a potent free radical scavenger which can lower excitatory amino acids and have a protective effect on the brain by decreasing levels of aspartic acid and taurine levels in brain tissue.[14] It may also protect from H_2O_2-induced damage while stimulating nitrous oxide

9   Liu, L.Y., *et al.* Protective effects of baicalin on oxygen/glucose deprivation- and NMDA-induced injuries in rat hippocampal slices. *Journal of Pharmacy and Pharmacology.* 2005; 57(8): 1019–1026.

10   Rudakewich, M., Ba, F., and Benishin, C.G. Neurotrophic and neuroprotective actions of ginsenosides Rb(1) and Rg(1). *Planta Medica.* 2001; 67(6): 533–537.

11   Joo, S.S., Won, T.J., and Lee, D.I. Reciprocal activity of ginsenosides in the production of proinflammatory repertoire, and their potential roles in neuroprotection in vivo. *Planta Medica.* 2005; 71(5): 476–481.

12   Marchetti, B. and Abbracchio, M.P. To be or not to be inflamed—is that the question in anti-inflammatory drug therapy of neurodegenerative disorders? *Trends in Pharmacological Sciences.* 2005; 26(10): 517–525.

13   Park, E., Kum, S., Wang, C., *et al.* Anti-inflammatory activity of herbal medicines: inhibition of nitric oxide production and tumor necrosis factor-alpha secretion in an activated macrophage-like cell line. *American Journal of Chinese Medicine.* 2005; 33(3): 415–424.

14   Tang, Hongmei, *et al.* Effects of Rhizoma Acori Tatarinowii on amino acids neurotransmitter in mice brain. *Traditional Chinese Drug Research and Clinical Pharmacology.* 2003; 15(5): 310–311.

production, 5-HT levels,[15] and phagocytic activity.[16] Chronic administration of acorus has shown an increase in alpha activity, along with an increase in norepinephrine levels in the cerebral cortex but a decrease in the midbrain and cerebellum. Serotonin levels were increased in the cerebral cortex but decreased in the midbrain. Similarly, dopamine level was increased in the caudate nucleus and midbrain but decreased in the cerebellum. From this it was concluded that acorus seems to exert its depressive action by changing electrical activity and by altering brain monoamine levels in different brain regions.[17] It's indication to "open the mind" has been verified by its ability to increase permeability of the blood–brain barrier.[18] This quality makes it particularly useful in cases of brain injury to direct other herbal medicines to the brain and allow for increased cerebral blood flow.

Ci Wu Jia (Radix Acanthopanacis Senticosi)

Animal studies have demonstrated the strong anti-inflammatory and antinociceptive activities of Acanthopanax Radix extract[19] and its effects as an agent in the prevention of multiple organ dysfunction.[20] Acanthopanax is also known to have healing and protective effects on stress-induced disturbances of mental status. Animal studies have suggested that Acanthopanax may act by regulating noradrenaline (NA) and dopamine (DA) levels in specific brain regions related to the stress response.[21]

Wu Wei Zi (Schizandra Sinensis)

Excites the central nervous system, increases brain efficiency, and regulates the cardiovascular system to improve circulation. It has shown some effect in enhancing impaired intelligence.[22]

Chuan Xiong (Ligusticum Wallichii)

Used to promote Blood circulation to remove stasis. Chuan Xiong has been proven to significantly increase cerebral blood flow and inhibit abnormalities (e.g. slow blood flow, granular and cotton-like

15   Xie, T-T., Wang, H., and Liu, P. The influence of Acorus tatarinowii Schott on level of 5-hydroxytryptamine in brain [J]. *Chinese Journal of Drug Application and Monitoring.* 2007; 3: 007.

16   Zhang, W., Song, D., Xu, D., *et al.* Purification, antioxidant and immunological activities of polysaccharides from Actinidia Chinensis roots. *International Journal of Biological Macromolecules.* 2014; 72.10.1016/j. ijbiomac.2014.09.056

17   Hazra, Rimi, and Guha, Debjani. Effect of chronic administration of Acorus calamus on electrical activity and regional monoamine levels in rat brain. *Biogenic Amines.* 2002; 17(3): 161–169.

18   Hu, Y., Yuan, M., Liu, P., *et al.* Effect of Acorus tatarinowii Schott on ultrastructure and permeability of blood–brain barrier. *China Journal of Chinese Materia Medica.* 2009; 34(3): 349–351.

19   Jung, H.J., Park, H.J., Kim, R., *et al. In vivo* antiinflammatory and antinociceptive effects of liriodendron isolated from the stem bark of *Acanthopanax senticosus. Planta Medica.* 2003 Jul; 69(7): 610–616.

20   Yokozawa, T., Rhyu, D.Y., and Chen, C.P. Protective effects of Acanthopanax Radix extract against endotoxemia induced by lipopolysaccharide. *Phytotherapy Research.* 2003 Apr; 17(4): 353–357.

21   Fujikawa, T., Soya, H., Hibasami, H., *et al.* Effect of Acanthopanax senticosus harms on biogenic monoamine levels in the rat brain. *Phytotherapy Research.* 2002 Aug; 16(5): 474–478.

22   Sinclair, S. Chinese herbs: clinical review of astragulus, ligusticum, and schizandrae. *Alternative Medicine Review.* 1998 Oct; 3(5): 338–344.

blood flow patterns, RBC aggregation, microembolus, and degeneration and necrosis of nerve tissue.[23, 24, 25]

Huang Qi (Astragalus Membranaceus)

Physiologically, astragalus's effects consist of tonifying, aiding diuretic functions, aiding blood flow as a cardiotonic and vasodilator, reducing hypotensive symptoms, antibacterial actions, promoting the immunological system, retarding the aging process (by lengthening telomeres), and adaptogen-like regulating. Its intellectual functions may be attributed to its ability to inhibit monoamine oxidase (MAO), thus increasing the transmitters which influence the excitation of the cerebral cortex and cerebral blood flow.[26]

He Shou Wu/Shou Wu Teng (Polygonum Multiflorum)

Polygonum is an outstanding herb for slowing the aging process, tonifying Liver and Kidney, Yin, and Blood. It has been shown to lower cholesterol, prevent atherosclerosis, and act as a cardiotonic. In the central nervous system, it has a stimulatory action and inhibits MAO.

She Xiang (Musk)

A series of studies have shown musk can markedly relieve brain edema, directly strengthen the tolerance of the CNS to hypoxia, and improve circulatory disturbance. These results furnish a new approach in the treatment of brain edema, ischemia, anoxia, and functional failure.

Lu Rong (Deer Antler)

A very effective herb for tonifying the Yang and Kidney. Among its important actions are promoting growth and development, enhancing hematopoietic and cardiotonic effects, improving the function of the nervous and muscular systems, and stimulating gonad function. It additionally inhibits MAO.

Tian Ma (Gastrodia Rhizome)

Tian Ma and Gou Teng are traditional Chinese herbs that are used to treat convulsive disorders such as epilepsy. Synergistic anticonvulsive effects were observed in animal studies.[27] Gastrodia is

23 Sinclair, S. Chinese herbs: clinical review of astragalus, ligusticum, and schizandrae. *Alternative Medicine Review.* 1998 Oct; 3(5): 338–344.

24 Li, M., Handa, S., Ikeda, Y., and Goto, S. Specific inhibiting characteristics of tetramethylpyrazine, one of the active ingredients of the Chinese herbal medicine "Chuanxiong," on platelet thrombus formation under high shear rates. *Thrombosis Research.* 2001 Oct 1; 104(1): 15–28.

25 Chen, K.J. and Chen, K. Ischemic stroke treated with Ligusticum chuanxiong. *Chinese Medical Journal.* 1992 Oct; 105(10): 870–873.

26 Jin, R., Zhang, X., Chen, C., *et al.* Studies on pharmacological junctions of hairy root of astragalus membranaceus. *China Journal of Chinese Materia Medica.* 1999 Oct; 24(10): 619–621.

27 Hsieh, C.L., Tang, N.Y., Chaing, S.Y., *et al.* Anticonvulsive and free radical scavenging actions of two herbs, uncaria rhynchophylla (MIQ) jack and gastrodia elata bl. in kainic acid-treated rats. *Life Sciences.* 1999; 65(20): 2071–2082.

widely used by TCM physicians to manage headache, dizziness, vertigo, dementia, and convulsions.[28] Pharmacological studies have shown that the anticonvulsive properties and brain neuronal protective effects of the constituents of Gastrodia are related to their free radical scavenging activities and modulator effects on neurotransmission.[29, 30, 31, 32] The cognitive beneficial effects of Gastrodia and its ability to improve learning and memory have been confirmed by animal studies.[33, 34, 35]

Other Herbal Indications Relevant to Brain Injury

Brain, increases brain flow: Bai Guo Ye, Ge Gen, Shu Di Huang

Cerebral atherosclerosis: Chuan Shan Long (two–three months of taking Saponin extract, 0.02–0.2g/day improved many symptoms), Dang Gui (injection), Jin Qian Cao (can help reduce cholesterol plaque), Ju Hua (Jin Yin Hua, Huai Hua, Shan Zha)

Brain concussion: Dang Gui (injection)

Head trauma: San Qi (good for mild-to-moderate cases)

Headache from brain concussion: Yan Hu Suo (60–120mg 1–4x/day of L-tetrahydropalmatine, active ingredient)

Headache, trauma induced: Xi Xin/Chai Hu

Trauma, head injuries: San Qi (3g orally, two–three times/day, three–ten days, maximum 21 days, accelerated recovery, 75% effective)

Brain, increases oxygen to: Zhi Shi

Brain: Hong Hua (protects from anoxia, ischemia, injury); Lu Rong (increases oxygen intake, other organs also)

Monoamine oxidase inhibitor: Rou Dou Kou

Memory, impaired: Wu Jia Pi

28   Huang, Z.L. Recent developments in pharmacological study and clinical application of gastrodia elata in China. *Chinese Journal of Modern Developments in Traditional Medicine.* 1985 Apr; 5(4): 251–254.

29   Ha, J.H., Shin, S.M., Lee, S.K., *et al.* In vitro effects of hydroxybenzaldehydes from gastrodia elata and their analogues on GABAergic neurotransmission, and a structure activity correlation. *Planta Medica.* 2001 Dec; 67(9): 877–880.

30   Kim, H.J., Moon, K.D., Oh, S.Y., *et al.* Ether fraction of methanol extracts of gastrodia elata, a traditional medicinal herb, protects against kainic acid-induced neural damage in the mouse hippocampus. *Neuroscience Letters.* 2001 Nov; 314(1–2): 65–68.

31   Hsieh, C.L., Chang, C.H., Chiang, S.Y., *et al.* Anticonvulsive and free radical scavenging activities of vanillyl alcohol in ferric chloride-induced epileptic seizures in Sprague-Dawley rats. *Life Sciences.* 2000; 67(10): 1185–1195.

32   Hsieh, C.L., Chiang, S.Y., Cheng, K.S., *et al.* Anticonvulsive and free radical scavenging activities of gastrodia elata Bl. in kainic acid-treated rats. *American Journal of Chinese Medicine.* 2001; 29(2): 331–341.

33   Hsieh, M.T., Wu, C.R., and Chen, C.F. Gastrodin and p-hydroxybenzyl alcohol facilitate memory consolidation and retrieval, but not acquisition, on the passive avoidance task in rats. *Journal of Ethnopharmacology.* 1997 Mar; 56(1): 45–54.

34   Hsieh, M.T., Peng, W.H., Wu, C.R., and Wang, W.H. The ameliorating effects of the cognitive-enhancing Chinese herbs on scopolamine-induced amnesia in rats. *Phytotherapy Research.* 2000 Aug; 14(5): 375–377.

35   Wu, C.R., Hsieh, M.T., Huang, S.C., *et al.* Effects of gastrodia elata and its active constituents on scopolamine-induced amnesia in rats. *Planta Medica.* 1996 Aug; 62(4): 317–321.

Memory, improves: Bai Gou Ye

Memory, poor: Fu Shen, He Huan Hua, Ren Shen, Shi Chang Pu, Yuan Zhi

Mental confusion: Lian Zi Xian (Heat in pericardium)

Herbs for cerebrovascular mechanism:
Dan Shen, Tao Ren, Bai/Chi Shao Yao, Dang Gui, Tu Bie Chong, Jiang Huang, Bi Cheng Qie, E Zhu, Hong Hua, Hu Zhong, Gui Zhi/Rou Gui

Herbs for transmitter's mechanism (MAO inhibitors):
He Shou Wu/Shou Wu Teng, Ci Wu Jia, Yuan Zhi, Jiao Gu Lan, Du Zhong, Dan Shen, Shan Zha

Appendix C

Brodmann's Areas of the Brain

Functions and Locations of Brodmann's Areas

Brodmann Area	Functional Area	Location	Function
1, 2, 3	Primary somatic sensory cortex	Postcentral gyrus	Touch
4	Primary motor cortex	Precentral gyrus	Voluntary movement control
5	Tertiary somatic sensory cortex	Superior parietal lobule	Stereognosis
6	Premotor and supplementary motor	Precentral gyrus	Limb and eye movement planning
7	Posterior parietal association area	Superior parietal lobule	Multimodal area for spatial body sense
8	Frontal eye lids	Posterior, superior, middle frontal gyri	Saccadic eye movements
9, 10, 11, 12	Prefrontal association cortex	Superior, middle frontal gyri	Thought, cognition, ethics, morals, movement, planning
13, 14, 15, 16	Part of the insular cortex		
17	Primary visual cortex	Banks of calcarine tissue	Vision
18	Secondary visual cortex	Medial and lateral occipital gyri	Vision, depth
19	Tertiary visual cortex	Medial and lateral occipital gyri	Vision, color, motion, depth
20, 21	Visual inferotemporal area	Middle and inferior temporal gyrus	Form vision
22	Higher order auditory cortex	Superior temporal gyrus	Hearing, speech

23, 24, 25, 26, 27	Limbic association cortex	Cingulate gyrus, subcallosal area, parahippocampal gyrus	Emotions, attention, detection of error, novelty
28	Olfactory and limbic cortex, sensory multimodal association cortex	Parahippocampal gyrus	Smell, emotions, memory
29, 30, 31, 32, 33	Limbic association cortex	Cingulate gyrus	Emotions
34, 35, 36	Olfactory cortex and limbic cortex	Parahippocampal gyrus	Smell, emotions
37	Occipital association cortex	Middle and inferior temporal gyri	Perception, vision, reading, speech, movement
38	Olfactory and limbic cortex	Temporal pole	Smell, emotions, language
39	Parietal association cortex	Inferior parietal lobule (angular gyrus)	Perception, vision, reading, speech
40	Parietal–temporal occipital association cortex	Inferior parietal lobule (supramarginal gyrus)	Reading, speech, movement
41, 42	Primary and secondary auditory cortex	Heschyl's gyri and superior temporal gyrus	Hearing
43	Gustatory cortex	Insular cortex, frontoparietal operculum	Taste, GI tract
44, 45	Lateral premotor cortex (dominant hemisphere)	Inferior frontal gyrus (frontal operculum)	Speech, movement, planning
45	Prefrontal association cortex	Inferior frontal gyrus (frontal operculum)	Thought, cognition, planning, behavior
46	Dorsolateral prefrontal cortex	Middle frontal gyrus	Thought, cognition, planning, behavior, eye movement
47	Prefrontal association cortex	Inferior frontal gyrus (frontal operculum)	Semantic speech area

Pharmaceuticals and Potential Herb–Drug Interactions

Individuals with brain injuries can be particularly prone to side effects and interactions between pharmaceuticals as well as interactions of herbal medications with pharmaceuticals. For this reason, it is particularly important to be aware of and attentive to potential herb–drug interactions. Included in this appendix are pharmaceuticals listed throughout this text, their potential uses relevant to this text, and potential herbal interactions according to the lectures of Dr. John Chen and the text *Integrated Pharmacology* by Dr. Greg Sperber with Bob Flaws. For further details on this material or other pharmaceuticals not included here, refer to these very informative sources.[1]

---

1   Chen, John. *Herb–Drug Interactions: An Advanced Class.* Web. www.elotus.org; Chen, John. *Integrating Chinese Herbology with Western Pharmacology: Clinical Applications and Safety Concerns, Part I.* Web. www.elotus.org; Chen, John. *Integrating Chinese Herbology with Western Pharmacology: Clinical Applications and Safety Concerns, Part II.* Web. www.elotus.org; Sperber, G. and Flaws, B. *Integrated Pharmacology: Combining Modern Pharmacology with Chinese Medicine.* Boulder, CO: Blue Poppy Press. 2007. Print.

Pharmaceutical	Possible Use	Category	Potential Herbal Interactions
Acamprosate (Campral)	Tinnitus, alcohol dependence	Drugs used in alcohol dependence	N/A
Acetaminophen (Amidrine, Anexsia, Darvocet, Duradin, Endocet, Esgic, Fiorcet, Hycet, Hycomine, Lorcet, Lortab, Maxidone, Medigesic, Migquin, Norco, Panlor, Percocet, Repan, Roxicet, Stagesic, Talacen, Tylenol with Codeine, Tylox, Ultracet, Vicodin, Zebutal, Zerlor, Zydone)	Migraine, headache, pain	Analgesic	• Da Suan (garlic): May prevent hepatotoxicity from acetaminophen. Aged garlic may prophylactically reduce it • Dang Gui: May treat liver damage caused by acetaminophen by promoting hepatocyte generation • Niu Bang Gen (burdock root): Hepatoprotective effects, alleviating toxicity and liver damage due to acetaminophen and carbon tetrachloride in rats
Acetaminophen-isomeptene-dichloralphenazone (Midrin)	Migraine	Antimigraine agent	• Da Suan (garlic): May prevent hepatotoxicity from acetaminophen. Aged garlic may prophylactically reduce it • Dang Gui: May treat liver damage caused by acetaminophen by promoting hepatocyte generation • Niu Bang Gen (burdock root): Hepatoprotective effects, alleviating toxicity and liver damage due to acetaminophen and carbon tetrachloride in rats
Almotriptan (Axert)	Migraine	Antimigraine agent	N/A
Amantadine (Symmetrel)	Impaired attention/ concentration, impaired memory, impaired executive function	Dopaminergic, antiviral	N/A
Amisulpride (Solian)	Schizophrenia	Atypical neuroleptic	• Bing Lang: May exacerabate extrapyramidal symptoms • Da Fu Pi: May exacerbate extrapyramidal symptoms • Man Jing Zi: Dopamine antagonists may be weakened due to dopaminergic effect

Pharmaceutical	Possible Use	Category	Potential Herbal Interactions
Amitriptyline (Elavil, Etrafon, Limbritrol)	Depression, pain, migraine, tinnitus, insomnia	Tricyclic antidepressant	• Ma Huang: Hypertensive effects of Ma Huang were blocked • Rou Cong Rong: May interect by increasing neurotransmitters such as norepinephrine, dopamine, and serotonin • Ying Su Ye: May exacerbate depressant and CNS suppressive effects of Ying Su Ye
Amoxapine	Depression	Tricyclic antidepressant	• Ma Huang: Hypertensive effects of Ma Huang were blocked • Rou Cong Rong: May interact by increasing neurotransmitters such as norepinephrine, dopamine, and serotonin • Ying Su Ye: May exacerbate depressant and CNS suppressive effects of Ying Su Ye
Aprepitant (Emend)	Nausea/vomiting	Antiemetic	N/A
Aripiprazole (Abilify)	Mania	Atypical neuroleptic	• Bing Lang: May exacerbate extrapyramidal symptoms • Da Fu Pi: May exacerbate extrapyramidal symptoms
Atomoxetine (Straterra)	Impaired attention/ concentration, impaired memory, impaired executive function	CNS stimulant	• Chen Pi: Stimulates sympathetic nervous system and should be used with caution • Ma Huang: May increase drug activity • Qing Pi: Stimulates sympathetic nervous system and should be used with caution • Rou Cong Rong: May interact by increasing neurotransmitters such as norepinephrine, dopamine, and serotonin • Zhi Ke: Stimulates sympathetic nervous system and should be used with caution • Zhi Shi: Stimulates sympathetic nervous system and should be used with caution
Baclofen (Lioresal, Gablofen)	Neuralgia, spasticity	Antispasmodic muscle relaxant	Shen calming herbs or those with sedative effects may exacerbate sedative effects of drug
Bromocriptine (Parlodel)	Impaired attention/ concentration, impaired memory, impaired executive function	Dopaminergic	• Ma Huang: May increase toxicity due to sympathomimetic effects

Buproprion (Wellbutrin, Budeprion, Buproban, Zyban)	Fatigue, neuralgia, impaired attention/concentration	Antidepressant: Dopamine reuptake inhibitor	N/A
Butalbital compound (Fioricet, Fiorinal)	Migraine, pain	Analgesic combination	• Da Suan (garlic): May prevent hepatotoxicity from acetaminophen. Aged garlic may prophylactically reduce it • Dang Gui: May treat liver damage caused by acetaminophen by promoting hepatocyte generation • Niu Bang Gen (burdock root): Hepatoprotective effects, alleviating toxicity and liver damage due to acetaminophen and carbon tetrachloride in rats
Carbamazepine (Carbatrol, Epitol, Equetro, Tegretol)	Seizure, pain, neuralgia, mania, bipolar	Anticonvulsant	• Yin Guo Ye: May precipitate epileptic seizures • Chen Pi: May contain constituents that stimulate the sympathetic nervous system and should be used with caution with anticonvulsive agents • Qing Pi: May contain constituents that stimulate the sympathetic nervous system and should be used with caution with anticonvulsive agents • Zhi Ke: May contain constituents that stimulate the sympathetic nervous system and should be used with caution with anticonvulsive agents • Zhi Shi: May contain constituents that stimulate the sympathetic nervous system and should be used with caution with anticonvulsive agents
Chlorpromazine (Thorazine)	Depression	Neuroleptic, 5 HT antagonist	• Bing Lang: May exacerbate extrapyramidal symptoms • Da Fu Pi: May exacerbate extrapyramidal symptoms
Citalopram (Celexa)	Depression, neuralgia	Antidepressant: Selective serotonin reuptake inhibitor	• Guan Ye Lian Qiao (St. John's wort): One case report of hypomanic episode when combined; inhibits serotonin reuptake • Rou Cong Rong: May interact by increasing neurotransmitters such as norepinephrine, dopamine, and serotonin • Yin Guo Ye: One case report of hypomanic episode when combined
Clomipramine (Anafranil)	Depression	Tricyclic antidepressant	• Ma Huang: Hypertensive effects of Ma Huang were blocked • Rou Cong Rong: May interact by increasing neurotransmitters such as norepinephrine, dopamine, and serotonin • Ying Su Ye: May exacerbate depressant and CNS suppressive effects of Ying Su Ye

Pharmaceutical	Possible Use	Category	Potential Herbal Interactions
Clonazepam (Klonopin)	Insomnia, vertigo, seizure, pain, neuralgia, myalgia, anxiety, mania	Benzodiazepine	• Bai Jiang Cao: May increase sedative effects • Bai Shao: May increase sedative effects of drugs • Chan Tui: May potentiate CNS inhibition • Dan Shen: May inhibit benzodiazepine receptor binding • Jiao Gu Lan (gynostemma): May increase sedative effects of drugs • Long Dan Cao: May increase sedative effects of drugs • Niu Huang: May increase sedative effects of drugs (mild effect) • Qin Jiao: May potentiate sedative effects through CNS inhibition • Suan Zao Ren: Sedative and hypnotic effects may potentiate sedative effects of drugs • Tian Ma: Potentiates sedative effect • Tian Nan Xing: May increase sedative effects of drugs • Wu Jia Pi: May increase sedative effects (mild) • Xie Cao (valerian): Potentiates sedative effect • Zhi Zi: May increase sedative effects • Shen calming herbs: May increase sedative effects
Clozapine (Clozaril, FazaClo)	Schizophrenia	Atypical neuroleptic	• Bing Lang: May exacerbate extrapyramidal symptoms • Da Fu Pi: May exacerbate extrapyramidal symptoms • Man Jing Zi: Dopamine antagonists may be weakened due to dopaminergic effect
Codeine (Brontex, Capital, Robafen, Robilar)	Pain	Opioid analgesic	• Bai Jiang Cao: May increase sedative effects • Bai Shao: May increase sedative effects of drugs • Chan Tui: May potentiate CNS inhibition • Jiao Gu Lan (gynostemma): May increase sedative effects of drugs • Long Dan Cao: May increase sedative effects of drugs • Niu Huang: May increase sedative effects of drugs (mild effect) • Qin Jiao: May potentiate sedative effects through CNS inhibition • Suan Zao Ren: Sedative and hypnotic effects may potentiate sedative effects of drugs • Tian Ma: Potentiates sedative effect • Tian Nan Xing: May increase sedative effects of drugs • Wu Jia Pi: May increase sedative effects (mild) • Xie Cao (valerian): Potentiates sedative effect • Zhi Zi: May increase sedative effects • Shen calming herbs: May increase sedative effects

Drug	Indication	Class	Interactions
Cyproheptadine (Periactin)	Allergies, migraine	Antihistamine	• Bai Shao: May increase sedative effects of drugs • Chan Tui: May potentiate CNS inhibition • Jiao Gu Lan (gynostemma): May increase sedative effects of drugs • Long Dan Cao: May increase sedative effects of drugs • Niu Huang: May increase sedative effects of drugs (mild effect) • Tian Nan Xing: May increase sedative effects of drugs • Wu Jia Pi: May increase sedative effects of drugs (mild effect) • Xi Jiao: May increase sedative effects of drugs • Zhi Zi: May increase sedative effects of drugs
Desipramine (Norpamin)	Depression, pain	Tricyclic antidepressant	• Ma Huang: Hypertensive effects of Ma Huang were blocked • Rou Cong Rong: May interact by increasing neurotransmitters such as norepinephrine, dopamine, and serotonin • Ying Su Ye: May exacerbate depressant and CNS suppressive effects of Ying Su Ye
Dexamethasone (Baycadron, Decadron, Dexpak, Taperpak, Maxidex)	Nausea/vomiting, pain	Glucocorticoid	• Gan Cao: May increase half-life of systemic corticosteroids • Ma Huang: May increase metabolism rate • Kidney supplement herbs/formulas: May treat and prevent dexamethasone-induced osteoporosis
Dextroamphetamine (Adderall, Dexedrin, Detrostat)	Impaired attention/ concentration, impaired memory, impaired executive function	Indirect adrenergic agonist	• Chen Pi: Stimulates sympathetic nervous system and should be used with caution • Ma Huang: May increase drug activity • Qing Pi: Stimulates sympathetic nervous system and should be used with caution • Rou Cong Rong: May interact by increasing neurotransmitters such as norepinephrine, dopamine, and serotonin • Zhi Ke: Stimulates sympathetic nervous system and should be used with caution • Zhi Shi: Stimulates sympathetic nervous system and should be used with caution

Pharmaceutical	Possible Use	Category	Potential Herbal Interactions
Diazepam (Valium, Diazepam, Diastat, Intensol)	Vertigo, seizure, anxiety, benzodiazepine withdrawal	Benzodiazepine anticonvulsant	• Bai Jiang Cao: May increase sedative effects • Bai Shao: May increase sedative effects of drugs • Chan Tui: May potentiate CNS inhibition • Dan Shen: May inhibit benzodiazepine receptor binding • Jiao Gu Lan (gynostemma): May increase sedative effects of drugs • Long Dan Cao: May increase sedative effects of drugs • Niu Huang: May increase sedative effects of drugs (mild effect) • Qin Jiao: May potentiate sedative effects through CNS inhibition • Suan Zao Ren: Sedative and hypnotic effects may potentiate sedative effects of drugs • Tian Ma: Potentiates sedative effect • Tian Nan Xing: May increase sedative effects of drugs • Wu Jia Pi: May increase sedative effects (mild) • Xie Cao (valerian): Potentiates sedative effect • Zhi Zi: May increase sedative effects • Shen calming herbs: May increase sedative effects
Difenoxin (Motofen)	Bowel incontinence	Antidiarrheal	This drug alters functioning of the small and large intestine and could affect the absorption of herbs. To minimize interactions, agents should be administered either four hours before or two hours after
Dihydroergotamine (D.H.E. 45 Injection, Migranal Nasal Spray)	Migraine, headache	Antimigraine agent	• Ma Huang: May cause hypertension when combined with ergot alkaloids or oxytocin
Diltiazem (Cardizem, Cartia XT, Dilacor, Diltia, Taztia, Tiazac)	Headache (cluster)	Calcium channel blocker	• Gan Cao: May reduce effects • Qing Hao: May interfere with effectiveness
Diphenhydramine (Benadryl)	Allergies, migraine	Antihistamine	• Bai Shao: May increase sedative effects of drugs • Chan Tui: May potentiate CNS inhibition • Jiao Gu Lan (gynostemma): May increase sedative effects of drugs • Long Dan Cao: May increase sedative effects of drugs (mild effect) • Niu Huang: May increase sedative effects of drugs • Tian Nan Xing: May increase sedative effects of drugs • Wu Jia Pi: May increase sedative effects of drugs (mild effect) • Xi Jiao: May increase sedative effects of drugs • Zhi Zi: May increase sedative effects of drugs

Diphenoxylate (Lomotil, Lonox)	Bowel incontinence	Antidiarrheal	This drug alters functioning of the small and large intestine and could affect the absorption of herbs. To minimize interactions, agents should be administered either four hours before or two hours after
Donepezil (Aricept)	Impaired attention/concentration, impaired memory, impaired executive function	Anticholinesterases (reversible)	N/A
Doxepin (Prudoxin, Zonalin)	Depression	Tricyclic antidepressant	• Ma Huang: Hypertensive effects of Ma Huang were blocked • Rou Cong Rong: May interact by increasing neurotransmitters such as norepinephrine, dopamine, and serotonin • Ying Su Ye: May exacerbate depressant and CNS suppressive effects of Ying Su Ye
Dronabinol (Marinol)	Nausea/vomiting	Antiemetic	N/A
Droperidol (Inapsine)	Nausea/vomiting	Miscellaneous CNS agents (sedative, tranquilizer, antiemetic)	• Bai Shao: May increase sedative effects of drugs • Chan Tui: May potentiate CNS inhibition • Jiao Gu Lan (gynostemma): May increase sedative effects of drugs • Long Dan Cao: May increase sedative effects of drugs • Niu Huang: May increase sedative effects of drugs (mild effect) • Tian Nan Xing: May increase sedative effects of drugs • Wu Jia Pi: May increase sedative effects of drugs (mild effect) • Xi Jiao: May increase sedative effects of drugs • Zhi Zi: May increase sedative effects of drugs
Duloxetine (Cymbalta)	Depression, pain	Antidepressant: serotonin/norepinephrine reuptake inhibitor	• Guan Ye Lian Qiao (St. John's wort): One case report of hypomanic episode when combined; inhibits serotonin reuptake • Rou Cong Rong: May interact by increasing neurotransmitters such as norepinephrine, dopamine, and serotonin • Yin Guo Ye: One case report of hypomanic episode when combined
Eletriptan (Relpax)	Migraine	Antimigraine agent	N/A

Pharmaceutical	Possible Use	Category	Potential Herbal Interactions
Ergotamine tartrate (Cafergot, Ergomar, Wigraine)	Migraine	Antimigraine agent	• Ma Huang: May cause hypertension when combined with ergot alkaloids or oxytocin
Escitalopram (Lexapro)	Depression	Antidepressant: Selective serotonin reuptake inhibitor	• Guan Ye Lian Qiao (St. John's wort): One case report of hypomanic episode when combined; inhibits serotonin reuptake • Rou Cong Rong: May interact by increasing neurotransmitters such as norepinephrine, dopamine, and serotonin • Yin Guo Ye: One case report of hypomanic episode when combined
Eszopiclone (Prosom)	Insomnia	Sedative, hypnotic	• Bai Jiang Cao: May increase sedative effects • Bai Shao: May increase sedative effects of drugs • Chan Tui: May potentiate CNS inhibition • Long Dan Cao: May increase sedative effects of drugs • Niu Huang: May increase sedative effects of drugs (mild effect) • Qin Jiao: May potentiate sedative effects through CNS inhibition • Suan Zao Ren: Sedative and hypnotic effects may potentiate sedative effects of drugs • Tian Nan Xing: May increase sedative effects of drugs • Wu Jia Pi: May increase sedative effects (mild) • Xie Cao (valerian): Potentiates sedative effect • Zhi Zi: May increase sedative effects • Shen calming herbs: May increase sedative effects
Ethosuximide (Zarontin)	Pain	Anticonvulsant	• Yin Guo Ye: May precipitate epileptic seizures • Chen Pi: May contain constituents that stimulate the sympathetic nervous system and should be used with caution with anticonvulsive agents • Qing Pi: May contain constituents that stimulate the sympathetic nervous system and should be used with caution with anticonvulsive agents • Zhi Ke: May contain constituents that stimulate the sympathetic nervous system and should be used with caution with anticonvulsive agents • Zhi Shi: May contain constituents that stimulate the sympathetic nervous system and should be used with caution with anticonvulsive agents

Drug	Indication	Class	Herb Interactions
Famotidine (Fluxid, Pepcid)	GERD (re: dysphagia)	H2 antagonist	• Aromatic and damp resolving herbs: May antagonize via increased stomach acid and peristalsis
Fentanyl (Actiq, Duragesic, Ionsys, Sublimaze)	Pain	Opioid analgesic	• Bai Jiang Cao: May increase sedative effects • Bai Shao: May increase sedative effects of drugs • ChanTui: May potentiate CNS inhibition • Jiao Gu Lan (gynostemma): May increase sedative effects of drugs • Long Dan Cao: May increase sedative effects of drugs • Niu Huang: May increase sedative effects of drugs (mild effect) • Qin Jiao: May potentiate sedative effects through CNS inhibition • Suan Zao Ren: Sedative and hypnotic effects may potentiate sedative effects of drugs • Tian Ma: Potentiates sedative effect • Tian Nan Xing: May increase sedative effects of drugs • Wu Jia Pi: May increase sedative effects (mild) • Xie Cao (valerian): Potentiates sedative effect • Zhi Zi: May increase sedative effects • Shen calming herbs: May increase sedative effects
Fluconazole (Diflucan)	Candidiasis (re: fatigue)	Antifungal	• Qing Hao: May interfere with effectiveness
Fluoxetine (Prozac, Sarafem, Symbyax)	Depression, pain, neuralgia, PTSD	Antidepressant: Selective serotonin reuptake inhibitor	• GuanYe Lian Qiao (St. John's wort): One case report of hypomanic episode when combined; inhibits serotonin reuptake • Rou Cong Rong: May interact by increasing neurotransmitters such as norepinephrine, dopamine, and serotonin • Yin GuoYe: One case report of hypomanic episode when combined
Frovatriptan (Frova)	Migraine	Antimigraine agent	N/A
Fruvoxamine (Luvox)	Depression	Antidepressant: Selective serotonin reuptake inhibitor	• GuanYe Lian Qiao (St. John's wort): One case report of hypomanic episode when combined; inhibits serotonin reuptake • Rou Cong Rong: May interact by increasing neurotransmitters such as norepinephrine, dopamine, and serotonin • Yin GuoYe: One case report of hypomanic episode when combined

Pharmaceutical	Possible Use	Category	Potential Herbal Interactions
Gabapentin (Neurontin)	Seizure, migraine, tinnitus, pain, neuralgia	Gamma-aminobutyric acid analogs	• Yin Guo Ye: May precipitate epileptic seizures • Chen Pi: May contain constituents that stimulate the sympathetic nervous system and should be used with caution with anticonvulsive agents • Qing Pi: May contain constituents that stimulate the sympathetic nervous system and should be used with caution with anticonvulsive agents • Zhi Ke: May contain constituents that stimulate the sympathetic nervous system and should be used with caution with anticonvulsive agents • Zhi Shi: May contain constituents that stimulate the sympathetic nervous system and should be used with caution with anticonvulsive agents
Galantamine (Razadyne)	Impaired attention/ concentration, impaired memory, impaired executive function	Anticholinesterases (reversible)	N/A
Guanfacine (Intuniv, Tenex)	Impaired attention/ concentration, impaired memory, impaired executive function	Direct antiadrenergic agent	• Chen Pi: Stimulates the sympathetic nervous system and should be used with caution • Ma Huang: May increase sympathomimetic activity • Qing Pi: Stimulates the sympathetic nervous system and should be used with caution • Rou Cong Rong: May interact by increasing activities of neurotransmitters such as norepinephrine, dopamine, and serotonin • Zhi Ke: Stimulates the sympathetic nervous system and should be used with caution • Zhi Shi: Stimulates the sympathetic nervous system and should be used with caution

| Hydrocordone (Anexsia, Bancap, Detuss, Endagen, Hitussin, Hydromet, Lorcet, Lortab, Maxidone, Pediatex, Tussafed, Tussigon, Vicodin, Vicoprofin) | Pain | Opioid analgesic | • Bai Jiang Cao: May increase sedative effects
• Bai Shao: May increase sedative effects of drugs
• Chan Tui: May potentiate CNS inhibition
• Jiao Gu Lan (gynostemma): May increase sedative effects of drugs
• Long Dan Cao: May increase sedative effects of drugs
• Niu Huang: May increase sedative effects of drugs (mild effect)
• Qin Jiao: may potentiate sedative effects through CNS inhibition
• Suan Zao Ren: Sedative and hypnotic effects may potentiate sedative effects of drugs
• Tian Ma: Potentiates sedative effect
• Tian Nan Xing: May increase sedative effects of drugs
• Wu Jia Pi: May increase sedative effects (mild)
• Xie Cao (valerian): Potentiates sedative effect
• Zhi Zi: May increase sedative effects
• Shen calming herbs: May increase sedative effects |
| Hydromorphone (Dilaudid) | Pain | Opioid analgesic | • Bai Jiang Cao: May increase sedative effects
• Bai Shao: May increase sedative effects of drugs
• Chan Tui: May potentiate CNS inhibition
• Jiao Gu Lan (gynostemma): May increase sedative effects of drugs
• Long Dan Cao: May increase sedative effects of drugs
• Niu Huang: May increase sedative effects of drugs (mild effect)
• Qin Jiao: May potentiate sedative effects through CNS inhibition
• Suan Zao Ren: Sedative and hypnotic effects may potentiate sedative effects of drugs
• Tian Ma: Potentiates sedative effect
• Tian Nan Xing: May increase sedative effects of drugs
• Wu Jia Pi: May increase sedative effects (mild)
• Xie Cao (valerian): Potentiates sedative effect
• Zhi Zi: May increase sedative effects
• Shen calming herbs: May increase sedative effects |

Pharmaceutical	Possible Use	Category	Potential Herbal Interactions
Imipramine (Tofranil)	Depression	Tricyclic antidepressant	• Ma Huang: Hypertensive effects of Ma Huang were blocked • Rou Cong Rong: May interact by increasing neurotransmitters such as norepinephrine, dopamine, and serotonin • Ying Su Ye: May exacerbate depressant and CNS suppressive effects of Ying Su Ye
Ketoconazole (Nizoral)	Candidiasis (re: fatigue)	Antifungal	• Qing Hao: May interfere with effectiveness
L-thyroxine (Levothroid, Synthroid, Levoxyl, Unithroid)	Hypothyroidism	Hormone	• Dan Dou Chi: May decrease drug effects
Lacosamide (Vimpat)	Seizure		
Lactulose (Constulose, Enulose, Generlac, Kristalose)	Constipation	Laxative	• Downward draining herbs such as Da Huang, Mang Xiao, Fan Xie Ye, etc. may act synergistically and should be used with caution • Gan Cao: May lead to increased potassium loss when used with laxatives
Lamotrigine (Lamictal)	Seizure, pain, neuralgia, impaired concentration/ attention, impaired memory, impaired executive function, mania, bipolar, PTSD	Anticonvulsant	• Yin Guo Ye: May precipitate epileptic seizures • Chen Pi: May contain constituents that stimulate the sympathetic nervous system and should be used with caution with anticonvulsive agents • Qing Pi: May contain constituents that stimulate the sympathetic nervous system and should be used with caution with anticonvulsive agents • Zhi Ke: May contain constituents that stimulate the sympathetic nervous system and should be used with caution with anticonvulsive agents • Zhi Shi: May contain constituents that stimulate the sympathetic nervous system and should be used with caution with anticonvulsive agents
Levetiracetam (Keppra)	Seizure, pain	Anticonvulsant	• Yin Guo Ye: May precipitate epileptic seizures • Chen Pi: May contain constituents that stimulate the sympathetic nervous system and should be used with caution with anticonvulsive agents • Qing Pi: May contain constituents that stimulate the sympathetic nervous system and should be used with caution with anticonvulsive agents • Zhi Ke: May contain constituents that stimulate the sympathetic nervous system and should be used with caution with anticonvulsive agents • Zhi Shi: May contain constituents that stimulate the sympathetic nervous system and should be used with caution with anticonvulsive agents

Drug	Indication	Class	Herb Interactions
Levodopa (Parcopa, Sinemet, Stalevo)	Impaired attention/concentration, impaired memory, impaired executive function	Dopaminergic	N/A
Lithium (Eskalith, Lithobid)	Mania, bipolar, headache	Antipsychotic	• Pu Gong Ying: Lithium toxicity may be worsened due to diuretic effect on sodium excretion
Lorazepam (Ativan)	Vertigo, seizure, insomnia, anxiety, alcohol dependence	Benzodiazepine anticonvulsant	• Bai Jiang Cao: May increase sedative effects • Bai Shao: May increase sedative effects of drugs • Chan Tui: May potentiate CNS inhibition • Dan Shen: May inhibit benzodiazepine receptor binding • Jiao Gu Lan (gynostemma): May increase sedative effects of drugs • Long Dan Cao: May increase sedative effects of drugs • Niu Huang: May increase sedative effects of drugs (mild effect) • Qin Jiao: May potentiate sedative effects through CNS inhibition • Suan Zao Ren: Sedative and hypnotic effects may potentiate sedative effects of drugs • Tian Ma: Potentiates sedative effect • Tian Nan Xing: May increase sedative effects of drugs • Wu Jia Pi: May increase sedative effects (mild) • Xie Cao (valerian): Potentiates sedative effect • Zhi Zi: May increase sedative effects • Shen calming herbs: May increase sedative effects
Maprotiline (Ludiomil)	Depression	Tricyclic antidepressant	• Ma Huang: Hypertensive effects of Ma Huang were blocked • Rou Cong Rong: May interact by increasing neurotransmitters such as norepinephrine, dopamine, and serotonin • Ying Su Ye: May exacerbate depressant and CNS suppressive effects of Ying Su Ye

Pharmaceutical	Possible Use	Category	Potential Herbal Interactions
Meclizine hydrochloride (Antivert)	Vertigo	Anticholinergic antiemetic	• Bai Jiang Cao: May increase sedative effect • Bai Shao: May increase sedative effects of drugs • Chan Tui: May potentiate CNS inhibition • Jiao Gu Lan (gynostemma): May increase sedative effects of drugs • Long Dan Cao: May increase sedative effects of drugs • Niu Huang: May increase sedative effects of drugs (mild effect) • Tian Nan Xing: May increase sedative effects of drugs • Wu Jia Pi: May increase sedative effects of drugs (mild effect) • Xi Jiao: May increase sedative effects of drugs • Zhi Zi: May increase sedative effects of drugs
Memantine (Namenda)	Impaired attention/concentration, impaired memory, impaired executive function	Miscellaneous CNS agent	N/A
Meperidine (Demerol, Meperitab)	Pain	Opioid analgesic	• Bai Jiang Cao: May increase sedative effects • Bai Shao: May increase sedative effects of drugs • Chan Tui: May potentiate CNS inhibition • Jiao Gu Lan (gynostemma): May increase sedative effects of drugs • Long Dan Cao: May increase sedative effects of drugs • Niu Huang: May increase sedative effects of drugs (mild effect) • Qin Jiao: May potentiate sedative effects through CNS inhibition • Suan Zao Ren: Sedative and hypnotic effects may potentiate sedative effects of drugs • Tian Ma: Potentiates sedative effect • Tian Nan Xing: May increase sedative effects of drugs • Wu Jia Pi: May increase sedative effects (mild) • Xie Cao (valerian): Potentiates sedative effect • Zhi Zi: May increase sedative effects • Shen calming herbs: May increase sedative effects

Methimazole (Tapazole)	Hyperthyroidism	Antithyroid medication	• Chen Pi: Stimulates the sympathetic nervous system and should be used with caution • Qing Pi: Stimulates the sympathetic nervous system and should be used with caution • Zhi Ke: Stimulates the sympathetic nervous system and should be used with caution • Zhi Shi: Stimulates the sympathetic nervous system and should be used with caution
Methylphenidate (Concerta, Daytrana, Metadate, Methylin, Ritalin)	Impaired attention/ concentration, impaired memory, impaired executive function	Indirect adrenergic agonist	• Chen Pi: Stimulates sympathetic nervous system and should be used with caution • Ma Huang: May increase drug activity • Qing Pi: Stimulates sympathetic nervous system and should be used with caution • Rou Cong Rong: May interact by increasing neurotransmitters such as norepinephrine, dopamine, and serotonin • Zhi Ke: Stimulates sympathetic nervous system and should be used with caution • Zhi Shi: Stimulates sympathetic nervous system and should be used with caution
Metoclopramide (Reglan)	Vertigo, nausea/ vomiting, GERD (re: dysphagia)	Antiemetic, GI stimulant	N/A

Pharmaceutical	Possible Use	Category	Potential Herbal Interactions
Morphine, methylmorphine (Astromorph, Avinza, Duramorph, Infumorph, Kadian, MS Contin, Oramorph, RMS, Roxanol)	Pain	Opioid analgesic	• Bai Jiang Cao: May increase sedative effects • Bai Shao: May increase sedative effects of drugs • Chan Tui: May potentiate CNS inhibition • Jiao Gu Lan (gynostemma): May increase sedative effects of drugs • Long Dan Cao: May increase sedative effects of drugs • Niu Huang: May increase sedative effects of drugs (mild effect) • Qin Jiao: May potentiate sedative effects through CNS inhibition • Suan Zao Ren: Sedative and hypnotic effects may potentiate sedative effects of drugs • Tian Ma: Potentiates sedative effect • Tian Nan Xing: May increase sedative effects of drugs • Wu Jia Pi: May increase sedative effects (mild) • Xie Cao (valerian): Potentiates sedative effect • Zhi Zi: May increase sedative effects • Shen calming herbs: May increase sedative effects
Naltrexone (Depade, ReVia, Vivitrol)	Alcohol dependence	Antidote	N/A
Naratriptan (Amerge, Naramig)	Migraine	Antimigraine agent	N/A
Nefazodone (Serzone)	Depression	Antidepressant: Selective serotonin reuptake inhibitor	• Guan Ye Lian Qiao (St. John's wort): One case report of hypomanic episode when combined; inhibits serotonin reuptake • Rou Cong Rong: May interact by increasing neurotransmitters such as norepinephrine, dopamine, and serotonin • Yin Guo Ye: One case report of hypomanic episode when combined
Nortriptyline (Pamelor)	Depression, migraine, pain	Tricyclic antidepressant	• Ma Huang: Hypertensive effects of Ma Huang were blocked • Rou Cong Rong: May interact by increasing neurotransmitters such as norepinephrine, dopamine, and serotonin • Ying Su Ye: May exacerbate depressant and CNS suppressive effects of Ying Su Ye
Odansetron (Zofran)	Vertigo, nausea/vomiting	Antiemetic	N/A

Drug	Indication	Category	Herb Interactions
Olanzapine (Zyprexa)	Mania, bipolar, schizophrenia, PTSD	Atypical neuroleptic	• Bing Lang: May exacerbate extrapyramidal symptoms • Da Fu Pi: May exacerbate extrapyramidal symptoms • Man Jing Zi: Dopamine antagonists may be weakened due to dopaminergic effect
Omeprazole (Prilosec, Zegerid)	GERD (re: dysphagia)	Proton pump inhibitor	• Bai Zhu: May potentiate • Cang Zhu: May potentiate • Aromatic and damp resolving herbs: May antagonize via increased stomach acid and peristalsis
Oxcarbazepine (Trileptal)	Seizure, pain, neuralgia	Anticonvulsant	• Yin Guo Ye: May precipitate epileptic seizures • Chen Pi: May contain constituents that stimulate the sympathetic nervous system and should be used with caution with anticonvulsive agents • Qing Pi: May contain constituents that stimulate the sympathetic nervous system and should be used with caution with anticonvulsive agents • Zhi Ke: May contain constituents that stimulate the sympathetic nervous system and should be used with caution with anticonvulsive agents • Zhi Shi: May contain constituents that stimulate the sympathetic nervous system and should be used with caution with anticonvulsive agents
Oxycodone (Combunox, Endocet, Endodan, OxyContin, Oxyfast, OxyIR, Percodan, Percocet, Roxicet, Roxicodon, Tylox)	Pain	Opioid analgesic	• Bai Jiang Cao: May increase sedative effects • Bai Shao: May increase sedative effects of drugs • Chan Tui: May potentiate CNS inhibition • Jiao Gu Lan (gynostemma): May increase sedative effects of drugs • Long Dan Cao: May increase sedative effects of drugs • Niu Huang: May increase sedative effects of drugs (mild effect) • Qin Jiao: May potentiate sedative effects through CNS inhibition • Suan Zao Ren: Sedative and hypnotic effects may potentiate sedative effects of drugs • Tian Ma: Potentiates sedative effect • Tian Nan Xing: May increase sedative effects of drugs • Wu Jia Pi: May increase sedative effects (mild) • Xie Cao (valerian): Potentiates sedative effect • Zhi Zi: May increase sedative effects • Shen calming herbs: May increase sedative effects

Pharmaceutical	Possible Use	Category	Potential Herbal Interactions
Pantoprazole (Protonix)	GERD (re: dysphagia)	Proton pump inhibitor	• Aromatic and damp resolving herbs: May antagonize via increased stomach acid and peristalsis
Paroxetine (Paxil, Pexeva)	Depression, anxiety, pain, neuralgia, PTSD	Antidepressant: Selective serotonin reuptake inhibitor	• Guan Ye Lian Qiao (St. John's wort): One case report of hypomanic episode when combined; inhibits serotonin reuptake • Rou Cong Rong: May interact by increasing neurotransmitters such as norepinephrine, dopamine, and serotonin • Yin Guo Ye: One case report of hypomanic episode when combined
Pergolide (Permax)	Impaired attention/concentration, impaired memory, impaired executive function	Dopaminergic	N/A
Phenobarbital (Donnatol, Luminal Sodium, Solfoton)	Seizure	Barbiturate Anticonvulsant/Hypnotic	• Yin Guo Ye: May precipitate epileptic seizures • Chen Pi: May contain constituents that stimulate the sympathetic nervous system and should be used with caution with anticonvulsive agents • Qing Pi: May contain constituents that stimulate the sympathetic nervous system and should be used with caution with anticonvulsive agents • Zhi Ke: May contain constituents that stimulate the sympathetic nervous system and should be used with caution with anticonvulsive agents • Zhi Shi: May contain constituents that stimulate the sympathetic nervous system and should be used with caution with anticonvulsive agents
Phenytoin (Dilatin, Phenytek)	Seizure, status epilepticus (intravenous), pain, neuralgia	Anticonvulsant	• Yin Guo Ye: May precipate epileptic seizures • Chen Pi: May contain constituents that stimulate the sympathetic nervous system and should be used with caution with anticonvulsive agents • Qing Pi: May contain constituents that stimulate the sympathetic nervous system and should be used with caution with anticonvulsive agents • Zhi Ke: May contain constituents that stimulate the sympathetic nervous system and should be used with caution with anticonvulsive agents • Zhi Shi: May contain constituents that stimulate the sympathetic nervous system and should be used with caution with anticonvulsive agents

Physostigmine (Eserine)	Impaired attention/concentration, impaired memory, impaired executive function	Acetylcholinesterase inhibitor	Unknown
Polyethylene glycol (Colyte, GoLYTELY, Gycolax, Miralax, NuLYTELY, Trylite)	Constipation	Laxative	• Downward draining herbs such as Da Huang, Mang Xiao, Fan Xie Ye, etc. may act synergistically and should be used with caution • Gan Cao: May lead to increased potassium loss when used with laxatives
Pramipexole (Mirapex)	Impaired attention/concentration, impaired memory, impaired executive function	Dopaminergic	N/A
Prednisone (Deltasone, Liquid Pred, Sterapred)	Headache, vertigo, pain	Adrenocorticosteroid hormone	• Gan Cao: May increase half life of systemic corticosteroids • Huang Qi: May stimulate T-cell activity and decrease immunosuppressant effects • Lu Hui: May increase potassium loss due to corticosteroid use • Ma Huang: May increase steroid metabolism (study using ephedrine, not whole herb) • Ren Shen: May have additive effects
Pregabalin (Lyrica)	Seizure, pain	Other analgesic	N/A
Primidone (Mysoline)	Seizure	Anticonvulsant	• Yin Guo Ye: May precipitate epileptic seizures • Chen Pi: May contain constituents that stimulate the sympathetic nervous system and should be used with caution with anticonvulsive agents • Qing Pi: May contain constituents that stimulate the sympathetic nervous system and should be used with caution with anticonvulsive agents • Zhi Ke: May contain constituents that stimulate the sympathetic nervous system and should be used with caution with anticonvulsive agents • Zhi Shi: May contain constituents that stimulate the sympathetic nervous system and should be used with caution with anticonvulsive agents

Pharmaceutical	Possible Use	Category	Potential Herbal Interactions
Prochlorperazine (Compazine, Compro™)	Migraine, nausea/vomiting	Antipsychotic, antiemetic	• Bing Lang: May exacerbate cholinergic extrapyramidal side effects • Ying Su Ye: Prochlorperazine may exacerbate depressive and CNS suppressive effects of herb
Promethazine (Phenergan, Phenadoz, Promethegan)	Migraine, vertigo, nausea/vomiting	Antihistamine	• Bai Shao: May increase sedative effects of drugs • Chan Tui: May potentiate CNS inhibition • Jiao Gu Lan (gynostemma): May increase sedative effects of drugs • Long Dan Cao: May increase sedative effects of drugs • Niu Huang: May increase sedative effects of drugs (mild effect) • Tian Nan Xing: May increase sedative effects of drugs • Wu Jia Pi: May increase sedative effects of drugs (mild effect) • Xi Jiao: May increase sedative effects of drugs • Zhi Zi: May increase sedative effects of drugs
Propranolol (Inderal, Innopran)	Migraine, PTSD	Non-cardioselective beta blocker	• Chen Pi: May contain constituents that stimulate the sympathetic nervous system and should be used with caution with antihypertensive agents • Gan Cao: May reduce antihypertensive effects • Ma Huang: Antagonizes antihypertensive effects • Qing Pi: May contain constituents that stimulate the sympathetic nervous system and should be used with caution with antihypertensive agents • Sheng Ma: May potentiate antihypertensive effect • Zhi Ke: May contain constituents that stimulate the sympathetic nervous system and should be used with caution with antihypertensive agents • Zhi Shi: May contain constituents that stimulate the sympathetic nervous system and should be used with caution with antihypertensive agents • Hei Hu Jiao (black pepper): Increases absorption kinetics

Drug	Indication	Classification	Interactions
Propylthiouracil	Hyperthyroidism	Antithyroid medication	• Chen Pi: Stimulates the sympathetic nervous system and should be used with caution • Qing Pi: Stimulates the sympathetic nervous system and should be used with caution • Zhi Ke: Stimulates the sympathetic nervous system and should be used with caution • Zhi Shi: Stimulates the sympathetic nervous system and should be used with caution
Protriptyline (Vivactil)	Depression	Tricyclic antidepressant	• Ma Huang: Hypertensive effects of Ma Huang were blocked • Rou Cong Rong: May interect by increasing neurotransmitters such as norepinephrine, dopamine, and serotonin • Ying Su Ye: May exacerbate depressant and CNS suppressive effects of Ying Su Ye
Psyllium seed (Fiberall, Metamucil)	Bowel incontinence, constipation	Antidiarrheal	This drug alters functioning of the small and large intestine and could affect the absorption of herbs. To minimize interactions agents should be administered either four hours before or two hours after
Quetiapine (Seroquel)	Insomnia (with paranoia or agitation), mania, schizophrenia	Atypical neuroleptic	• Bing Lang: May exacerbate extrapyramidal symptoms • Da Fu Pi: May exacerbate extrapyramidal symptoms • Man Jing Zi: Dopamine antagonists may be weakened due to dopaminergic effect
Ranitidine (Taladine, Zantac)	GERD (re: dysphagia)	H2 antagonist	• Aromatic and damp resolving herbs: May antagonize via increased stomach acid and peristalsis
Risperidone (Risperdal)	Insomnia (with psychosis), mania, schizophrenia	Atypical neuroleptics	• Bing Lang: May exacerbate extrapyramidal symptoms • Da Fu Pi: May exacerbate extrapyramidal symptoms • Man Jing Zi: Dopamine antagonists may be weakened due to dopaminergic effect
Rivastigmine (Exelon)	Impaired attention/ concentration, impaired memory, impaired executive function	Anticholinesterases (reversible)	N/A
Rizatriptan (Maxalt)	Migraine	Antimigraine agent	N/A

Pharmaceutical	Possible Use	Category	Potential Herbal Interactions
Ropinirole (Requip)	Impaired attention/ concentration, impaired memory, impaired executive function	Dopaminergic	N/A
Rufinamide (Banzel)	Seizure	Anticonvulsant	• Yin Guo Ye: May precipitate epileptic seizures • Chen Pi: May contain constituents that stimulate the sympathetic nervous system and should be used with caution with anticonvulsive agents • Qing Pi: May contain constituents that stimulate the sympathetic nervous system and should be used with caution with anticonvulsive agents • Zhi Ke: May contain constituents that stimulate the sympathetic nervous system and should be used with caution with anticonvulsive agents • Zhi Shi: May contain constituents that stimulate the sympathetic nervous system and should used with caution with anticonvulsive agents
Scopolamine (Donnatal, Isopto, Hyoscine, Maldemar, Murocoll, Scopace, Transderm-Scop)	Vertigo (transdermal patch)	Antimuscarinic agent	• Fu Ling: May decrease memory impairment • Dang Gui: May relieve amnesia caused by scopolamine • Ren Shen: May decrease memory impairment • Shi Chang Pu: May decrease memory impairment • Yuan Zhi: May decrease memory impairment
Selegiline (Eldepyrl, Emsam, Zelapar)	Impaired attention/ concentration, impaired memory, impaired executive function	Dopaminergic	N/A
Sertraline (Zoloft)	Depression, PTSD	Antidepressant: Selective serotonin reuptake inhibitor	• Guan Ye Lian Qiao (St. John's wort): One case report of hypomanic episode when combined; inhibits serotonin reuptake • Rou Cong Rong: May interact by increasing neurotransmitters such as norepinephrine, dopamine, and serotonin • Yin Guo Ye: One case report of hypomanic episode when combined

Sumatriptan (Imitrex)	Migraine	Antimigraine agent (narrows blood vessels around the brain)	N/A
Temazepam (Restoril)	Insomnia, anxiety	Benzodiazepine hypnotic	• Bai Jiang Cao: May increase sedative effects • Bai Shao: May increase sedative effects of drugs • Chan Tui: May potentiate CNS inhibition • Dan Shen: May inhibit benzodiazepine receptor binding • Jiao Gu Lan (gynostemma): May increase sedative effects of drugs • Long Dan Cao: May increase sedative effects of drugs • Niu Huang: May increase sedative effects of drugs (mild effect) • Qin Jiao: May potentiate sedative effects through CNS inhibition • Suan Zao Ren: Sedative and hypnotic effects may potentiate sedative effects of drugs • Tian Ma: Potentiates sedative effect • Tian Nan Xing: May increase sedative effects of drugs • Wu Jia Pi: May increase sedative effects (mild) • Xie Cao (valerian): Potentiates sedative effect • Zhi Zi: May increase sedative effects • Shen calming herbs: May increase sedative effects
Thyroid (Armour Thyroid, Nature-thyroid, Westhroid)	Hypothyroidism	Hormone	N/A
Tiagabine (Gabitril)	Seizure	GABA reuptake inhibitor	• Yin Guo Ye: May precipitate epileptic seizures • Chen Pi: May contain constituents that stimulate the sympathetic nervous system and should be used with caution with anticonvulsive agents • Qing Pi: May contain constituents that stimulate the sympathetic nervous system and should be used with caution with anticonvulsive agents • Zhi Ke: May contain constituents that stimulate the sympathetic nervous system and should be used with caution with anticonvulsive agents • Zhi Shi: May contain constituents that stimulate the sympathetic nervous system and should be used with caution with anticonvulsive agents

Pharmaceutical	Possible Use	Category	Potential Herbal Interactions
Topiramate (Topamax)	Seizure, migraine, headache, mania, bipolar	Carbonic anhydrase inhibitor anticonvulsant	• Yin Guo Ye: May precipitate epileptic seizures • Chen Pi: May contain constituents that stimulate the sympathetic nervous system and should be used with caution with anticonvulsive agents • Qing Pi: May contain constituents that stimulate the sympathetic nervous system and should be used with caution with anticonvulsive agents • Zhi Ke: May contain constituents that stimulate the sympathetic nervous system and should be used with caution with anticonvulsive agents • Zhi Shi: May contain constituents that stimulate the sympathetic nervous system and should be used with caution with anticonvulsive agents
Tramadol (Ultracet, Ultram)	Pain	Analgesic	N/A
Trazodone (Desyrel)	Insomnia, depression, anxiety	Antidepressant: Selective serotonin reuptake inhibitor	• Guan Ye Lian Qiao (St. John's wort): One case report of hypomanic episode when combined; inhibits serotonin reuptake • Rou Cong Rong: May interact by increasing neurotransmitters such as norepinephrine, dopamine, and serotonin • Yin Guo Ye: One case report of hypomanic episode when combined
Triazolam (Halcion)	Insomnia, anxiety	Benzodiazepine hypnotic	• Bai Jiang Cao: May increase sedative effects • Bai Shao: May increase sedative effects of drugs • Chan Tui: May potentiate CNS inhibition • Dan Shen: May inhibit benzodiazepine receptor binding • Jiao Gu Lan (gynostemma): May increase sedative effects of drugs • Long Dan Cao: May increase sedative effects of drugs • Niu Huang: May increase sedative effects of drugs (mild effect) • Qin Jiao: May potentiate sedative effects through CNS inhibition • Suan Zao Ren: Sedative and hypnotic effects may potentiate sedative effects of drugs • Tian Ma: Potentiates sedative effect • Tian Nan Xing: May increase sedative effects of drugs • Wu Jia Pi: May increase sedative effects (mild) • Xie Cao (valerian): Potentiates sedative effect • Zhi Zi: May increase sedative effects • Shen calming herbs: May increase sedative effects

Drug	Classification	Indication	Herb Interactions
Trimipramine (Surmontil)	Tricyclic antidepressant	Depression	• Ma Huang: Hypertensive effects of Ma Huang were blocked • Rou Cong Rong: May interact by increasing neurotransmitters such as norepinephrine, dopamine, and serotonin • Ying Su Ye: May exacerbate depressant and CNS suppressive effects of Ying Su Ye
Valproic acid (Depacon, Depakene, Depakote, Sprinkle)	Fatty acid derivative anticonvulsant	Seizure, migraine, headache, status epilepticus, pain, mania, bipolar	• Yin Guo Ye: May precipitate epileptic seizures • Chen Pi: May contain constituents that stimulate the sympathetic nervous system and should be used with caution with anticonvulsive agents • Qing Pi: May contain constituents that stimulate the sympathetic nervous system and should be used with caution with anticonvulsive agents • Zhi Ke: May contain constituents that stimulate the sympathetic nervous system and should be used with caution with anticonvulsive agents • Zhi Shi: May contain constituents that stimulate the sympathetic nervous system and should be used with caution with anticonvulsive agents
Venlafaxine (Effexor)	Antidepressant: Serotonin/norepinephrine reuptake inhibitor	Depression	• Guan Ye Lian Qiao (St. John's wort): One case report of hypomanic episode when combined; inhibits serotonin reuptake • Rou Cong Rong: May interact by increasing neurotransmitters such as norepinephrine, dopamine, and serotonin • Yin Guo Ye: One case report of hypomanic episode when combined
Verapamil (Calan, Covera, Isoptin, Tarka, Verelan)	Calcium channel blocker	Migraine, mania	• Gan Cao: May reduce effects • Qing Hao: May interfere with effectiveness
Zaleplon (Sonata)	Sedative, hypnotic	Insomnia	• Bai Jiang Cao: May increase sedative effects • Bai Shao: May increase sedative effects of drugs • Chan Tui: May potentiate CNS inhibition • Long Dan Cao: May increase sedative effects of drugs • Niu Huang: May increase sedative effects of drugs (mild effect) • Qin Jiao: May potentiate sedative effects through CNS inhibition • Suan Zao Ren: Sedative and hypnotic effects may potentiate sedative effects of drugs • Tian Nan Xing: May increase sedative effects of drugs • Wu Jia Pi: May increase sedative effects (mild) • Xie Cao (valerian): Potentiates sedative effect • Zhi Zi: May increase sedative effects • Shen calming herbs: May increase sedative effects

Pharmaceutical	Possible Use	Category	Potential Herbal Interactions
Zolmitriptan (Zomig, Zomig ZMT)	Migraine	Antimigraine agent (narrows blood vessels around the brain)	N/A
Zolpidem (Ambien)	Insomnia	Sedative, hypnotic	• Bai Jiang Cao: May increase sedative effects • Bai Shao: May increase sedative effects of drugs • Chan Tui: May potentiate CNS inhibition • Long Dan Cao: May increase sedative effects of drugs • Niu Huang: May increase sedative effects of drugs (mild effect) • Qin Jiao: May potentiate sedative effects through CNS inhibition • Suan Zao Ren: Sedative and hypnotic effects may potentiate sedative effects of drugs • Tian Nan Xing: May increase sedative effects of drugs • Wu Jia Pi: May increase sedative effects (mild) • Xie Cao (valerian): Potentiates sedative effect • Zhi Zi: May increase sedative effects • Shen calming herbs: May increase sedative effects
Zonisamide (Zonegran)	Seizure	Anticonvulsant	• Yin Guo Ye: May precipitate epileptic seizures • Chen Pi: May contain constituents that stimulate the sympathetic nervous system and should be used with caution with anticonvulsive agents • Qing Pi: May contain constituents that stimulate the sympathetic nervous system and should be used with caution with anticonvulsive agents • Zhi Ke: May contain constituents that stimulate the sympathetic nervous system and should be used with caution with anticonvulsive agents • Zhi Shi: May contain constituents that stimulate the sympathetic nervous system and should be used with caution with anticonvulsive agents

Bibliography

Chen, John and Chen, Tina. *Chinese Herbal Formulas and Applications: pharmacological effects and clinical research.* City of Industry, CA: Art of Medicine Press. 2009. Print.

Chen, John, Chen, Tina, and Crampton, Laraine. *Chinese Medical Herbology and Pharmacology.* City of Industry, CA: Art of Medicine Press. 2004. Print.

Flaws, Bob and Lake, James. *Chinese Medical Psychiatry: a textbook and clinical manual: including indications for referral to Western medical services.* Boulder, CO: Blue Poppy. 2003. Print.

Joseph, R. *Neuropsychiatry, Neuropsychology and Clinical Neuroscience: emotion, evolution, cognition, language, memory, brain damage, and abnormal behavior.* Baltimore: Williams and Wilkins. 1996. Print.

Kastner, Joerg. *Chinese Nutrition Therapy: dietetics in traditional Chinese medicine.* 2nd ed. New York: Thieme. 2009. Print.

Kidwell, Martin. "TCM Pathology," Lecture. Oregon College of Oriental Medicine, Portland, OR, 2009–2011.

Lash, Marilyn. *The Essential Brain Injury Guide.* 5th ed. Vienna, VA: Academy of Certified Brain Injury Specialists, Brain Injury Association of America. 2016. Print.

Maciocia, Giovanni. *The Psyche in Chinese Medicine: treatment of emotional and mental disharmonies with acupuncture and Chinese herbs.* Edinburgh: Churchill Livingstone. 2009. Print.

Marz, Russell. *Medical Nutrition from Marz: a textbook in clinical nutrition.* Portland, OR: Omni-Press. 1999. Print.

Morgan, Cara. *Concussion and Traumatic Brain Injury: a Chinese medical approach.* Portland, OR: National College of Naturopathic Medicine. 2005. Print.

Shi, Anshen, Shih-Shun Lin, and Caldwell, Leigh. *Essentials of Chinese Medicine: internal medicine.* Walnut, CA: Bridge Pub. Group. 2003. Print.

Silver, Jonathan, Yudofsky, Stuart, and McAllister, Thomas. *Textbook of Traumatic Brain Injury.* Washington, DC: American Psychiatric Pub. 2011. Print.

Soulié de Morant, George and Zmiewski, Paul. *Chinese Acupuncture.* Brookline, MA: Paradigm Publications. 1994. Print.

Ward, Jamie. *The Student's Guide to Cognitive Neuroscience.* London: Taylor and Francis. 2015. Print.

Yan, Wu, Fratkin, Jake, and Fischer, Warren. *Practical Therapeutics of Traditional Chinese Medicine.* Brooklyn, MA: Paradigm. 1997. Print.

Yang, Joseph. *Shen Disturbance: a guideline for psychiatry in traditional Chinese medicine.* Los Angeles. 2005. Print.

Zasler, Nathan, Katz, Douglas, and Zafonte, Ross. *Brain Injury Medicine: principles and practice.* New York: Demos Medical Pub. 2013. Print.

Subject Index

Author Index